Medical Management of HIV Infection
2012 Edition

John G. Bartlett, M.D.

Professor of Medicine
Director, Johns Hopkins AIDS Service
Division of Infectious Diseases
Department of Medicine
Johns Hopkins University School of Medicine

Joel E. Gallant, M.D., M.P.H.

Professor of Medicine and Epidemiology
Associate Director, Johns Hopkins AIDS Service
Division of Infectious Diseases
Department of Medicine
Johns Hopkins University School of Medicine

Paul A.Pham, Pharm. D.

Research Associate
Division of Infectious Diseases
Department of Medicine
Johns Hopkins University School of Medicine

i

Medical Management of HIV Infection

Some of the information contained in this book may cite the use of a particular drug in a dosage, for an indication, or in a manner other than recommended or FDA-approved. Therefore, the manufacturers' package inserts should be consulted for complete prescribing information.

ISBN: 978-0-9837111-0-0
10-digit ISBN: 0-9837111-0-x

Address of the publisher:

Knowledge Source Solutions

2011 MMHIV
Knowledge Source Solutions
762 9th Street #624
Durham, NC 27705-4803
www.knowledgesourcesolutions.com
info@knowledgesourcesolutions.com

Contents

Medical Management of HIV Infection: CME

Contents

1 | Natural History and Classification

Stages

The natural history of untreated HIV infection is divided into the following stages:

Viral transmission $\xrightarrow{\text{2-3 wks}}$ Acute retroviral syndrome $\xrightarrow{\text{2-3 wks}}$ Recovery + seroconversion $\xrightarrow{\text{2-4 wks}}$ Asymptomatic chronic HIV infection $\xrightarrow{\text{Avg. 8 yrs}}$ Symptomatic HIV infection/AIDS $\xrightarrow{\text{Avg. 1.3 yrs}}$ Death

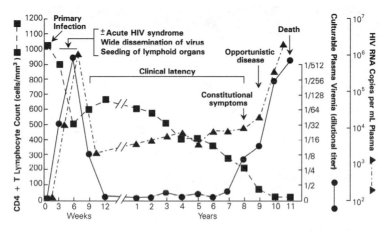

■ FIGURE 1-1: **Natural history of HIV infection in an average patient without antiretroviral therapy from the time of HIV transmission to death at 10-11 years.**

Life cycle and natural history of HIV: The external glycoprotein gp120 attaches to the CD4 cell receptor. This allows binding of gp120 to coreceptors (CCR5 and CXCR4) on the cell surface. Binding is followed by insertion of gp41 into the CD4 cell, resulting in membrane fusion and fusion within pores followed by release of viral core into the CD4 cell cytoplasm (*Lancet* 2006;368:489). The HIV genome is then reverse transcribed to DNA by reverse transcriptase. Viral DNA is then carried into the nucleus and inserted into host DNA by the viral integrase enzyme. Finally, translated viral proteins are processed by viral proteases, allowing assembly of new virions, which are released from the cell to infect other targets, completing the viral life cycle.

Immediately after infection, the virus is harbored in the gut-associated lymphoid tissue (GALT), the lymphatic tissue of the small bowel. The early phase of infection is characterized by viral amplification in GALT and peak viremia ($10^6 - 10^7$ copies/mL) that is often associated with symptoms of the "acute retroviral syndrome" and massive depletion of activated and memory cells primarily from GALT (*J Exp Med* 2004;200:761). The preferential depletion of CD4 cells from GALT persists despite antiretroviral therapy (ART), which often produces normal CD4 counts in peripheral blood. HIV replication persists throughout the disease despite absence of symptoms for years during most of the chronic infection phase (Figure 1.1). The half-life of the virus is about 30 minutes, the number of virions produced daily is estimated at 10^{10} and lymphocyte turnover is rapid. This is attributed to viremia in the early phase of infections, but it is sustained by immune activation during the chronic stage and this appears to dictate the rate of progression (*J Immun* 2003;170:2479; *JAMA* 2006;296:1498). The population of HIV is relatively homogeneous initially, but the virus is error-prone and multiple quasi-species are produced that facilitate evasion of viral control by immune mechanisms and antiretroviral agents. Common observations in the average patients are shown in Table 1-1.

■ TABLE 1-1: **Natural History of HIV Infection (*Lancet* 2006;368:489)**

	Acute Wk 0-6	Chronic Year 1-10	Late Year > 10
Symptoms	Variable	Asymptomatic	Opportunistic infections Table 1-2
Viral load (c/mL)	10^6 –10^7 (c/mL)	10^5 –10^6 (c/mL)	10^5 –10^7 (c/mL)
Transmission	+ + + +	+ +	+ + +
Cytotoxic T cells and antibody	0	+ +	+ +
CD4 count (cells/mm³)	> 600	300–500	< 200
GALT depletion	severe	severe	severe
Viral diversity	none	modest	great

DEFINITIONS OF HIV STAGES AND COURSE

Primary HIV Infection: Evidence of HIV (HIV RNA or p24 antigen) prior to seroconversion (See below)

Chronic HV Infection:

* Chronic progressor: "Typical" disease progression as illustrated in Figure 1, usually with VL >10,000 c/mL and CD4 decline of 50-100 cells/mm³/yr.

* Chronic nonprogressors (or "long-term nonprogressors"): HIV infection without opportunistic infections and a CD4 count >500 cells/mm³ >10 years. This includes subsets of "slow progressors" who have slow CD4 loss, usually with VL 1,000-10,000 c/mL (*PLoS Med* 2009;4:e5474; *PNAS* 2000;97:2709) and "elite controllers" defined by a VL <50 c/mL in the absence of therapy (see pg. 29). However, not all elite controllers are non-progressors; a small proportion experience progression, as defined by decline in CD4 count.

* AIDS: Defined by an AIDS-defining diagnosis or a CD4 count <200 cells/mm³ (Tables 1-3 and 1-4).

Primary HIV Infection

Acute HIV infection refers to the period from HIV transmission to seroconversion. Laboratory testing shows presence of HIV RNA in the absence of HIV antibody

CD4 Cell Count*	Infectious Complications	Noninfectious† Complications
>500 cells/mm³	■ Acute retroviral syndrome ■ Candidal vaginitis	■ Persistent generalized lymphadenopathy (PGL) ■ Guillain-Barré syndrome ■ Myopathy ■ Aseptic meningitis
200-500 cells/mm³	■ Pneumococcal and other bacterial pneumonia ■ Pulmonary tuberculosis ■ Herpes zoster ■ Oropharyngeal candidiasis (thrush) ■ Cryptosporidiosis, self-limited ■ Kaposi's sarcoma† ■ Oral hairy leukoplakia	■ Cervical and anal dysplasia† ■ Cervical and anal cancer† ■ B-cell lymphoma ■ Anemia ■ Mononeuronal multiplex ■ Idiopathic thrombocytopenic purpura ■ Hodgkin lymphoma ■ Lymphocytic interstitial pneumonitis
<200 cells/mm³	■ *Pneumocystis* pneumonia ■ Disseminated histoplasmosis and coccidioidomycosis ■ Miliary/extrapulmonary TB ■ Progressive multifocal leuko-encephalopathy (PML)	■ Wasting ■ Peripheral neuropathy ■ HIV-associated dementia ■ Cardiomyopathy ■ Vacuolar myelopathy ■ Progressive polyradiculopathy ■ Non-Hodgkin's lymphoma
<100 cells/mm³³	■ Disseminated herpes simplex ■ Toxoplasmosis ■ Cryptococcosis ■ Cryptosporidiosis, chronic ■ Microsporidiosis ■ Candidal esophagitis	
<50 cells/mm³	■ Disseminated cytomegalovirus (CMV) ■ Disseminated *Mycobacterium avium* complex	■ Primary central nervous system lymphoma (PCNSL)

* Most complications occur with increasing frequency at lower CD4 cell counts.

† Some conditions listed as "noninfectious" are associated with transmissible microbes. Examples include lymphoma (Epstein-Barr virus [EBV]) and anal and cervical cancers (human papillomavirus [HPV]).

Natural History and Classification

1

Indicator Conditions
Candidiasis of esophagus, trachea, bronchi, or lungs – 3,846 (16%)* [12.6 → 5.2]§
Cervical cancer, invasive†† – 144 (0.6%)* [3.5 → 3.5]§
Coccidioidomycosis, extrapulmonary† – 74 (0.3%)* [–]
Cryptococcosis, extrapulmonary – 1,168 (5%)* [2.6 → 0.8]§
Cryptosporidiosis with diarrhea >1 month – 314 (1.3%)* [7.3 → 0.8]§
CMV of the eye or any organ other than liver, spleen, or lymph nodes; eye – 1,638 (7%)* [33.0 → 1.8]§
Herpes simplex with mucocutaneous ulcer >1 month; or bronchitis, pneumonitis, esophagitis – 1,250 (5%)* [1.6 → 1.0]§
Histoplasmosis, extrapulmonary† – 208 (0.9%)* [–]
HIV-associated dementia†: Disabling cognitive and/or other dysfunction interfering with occupation or activities of daily living – 1,196 (5%)* [5.4 → 1.4]§
HIV-associated wasting†: Involuntary weight loss >10% of baseline plus chronic diarrhea (≥2 loose stools/day lasting ≥30 days) or chronic weakness and documented enigmatic fever ≥30 days – 4,212 (18%)* [–]
Isosporiasis with diarrhea >1 month† – 22 (0.1%)* [–]
Kaposi's sarcoma in patient under 60 yrs (or over 60 yrs)† – 1,500 (7%)* [16.4 → 1,2]§
Lymphoma, Burkitt's – 162 (0.7%), immunoblastic – 518 (2.3%), primary CNS – 170 (0.7%)* [5.5 → 1.6]§
Mycobacterium avium complex or _M. kansasii_ – disseminated or extrapulmonary disease – 1,124 (5%)* [26.9 → 2.5]§
Mycobacterium tuberculosis, pulmonary – 1,621 (7%), extrapulmonary – 491 (2%)* [5.0 → 0.8]§
Pneumocystis pneumonia – 9,145 (38%)* [29.9 → 3.9]§
Pneumonia, recurrent bacterial (≥2 episodes in 12 months)†‡ – 1,347 (5%)* [–]
Progressive multifocal leukoencephalopathy – 213 (1%)* [2.7 → 0.7]§
Salmonella septicemia (nontyphoid), recurrent† – 68 (0.3%)* [–]
Toxoplasmosis of internal organ – 1,073 (4%)* [4.1 → 0.7]§

*   Indicates frequency as the AIDS-indicator condition among 23,527 reported cases in adults for 1997. The AIDS diagnosis was based on CD4 count in an additional 36,643 or 61% of the 60,161 total cases. Numbers indicate sum of definitive and presumptive diagnoses for stated condition. The number in parentheses is the percentage of all patients reported with an AIDS-defining diagnosis; these do not total 100% because some had a dual diagnosis. This is the last year the CDC systematically collected these data and reflects the pre-HAART experience.

§   Data are for the HIV Oupatient Study (HOPS) which is a prospective cohort study of 7,155 patients in 10 US Clinics. The numbers show the rate (/1000 person-years for AIDS-defining conditions for 1994-97 (pre HAART) – 2003-07 (post HAART). [–] indicates data not provided (_AIDS_ 2008;22:1345).

†   Requires positive HIV serology.

‡   Added in the revised case definition, 1993.

- TABLE 1-4: **CDC Revised Case Definition for HIV in Adults***
  (*MMWR* 2008;RR10:1-8)

Stage	CD4 data		Clinical
	Count	%	
1	≥ 500	≥ 29	No AIDS-defining dx
2	200-499	14-28	No AIDS-defining dx
3	< 200	14	or Documentation of AIDS-defining dx
Unknown	No information		No information

* HIV infection (>13 years)

Laboratory criteria: 1) Positive screening test (EIA) confirmed by a) Western blot, b) indirect immunofluorescent test, or c) supplemental HIV Ab test; or 2) Detectable quantity within established laboratory limits for: a) HIV RNA or DNA, b) HIV p24 antigen test with neutralization assay, or c) HIV culture (*PNAS* 2008;105:75552; *JID* 2010;202 Suppl 2:S270). It is important to make the diagnosis at this stage because it is associated with high rates of HIV transmission (*JID* 2004;189:1785; *JID* 2007;195:951), is a time when standard serologic tests for HIV antibody are deceptively negative, and diagnosis may explain an otherwise enigmatic illness. The ability to detect this stage of disease is facilitated by the availability of "fourth generation" HIV tests that detect both antigen and antibody (Chapter 2) (*JAIDS* 2009;52:121; *JCM* 2009;47:2639). See pg. 15, 19.

Elite Controller

The usual definition is: 1) positive HIV serology; 2) no opportunistic conditions; and 3) HIV VL <50 c/mL without ART (*JAMA* 2010;302:194; *AIDS* 2008;22:541). Elite controllers make up <0.5% of persons with HIV infection (*CID* 2005;41:1053; *JID* 1999;180:526; *Top HIV Med* 2007;15:134; *CID* 2010;50:1187). Differences between elite controllers and "slow progressors" are that the latter usually have VLs of 1,000-10,000 c/mL, CD4 depletion over time and eventual development of opportunistic conditions (*Blood* 1997;90:1133; *Immunity* 2008; 29:1009). A review of 14 elite controllers with known HIV infection for a median of 13 years showed a median CD4 count of 812 cells/mm^3, and all had a VL <50 c/mL. Nine (64%) had VLs <1 c/mL, and the median VL in the other 6 was 26 c/mL (*CID* 2008;47:102). The variation in VL is significantly greater than in patients receiving ART with viral suppression. The virus in elite controllers is replication competent, and there may be viral evolution with sequential testing (*CID* 2009;49:1763). Virologic control in elite controllers may be immunologically mediated as suggested by the fact that the HLA-B*57 allele is highly overrepresented (*PNAS* 2000;97:2709). Of interest is the observation that ART in elite controllers with stable low viral loads and high CD4 counts further reduces markers of immune activation (*CID* 2009;49:1763).

Natural History and Classification

1

2 | Laboratory Tests

Laboratory tests recommended for initial evaluation and follow-up of all patients are summarized in Table 2-17, pg. 51.

HIV Types and Subtypes

HIV-1

HIV infection is established by detecting antibodies to the virus, viral antigens, viral RNA/DNA, or by culture (*Lancet* 1996;348:176). The standard test is serology for antibody detection. Two HIV types are HIV-1 and HIV-2, which show 40-60% amino acid homology. HIV-1 accounts for nearly all cases except a minority of strains that originate in West Africa. HIV-1 is divided into subtypes designated A through K (collectively referred to as Group M with subtypes designated A, B, C, D, F, G, H, J and K) and 15 circulating recombinant forms (CRFs) (*AIDS* 2000;14:S31). These CRFs include CRF01_AE (a mosaic with sequences from clades A and E), and CRF02_AG. Subtype O shows 55-70% homology with the M subtypes. Six strains account for most infections: subtype A, B, C, D and CRFs – CRF01_AE and CRF02_AG (Table 2-1). Another group of viruses is labeled "N" for "new," first reported in 1998 (*Nat Med* 1998;4:1032; *Science* 2000;287:607). The O and N Groups are now thought to represent divergent evolution or distinctive cross-species transmission. Group O strains were once common in Cameroon, and HIV-2 was prominent in West Africa in the mid 1990s, but both have been largely displaced by HIV-1. Over 98% of HIV-1 infections in the United States are caused by subtype B; most non-B subtypes in the United States were acquired in other countries (*JID* 2000;181:470); the relatively rare O and N subtypes are still found primarily in West Africa. In a review of subtypes from 196 immigrants in New York City in 2005, subtype B accounted for 111 (55%), subtype A for 54 (27%), and subtype C for 8 (4%) (*JID* 2006;41:399).

HIV-2

HIV-2 is another human retrovirus that causes immune deficiency due to depletion of CD4 cells. It is found primarily in West Africa.*

---

* Endemic areas in West Africa – Benin, Burkina Faso, Cape Verde, Cote d'Ivoire, Gambia, Ghana, Guinea Guinea-Bissau, Liberia, Mali, Mauritania, Niger, Nigeria, São Tome, Senegal, Sierra Leone, and Togo; other African countries – Angola and Mozambique (*MMWR* 1992;4[RR-12]:1).

■ TABLE 2-1: **Global Distribution of HIV-1 by Subtype (***Lancet* **2007;368:489)**

Regions	Total Infected	Subtypes
N. America	1,200,000	B
Caribbean	300,000	B
Latin America	1,800,000	B, BF
Western Europe	720,000	B
N. Africa, Mid East	510,000	B, C
Sub-Saharan Africa	25,800,000	A, C, D, F,G, H, J, K, CRF
East Europe, central Asia	1,600,000	A, B
East Asia	870,000	B, C, BC, CRF 01
Southeast Asia	7,400,000	B, AE

CLINICAL FEATURES OF HIV-2: Compared with HIV-1, HIV-2 infections are characterized by low VL, slow rates of clinical progression, low rates of transmission (vertically or sexually) and unique treatment recommendations due to intrinsic resistance to NNRTIs (*JAIDS* 2004;37:1543; *Retrovirology* 2010;7:46; *AIDS* 2003;17:2591; *AIDS Res Ther* 2008;5:18; *AIDS* 2008;22:2069; *Lancet* 1994;344:1380; *AIDS* 1994;8 [suppl 1]:585; *JID* 1999;180:1116; *JAIDS* 2000;24:257; *Arch Intern Med* 2000;160:3286; *AIDS* 2000;14:441; *JID* 2002;185:905; *AIDS* 2008;22:211; *CID* 2010;51:1334). Despite slow rates of progression, mortality rates for HIV-1 and HIV-2 infection are similar when adjusted for VL (*JAIDS* 2005;38:335). HIV-2 has less homology with HIV-1 than HIV-1 subtypes (*Nature* 1987;328:543), and serology can be negative in 20-30% depending on which enzyme immunosorbent assay (EIA) is used. Several FDA-cleared rapid tests detect HIV-2 (see below). A review of 40,300 cases of HIV infection in New York City for 2000-08 showed 62 (0.15%) were caused by HIV-2. Sixty of the 62 were foreign-born (Africa-58, Central America-2), one was white, 11 (18%) had CDC-defined AIDS, 33 (62%) had a CD4 count <500 cells/mm^3, 40 (65%) were initially diagnosed with HIV-1 infection, and none had dual infection (*CID* 2010;51:1334). HIV-2 should be suspected: 1) in patients who are of West African origin; 2) in patients who have undetectable virus without therapy; 3) in a patient epidemiologically linked to HIV-2 infection; and 4) in cases where the HIV-1 WB is negative, indeterminant, or atypical. In such cases, diagnostic testing for HIV-2 should be requested (see below). HIV-2 infection is associated with immune activation that is comparable to that seen with HIV-1 infection when adjusted for VL (*JID* 2010;201:114). There are no treatment guidelines for HIV-2 infection based on comparative trials, but PI-based ART treatment is generally recommended (*AIDS* 2009;23:1171; *BMC Infect Dis* 2008;8:21). See pg. 94-95.

Several issues affect the management of HIV-2-infected patients:

1) Many patients are co-infected with HIV-1 (*AIDS* 2002;16:1775).

2) Doubling time is 6-fold longer than HIV-1, leading to low VL,

decreased transmission, and long period of asymptomatic infection (*JAMA* 1993;270:2083).

3) Laboratory confirmation of infection may be difficult (see below).

4) There are no commercially available VL assays or resistance testing (*Arch Intern Med* 2000;160:3286), although these tests can be performed by some specialty laboratories (*J Virol Methods* 2000;88:81; *CID* 2004;38:1771; *JAIDS* 2000;24: 257). One report suggested RT-DNA (*AIDS Res Ther* 2008;15:18).

5) Antiretroviral treatment: See pg. 94-95.

SEROLOGY: An HIV-2 EIA was licensed by the FDA in 1990 and became mandatory for screening blood donors in 1992. Suspected cases of HIV-2 infection should undergo diagnostic testing. The testing advocated by the New York City Public Health Laboratories and most commercial labs is screening for HIV-1, HIV-2 and group O. HIV-2 is suspected if the WB for HIV-1 is negative, indeterminate or atypical. Supplemental HIV-2 testing includes EIA (FDA-approved) tests that differentiate HIV-1 and HIV-2 and tests for HIV-2 qualitative DNA PCR (*CID* 2010;51:1334; *JCM* 2010;48:2902). There is no standardized diagnostic algorithm to detect dual infection, but findings that suggest HIV-2 are an indeterminant band pattern of gag (p66, p51, p32) and absence of env (gp 160, gp 120 and gp 41). Of the FDA-approved rapid tests, *OraQuick*, *Multispot*, *VITROS* and *Clearview* detect HIV-1 and -2. *Reveal G2* and *Uni-Gold Recombigen* are approved for detection of only HIV-1. For more information see pg. 17. A new HIV-2 strain was recently reported that is not detected by PCR for endemic HIV-2 (*Retrovirology* 2008;5:103).

HIV Serology

INDICATIONS: Recommendations for HIV testing in the US were changed in 2006 (*MMWR* 2006;55 RR14) to favor "opt-out" testing. The rationale for the change included the following: 1) remarkable changes in the HIV field making HIV treatable and less stigmatizing; 2) the failure of risk-based testing indicated by the fact that an estimated 210,000 in the US were unaware of having HIV infection; 3) the average patient was diagnosed with a CD4 count below the threshold for ART initiation (*CID* 2010;50:1512); and 4) delayed diagnosis resulted in delayed treatment (an individual health concern) and promoted HIV transmission by delaying precautions that usually accompany knowledge of HIV infection (a public health concern) (*MMWR* 2006;55:1269; *MMWR* 2010;59:1550; *CID* 2010;50:1512). It was estimated that if the 210,000 Americans with undiagnosed HIV infection were diagnosed, the rate of new infections would decrease by >30% (*AIDS* 2006;20:1447). See pg. 12, 17.

The revised CDC recommendations advocate:

- Testing for all persons ages 13-64 years
- Testing should be performed in all healthcare settings including

emergency rooms, clinics, hospital admissions, STD clinics, family planning clinics, etc.

- There should be no requirement for signed, informed consent and no requirement for pre- or post-test counseling. (Counseling should be done as it is with any transmissible disease, and consent for the test is implied with the consent for care).
- The patient should be aware of the test and be given the option to "opt-out" (the patient may refuse this test just as they can refuse any test). Refusal should be documented in the medical record.
- Patients with positive tests should be informed of their results as they would for any other significant lab test, and they should be referred to an HIV provider.
- Frequency of testing: 1) Patients in high risk categories should be tested at least annually; 2) low risk patients should be tested once and retested if there is a new potential risk such as a new sex partner; and 3) areas with a HIV prevalence <0.1% should revert to risk-based testing, because the test is not cost effective with that prevalence (*NEJM* 2005;353:570). (The prevalence of HIV in the US is about 0.3%).
- State laws: All but four states changed their laws by 2011 to be in compliance with the revised 2006 CDC guidelines on HIV testing. For state specific information:

  www.mmhiv.com/link/State-HIV-Testing-Laws

Standard HIV Test

The standard serologic test consists of a screening enzyme-linked immunoassay (EIA) performed in the lab with whole blood. This test accounts for the majority of HIV screening tests in the US, with finger stick blood (or saliva) done as a "rapid test" at the point-of-care (POC). The EIA tests are screening tests and require a confirmatory Western blot (WB). Fourth generation tests combine anti-HIV and p24 antigen in one assay to reduce "the window period." EIA screening for anti-HIV requires a "repeatedly reactive" test, which is the criterion for WB testing. WB detects antibodies to HIV-1 proteins, including core (p17, p24, p55), polymerase (p31, p51, p66), and envelope (gp41, gp120, gp160). WB testing should be coupled with EIA screening due to a 2% rate of false positive EIA tests. Results of WB are interpreted as follows (*Am J Med* 2000;109:568):

- **Negative:** No bands.
- **Positive:** Reactivity to gp120/160 plus gp41 and p24.
- **Indeterminate:** Presence of any band pattern that does not meet criteria for positive results.

ACCURACY: Standard serologic assays (EIA and WB or immuno-fluorescent assay) show sensitivity in patients with established disease

(>3 mos after transmission) of 99.5%(CI 98-99.9%) and a specificity of 99.994% (*NEJM* 2005;352:570; *JAMA* 1991;266:2861; *Am J Med* 2000;109:568). Positive tests should be confirmed with repeat tests or with corroborating clinical or laboratory data.

FALSE NEGATIVE RESULTS: False negative results are usually due to testing in the "window period." The rate of false negatives ranges from 0.3% in a high-prevalence population (*JID* 1993;168:327) to <0.001% in low-prevalence populations (*NEJM* 1991;325:593). The largest review of unexplained persistently seronegative HIV infection includes 25 patients (median age 30 years) who generally presented with late stage disease with CD4 counts <200 cells/mm^3 (20 patients), an AIDS-defining condition at presentation (14), high VL (median 600,000 c/mL) and clade B virus (11/17) (*AIDS* 2010;1407). The authors speculated that failure to mount an immune response contributed to the rapid course. Causes of false-negative results include:

- **Window period:** The time delay from infection to positive EIA averages 3-4 wks (Fig 1; Table 1-1). Some do not seroconvert for 3-12 wks or more (*J Med Virol* 2000;60:43; *NEJM* 1997;336:919), and case reports document seroconversion delayed 3-8 mos (*Internat J STD & AIDS* 2009;20:205), but nearly all patients seroconvert within 6 mos (*Am J Med* 2000;109:568). Newer fourth generation tests detect HIV RNA as well as HIV antibody and should correct for this, although many labs still use 3rd generation tests. One clinic reported the p24 screening with negative antibody accounted for 3% of their cases (*J Med Virol* 2007;79:S23).

- **Seroreversion:** Seroreversion is rare: one report found no cases in a review of 2.5 million HIV-infected persons (*JAMA* 1993;269:2876). Nevertheless, there are at least 24 reported cases of seroreversion. These reports suggest that seroreversion is most common in infants, patients treated prior to seroconversion and patients with late stage disease (*AIDS* 2010;24:2760; *STD* 2007;34:627; *AIDS* 2006; 20:1460; *CID* 2005;40:368; *CID* 2006;42:700; *AIDS* 2004;18:1607; *JAMA* 1993;269:2786; *Path Onc Res* 1997;3:224; *JAMA* 1993;269: 2786; *Ann Intern Med* 1988;108:785; *J Med Virol* 2008;80:1515; *Ann Intern Med* 2008;149:71). For infants it is important to distinguish between those with passive transfer of maternal antibody who were never infected (common) and those infected with true seroreversion (rare).

- **Unexplained or "atypical response":** There are several well-confirmed cases of HIV-1 infection that have negative serologies using standard test methods. These include one patient with AIDS who had 35 negative EIA tests over a four year period (*CID* 1997;25:98). A total of 16 patients have been reported with inexplicable false negative standard serologic tests outside the "window" (*AIDS* 1995;9:95; *Vox Sang* 1994;67:410; *AIDS* 1999;13:89; *JID* 1997; 175;1352; *JID* 1997;175:955; *CID* 2008;46:785; *JID* 2010;201:341).

- **"Atypical host response"** accounts for rare cases of false negative serology and is largely unexplained (*AIDS* 1995;9:95; *MMWR* 1996; 45:181; *CID* 1997;25:98; *JID* 1997;175:955; *AIDS* 1999;13:89; *CID* 2008;46:785). The diagnosis in these cases is made with VL testing, but the potential for false positives at titers <10,000 c/mL should be noted (*Ann Intern Med* 2001; 134:25).

- **Failure to mount an immunologic response:** Most common in patients with agammaglobulinemia (*NEJM* 2005;353:1074), but this is not always the explanation (*JID* 1999;180:1033). Rare cases of false negative tests in advanced disease have seroreverted with immune reconstitution following ART (*JID* 2010;201:341; *AIDS* 2010;24:327; *CID* 2009;48:229; *JID* 1999;180:1033). These can be confirmed with VL testing.

- **Type N or O strains or HIV-2:** Standard serologic tests detect M subtypes (subtypes A-K) of HIV-1, and some now detect both HIV-1 and -2 and some also detect type O. Nevertheless, most may fail to detect the O subtype, and none detect N subtypes (*Lancet* 1994;343:1393; *Lancet* 1994;344:1333; *MMWR* 1996;45:561; *JCM* 2006;44:1856; *JCM* 2006;44:662; *JCM* 2008;6:2453; *CID* 2008; 46:1936; *JCM* 2009; 47:2906). Only two patients with subtype O HIV infection were detected in the United States through March, 2000 (*MMWR* 1996;45:561; *Emerg Infect Dis* 1996;2:209; *AIDS* 2002;18:269). The N group is another rare variant that causes false-negative EIA screening tests but may be positive by WB (*Nat Med* 1998;4:1032). There have been no recognized infections with the N strain in the United States through March 2000 (*JID* 2000; 181:470). One case of seronegative AIDS caused by an A2 subtype of HIV-1 has been reported (*AIDS* 2004;18:1071). Most important is HIV-2, which requires specific tests and accounted for 0.15% of HIV infections in New York City (*CID* 2010;51:1334), almost exclusively in patients from West Africa (see pg. 8). Several screening tests now detect both HIV-1 and HIV-2, summarized above.

- **Rapid tests:** False negative tests are occasionally reported for rapid tests that are positive with "conventional" serology, although this is unusual (*Ann Intern Med* 2008;149:71; *JCM* 2003;41:2153).

- **Technical or clerical error:** One report from US Army HIV Data System reviewed 4,911 positive tests with 6 "seroreverters." Review of these 6 cases found that 5 were due to misidentified blood sources, indicating "human error" in the lab or in reporting (*JAMA* 1993;269:2876).

FALSE POSITIVE RESULTS: The frequency of false positive HIV serology (both EIA and WB) was reported to range from 0.0004-0.0007% (*JAMA* 1998;280:1080; *Arch Intern Med* 2003;163:1857; *Arch Intern Med* 2000;160:2386). The 0.0004% rate is based on a report from the Red Cross showing 20 false positives among 5.02 million donations from 1991-95 or 1/251,000 (*JAMA* 1998;280:1081). Of the 20,18 (90%) had

Laboratory Tests

a WB pattern showing envelope +/- one additional band only. Important clues to possible false positive tests are lack of risk factors, an undetectable VL, and a normal CD4 count (*Arch Intern Med* 2003;163:1857). The serologic test should be repeated in patients without other laboratory evidence of infection. VL testing is especially important here. Causes of false-positive results include:

- **Autoantibodies:** A single case was reported in which a false-positive serology was ascribed to autoantibodies (*NEJM* 1993;328: 1281), but a subsequent report indicated that this patient did have HIV infection as verified by positive cultures (*NEJM* 1994;331:881).

- **HIV vaccines:** Investigational HIV vaccines are the most common cause of false positive HIV serology. A review of 2,176 participants in HIV vaccine trials with 25 vaccine products showed 908 (42%) had vaccine-induced seropositive results using 3 common EIA screening tests (*JAMA* 2010;304:275). WB results in the vaccine recipients with positive EIA tests were positive in 10%, indeterminant in 66% and negative in 24%. VL testing and WB will help exclude active infection.

- **False positive oral fluid *OraQuick* test:** This test has shown sporadic reports of false positive results, sometimes in substantial numbers (*PLoS One* 2007;2:e185; *MMWR* 2008;57:660; *Ann Intern Med* 2008;149:153; *AIDS* 2006;20:1661). The false positive tests were corrected in most cases by negative confirming WB testing, the *OraQuick* rapid test using finger stick blood or other alternative test platform. See pg. 18.

- **Factitious HIV infection:** This refers to patients who report a history of a positive test that is erroneous, due to either misunderstanding or an intent to deceive (*Ann Intern Med* 1994;121: 763). It is important to confirm anonymous tests and to repeat laboratory reports that cannot be verified, using either repeat serology or VL testing. Note that 2-9% of VL tests are falsely positive, usually with low viral titers (*Ann Intern Med* 1999;130:37).

- **Influenza vaccination:** Any brand of influenza vaccine may cause false positive screening results for HIV-1, presumably due to homology in their envelope proteins (*Am J Epidemiol* 1995;141: 1089; *NEJM* 2006;354:1422; *Cell* 1997;89:263). Confirmatory tests are negative.

- **False positive screening rapid tests:** The cause of false positives is usually unknown but sometimes attributed to other infections, especially parasitic infection (malaria, dengue, trypanosomiasis, and shistosomiasis) possibly due to polyclonal B cell activation (*JCM* 2010; 48:2836; *JCM* 2010;48;1570; *JCM* 2006;44:3024; *CID* 2007;45:139; *CID* 2000;30:819; *JAIDS* 2010;54:641). The frequency of a single positive rapid test that is not confirmed by a second test and shows a negative WB ("false positive screening test") is reported in one review at 6/17,304 (0.03%) (*CID* 2011;52:257), but the

Laboratory Tests

2

positive predictive value depends on the prevalence of HIV in the population tested (Table 2-4). Confirmatory tests are critical. See Table 2-4, pg. 17.

- **Technical or clerical error** (*Arch Intern Med* 2003;163:1857).

INDETERMINATE RESULTS: Indeterminate test results account for 4-20% of WB assays with positive bands for HIV-1 proteins. Tests with this result should be repeated at one month or later (*MMWR* 2001;50 RR-19:1). Causes of indeterminate results include:

- **Serologic tests in the process of seroconversion**; anti-p24 is usually the first antibody to appear.

- **Late-stage HIV infection**, usually with loss of core antibody.

- **Cross-reacting nonspecific antibodies**, as seen with collagen-vascular disease, autoimmune diseases, lymphoma, liver disease, injection drug use, multiple sclerosis, parity, or recent immunization. A review of 46 dialysis patients with false positive EIA screening tests showed 23 were "indeterminant" by WB (*Am J Kidney Dis* 1999;34:146; *Pediatr Nephrol* 2004;19:547).

- **Infection with O strain or HIV-2**

- **HIV vaccine recipients** (see above)

- **Pregnancy:** Positive screening EIA tests with negative or indeterminate WB appear over-represented in pregnancy; those with indeterminate tests usually revert to negative after delivery suggesting pregnancy per se may cause these results (*Am J Perinatol* 2011;28:467).

- **Technical or clerical error:** The most important factor in evaluating indeterminate results is risk assessment and VL measurement. Patients in low-risk categories with indeterminate tests are almost never infected with either HIV-1 or HIV-2; repeat testing often continues to show indeterminate results, and the cause of this pattern is infrequently established (*NEJM* 1990;322:217). For this reason, such patients should be reassured that HIV infection is extremely unlikely, although follow-up serology at 1-3 mos and VL testing is recommended to provide absolute assurance (*MMWR* 2001;50 RR-19:1). Patients with indeterminate tests who are in the process of seroconversion usually have a very high VL at the time of the intermediate result and positive WBs within 1 mo (*J Gen Intern Med* 1992;7:640; *JID* 1991;164:656; *Arch Intern Med* 2000; 160: 2386; *JAIDS* 1998;17:376).

ACUTE HIV INFECTION: Acute HIV infection is defined as the time from HIV transmission to seroconversion. Detection of infection during this early stage is a priority because: 1) it may be accompanied by symptoms of an otherwise unexplained illness; 2) ART may be important at this stage to reduce symptoms and possibly to slow the subsequent course of disease (although this is unproven); and 3)

Laboratory Tests

14

undiagnosed individuals with acute infection are at high risk of further transmission due to high levels of viremia combined with ongoing high-risk behavior (*JID* 2005;191:1403; *JID* 2004; 189:1785).

The natural history of HIV infection dictates the utility of various tests in early stage disease. Studies in macaques show that transmission can be detected 3 days after exposure (*Science* 1999;286:1353); viral homology suggests single virion transmission (*PNAS* 2008;105:7552); HIV then becomes established over 8-10 days ("eclipse stage") followed by a sequence of 6 stages described by Fiebig (*AIDS* 2003; 17:1871) and illustrated by Cohen M, et al, Figure 1 from (*JID* 2010;202 Suppl 2: S270). These 6 stages define the approximate time of positive tests, which follows the eclipse stage and viral dissemination.

The acute retroviral syndrome (pg 3) is characterized by high VL and negative or indeterminate HIV serology. This syndrome should be suspected in patients with typical symptoms (fever, pharyngitis, adenopathy, rash, etc.) preceded by a high risk exposure within 3-4 wks that may or may not be easily recalled or revealed by the patient (*NEJM* 2005;352:1873).The recommended diagnostic is a test that detects HIV, including the rapid Ag/Ab test.

■ TABLE 2-2: **Time of HIV Detection Following Transmission Using Various Test Methods***

Fiebig	Test	Positive from transmission in days†
1	Viral load	17 (13-28)
2	p24 antigen	22 (18-34)
3	EIA positive	25 (22-37)
4	WB positive or negative	31 (27-43)
5	WB positive, p31 Ag negative	101 (71-154)
6	WB positive, p31 Ag positive	--

*   Based on classification of Fiebig, et al. (*AIDS* 2003;17:1871) and adapted from Cohen et al. (*JID* 2010;202 [Suppl 2]:S271)

†   Time in days with mean (range)

ALTERNATIVE HIV SEROLOGIC TESTS

IMMUNOFLUORESCENCE ASSAY (IFA): This is an alternative to the WB to confirm a positive screening test (rapid test or EIA). Possible advantages of the IFA are that it is technically simple, less expensive and more rapid than WB (*Internat J Infect Dis* 2010; 14:e10930. The major use is in resource-limited settings.

HOME KITS: The *Home Access* HIV self test kit: (Home Access Health Corp., Hoffman Estates, IL; 800-HIV-TEST) is sold in retail pharmacies, online (www.HomeAccess.com), and by phone order (1-800-448-8378). Cost of the test is $60 for a 5-day report service or $66 for next

2 Laboratory Tests

day report service. Blood is obtained with a lancet, and blotted blood collected on a filter strip is mailed in a protected envelope using an anonymous code. The *Home Access* test uses a double EIA with a confirmatory IFA. Sensitivity and specificity approach 100%. The results are confidential, and counseling plus referral is available by phone. In a study of 174,316 HIV home sample collection tests in 1996-1997, 0.9% were positive and 97% of users called for their results (*JAMA* 1998;280:1699). Merits of this type of home testing are debated (*NEJM* 1995;332:1296), but opinion is changing toward more general acceptance (*NEJM* 2006;354: 437). The FDA has subsequently reviewed another home test in which results are interpreted by the user, which would make home testing available to consumers in a fashion similar to the OTC pregnancy test. The initial review was favorable (*JCM* 2006; 44:3472)

RAPID TESTS: There are eight FDA-approved rapid serologic tests, listed in Table 2-3, which show variations in the specimen type and CLIA category (www.mmhiv.com/link/CDC-Rapid-HIV-Testing).

Performance is regulated by the Clinical Laboratory Improvement Amendment of 1988 (CLIA). The tests are categorized as CLIA "waived" or "moderate complexity." *OraQuick, Clearview* and *Uni-Gold* are CLIA waived tests, which means there are no federal restrictions for personnel, quality assessment or proficiency testing. The tests can be performed in laboratories, clinical settings, mobile vans, physicians' offices, etc. The requirement is to obtain a certificate of waiver and follow manufacturer's instructions (www.mmhiv.com/link/CDC-CLIA-Waiver). *ARCHITECT Ag/Ab Combo, Reveal, VITROS Anti-HIV-1 & -2* and *Multispot HIV-1/HIV-2* are "moderately complex," which requires registering with CLIA, and satisfying CLIA standards for personnel, quality assessment, proficiency testing and inspections. The retail cost is $15-25/test or $8-9 for CDC funded expanded access sites, but the cost to a consumer may be much more. *Reveal, VITROS* and *Multispot* require plasma or serum, and thus a centrifuge. Common features for all of these tests:

- The positive predictive value depends on the prevalence of HIV in the population sampled (Table 2-4, pg. 17).
- Persons receive a "Subject Information Notice" with the test.
- A negative test is a definitive negative unless tested in the "window period" (first 3 mos post-exposure).
- Positive tests are considered preliminary positive results and must be confirmed with a Western blot or IFA.
- Indeterminate tests should be repeated in 1 mo.
- There are multiple test methods to detect HIV that vary greatly in sensitivity, specificity, cost and availability (Table 2-5, pg. 22).
- The rapid test is considered slightly more cost effective compared to conventional tests (*Public Health Reports* 2008; Supple 3, 123:51).

Laboratory Tests

Test	Source	Specimen*	CLIA†	Sens %‡	Spec %‡	Comment
OraQuick	OraSure Technologies www.orasure.com	Blood	Waived	100	99.8	HIV-1 & -2 20 minutes
		Oral Fluid		99.6	99.7	20-40 min
Uni-Gold Recombigen	Trinity BioTech www.unigoldhiv.com	Blood	Waived	100	99.7	HIV-1 10 minutes
		Plasma		100	99.8	
		Serum		100	99.8	
Clearview	Inverness Medical www.inverness medicalpd.com	Blood	Waived	99.7	99.9	HIV-1 & -2 15-20 minutes
Reveal G2	MedMira Inc. www.reveal-hiv.com	Plasma	Mod Complex	99.8		HIV-1 5 min
		Serum		99.8	98.6	
Multispot HIV-1/HIV-2	Bio-Rad Labs 1-800-224-6723 www.biorad.com	Serum	Mod Complex	100	99.9	HIV-1 & -2 15 minutes
Multispot HIV-2		Serum		100		
VITROS Anti-HIV-1 & -2	Ortho Clinical Diagnostics www.orthoclinical.com	Serum	Mod Complex	100	99.5	HIV-1 & -2 50 minutes
Architect Ag/Ab Combo	Abbott Diagnostics www.abbott.com	Serum	High Complex	99.7	98.5	HIV-1 & -2 29 minutes Ag + Ab
Insti HIV-1 Test	bioLytical Labs www.biolytical.com	Blood	Mod complex	99.8	99.5	60 seconds

* Use of whole blood avoids the need for a centrifuge or any other equipment.

† CLIA requirements include registration with CLIA and compliance with their standards for testing, inspection, etc.

‡ Sensitivity and specificity of the Ag (Package insert)

■ TABLE 2-4: **Positive Predictive Value of a Single Test***

HIV prevalence	Predictive Value, positive test		
	OraQuick	Uni-Gold	Single EIA
10%	99%	97%	98%
2%	95%	87%	91%
1%	91%	77%	83%
0.5%	83%	63%	71%
0.1%	50%	25%	33%
Specificity	99.9%	99.7%	99.8%

* Branson B, www.mmhiv.com/link/CDC-Rapid-HIV-Testing

Note: The prevalence of HIV in the US is about 0.3%. With 1000 tests in a population with a prevalence of 0.1% there would be 1 true positive test and 2 false positives (Branson)

Laboratory Tests

2

- Note that up to 35-50% of people with positive rapid tests never return for confirmatory test results (*Expert Rev Anti Infect Ther* 2010;8:631).
- Resource-limited countries confirm positive tests with a second rapid test from a different supplier and a different antigen. A major advantage of this double test method in the clinic or emergency room is that it allows for definitive results with positive as well as negative tests.
- *Uni-Gold* detects IgM as well as IgG and consequently may give more positive tests in early stage disease.

Sensitivity and specificity of a single rapid test: A study of six rapid tests with 6,282 specimens showed sensitivities of 97.2-100% and specificities of 94.5-99.4% (*CID* 2011;52:257). The positive predictive value is dependent on HIV prevalence, an observation that emphasizes the need for a confirmatory test as shown in Table 2-4.

INDICATIONS: Rapid tests are recommended for HIV screening as an alternative to EIA. The rapid tests may be especially useful where rapid results are important, as with occupational exposure, in pregnant women who present in labor without prior testing, in outreach settings (*MMWR* 2006;55: 673), and in settings where patients are unlikely to return for test results, including emergency rooms and STD clinics. With provider-read (CLIA-waived) tests the average turnaround time is 45 minutes, but it may be as short as 10 minutes (www.mmhiv.com/link/CDC-Rapid-HIV-Testing and Table 2-2; pg. 15).

RAPID TESTS IN RESOURCE-LIMITED COUNTRIES: The WHO recommends a rapid screening test followed by a confirmatory rapid test in positives using an assay from an alternative commercial source (and alternative antigen). The Rapid HIV Test Evaluation Work Group from WHO and CDC has reported a median specificity of 100% using *Determine, OraQuick, Uni-Gold* and 6 other commercial sources (*AIDS Res Hum Retrovir* 2007;23:1491). With field testing of 735,000 patients with a seroprevalence of 28%, the rate of concordance was 96.8-99.3% for positive specimens and 98.1-99.7% for negative specimens. A more recent report with 10,819 tests in adults using two rapid tests in the field (home-based testing) for comparison with lab-based testing showed 99.6% sensitivity and 100% specificity (*JAIDS* 2010;55:245).

SALIVA TEST: *OraSure* (OraSure Technologies, Inc.; Bethlehem, Pa; 800-672-7873; www.orasure.com), is an FDA-approved device for collecting saliva and concentrating IgG for application of EIA tests for HIV antibody. The test consists of a specially treated pad used to swab the gums; the swab is then inserted into a vial for 20 minutes and read at 20-40 minutes. The amount of IgG obtained from saliva is far higher than in plasma and is well above the 0.5 mg/L level necessary for detection of HIV antibodies. Specimens from 26,066 patients showed a sensitivity of 99.24% and specificity of 99.89% compared to blood tests; there were 56 (0.22%) discordant results (*AIDS* 2006;20:1661).

Laboratory Tests

There are several reports of false positive tests, often in clusters; the error can be detected by alternative test for antibody (including *OraQuick* using blood samples, WB or VL testing (see pg. 12). Potential advantages over standard serologic testing is the use of saliva instead of blood, providing better patient acceptance, reduced risk of occupational exposure and availability in places that do not normally draw blood. However, there is no advantage if blood is to be drawn anyway, and the high rate of false positives is bothersome. The recommendation is to use fingerstick blood initially or to confirm a positive oral fluid test with a rapid test using blood or standard serology. There is a proposal before the FDA to market an over-the-counter home test that can be interpreted by the user like a home pregnancy test (*NEJM* 2006;354:437). This is different than the currently available home test (*Home Access*, see above) which is read and accompanied by a telephoned result with counseling and referral to a regional provider.

NAAT TESTING: Nucleic acid amplification testing (NAAT) is used to detect HIV and may be used to detect acute HIV, as the test is positive about 11 days before 3rd generation assays and 6 days before 4th generation EIAs (*AIDS* 2003;17:1871). A common use is pooling of EIA-negative specimens to more efficiently detect acute HIV. The limit of detection with 1:16 pooling is estimated at 30 c/mL (*Arch Intern Med* 2010;170:60). One report from 14 STD clinics used this method to screen 54,948 seronegative specimens with various 3rd generation rapid tests and detected 27 additional cases (1.4%). The Abbott *ARCHITECT HIV Ag/Ab Combo* (4th generation) test was positive in 23 of the 27 (85%) (*Arch Intern Med* 2010;170:66). In another report of 14,005 tests in a high incidence population (MSM), 328 (2.3%) were antibody-positive, and 36 (0.3%) of the 13,677 antibody-negative men were NAAT positive (*CID* 2009;49:444). The median VL in this population was >1,000,000 c/mL. All specimens positive in the NAAT pooling were also positive in the Abbott *ARCHITECT HIV Ag/Ab Combo*.

ABBOTT *ARCHITECT* 4TH GENERATION AG/AB COMBO ASSAY: The enzyme immunoassays to detect HIV have evolved through four generations. The first and second generation detected IgG antibody to HIV and are no longer used. The third generation test is a "sandwich" immunoassay that detects IgM and IgG antibody to HIV and is standard in most labs with the advantage that it detects HIV infection somewhat earlier. The Abbott 4th generation *Combo* test detects HIV Ab but also detects p24 antigen. The advantage is detection of acute HIV infection with an 8-10 day reduction in the window period compared to the 3rd generation tests and detection of 80% of acute HIV infections (*Expert Rev Anti-Infect Ther* 2010;8:63). See pg. 14-15. The test is FDA-cleared as a highly complex test (not CLIA-waived), eg requires a lab technician for detecting HIV-1 and HIV-2 and takes 29 minutes to perform. Use in high prevalence populations (South Africa, MSM-US, STD clinics) shows positive results in 0.08-0.3% of antibody-negative specimens (*JCM* 2010;48:3407; *JAIDS* 2009;52:121; *CID* 2009;49:444; *MMWR* 2009;58:1296). The rate of positive assays for p24 antigen compared to NAAT pooling is 84-100% (*Expert Rev Anti-Infect Ther* 2010;8:631). Acute seroconverters with negative Ab screening tests showed 13/21 (62%) were positive for Ag with the *ARCHITECT* test; false negatives had VL values of 700-15,000 c/mL (*JAIDS* 2009;52:121).

THE 60 *SECOND TEST* (BIOLYTICAL LABORATORIES): This test is FDA-cleared and is similar to other FDA-cleared point-of-care HIV tests except that it can be read in 60 seconds. Sensitivity with finger stick blood is 99.9%. Positive tests require WB confirmation. It is "moderately complex" and not CLIA-waived, meaning it requires a laboratory technician.

RNA QUALITATIVE TEST: The *Aptima* HIV-1 RNA Qualitative Assay (GenProbe, San Diego, CA) detects HIV-1 RNA in plasma and can be used to detect acute HIV or it can be used to confirm a standard serologic test. *Aptima* is FDA-cleared, (October, 2006) and is the only FDA cleared test for detecting acute HIV infection (*JCM* 2008; 46:1588). However, most would conclude that the standard VL tests can easily be used for this purpose at no extra cost and with far greater experience. An alternative use is for detecting HIV in pooled samples to detect acute HIV infection (*JCM* 2010;48:3343; *JAIDS* 2009;52:121) (although it is FDA-cleared for single specimen analysis only).

Viral Detection

Other methods to establish HIV infection include techniques to detect DNA (HIV-1 DNA PCR) or RNA (HIV-1 RNA) by bDNA or RT-PCR (Table 2-4, pg. 17). HIV-1 DNA PCR is the most sensitive and can detect 1-10 copies/mL of HIV proviral DNA, but the reagents are not well standardized nor FDA-approved. None of these tests is considered to be more accurate than routine serology, but some may be useful in patients with confusing serologic test results, and for HIV detection when routine serologic tests are likely to be misleading, as in patients with agammaglobulinemia, acute retroviral infection, neonatal HIV infection, and patients in the window period following viral exposure. In most cases, confirmation of positive serology is accomplished simply by repeat serology or VL testing.

Quantitative Plasma HIV RNA (Viral Load)

TECHNIQUES: See Table 2-5, pg. 22.

- **HIV RNA PCR:** *Amplicor HIV-1 Monitor Test* version 1.5, and *COBAS TagMan HIV-1* test, Roche; 800-526-1247.
- **Branched chain DNA or bDNA:** *Versant* HIV-1 RNA 3.0 Assay, Seimans Diagnostics (formerly Bayer);800-434-2447.
- **Nucleic acid sequence-based amplification (NASBA):** *NucliSens*

20

HIV-1 QT (bioMérieux), 800-682-2666.

REPRODUCIBILITY: Commercially available assays vary based on the lower level of detection and dynamic ranges, as shown in Table 2-6, pg. 24 (*JCM* 1996;34:3016; *J Med Virol* 1996;50:293; *JCM* 1996;34:1058; *JCM* 1998;36:3392). Two standard deviations (95% confidence limits) with this assay is 3-fold or 0.5 $\log_{10}$ c/mL (*JID* 1997;175:247; *AIDS* 1999;13:2269). This means that the 95% confidence limit for a value of 10,000 c/mL ranges from 3,100-32,000 c/mL. Quantitative results with the *Amplicor* (Roche) assay version 1.5 and bDNA assay (*Versant* 3.0) are comparable except at the low end of the linear range (<1,500 c/mL) (*JCM* 2000;38: 2837; *JCM* 2000;38:1113). Comparative testing for the *NucliSens* (bioMérieux) assay is less extensive but appears comparable (*JCM* 2000;38:3882; *JCM* 2000;38: 2837). The *COBAS TagMan HIV-1* test is similar to the *HIV-1 Monitor* but uses RT-PCR to detect a conserved region in HIV-1 gag, has a greater dynamic range (40-10^7 c/mL) and performance comparison shows a strong correlation with *HIV-1 Monitor* results (correlative R^2=0.99) with the greater deviation at the lowest and highest ends of the linear curve (*J Clin Virol* 2007;38:304; *JCM* 2007;45:3436). Sensitivity of this assay was subsequently improved by a dual target strategy that includes the long terminal repeat region (5' LTR, U5) as well as gag. This is version 2.0 with a lower limit of quantitation of 20 c/mL (*J Clin Virol* 2010;49:41). A concern with this assay is an apparent reduced accuracy with persistently detectable levels (>50 c/mL) reported in patients who do not have evidence of failure with sequential testing and have <50 c/mL with duplicate *Amplicor* monitor tests (*HIV Clin Trials* 2008;9:283). This has prompted concern for the need to repeat the test or change treatment with low level viremia using that assay.

SUBTYPES: There is greater performance variation with non-subtype B. In tests with subtypes A-D,F,G,CRF 01_AE and CRF 02_AG, inter-subtype recombinants and group O, bDNA (*Versant* 3.0) was somewhat superior, with 83% within 0.5 $\log_{10}$ c/mL. The result for *Amplicor Monitor* 1.5 was 74% and 61% for *NucliSens* (*JCM* 2005;43:3860). Other studies support these findings (*J Med Virol* 2006; 78:883; *JAIDS* 2002;29:330).

COST: $100-150 per assay (Medicare reimbursement $111-130).

USES OF VIRAL LOAD TESTING

- **Treatment goal:** The major goal of ART is HIV viral suppression to <50 c/mL. Concerns for variations in test results resulted in use of a >200 c/mL threshold to define failure in clinical monitoring to avoid unnecessary expense and concern with repeat visits, and resistance testing due to erroneous lab tests. This is now policy for the ACTG and 2011 DHHS Guidelines (*CID* 2009;48:260; *JAIDS* 2010;54:42).

- **Diagnosis of primary infection:** VL testing can be used to establish the diagnosis of HIV infection in patients with confusing serology (see pg. 15). Most studies show high levels of virus (10^5-10^6 c/mL)

2 Laboratory Tests

■ TABLE 2-5: **Comparison of FDA-approved Assay Methods for Viral Load**

	Roche	Siemens	bioMérieux	TaqMan
Trade name	*Amplicor HIV Monitor* 1.5	*Versant* HIV-1 RNA 3.0	*NucliSens* HIV-1 QT	*COBAS TaqMan V₂*
Technique	RT-PCR	bDNA	NASBA	RT-PCR
Comparison of results	Results are similar to bDNA (*Versant*) results using version 2.0 or 3.0.	Results with are comparable with RT-PCR (*Amplicor*) assays.	Results appear comparable with RT-PCR and bDNA assays, but supporting data are less robust.	Results are similar to Abbott *RealTime* assay
Advantages/ disadvantages	Fewer false-positives in patients without HIV infection compared with bDNA.	Less technician time. Good dynamic range, but higher threshold for undetectable virus.	May be used with tissue or body fluids such as genital secretions. Greatest dynamic range.	Increased sensitivity Broad linear range Poor specificity at lower threshold giving false positives
Dynamic range	*Amplicor* 1.5: 400-750,000 c/mL *Ultra-Direct* 1.5: 20-100,000 c/mL	75-500,000 c/mL*	176-3,500,000 c/mL depending on volume	20-10,000,000 c/mL
Subtype amplified	Version 1.5: A to H	A to H	A to H	A-H and O
Specimen volume	*Amplicor*: 0.2 mL *Ultra-Direct*: 0.5 mL	1 mL	10 µL to 2 mL	1 mL
Tubes	EDTA (lavender top)	EDTA (lavender top)	EDTA, heparin, whole blood, any body fluid, PBMC, semen, tissue, etc.	EDTA
Requirement	Separate plasma <6 hrs and freeze prior to shipping at -20°C or -70°C.	Separate plasma <4 hrs and freeze prior to shipping at -20°C or -70°C.	Separate serum or plasma <4 hrs and freeze prior to shipping at -20°C or -70°C.	Plasma
Contact	800-526-1247	800-434-2447	800-682-2666	800-526-1247

* The FDA-cleared lower threshold is 75 c/mL.
Outside the US the lower threshold is 50 c/mL.

Laboratory Tests

during acute infection. Note that 2-9% of persons without HIV infection have false-positive results, virtually always with low level HIV RNA titers (<10,000 c/mL) (*Ann Intern Med* 1999;130:37; *JCM* 2000;38:2837; *Ann Intern Med* 2001;134:25).

- **Prognosis:** VL correlates with the rate of CD4 decline or CD4 slope (*JID* 2002;185:908), but this association is not as strong as once thought (*JAMA* 2006;296:1523). The most comprehensive study to assess the association between VL and natural history is the analysis of stored sera from the Multicenter AIDS Cohort Study (MACS), which found a strong association between "set point" and rate of progression that was independent of the baseline CD4 count (*Ann Intern Med* 1995;122:573; *Science* 1996;272:1167; *JID* 1996;174:696; *JID* 1996;174:704; *AIDS* 1999;13:1305; *NEJM* 2001;349,720; *AIDS* 2002;16:2455; *Lancet* 2003;362:679; *JAIDS* 2005;38:289). This has changed in the HAART era, when outcome is determined primarily by therapy and is less dependent on baseline VL (*AIDS* 2006;20:1197; *CID* 2006;42:136; *JID* 2004;190: 280). Even without ART the CD4 slope appears to be influenced by other factors that influence immune activation (*Nat Med* 2006;12:1365). A strong association between CD4 count and VL is supported by the rapid CD4 decline that accompanies rapid return of viremia to pretreatment levels when ART is discontinued (*NEJM* 2003;349:837) and the sustained normal CD4 counts in most "elite controllers" (*JID* 2008;197:563).

- **Copy years viremia:** The term refers to the cumulative viral burden based on VL from the time of HIV transmission. One report showed each $\log_{10}$ increase in copy-years was associated with a 1.7-fold increase in AIDS or death (*Am J Epid* 2010;171:198). An association has also been noted with AIDS-related lymphoma (*JID* 2009;200:79). There is speculation that this may also correlate with immune activation and its consequences. The utility of this metric for clinical monitoring is being investigated.

- **Risk of opportunistic infection:**The VL appears to predict OIs independently of CD4 count when counts are <200 cells/mm^3 (*JAMA* 1996;276:105; *AIDS* 1999;13:341; *AIDS* 1999;13:1035; *JAIDS* 2001;27:44), *JID* 2006; 194:633). The major prospective study examining this association was ACTG 722, which found that the failure to decrease VL by ≥ 1 $\log_{10}$ c/mL in patients with a baseline CD4 count of <150 cells/mm^3 increased the risk of an OI 15-fold (*JAIDS* 2002;30:154). A retrospective review of over 12,000 patients found that CD4 counts are the best predictors of progression to an AIDS-defining complication (*Lancet* 2002;360:119). See pg. 3.

- **Probability of transmission:** The probability of HIV transmission with nearly any type of exposure is directly correlated with VL (*NEJM* 2000;342:921; *JAIDS* 1996;12:427; *JAIDS* 1998;17:42; *JAIDS* 1999;21:120; *JID* 2002;185:428; *Lancet* 2001;357:1149; *AIDS* 2001;

■ TABLE 2-6: **Tests for HIV-1**

Assay	Sensitivity	Comments
Routine serology	99.7%	Readily available and inexpensive. Sensitivity >99.7% and specificity >99.9% (*MMWR* 1990;39:380; *NEJM* 1988;319:961; *JAMA* 1991;266:2861).
Rapid test See pg. 16 and Table 2-2	99.6%	Results are available in 20 min. Advantages with CLIA-waived tests (*OraQuick, Clearview* and *Uni-Gold Recombigen*) are that the test requires no lab equipment, results are available in ≤20 minutes, and interpretation may be done by the provider. Negative tests are definitive for patient care purposes unless "in the window" that precedes seroconversion; positive tests must be confirmed with a WB. Table 2-2 lists the FDA-approved rapid tests in the U.S. (www.mmhiv.com/link/CDC-Rapid-HIV-Testing). Other rapid tests are available but are not FDA-approved (*Int J STD AIDS* 2006;17:357; *Vox Sang* 1997;72:11; *JCM* 2004;42:3850).
Salivary test (*OraSure*) See pg. 18	99.6%	Salivary collection device to collect IgG for EIA and WB. Advantage is avoidance of the need for blood. Some reports of poor specificity with rapid tests using blood if properly interpreted (*JAMA* 1997; 227:254), but specificity is a problem in some studies (see text).
PBMC culture	95-100%	Viral isolation by co-cultivation of patient's PBMC with phytohemagglutinin-stimulated donor PBMC with IL-2 over 28 days. Expensive and labor-intensive. May be qualitative or quantitative. Main use of qualitative technique is viral isolation for further study such as sequence analysis. Studies prior to availability of quantitative HIV RNA PCR showed quantitative culture results correlated with stage of disease: Mean titer was 2000/10^6 cells in patients with AIDS (*NEJM* 1989;321:1621).
DNA PCR assay	>99%	Qualitative DNA PCR is used to detect cell-associated proviral DNA, including HIV reservoirs in peripheral CD4 cells in patients responding to ART with a sensitivity of about 5 copies/10^6 cells (*J Virol Methods* 2005;124:157). This is not considered sufficiently accurate for diagnosis without confirmation and is not FDA approved (*Ann Intern Med* 1996;124:803), although it is occasionally used when other tests are disputed or serology is indeterminate.
HIV RNA PCR	95-98%	False positive tests in 2-9%, usually at low titer (<10,000 c/mL). Sensitivity depends on VL, threshold of assay, and ART status. Sensitivity approaches 100% with acute HIV infection; specificity is 97%, but nearly 100% with viral load >10,000 c/mL.
p24 antigen	30-90%	Sometimes used as an alternative to VL test to detect acute HIV infection due to reduced cost. Specificity is 100%, but sensitivity is about 30-90%, much less than quantitative VL tests (*Ann Intern Med* 2001;134:25). Another use is as a lower-cost alternative to VL testing in resource-limited countries (*JCM* 2005;43:506).
Nucleic acid amplification test (NAAT)	>99%	Detects HIV, not HIV antibody. Use with early infection (pre-seroconversion).

Laboratory Tests

15:621; *CID* 2002;34:391; *JID* 2005;191:1403; *AIDS* 2006 ;20:895). Evidence was based on: Multiple discordant couple studies show no seroconversions when the positive partner had an undetectable VL (*NEJM* 2000; 342:921; *JAIDS* 2005;40:96; *STD* 2008;35:912; *AIDS* 2011;20:25; *AIDS* 2009;23:1397; *JAIDS* 2010;55 [Suppl 1]:1; *JAIDS* 2006;43: 324); and lack of functional HIV virions in male and female genital secretions in patients with viral suppression (*AIDS* 2000; 14:117; *AIDS* 2000;14:415; *JID* 2006;52: 290; *JAIDS* 2006;42: 584; *JAIDS* 2007;44:38). There is agreement that risk is substantially decreased but disagreement as to whether it can be concluded that there is no risk based on discrepancies sometimes noted between VL in plasma vs genital secretions, the small sample sizes of discordant couple studies, lack of data for anal intercourse, and the fact that VL could become detectable between measurements (*STD* 2008; 35:55).

- **Community viral load (CVL):** Sequential mean and total VL in HIV-infected persons has been found to predict HIV incidence in seronegative persons within the population sampled for geographic areas (*PLoS One* 2010;5:e11068) and populations at risk (*BMJ* 2009;338:b1649; Kirk G. 2011 CROI:Abstr. 484). This is the scientific rationale for the Test and Treat hypothesis proposed by WHO (*Lancet* 2009;373:48) and undergoing large trials (*CID* 2010;51:725). One method to determine the mean CVL is the average of the most recent VL of all HIV-positive persons in a specified time period. A median VL could also be used but it lacks a direct relation with transmission rates (*PLoS Med* 2010;6:e11068). The total CVL is the sum which determines risk based on the number with infections as well as VL.

- **Therapeutic monitoring:** Following initiation of ART, there is a rapid initial decline in VL over 2-4 wks (alpha slope), reflecting activity against free plasma HIV virions and HIV in acutely infected CD4 cells. This is followed by a second decline (beta slope) that is longer in duration (months) and more modest in degree (see quantitation, below, under "Frequency and therapeutic monitoring"). The beta slope reflects activity against HIV-infected macrophages and HIV released from other compartments, especially those trapped in follicular dendritic cells of lymph follicles. The maximum antiviral effect is expected by 4-6 mos. VL is accepted as the most important barometer of therapeutic response, although CD4 count best predicts clinical progression (*NEJM* 1996; 335:1091; *Ann Intern Med* 1996;124:984; *JID* 2002; 185:178). The most important long-term goal of treatment is achieving a VL <50 c/mL, because some authorities note that clonal sequence analyses show no viral evolution with resistance mutations at that level (*JID* 2004;189:1452; *JID* 2004;189:1444), and some studies show that VL of <1 c/mL is common (*AIDS* 2011;25:341).The implication is that there is no viral replication and little likelihood of developing resistance or disease

2 Laboratory Tests

progression. Nevertheless, some blips are associated with lapses in adherence, which could lead to drug failure and resistance (*JID* 2007;193:1773). Given the variability in VL assays and results with long term outcome, most authorities endorse a therapeutic goal of maintaining the VL <50 c/mL defines failure since most of the reports from 50-200 c/mL appear to be lab errors (*JAMA* 2005;293:817).

- **Unexpectedly low VL:** A minority of patients are long-term non-progressors, with persistently high CD4 cell counts. Another even more uncommon group are the "elite controllers" defined as those having VL <50 c/mL without therapy (see pg. 5).

- **Subtype variations:** The standard assays are most accurate for sub-type B but are FDA-cleared for quantitation of subtypes A-G. A study of performance characteristics of non-subtype-B specimens found that the frequency of undetectable VL or discordance by >1 log_{10} c/mL was 3% for *Amplicor Monitor* 1.5, 9% for *Versant* 3.0, and 15% for *NucliSens* (*JCM* 2005;43:3860). There is no commercially available quantitative test for HIV-2.

- **Reservoirs:** HIV resides in some anatomical sites that may be differentially affected by antiretroviral drugs and may be the source of archived strains resistant to these drugs. The most important and best characterized reservoirs are resting CD4 cells; others are cells in the CNS, GI tract (GALT) and genital tract (*AIDS* 2002;16:39; *JCM* 2000;38:1414; *Ann Intern Med* 2007;146:591; *Top HIV Med* 2010;18:104; *PNAS* 2008;105: 3879; *Ann Rev Med* 2008;59:487).

RECOMMENDATIONS: Adapted from the International AIDS Society–USA (*JAMA* 2006;296:827) and January 10, 2011 DHHS Guidelines (www.mmhiv.com/link/2011-DHHS-HIV). Some of the commercially available tests are summarized and compared in Table 2-6.

- **Quality assurance:** Assays on individual patients should preferably be obtained at times of clinical stability, at least 4 wks after immunizations or intercurrent infections, and with use of the same lab and same technology over time.

- **Frequency and therapeutic monitoring:** Tests should be performed at baseline and followed by routine testing at 3-6 mo intervals (*CID* 2001;33:1060). With new therapy and changes in therapy, assays should be obtained at 2-4 wks, then at 4-8 wk intervals until VL <50 c/mL is achieved. An expected response to therapy is a decrease of 0.75-1.0 log_{10} c/mL at 1 wk (*Lancet* 2001;358:1760; *JAIDS* 2002;30:167), a decrease of 1.5-2 log_{10}-<5,000 c/mL at 4 wks (*JAIDS* 2000;25:36; *AIDS* 1999;13:1873; *JAIDS* 2004;37: 1155), <500 c/mL at 8-16 wks (*Ann Intern Med* 2001;135:945; *JAIDS* 2000;24:433), and <50 c/mL at 24-48 wks. The 2003 Swiss guidelines define treatment failure by the failure to decrease VL by 1.5 log_{10} c/mL within 4 wks or to achieve undetectable virus by 4 mos (*Scand JID* 2003;35:155). The time to VL nadir is dependent on pretreatment VL as well as potency of the regimen, adherence, pharmacology, and resistance. Patients with high baseline VL take longer to achieve maximum suppression. Failure to reduce VL by 1 $\log_{10}$ c/mL (90%) at 4 wks suggests virologic failure due to non-adherence, pre-existing resistance, or inadequate drug exposure. The expectation is to reduce the VL to <50 c/mL by 16-24 wks (*JAMA* 2006;296:827; *JCI* 2000;105:777). The VL should then be measured in patients on treatment every 3-6 mos to assure a VL <50 c/mL (*JID* 1999; 180:1347). Blips (see pg. 106) are usually inconsequential but can also indicate non-adherence (*JID* 2007;196:1773) and sustained levels >50 c/mL indicate virologic failure (*JAMA* 2005;293:817; *JAC* 2008;61:699). Virologic failure is now defined by the 2011 DHHS Guidelines panel as confirmed VL >200 c/mL.

- **Interpretation:** Changes of ≥50% (0.3 $\log_{10}$ c/mL) are considered significant.

- **Factors that correlate with increase VL**
  - Switch from R5-tropic to X4-tropic HIV
  - Progression of disease
  - Failure of ART due to inadequate potency, inadequate drug levels, nonadherence, and/or resistance.
  - HIV superinfection (*JID* 2005;192:438)
  - Active infections; active TB increases VL 5- to 160-fold (*J Immunol* 1996;157:1271); pneumococcal pneumonia increases VL 3- to 5-fold.
  - Immunizations such as influenza or pneumococcal vaccine (*Blood* 1995;86:1082; *NEJM* 1996;335:817; *NEJM* 1996;334:1222). Increases are modest and last 2-4 wks.

- **Relative merit of tests:** The *COBAS TaqMan HIV-1* test has advantages of increased sensitivity and a very broad dynamic range (20-10 million c/mL). A concern is an increased frequency of false positive blips (*Pathology* 2011;43:275; *J Clin Virol* 2010;49:249). The *Versant* version 3.0 assay has good reproducibility for VL levels of 75-500,000 c/mL. The linear range for *Amplicor* is 50-100,000 c/mL for the ultrasensitive test. It should not be used in patients expected to have higher VL (*JCM* 2000;38:2837). The *NucliSens* assay has a broad dynamic range (176-3,500,000 c/mL) and can be used for HIV quantification on blood or on various body fluids or tissue such as seminal fluid, CSF, breast milk, saliva, and vaginal fluid (*JCM* 2000;38:1414). Comparison tests show discrepancies between techniques based on HIV-1 subtype. The recommendation is to use the same assay to monitor patients (*JCM* 2011;49:292).

CD4 Cell Count

This is a standard test to assess prognosis for progression to AIDS or death, to formulate the differential diagnosis in a symptomatic patient (Table 1-2, pg. 3), and to make therapeutic decisions regarding antiviral treatment and prophylaxis for opportunistic infections. It is the most reliable indicator of prognosis (*Ann Intern Med* 1997;126:946; *Lancet* 2002;360:119; *Lancet* 2003;362:679). An analysis of 13 cohorts with 16,214 patients found that the CD4 count was by far the most important predictor of death (*Lancet* 2004; 364:51). CD8 cell counts have not been found to predict outcome (*NEJM* 1990;322:166), but a prolonged time from HIV seroconversion to inversion of the CD4/CD8 ratio predicts slow progression (*JAIDS* 2006;42:620). HIV-specific CD8 cells (CD38 cells) are important for controlling HIV levels but cannot be routinely measured (*Science* 1999;283:857; *JAIDS* 2002;29:346).

- **Technique:** The standard method for determining CD4 count uses flow cytometers and hematology analyzers. The test requires fresh blood (<18 hrs old) and generally costs $50-150. There is great need for rapid, simple, and affordable CD4 tests in resource-limited countries. The PIMA POC (point-of-care) CD4 test is an example of a test that uses finger stick blood, does not require laboratory equipment and provides results in 20 minutes that correlate well with standard methods (*JAIDS* 2010;55:1).

- **Normal Values:** Normal values for most laboratories are a mean of 800-1050 cells/mm³, with a range of two standard deviations of approximately 500-1400 cells/mm³ (*Ann Intern Med* 1993;119:55).

- **Frequency of Testing:** The CD4 count should be measured at baseline, and some recommend two measurements before levels starting treatment (2011 DHHS Guidelines).The CD4 count should be repeated every 3-6 mos in most patients but can be at 6-12 mo intervals in patients with good virologic control and relatively high CD4 counts (2011 DHHS Guidelines). The test should be repeated when results are inconsistent with prior trends.

- **Reproducibility:** Both clinicians and patients must be aware of the variability in CD4 test results, especially if they will be used to make clinical decisions, such as initiation of ART or opportunistic infection prophylaxis. The 95% confidence range for a true count of 200 cells/mm³, for example, is 118-337 cells/mm³ (*JAIDS* 1993;6:537). Results that are inconsistent with prior trends should be repeated. A significant change between two CD4 counts (two standard deviations) is approximately 30% of the absolute count or a CD4 % change of 3% (2011 DHHS Guidelines).

- **Factors that Influence CD4 Cell Counts:** Factors include analytical variation, seasonal and diurnal variations, some intercurrent illnesses, and corticosteroids. Substantial <u>analytical variations</u> account for the wide range in normal values (usually about 500-1400 cells/mm³) and reflect the fact that the CD4 cell count is the product of three variables: the white blood cell count, percent lymphocytes, and the CD4 percentage. There are also <u>seasonal changes</u> (*Clin Exp*

Immunol 1991;86:349) and diurnal changes, with the lowest levels at 12:30 PM and peak values at 8:30 PM (*JAIDS* 1990;3:144); these variations do not clearly correspond to the circadian rhythm of corticosteroids. Modest decreases in the CD4 cell count have been noted with some acute infections and with major surgery. Corticosteroid administration may have a profound effect, with decreases from 900 cells/mm^3 to <300 cells/mm^3 during acute administration; chronic administration has a less pronounced effect (*Clin Immunol Immunopathol* 1983;28:101). Interferon treatment causes severe decreases in CD4 counts. Medical conditions associated with low CD4 counts include Sjögren syndrome, sarcoidosis, radiation, atopic dermatitis, collagen-vascular disease, lymphoma, stem cell transplant recipients, interferon treatment and idiopathic CD4 lymphocytopenia (see pg. 32). Acute changes are probably due to a redistribution of leukocytes between the peripheral circulation and the marrow, spleen, and lymph nodes (*Clin Exp Immunol* 1990;80: 460).

Deceptively high CD4 counts may occur with HTLV-1 co-infection or splenectomy. HTLV-1 is closely related to HTLV-2, and most serologic assays do not distinguish between the two, but only HTLV-1 causes deceptively high CD4 cell counts. Serologic studies in the United States show HTLV-1 or -2 seroprevalence of 7-12% in injection drug users and 2-10% in commercial sex workers (*NEJM* 1990;326:375; *JAMA* 1990;263:60; *STD* 2000;27:87); 80-90% of these are a result of HTLV-2 infection in both populations. High rates of concurrent HIV and HTLV-1 have been reported in Brazil (*JAMA* 1994;271:353) Peru and Haiti (*JCM* 1995;33: 1735). Analysis of patients with co-infection suggests that CD4 counts are 80-180% higher than in controls for comparable levels of immunosuppression (*JAMA* 1994;271:353). Some work suggests that HTLV-2/HIV-1 co-infection has a favorable effect on the natural history of HIV infection (*AIDS Rev* 2007;9:140). Splenectomy results in a prompt, sustained increase in CD4 count. The CD4 percentage more accurately reflects immunocompetence with HTLV-1 co-infection or splenectomy (*CID* 1995;20:768; *Arch Surg* 1998;133:25). The following have minimal effect on the CD4 cell count: gender, age in adults, risk category, psychological stress, physical stress, and pregnancy (*Ann Intern Med* 1993;119:55).

- **CD4 Slope:** The term refers to the rate of decline of CD4 counts Sequentially collected data for 8,729 untreated HIV-infected patients from 20 cohorts in CASCADE (Europe and Australia) showed that the median CD4 count at about 8 mos post-seroconversion was approximately 610 cells/mm^3 with a negative slope at 2 years of -130 cells/mm^3/year and a 5-year slope of -70 cells/mm^3/year (*JAIDS* 2003;34:76). The median baseline CD4 count post-seroconversion was about 40 cells/mm^3 higher in women vs. men and in persons <40 years vs. >40 years. The CD4 slope was significantly steeper by a mean of -40 cells/mm³/yr for persons >40 years vs. 16-20 years. The CD4 slope was not significantly different by sex or risk category. A sequel report from CASCADE (*JID* 2007;195:525) showed a significant decrease in the median initial CD4 cell count (median − 570 cells/mm³).

- **CD4 Percentage:** The CD4 percentage is sometimes used because it reduces variability to that of a single measurement (*JAIDS* 1989;2: 114) and corrects for deceptive CD4 counts due to splenectomy, HTLV-1 co-infection and medication factors such as interferon. In the ACTG laboratories, the within-subject coefficient of variation for CD4 percentage was 18% compared with 25% for the absolute CD4 count (*JID* 1994;169:28). Data from a large observational database suggested that the CD4 count is the most useful predictor of the risk for development of opportunistic infections (*JAIDS* 2004;36:1028). More recent analyses based on cohort studies suggest that the CD4 percentage may be better for predicting disease progression with a CD4 count >350 cells/mm³ (*JID* 2005;192:950), and for determining the time to initiate ART (*JID* 2007;195:425). Others conclude that the absolute count may be preferred for levels below the 350 cells/mm³ threshold (*JID* 2005;192: 945; 2004;36:1028). Corresponding CD4 cell counts and percentages for major CD4 thresholds are summarized in Table 2-7.

■ TABLE 2-7: **Approximate CD4/CD4% Equivalents**

CD4 Cell Count	% CD4
>500 cells/mm³	>29%
200-500 cells/mm³	14-28%
<200 cells/mm³	<14%

- **Response to ART:** The CD4 count typically increases by ≥50 cells/mm³ at 4-8 wks after viral suppression with ART and then increases at a rate that correlates with time, baseline CD4 count and virologic suppression (*CID* 2009;48:787). With good virologic response the increase at one year averages 100-150 cells/mm³, at 3-5 years it averages 20-50 cells/mm³/yr and at ≥5 years it averages 20-30 cells/mm³/yr. (*Lancet* 2007;370:407). Some cohort studies show sustained incremental gains to normal levels (*Lancet* 2007;370:366); other long term studies show that about half of the patients with a baseline CD4 count <100 cells/mm³ never achieve a count >500 cells/mm³ with ART (*CID* 2009;48:787), suggesting limited immunologic reserve (*CID* 2007; 44:441; *AIDS* 2003;17:1707; *AIDS* 2003;13:963). The cause of this blunted immune response is unknown (*CID* 2009;48:787). The CD4 response generally correlates with virologic control, but VL <10,000 c/mL is usually associated with CD4 stability or modest increases and protection from opportunistic infections (*NEJM* 2003; 2175; *JAIDS* 2005; 40:404; *Lancet* 2007; 369:1169; *Lancet* 2006; 368:466).

Laboratory Tests

Although viral suppression is usually associated with a CD4 response (*JID* 2004;190:148), discordant results are common in both directions (*Antiviral Ther* 1999;4(Suppl 3):7; *JID* 2001;183:1328). The CD4 count usually declines rapidly, up to 100-150 cells/mm³ in 3-4 mos, when ART is discontinued (*CID* 2001;33:344; *CID* 2001;32:1231; *NEJM* 2003;349: 837). When the CD4 count fails to increase appropriately with viral suppression there is often concern for alternative methods to boost the CD4 count including changes in the ART regimen. This type of discordant immune response was reviewed by the ClinSurv Study, in which the CD4 increase was considered discordant if it was <200 cells/mm³ before ART and failed to increase to >200 cells/mm³ at least once and were grouped by time of discordance at 0-6 mo, 7-12 mo, 13-24 mo or >24 mo despite ART with persistent VL <50 c/mL (*JID* 2011;203:364). In those with discordant CD4 responses: 1) most new AIDS events occurred within 6 mos (54%); 2) the incidence of AIDS events decreased by 65%/yr. However, the main finding was the remarkably low rate of AIDS events despite a CD4 count <200 cells/mm³ when the VL was <50 c/mL: 42 AIDS events with follow-up of over 5000 person-years.

Attempts to improve immune recovery include changes in antiretroviral regimens despite viral suppression, but that has generally not been successful (*CID* 2008;47:1093). Intensification by adding RAL or MVC to a regimen with good viral suppression, but suboptimal CD4 recovery has also failed (*JID* 2011;203:960; Rusconi S. 2010 Glasgow:Abstr. 0421). An ambitious study to increase CD4 counts was attempted with two placebo-controlled trials using IL-2: ESPRIT included 4,111 patients receiving ART with CD4 counts >300 cells/mm³ (*NEJM* 2009;361:1548). SILCATT included 1,695 patients receiving ART with CD4 counts of 50-299 cells/mm³. Pooled analyses from these trials demonstrated that IL-2 therapy significantly increased CD4 counts but conferred no clinical benefit and was associated with side effects (gastrointestinal, psychiatric disorders and deep vein thrombosis).

- **CD4 count as a surrogate for virologic failure.** CD4 decline is recommended by WHO as a surrogate for VL to detect virologic failure. This has not proven to be successful for several reasons: 1) the CD4 measurement has substantial variation (30% for the 95% CI); 2) The CD4 count is generally measured only at 6 mo intervals; 3) CD4 counts are often stable or they increase with a slow positive slope during virologic failure according to data from large salvage trials (TORO, RESIST, POWER, BENCHMRK, TITAN, etc) (see pg. 115). Pharmacy records appear to be better predictors of virologic failure in some settings (*PLoS Med* 2008;5:e109).

- **Total Lymphocyte Count (TLC):** The TLC is sometimes used as a surrogate for CD4 count to facilitate clinical decisions when the CD4 test is pending (*JAMA* 1993;269: 622; *Am J Med Sci* 1992;304:79). A TLC of <1200 cells/mm³ is consistent with a CD4 count <200

Laboratory Tests

2

cells/mm^3, but confirmation is needed (*JAIDS* 2007;46:338).

- **CD4 Repertoire:** Progressive immunodeficiency in HIV infection is associated with both quantitative and qualitative changes in CD4 cells. The two major categories of CD4 cells are naïve cells and memory cells. In early life, all cells are naïve and express the isoform of CD45RA+. Memory cells (CD45RA—) represent the component of the T-cell repertoire that has been activated by exposure to antigens. These are the CD4 cells with specificity for most opportunistic infections, such as *P. jiroveci*, cytomegalovirus (CMV), and *Toxoplasma gondii*. It is the depletion of these cells that accounts for the inability to respond to recall antigens, a defect noted relatively early in the course of HIV infection. Studies of HIV-infected patients show a preferential decline in naïve cells. With ART, there is a three-phase component to the CD4 rebound. The initial increase is due primarily to redistribution of CD4 cells from lymphatic sites. The second phase is characterized by an influx of CD4 memory cells with reduced T-cell activation and improved response to recall antigens. In the third phase there is an increase in naïve cells following at least 12 wks of ART (*Nat Med* 1997;5:533; *Science* 1997;277:112). By 6 mos the CD4 repertoire is diverse. The competence of these cells is evidenced by favorable control of selected chronic infections such as cryptosporidiosis, microsporidiosis, and molluscum contagiosum, the ability to discontinue maintenance therapy for disseminated MAC and CMV, and the ability to safely discontinue primary prophylaxis for PCP and MAC in responders. Nevertheless, some patients with immune reconstitution have deficits in CTL responses to specific antigens that may result in PCP or relapses in CMV retinitis despite CD4 counts >300 cells/mm^3 (*JID* 2001;183: 1285).

- **Idiopathic CD4 Lymphocytopenia (ICL):** ICL is a syndrome characterized by a low CD4 cell count that is unexplained by HIV infection or other medical conditions as described in 1993 (*NEJM* 1993;328:386). Case definition criteria include: 1) CD4 <300 cells/mm^3 or a CD4 percent <20% on two or more measurements; 2) lack of laboratory evidence of HIV infection; and 3) absence of alternative explanation for the CD4 cell lymphocytopenia including Sjögren syndrome, sarcoidosis, radiation therapy, atopic dermatitis, collagen vascular disease, steroid therapy, or lymphoma (*NEJM* 1993;328:373). Transient, unexplained decreases in CD4 cells may occur in healthy persons (*Chest* 1994;105:1335; *Eur J Med* 1993;2:509; *Am J Med Sci* 1996;312:240). One study of 430 HIV-negative TB patients found that 62 (14%) had ICL (*JID* 2000;41:167). The CDC receives a report of about one ICL case/mo (Dr. T.J. Spira, personal communication). There is speculation that persistent CD4 lymphopenia may be due to diminished stem cell precursors (*Int Arch Allergy Immunol* 2005;136:379). Conclusions from the experience with patients with ICL are: 1) they typically lack risk factors for HIV infection; 2) there is no evidence of an infectious etiology based on clustering or contact evaluations; 3) they have fewer OIs than HIV-infected patients for a given CD4 count level; 4) the predominant OIs associated with ICL are cryptococcosis, zoster, molluscum, and histoplasmosis; infections with *P. jiroveci, Candida,* and HHV-8 (KS) are unusual; and 5) their CD4 counts tend to remain stable. One review of 53 cases found that the median age was 41 years; there was a predominance of cryptococcal meningitis, a median CD4 count of 82 cells/mm^3 and only a single case of PCP (*Medicine* 2007; 86:78). Nevertheless, some have recommended PCP prophylaxis for those with persistent counts <200 cells/mm^3. Another more recent review included 39 cases followed at the NIH for a median of 50 mos and found that: 1) cryptococcal meningitis and non-tuberculous mycobacteria were the major presenting infections; 2) the CD4 count remained <300 cells/mm^3 in 32 and returned to normal in 7; 3) there were 15 infections including 5 AIDS-defining infections – 4 developed autoimmune diseases; and 4) 7 died within 42 mos, including 4 due to opportunistic infections (*Blood* 2008;112:287). Numerous attempts with various forms of treatment have been unsuccessful (*Lancet* 1992;340:273; *NEJM* 1993;328:373; *NEJM* 1993; 328:380; *NEJM* 1993;328:386; *NEJM* 1993;328:393; *Clin Exp Immunol* 1999;116:322; *CID* 2000:3:e20; *CID* 2001;33:e125; *CID* 2006;42: e53; *FEMS Immunol Med Microbiol* 2008;54:283; *Clin Chim Aeta* 2011;412:7; *Am J Med Sci* 2010;340:158). Cases of this syndrome should be reported to local/state health departments rather than directly to the CDC as originally advocated.

Resistance Testing

Resistance tests are intended to facilitate the selection of antiretroviral agents in patients with HIV infection. There are two standard commercially-available methods, genotype and phenotype resistance tests, that provide information relevant to selection of NRTIs, NNRTs and PIs; testing for resistance to ENF, CCR5 antagonists and integrase inhibitors is also available but requires separate tests. There is a genotype assay of the V-3 coding region to detect CCR5 antagonist resistance, but the *Trofile* phenotypic assay is preferred due to better sensitivity (2011 DHHS Guidelines). The following resources are recommended for information relevant to genotypic, phenotypic and integrase inhibitor resistance:

- International Antiviral Society – USA: http://iasusa.org
- Stanford University HIV database: http://hivdb.stanford.edu

INDICATIONS: Most guidelines recommend resistance testing at the time of diagnosis of either acute or chronic HIV infection, regardless of intent to start ART. Resistance testing is also recommended in patients with virologic failure. (*JAMA* 2010;304:321, 2011 DHHS Guidelines; *Top HIV Med* 2009;18:132).

Laboratory Tests

2

- **Primary HIV Infection:** A genotypic resistance test is recommended in all patients at the time of diagnosis. This is the optimal time to test the transmitted strain because resistant mutants may later become undetectable minority strains that then emerge with selective pressure (*J Virol* 2008;82:5510; *JID* 2010;65:548). If ART is to be initiated during acute infection the regimen may need to be chosen and initiated before test results are available. In this case the regimen should be based on anticipated resistance patterns for treatment-naïve patients (Table 2-8), local resistance patterns or data from the transmission source if this information is available. In most cases, the use of a ritonavir-boosted PI-based regimen is preferred in this setting, since transmitted NNRTI resistance is more common than transmitted PI resistance.

- **Chronic HIV Infection:** Genotypic resistance testing is recommended at the time of diagnosis regardless of the intention to initiate ART. The baseline genotype should be considered when selecting the initial ART regimen (*CID* 2005;40:468; *JID* 2010;65:548; *PLoS Med* 2008;5:e158; *JID* 2009;199:693). Waiting to test until the decision has been made to start ART may decrease the yield of testing due to time-dependent reversion to wild-type virus. Despite this limitation, baseline genotypic resistance testing is also recommended at the time ART is initiated based on studies showing better virologic responses when these results are considered (*NEJM* 2002;347:385; *JID* 2008;197:867; *HIV Clin Trials* 2002;3:1; *AIDS* 2006;20:21; *JAIDS* 2010;53:633).

- **Virologic Failure:** Genotypic resistance testing is recommended with virologic failure assuming a sufficient VL for the test (>500-1000 c/mL). Suboptimal response is also considered an indication as defined by the failure to achieve a decrease in VL of: 1) $0.5-0.7 \log_{10}$ c/mL by 4 wks; 2) reduction by $1 \log_{10}$ c/mL (10-fold reduction) by 8

■ TABLE 2-8: **Resistance Test Results in Patients with Acute or Recent HIV Infection**

Source	Year	N	Any	NRTI	NNRTI	PI
CPCRA-US [1]	1999-01	491	11.6%	7.8%	3.0%	0.7%
Europe Commission [2]	2002-05	2793	8.4%	4.7%	2.3%	2.9%
Canada [3]	2000-01	494	6.1%	3.1%	1.2%	1.2%
10 N. American cities [4]	1995-01	377	11.6%	7.8%	3.0%	0.7%
U.K. [5]	2002-03	171	19.2%	12.4%	8.1%	6.6%
CDC survey [6]	2003-06	3130	10.4%	3.6%	6.9%	2.4%
UK CHIC [7]	1997-07	7994	9.0%	5.3%	2.9%	1.5%
France [8]	2006-07	530	9.5%	5.8%	2.8%	4.7%

1. *CID* 2005;40:468
2. *JID* 2009;200:1503
3. *JAIDS* 2006;42:86
4. *NEJM* 2002;347:385
5. *BMJ* 2005;331:1368
6. *Topics HIV Med* 2007;15:150
7. *AIDS* 2010;24:1917
8. *JAC* 2010;65:2620

Laboratory Tests

wks and 3) VL >1000 c/mL at 16-24 wks. Possibly the most important studies of the value of resistance testing with therapeutic failure were TORO-1 and TORO-2 (*NEJM* 2003;348:2175 and 2293) and other salvage trials, which found a strong correlation between the number of active drugs in the background regimen (by genotype or phenotype analysis) and virologic response. Multiple salvage trials have confirmed this observation (see pg. 258).

The currently available tests are standardized for clade B strains; utility for the other clades is less well established (*Scand JID* 2003;35[Suppl 106]:75; *J Med Virol* 2007;80:1).

- **Baseline testing in patients with chronic HIV infection.** Baseline genotypic resistance testing is now considered the standard of care (see pg. 88), because mutations in transmitted strains tend to persist. Testing should be performed at the time of diagnosis, regardless of the duration of infection and whether therapy will be initiated immediately (*JAIDS* 2006;41:573; *JAIDS* 2004;37:1665; 2011 DHHS Guidelines). Resistance testing may fail to detect mutations present at low levels, which is most likely to be a problem in patients with acquired resistance from failed ART rather than in those with transmitted resistance. In either case this testing is best for defining what drugs not to use. Detection of minority variants is not currenlty possible with commercially available assays. The more complete baseline data requires testing for resistance in the "minority pool" that is technically possible but not commercially available (*JAMA* 2011;305:1327).

Test Methods: There are two types of tests, genotypic and phenotypic assays. These are compared in Table 2-9 (*JAC* 2004;53:555; *Top HIV Med* 2008;16:89).

GENOTYPIC ASSAYS: Genotype analysis identifies mutations associated with phenotypic resistance. Testing may be performed using commercial kits or "home brews." Assays vary in cost and method of reporting, but there is 98% concordance when two commercial kits are tested by the same laboratory (*Antiviral Ther* 2000;5 suppl 4:60; *Antiviral Ther* 2000; suppl 3:53). Another study found a 0.3% frequency of false positive results and a 6.4% frequency of false negative results (*Antiviral Ther* 2001;6 suppl 1:1). The methodology involves: 1) amplification of the reverse transcriptase (RT) and protease (Pr) genes, by RT PCR. 2) DNA sequencing of amplicons generated for the dominant species (mutations are limited to those present in >20% of plasma virions). 3) Reporting of mutations for each gene using a letter-number-letter standard, in which the first letter indicates the wild-type amino acid at the designated codon, the number is the codon position, and the second letter indicates the amino acid substituted in the mutation. Thus, the RT mutation K103N indicates that asparagine (N) has replaced lysine (K) on codon 103.

2 Laboratory Tests

Table 2-10 (see pg. 37) shows the amino acids and corresponding letter codes used to describe mutations in genotype analyses. Interpretation is based on lists of drug resistance mutations or computerized rules-based algorithms.

Mutations associated with HIV resistance are summarized in Table 2-11–Table 2-14 (see pg. 38-45). Interpretation of genotype resistance patterns in drug selection may be improved by consultation with an expert (*AIDS* 2002;16:209; *Curr Opin HIV AIDS* 2009;4:474) and by use of a genotypic interpretation scores (GIS) that are available from:

- Stanford University HIV data base: http://hivdb.stanford.edu or
- International Antiviral Society-USA: http://iasusa.org

Genotypic Susceptibility Scores (GSS) are derived GIS and used to predict virologic response (*NEJM* 2008;359:355; *NEJM* 2008; 359:1442; *AIDS* 2007;21:2033).

PHENOTYPIC ASSAYS: Phenotype analysis measures the ability of HIV to

■ TABLE 2-9: Comparison of Genotypic and Phenotypic Assays

Genotypic Assays	
Advantages	**Disadvantages**
<ul><li>Less expensive ($300-480/test).</li><li>Short turn-around of 1-2 weeks.</li><li>Well standardized</li><li>Good reproducibility</li><li>Possibility of virtual phenotype*</li><li>More sensitive for detection of mixtures, which can occur with emerging or disappearing resistance</li><li>Favored in comparative studies with failure of first or second regimens.</li></ul>	<ul><li>Detect resistance only in dominant species (>20%).</li><li>Interpretation requires expertise or use of algorithms that vary in their ability to predict susceptibility.</li><li>Algorithms may be incomplete, especially for new drugs.</li><li>Require VL >500-1000 c/mL.</li><li>Limited data on non-clade B virus</li><li>Separate test required for integrase or fusion inhibitor resistance</li></ul>
Phenotypic Assays	
Advantages	**Disadvantages**
<ul><li>Interpretation more straight forward and familiar.</li><li>Assess total effect, including mutational interactions.</li><li>Do not require data on genotypic correlates of resistance (advantageous with newer agents).</li><li>Reproducibility is good.</li><li>Advantage over genotype when there are complex mutation patterns, especially with PIs.</li><li>Provide quantitative assessment of susceptibility</li></ul>	<ul><li>More expensive (usually $800-1000). High cost may affect reimbursement.</li><li>Report takes longer than genotypic assay.</li><li>Clinically determined thresholds not available for all drugs.</li><li>Detect resistance only in dominant species (>20%).</li><li>Require VL >500-1000 c/mL.</li><li>Separate test required for integrase inhibitor or fusion inhibitor resistance</li></ul>

* *VircoTYPE*, a genotype that estimates phenotype, is rapid, easily done, and less expensive than phenotypic assays; the disadvantage is that its ability to predict phenotype is dependent on the accuracy of algorithms derived from the database.

Laboratory Tests

36

■ TABLE 2-10: **Letter Designations for Amino Acids***

A	Alanine	I	Isoleucine	R	Arginine
C	Cysteine	K	Lysine	S	Serine
D	Aspartate	L	Leucine	T	Threonine
E	Glutamate	M	Methionine	V	Valine
F	Phenylalanine	N	Asparagine	W	Tryptophan
G	Glycine	P	Proline	Y	Tyrosine
H	Histidine	Q	Glutamine		

* Single-letter codes are used in describing genotypes.

replicate at different concentrations of tested drugs. The test involves insertion of the RT and protease genes from the patient's strain into a backbone laboratory clone by cloning or recombination. Replication is monitored at various drug concentrations and compared with a reference wild-type virus. This assay is comparable with conventional *in vitro* tests of antimicrobial sensitivity, in which the microbe is grown in serial dilutions of antiviral agents. Results are reported as the IC_{50} for the test strain relative to that of a reference or wild-type strain. The interpretation uses either biologic thresholds based on the normal distribution of wild-type virus from untreated patients or, for most drugs, clinical thresholds based on data from clinical trials. Two cutoffs are provided for most drugs: a lower cutoff that indicates the fold-change for declining activity and an upper cut-off that indicates the threshold for total loss of activity as reported by two commercial suppliers, Monogram (*PhenoSense*) and Virco (*Antivirogram*) (see Table 2-15). A "virtual phenotype" (*VircoTYPE*) is also provided by Virco and uses the genotype to predict phenotype based on a large database with genotype-phenotype pairs. It is unclear whether this provides additional advantage beyond standard genotype testing (*JID* 2003;126:194; *Curr Opinion HIV AIDS* 2009;4:474) (Table 2-15, pg. 47).

RELATIVE MERITS: Genotypic resistance tests are generally preferred for baseline (pretreatment) testing, with early failures of initial regimens in which multiple mutations are not expected, and in patients who have discontinued therapy. Arguments for this approach are that genotypes are easy to interpret at early stages of failure and are more sensitive for detecting wild-type/mutant mixtures, which may be present in treatment-naïve patients or in patients who have discontinued therapy. In addition, clinical trials demonstrated better outcomes in this setting when compared to the standard of care (GART [*AIDS* 2000;14:F83], VIRADAPT [*Lancet* 1999;353:2195]; HAVANA [*AIDS* 2002;16:209]) or when compared to phenotypic testing (REALVIRFEN [*Antiviral Ther* 2003;8:577]; NARVAL [*Antiviral Ther* 2003;8: 427]). Genotypic testing is less expensive and appears cost-effective when used for first or second regimen failures (*Ann Intern Med* 2001;134:440; *JAIDS* 2000; 24:227). Phenotype resistance may supplement genotypic test results

2 | Laboratory Tests

Drug	Mutations* selected	Comments
Nucleoside Reverse Transcriptase Inhibitors (NRTIs): RT gene mutations		
AZT	41L, 67N, 70R, 210W, 215Y/F, 219Q/E	Thymidine analog mutations (TAMs): reduce susceptibility to all NRTIs (see TAMs below). Most frequent TAMs are 41L, 210W, 215Y, which have greatest impact on NRTI susceptibility. 184V increases AZT susceptibility and reduces the emergence of TAMs. 44D and 118I further decrease susceptibility when present with TAMs. Some NRTI mutations may mutate to produce hypersensitivity to NNRTIs. The 118Y, 208Y and 215Y mutations are examples and have shown improved response with EFV or NVP treatment (*AIDS* 2002;16:F33; *JID* 2004;189:F33; *HIV Clin Trials* 2008;9:11). TAMs infrequently coexist with 65R.
d4T	41L, 65R, 67N, 70R, 210W, 215Y/F, 219Q/E	Most d4T resistance is due to TAMs (see AZT). 65R causes low-level resistance, occasionally selected by d4T. 75T/M/A seen infrequently (see TAMs below).
3TC	65R,184V	184V/I: high-level 3TC and FTC resistance, with increase in activity of AZT, d4T, and TDF, and partial reduction of resistance due to TAMs. Also delays emergence of TAMs. Reduces susceptibility to ddI, ABC, though not clinically significant with 184V alone. 44D and 118I not selected by 3TC, but they confer moderate 3TC resistance. 65R not selected by 3TC, but can cause intermediate resistance to 3TC.
FTC	65R,184V	See 3TC.
ddI	65R, 74V	ddI resistance is seen with any three of the following: 41L, 67N, 210 W, 215Y/F, 219Q/E (*AAC* 2005;49:1739. the 70R and 184V mutations alone did not reduce viral response (*JID* 2005;191:840). 74V or 65R mutations alone or combined with 184V are associated with ddI resistance and cross-resistance to ABC (74V, 65R) and TDF (65R).
ABC	65R, 74V, 115F, 184V	Resistance with 65R or 74V, increased if 184V/I also present. 74V more commonly selected by ABC then 65R. TAM-mediated resistance depends on number of TAMs and TAM-pathway. 184V alone does not confer clinically significant resistance but further decreases *in vivo* response when in combination with TAMs or ABC mutations (*JID* 2000;181:912; *Antivir Ther* 2004;9:37).
TDF	65R, 70E	Reduced activity with 65R or with ≥3 TAMs that include 41L and 210W. 184V/I increases TDF activity, partially compensating for 65R or TAMs. 70E uncommon, but reduces TDF susceptibility.

* The distinction between primary and secondary mutations has been eliminated for NRTIs and NNRTIs by the IAS-USA Expert Committee; this distinction has been retained for PIs, but with the terms have been replaced by "major" or "minor" muations.

(continued)

Laboratory Tests

Drug	Mutations* selected	Comments
Multi Nucleoside Resistance		
Multi-nucleoside resistance: Q151M complex	151M plus 62V, 75I, 77L, 116Y, 151M	Uncommon with 3TC- or FTC-containing regimens. Occurs with or without TAMs. The 151M complex confers high-level resistance to AZT, d4T, ABC, ddI, intermediate resistance to TDF, and low-level resistance to 3TC, FTC. TDF has activity against Q151M mutant strains (*JID* 2004;189:837).
Multi-nucleoside resistance: T69 insertion	69 insertion 41L, 62V, 70R, 210W, 215Y/F, 219Q/E	The 69 insertion complex confers resistance to all NRTIs when combined with a TAM at codons 41, 210 or 215.
Multi nucleoside resistance: multiple TAMs	41L, 67N, 70R, 210W, 215Y/F, 219Q/E	TAMs reduce in vitro susceptibility of all NRTIs, but the clinical significance of the *in vitro* findings is unclear (*CID* 2010;51:620; *JID* 2010;201:1054). Most common cause of multinucleoside resistance. Only AZT and d4T select for TAMs. 44D and 118I further decrease NRTI susceptibility.
Non-Nucleoside Reverse Transcriptase Inhibitors (NNRTIs): RT gene mutations		
NVP	100I:101P, 103N, 106A/M, 108I, 181C/I, 188C/L/H, 190A	181C is favored mutation with NVP unless combined with AZT, in which case 103N favored. 103N, 106M, 188L/C cause high-level NVP resistance. 188H causes low-level NVP resistance.
DLV	103N, 106M, 181C, 188L, 236L	Some NNRTI mutations (190A/S, 225) decrease susceptibility to NVP and EFV but cause DLV hypersusceptibility; clinical significance unknown.
EFV	100I, 101P, 103N, 106M, 108I, 181CI, 188L, 190S/A, 225H	103N is favored mutation with EFV, causing high-level NNRTI resistance. 188L and 106M also cause high-level EFV resistance. Although 181C (and some other NNRTI mutations) cause only low-level EFV resistance phenotypically, response to EFV is generally poor, and other NNRTI mutations may be present in sub-populations.
ETR	90I, 98G, 100I, 181V/I, 101P, 106I, 138AGK, 179DFT, 181C/I/V, 106I, 138AGK, 179DFT	Weighted resistance score Score **3:** 181/V/I **2.5:** 101P, 100I, 181C, 230L **1.5:** 138A, 106I, 190S, 179F **1.0:** 90I, 179D, 101E, 101H, 98G, 190A, 179T *Failure* 0-2: 38%; 2.5-3.5: 52%; ≥4: 74%. The IAS-USA December 2010 update on drug resistance mutations did not provide a weighted ETR resistance ETR resistance score but noted that the most important mutations are 181C/I/C, 101P and 100L.

* The distinction between primary and secondary mutations has been eliminated for NRTIs and NNRTIs by the IAS-USA Expert Committee; this distinction has been retained for PIs, but with the terms have been replaced by "major" or "minor" muations.

(continued)

2   Laboratory Tests

Drug	Major† mutations	Minor‡ mutations	Comments
Protease Inhibitors (PIs): Protease gene mutations			
IDV and IDV/r	46I/L, 82A/F/T, 84V	10I/R/V, 20M/R, 24I, 32I, 36I, 54V, 71V/T, 73S/A, 76V, 77I, 90M	At least 3 mutations required for resistance to unboosted IDV (>4-fold decrease in susceptibility).
NFV	30N, 90M	10F/I, 36I, 46I/L, 71V/T, 77I, 82A/F/T/S, 84V, 88D/S	30N most common mutation, causing no PI cross-resistance. 90M occurs in some (especially non-B subtypes), causing greater PI cross-resistance.
SQV and SQV/r	48V, 90M	10I/R/V, 24I, 54L/V, 62V, 71V/T, 73S, 77I, 82A/F/T/S, 84V	With unboosted SQV 90M is typically first mutation, then 48V. 48V is unique to SQV, but 90M causes PI cross-resistance. Selection of PI mutations is unlikely with SQV/r in PI-naïve patients.
FPV and FPV/r	50V, 84V	10F/I/R/V, 32I, 46I/L, 47V, 54L/V/M, 73S, 76V, 82A/F/T/S, 90M	50V associated with cross-resistance to LPV. 50V, 84V, 32I, 54L/M, 47V decrease DRV susceptibility. 10V, 47V, 54M, 84V decrease TPV susceptibility. PI mutations unlikely to be selected by FPV/r in PI-naïve patients.
LPV/r	32I, 47V/A, 76V, 82A/F/T/S	10F/I/R/V, 20M/R, 24I, 33F, 46I/L, 50V, 53L, 54V/L/A/M/T/S, 63P, 71V/T, 73S, 84V, 90M	Most PI-naïve patients failing LPV/r as first PI have no PI mutations. 47A, 32I and possibly 47V confer intermediate-to-high level LPV resistance. It is usually thought that >6 mutations are required for LPV resistance (package insert; *AAC* 2002;46:2926; *J Virol* 2001;75:7462), but more recent data suggests 147 V, 32I and possibly 147V produce high level resistance and the combination of 76V and 3PI resistances LPV resistance (*J Virol* 2005;79:333; *Protein Sci* 2005;15:1870).
TPV/r	47V, 74P, 82L/T, 83D, 84V	10V, 33F, 36I/L/V, 46L, 54A/M/V, 69K/R, 89I/M/V	Best response seen with 0-1 TPV mutations. Intermediate response with 2-7 mutations. Minimal response with 8 or more mutations. However, the validity of these scores in terms of clinical correlates is not well established with limited clinical experience. (*TOP HIV Med* 2010;18:156).
DRV/r	47V, 50V, 54M/L, 84V	11I, 32I, 33F, 74P, 76V, 89V	Reduced response with increasing DRV mutations; poor response with ≥3 mutations.

† **Major mutations** emerge first or are associated with decreased drug binding or reduced viral activity; these effect phenotype resistance.

‡ **Minor mutations** appear later and, by themselves, do not significantly change phenotypic resistance, but they may further decrease susceptibility in combination with major mutations, or help to compensate for loss of fitness caused by major mutations.

(continued)

Laboratory Tests

Drug	Major mutations	Minor mutations	Comments
Protease Inhibitors (PIs): Protease gene mutations (continued)			
ATV and ATV/r	50L, 84V, 88S	10I/F/V/C, 16E, 20R/M/I/T/V, 24I, 32I, 33I/F/V, 34Q, 36I/L/V, 46I/L, 48V, 53L/Y, 54L/V/M/T/A, 60E, 62V, 64L/M/V, 71V/I/T/L, 73C/S/T/A, 82A/T/F/I, 85V, 90M, 93L/M	50L causes no PI cross-resistance, and possible hypersusceptibility to other PIs. Reduced *in vivo* activity associated with ≥3 of the following: 10F/V/I, 16E, 33F/I/V, 46I/L, 60E, 84V, 85V. Boosted ATV increases the number of mutations necessary to reduce activity. Selection of PI mutations uncommon with ATV/r in PI-naïve patients. Another report showed 75% or 0% response with 2 or > 3 of the following: 10V/I/C, 32I, 34Q, 46I/L, 53L, 54 A/M/V, 82A/F/I/T and 184 V. Mutations 46I + 76V may increase activity of ATV.
Fusion inhibitors: gp41 mutations			
ENF		36D/S, 37V, 38A/M/E, 39R, 40H, 42T, 43D	Mutations in other envelope regions may affect sensitivity. Resistance correlates with mutations at the HR1 region of gp41. Mutations in other parts of the envelope gene may be associated with reduced activity (*PNAS* 2002;99:16249; *AAC* 2005;49:113).
CCR5 antagonists: gp120 mutations			
MVC	92Q, 143R/H/C, 148 H/K/R, 155H		Activity is limited to patients with purely R5-tropic virus. Resistance is most common with selection of X4 or D/M virus. Mutations in gp120 that allow viral binding of the drug-bound form have been reported with virologic failure despite R5 virus. Most mutatons are in the V3 loop, which is the major determinant of HIV tropism. There is no consensus on the specific mutations associated with MVC resistance. Resistance has also been noted with gp41 mutations without involving the V3 loop (*Top HIV Med* 2010;18:156).
Integrase inhibitors: integrase gene mutations			
RAL	92Q, 143R/H/C, 148H/K/R, 155H		There are 3 genetic resistance pathways with a signature mutation at 148 H/K/R, 155H or 143R/H/C, each combined with minor mutations. The combination of 148H and 140S is most common and causes the greatest loss of activity. Other signficant mutations with 148H/K/R include 74M + 138A, 138K or 140S. Significant mutations in the 155H pathway are 74M, 92Q, 97A and 92Q + 97A and 92Q = 97A, 143H, 163 K/R, 151I or 232N (*Antiviral Ther* 2007;12:S10). The 143 R/H/C pathway is rare.

2 Laboratory Tests

■ TABLE 2-12: Nucleoside and Nucleotide Analog Resistance Mutations by Category

Mutation Category	Mutation	Comments
Thymidine analog mutations (TAMs)	M41L, D67N/G, K70R, L210W, T215F/Y, K219E/Q/N	Selected by thymidine analogs (AZT, d4T) but cause resistance to all NRTIs. M41L, L210W, T215F/Y pattern more common in subtype B virus and causes higher-level NRTI resistance than D67N/G, K70R, K219E/Q/N. T215C/D/E/S/I/V are "revertants" that typically indicate "back mutation" after initial infection with NRTI-resistant virus. Revertants do not cause resistance themselves, but may indicate presence of archived resistant virus.
Accessory mutations	E44D, VI118I	Contribute to NRTI resistance when accompanied by multiple TAMs.
Non-TAM nucleoside analog mutation	K65R	Selected by TDF, ABC, ddI. Causes variable decrease in susceptibility to those drugs and to d4T, 3TC, and FTC, but hypersusceptibility to AZT. Rarely occurs in patients on AZT-containing regimens or in setting of TAMs. Can also be selected by d4T. Selection appears less common with TDF/FTC than with TDF/3TC.
Non-TAM nucleoside analog mutation	L74V	Selected by ABC, ddI. (More common than K65R with ABC/3TC-containing regimens). Causes variable decrease in susceptibility to ABC and ddI, but hypersusceptibility to AZT, TDF. Rarely occurs in patients on AZT-containing regimens or in setting of TAMs.
3TC/FTC resistance mutation	M184V/I	Selected by 3TC, FTC. Causes high-level resistance to both drugs and modest decrease in susceptibility to ABC and ddI (not clinically significant when present alone). Increases susceptibility to AZT, d4T, TDF. Delays emergence of TAMs in thymidine analog-containing regimens.
Multi-nucleoside resistance mutations	T69 insertion	Selected by thymidine analogs, but rare in HAART era, especially with 3TC- or FTC-containing regimens. Causes high-level resistance to all NRTIs and TDF.
Multi-nucleoside resistance mutations	Q151M complex	Selected by thymidine analogs, but rare in HAART era, especially with 3TC- or FTC-containing regimens. Causes high-level resistance to all NRTIs when combined V75I, F77L, F116Y. TDF may retain activity.
d4T mutation	V75T/M/A	Selected by d4T *in vitro* and results in decreased d4T susceptibility, but uncommon with clinical use of d4T.
ABC mutation	Y115F	Selected by ABC, resulting in ~3-fold decrease in ABC susceptibility.

Laboratory Tests

■ TABLE 2-13: **Non-nucleoside Reverse Transcriptase Inhibitor (NNRTI) Resistance Mutations**

Mutation	Comments
V90I	Associated with decrease ETR susceptibility in combination with other ETR mutations
A98G	Selected by NVP (uncommon), resulting in minimal decrease in NVP susceptibility. Associated with decreased ETR susceptibility in combination with other ETR mutations.
L100I	Causes intermediate resistance to DLV, NVP, and EFV. Usually occurs with K103N, resulting in further loss of NNRTI susceptibility especially to EFV and DLV. Associated with decreased ETR susceptibility in combination with other ETR mutations. Increases susceptibility to AZT and possibly d4T.
K101E/H/P	**K101E:** Selected by NVP and EFV (uncommon), resulting in intermediate-level resistance to NVP and DLV, and low-level resistance to EFV. **K101P:** Associated with intermediate resistance. to DLV, NVP, and EFV, but usually occurs in combination with K103N, resulting in high-level resistance. **K103E/H/P** is associated with decreased ETR susceptibility in combination with other ETR mutations.
K103N/S/R	**K103N:** Commonly selected by all NNRTIs, resulting in high-level resistance to DLV, NVP, EFV. Does not affect ETR susceptibility. **K103S** less common, resulting in lower degree of resistance to DLV and EFV, but moderate resistance to NVP. **K103R:** Polymorphism with minimal effect on NNRTI susceptibility, unless combined with V179D.
V106M/A	**V106M:** Selected by NVP (common with subtype C), resulting in high-level resistance to DLV, NVP, and EFV. Does not affect ETR susceptibility. **V106A:** Selected by NVP (uncommon), resulting in high-level NVP resistance, intermediate DLV resistance, and low-level EFV resistance. **V106I** was considered a polymorphism that does not cause NNRTI resistance; however, in the DUET studies it was associated with decreased ETR susceptibility in combination with other ETR mutations.
V108I	Selected by NVP and EFV (uncommon), resulting in minimal decrease in DLV, NVP and EFV susceptibility. Does not affect ETR susceptibility.
E138A/G/K	Included in Monogram (**A/G**) and Tibotec (**A**) scoring systems as ETR mutations, reducing ETR susceptibility in combination with other mutations. **E138K** selected by RPV, and causes cross-resistance to ETR.
V179 D/E/F/M/T	**V179D:** Selected by NNRTIs (uncommon), resulting in low-level resistance to DLV, NVP, and EFV. Greater resistance with V179D + K103R. Associated with decreased ETR susceptibility in combination with other ETR mutations. **V179E:** Low-level resistance to DLV, NVP, and EFV. **V179F:** Associated with intermediate resistance to NVP and DLV, low-level resistance to EFV, and decreased ETR susceptibility in combination with other ETR mutations. Usually occurs in combination with Y181C, resulting in high-level ETR resistance. **V179D:** Decreases susceptibility to ETR in combination with other ETR mutations.

(continued)

Mutation	Comments
Y181C/I/V	Selected by NVP and DLV, causing resistance to both. Causes only low-level resistance to EFV, but clinical response to EFV unlikely, possibly because of presence of viral subpopulations with other resistance mutations. Increases susceptibility to AZT. Associated with decreased ETR susceptibility in combination with other ETR mutations. Alone, it causes 5-10 fold decrease in ETR susceptibility.
Y188 L/H/C	**Y188L:** Selected by NVP, DLV, and EFV (uncommon) resulting in high-level resistance to NVP and EFV and low-level resistance to DLV. Decreased ETR susceptibility in combination with other mutations. **Y188C:** Selected by NVP; causes high-level NVP resistance and low-level EFV and DLV resistance. **Y188H:** Low-level NNRTI resistance. **Y188H/C** Effects on ETR susceptibility unknown.
G190 S/A/E/Q	**G190A:** Selected by NVP and EFV, causing high-level resistance to NVP and intermediate resistance to EFV. Associated with decreased ETR susceptibility in combination with other ETR mutations. Increases DLV susceptibility (clinical relevance unknown). **G190S** cause high-level resistance to NVP and EFV and hypersusceptibility to DLV. Associated with decreased ETR susceptibility in combination with other ETR mutations. **G190E/Q:** Causes high-level resistance to EFV and NVP, low-level resistance to DLV. Associated with decreased ETR susceptibility in combination with other ETR mutations.
P225H	Usually occurs with K103N, resulting in further loss of EFV susceptibility. Decreased ETR susceptibility in combination with other mutations.
F227L	Sometimes seen in combination with V106A, resulting in further loss of NVP susceptibility.
M230L	Selected by NNRTIs (uncommon), resulting in high-level resistance to DLV and NVP and intermediate resistance to EFV. Decreased ETR susceptibility in combination with other mutations.
P236L	Selected by DLV (uncommon), resulting in high-level DLV resistance .
K238T/N	Selected by NNRTIs (uncommon), usually in combination with K103N or other NNRTI mutations. Causes intermediate resistance to DLV and NVP and low-level resistance to EFV.
Y318F	Selected by NNRTIs (uncommon), resulting in intermediate-to-high-level DLV resistance and low-to-intermediate NVP resistance.

Laboratory Tests

■ TABLE 2-14: Protease Inhibitor (PI) Resistance Mutations

Mutation	Comment
L10 **I/V/F/R/V**	Accessory mutations that can contribute to reduced susceptibility in the presence of other PI mutations. **L10V:** Contributes to TPV resistance in presence of other TPV mutations.
V11I	Contributes to DRV resistance in presence of other DRV mutations
I13V	Contributes to TPV resistance in presence of other TPV mutations.
K20 **R/I/M/T/V**	Accessory mutations/polymorphisms that may contribute to reduced susceptibility in the presence of other PI mutations. **K20M/R/V:** Contribute to TPV resistance in presence of other TPV mutations.
L23I	Uncommon mutation; low-level NFV resistance.
L24I/F	**L24I:** PI resistance, especially to IDV, when combined with other PI mutations. **L24F:** Rare mutation with unknown effect on PI susceptibility.
D30N	Primary PI mutation selected only by NFV, especially with subtype B virus; intermediate NFV resistance; further loss of susceptibility with N88D/S.
V32I	Accessory mutation that confers low-level resistance to IDV, RTV, APV, LPV. Contributes to DRV resistance in presence of other DRV mutations.
L33F/I/V	**L33F:** decreases susceptibility to RTV, APV, LPV, ATV, TPV, and DRV in presence of other PI mutations. **L33I/V:** Polymorphisms not known to be associated with drug resistance.
E35G	Contributes to TPV resistance in presence of other TPV mutations.
M36I/V/L	**M36I/V:** Accessory mutations that contribute to reduced PI susceptibility in the presence of other PI mutations. **M36I:** Contributes to TPV resistance in presence of other TPV mutations. **M36L:** Unknown effect on PI susceptibility.
K43T	Contributes to TPV resistance in presence of other TPV mutations.
M46I/L/V	**M46I/L:** Accessory mutation that contributes to reduced PI susceptibility in the presence of other PI mutations. **M46L:** Contributes to TPV resistance in presence of other TPV mutations. **M46V:** Uncommon mutation with unknown effect on PI susceptibility.
I47A/V	**I47V:** Reduced susceptibility to APV, IDV, RTV, LPV, TPV, and DRV in combination with other PI mutations. **I47A:** Moderate to high-level LPV resistance.
G48V/M	**G48V:** selected by SQV; intermediate SQV resistance; low-level resistance to other PIs. **G48M:** Effect on PI susceptibility unknown.
I50V/L	**I50V:** Selected by APV in PI-naïve patients; intermediate APV resistance; low to intermediate resistance to RTV, LPV. Contributes to DRV resistance in presence of other DRV mutations. **I50L:** Selected by ATV in PI-naïve patients; moderate to high-level ATV resistance; susceptibility to other PIs maintained or increased.

(continued)

Mutation	Comment
F53L	Associated with PI resistance when combined with other PI mutations.
I54V/M/L/T/S/A	**I54V:** Increases resistance to PIs when combined with other PI mutations. **I54M/L:** Selected by APV or FPV, causing low to intermediate resistance. Contributes to DRV resistance in presence of other DRV mutations. **I54T/S/A:** Effect on PI susceptibility unknown. **I54A/M/V:** Contribute to TPV resistance in presence of other TPV mutations.
Q58E	Contributes to TPV resistance in presence of other TPV mutations.
L63A/C/E/H/P/Q/R/S/T/V/I	**L63P:** Common polymorphism that increases PI resistance when combined with other PI mutations. **Others:** Effect on PI susceptibility unclear.
H69K	Contributes to TPV resistance in presence of other TPV mutations.
A71V/T/I	**A71V/T:** Decreases susceptibility to all PIs when combined with other mutations. **A71I:** Effect on PI susceptibility unknown.
G73S/C/T/A	**G73S/C/T:** Resistance to NFV, IDV, SQV, ATV in combination with other PI mutations. **G73A:** Uncommon variant.
T74P	Contributes to TPV and DRV resistance in presence of other mutations.
L76V	Decreases LPV susceptibility to unknown degree. Contributes to DRV resistance in presence of other DRV mutations.
V77I	Polymorphism associated with slight decrease in NFV susceptibility.
V82A/T/F/S/I/G/L	**V82A/T/F/S:** Primary PI mutation that reduces susceptibility to LPV, IDV, RTV, and also to NFV, SQV, APV, ATV when combined with other PI mutations. **V82I:** Polymorphism with minimal effect on PI susceptibility. **V82M:** Seen with subtype G infection; reduces IDV susceptibility. **V82L/T:** Contribute to TPV resistance in presence of other TPV mutations.
N83D	Contributes to TPV resistance in presence of other TPV mutations.
I84V/A/C	**I84V:** Decreases susceptibility to all PIs: greatest effect on APV, NFV, SQV, lowest on LPV. Contributes to TPV and DRV resistance in presence of other mutations. **I84A/C:** Effects similar to I84V, but rare.
N88S/D	**N88D:** Intermediate resistance to NFV; low-level resistance to SQV, ATV. **N88S:** Intermediate resistance to NFV, ATV; low-level resistance to IDV; hypersusceptibility to APV.
L89V	Contributes to DRV resistance in presence of other DRV mutations.
L90M	By itself, causes intermediate resistance to SQV and NFV and low-level resistance to other PIs. Contributes to TPV resistance in presence of other TPV mutations.
I93L/M	**I93L:** Common polymorphism that increases PI resistance when combined with other PI mutations. **I93M:** PI mutation with unknown effect on PI susceptibility.

Laboratory Tests

■ TABLE 2-15: **Fold Change Cutoffs for Phenotype and *VircoTYPE* Assays**

Drug		Monogram *PhenoSense*				Virco *Antivirogram*			Virco *VircoTYPE*		
		LCO	UCO	SCO	B/C	LCO	UCO	BCO	CCO1	CCO2	BCO
abacavir	ABC	4.5	6.5		C	3.2	7.5	2.2	0.9	3.5	
didanosine	ddl	1.3	2.2		C			2.2	0.9	2.6	
emtricitabine	FTC			3.5	B			3.5			3.1
lamivudine	3TC			3.5	C			2.4	1.2	4.6	
stavudine	d4T			1.7	C			2.3	1.0	2.3	
tenofovir DF	TDF	1.4	4.0		C			2.1	1.0	2.3	
zidovudine	AZT			1.9	B			2.7	1.5	11.4	
delavirdine	DLV			6.2	B						
efavirenz	EFV			3.0	B			3.4			3.3
etravirine	ETR								1.6	27.6	
nevirapine	NVP			4.5	B			5.5			6.0
amprenavir	APV							2.2			
amprenavir/ritonavir	APV/r										
atazanavir	ATV			2.2	C			2.4			
atazanavir/ritonavir	ATV/r			5.2	C				2.5	32.5	
darunavir/ritonavir	DRV/r	10.0	90.0		C	10	40.0	2.4	10.0	106.9	
fosamprenavir	FPV			2.0	B						
fosamprenavir/ritonavir	FPV/r	4.0	11.0		C				1.5	19.5	
indinavir	IDV			2.1	B			2.4	1.0	5.4	
indinavir/ritonavir	IDV/r			10	C				2.3	27.2	
lopinavir/ritonavir	LPV/r	9.0	55.0		C	10	40.0	1.7	6.1	51.2	
nelfinavir	NFV			3.6	B			2.2	1.2	9.4	
ritonavir	RTV			2.5	B						
saquinavir	SQV			1.7	B			1.8			
saquinavir/ritonavir	SQV/r	2.3	12.0		C				3.1	22.6	
tipranavir/ritonavir	TPV/r	2.0	8.0		C	3.0	10.0	1.8	1.5	7.0	

LCO = lower cutoff
UCO = upper cutoff
SCO = single cutoff

B = biological
C = clinical

CCO1 = lower clinical cutoff
CCO2 = upper clinical cutoff
BCO = biological cutoff

2 Laboratory Tests

in patients with more extensive resistance after multiple regimen failures (*CID* 2004;38:723) and TORO (*NEJM* 2003; 348:2175). Phenotypes provide quantitative results, allowing comparison of relative susceptibility and resistance. They assess interactions among mutations, and may be preferable for the assessment of susceptibility to new drugs for which genotypic correlates of resistance have not been completely determined. In the POWER studies, phenotypic susceptibility to darunavir was the best predictor of response to therapy (*Antiviral Ther* 2006;11:S83.)

Tropism Assay

Tropism assays are used to determine whether patients are candidates for therapy with CCR5 antagonists, which are indicated only in patients with exclusively R5-tropic virus (see pg. 317-323).

Background: HIV binds to the host CD4 cell by attachment of gp120 to a CD4 receptor. This results in a conformational change in gp120 that allows binding to one of two chemokine co-receptors on the CD4 cell surface: CCR5 or CXCR4. There are four categories of tropism:

- **R5-tropism:** Viruses that bind only to the CCR5 co-receptor
- **X4-tropism:** Viruses that bind only to the CXCR4 co-receptor
- **Dual-tropism:** Viruses that can bind to either co-receptor
- **Mixed-tropism:** Mixed populations that include both R5-tropic and X4-tropic viruses.

Tropism assays cannot distinguish between dual- and mixed-tropic virus; therefore, these viruses are collectively referred to as dual/mixed (D/M)-tropic virus.

Sequential data show that transmitted virus is almost always R5 virus, even when the source has D/M-tropic virus (*Ann Rev Immunol* 2003; 21:265). Therefore, patients with early HIV infection typically have R5 virus exclusively. With progressive disease, a shift to D/M-tropic virus can occur (*CID* 2007;44:591). Patients with extensive treatment experience or rapid progression have a higher frequency of X4 virus, but pure X4 populations are rare (*JID* 2005;191:806; *CID* 2007;44:591; *JID* 2006;194:926). The presence of X4 virus is associated with more

■ TABLE 2-16: **Prevalence of R5, D/M, and X4 viruses in patients with HIV-infection**

Source	Treatment	N	R5	D/M	X4
JID 2005; 192:466	Naïve	979	82%	18%	<1%
JID 2005; 191:866	Naïve	462	81%	18%	<1%
CID 2007; 44:591	Experienced	391	50%	46%	4%
Viral Entry 2007;3:10	Experienced	2,560	56%	41%	3%
NEJM 2008;359:1429	Experienced	3,244	61%	–	–

Laboratory Tests

rapid clinical progression but this does not alter response to standard therapy (*CID* 2008;46:1617).

Available Assays: There are two high-throughput phenotypic assays: *Phenoscript* (VIRalliance, Paris, France) and *Trofile* (Monogram Biosciences, Inc., San Francisco CA). The *Trofile* test requires, a VL of ≥1000 c/mL, the cost $1,960/test and the turnaround time is about 2 wks (see www.trofileassay.com or 1-800-777-0177). The indication for the test is consideration of use of a CCR5 antagonist, because the drug should be used only in patients with exclusive R5 virus. In MOTIVATE -1 and -2, the *Trofile* test was used to screen treatment-experienced patients with 3-class resistance; 61% of 3,244 potential participants had R5 virus. A subsequent report showed that some of the failures had D/M virus detected only with the more recent and more sensitive *Trofile* ES (Enhanced Sensitivity) that has the ability to detect X4 virus with 100% sensitivity when X4 or D/M virus accounted for >0.3% of the viral population (*JCM* 2009;47:2604). Disadvantages of the *Trofile* assay include cost, requirement for a VL of >1000 c/mL, occasional cases of "non-reportable" results and the 2-3 wk wait time. An alternative to the *Trofile* is the tropism coreceptor assay information or "TROCAI" assay based on the virologic response to short term exposure to the CCR5 antagonist (MVC). Results of this tests have correlated well with the *Trofile* (*JCM* 2010;48:4453). There is also a genotypic assay of the HIV-1 env V3 loop to determine coreceptor tropism (*AIDS* 2010;24:2517). This assay is less expensive and does not require a VL >1000 c/mL (*JCM* 2010;48:4453), but it is less sensitive for detecting X4 virus (*Antiviral Res* 2011;89:182) and is consequently not recommended in the 2011 DHHS Guidelines. *Trofile* is preferred for cases with VL >1000 c/mL.

SCREENING LABORATORY TESTS

The usual screening battery advocated for patients with established HIV infection is summarized in Table 2-17, pg. 51-53 (Primary Care Guidelines IDSA, *CID* 2004;39:609).

Complete Blood Count: The CBC is important, because anemia, leukopenia, lymphopenia and thrombocytopenia are common due to HIV per se or to medications (*JAIDS* 1994;7:1134; *JAIDS* 2001;28:221). Repeat at 3- to 6-mo intervals and more frequently in patients with symptoms (headache, fatigue), those receiving marrow-suppressing drugs such as AZT, and in those with marginal or low counts.

Serum Chemistry Panel: This panel is advocated in the initial evaluation of HIV infection due to high rates of baseline hepatic disease (*JID* 2002;186:231),to assess renal function and nutritional status, and to obtain baseline values in patients who are likely to have multisystem disease due to HIV or its treatment.

Syphilis Serology (*MMWR* 2010;59:RR-12): Screen with a nontreponemal test (VDRL or RPR) at baseline and annually thereafter in sexually active patients due to high rates of co-infection. The screening test is confirmed with a treponemal test: fluorescent treponemal antibody absorbed (FTA-ABS), the *T. pallidum* passive partical agglutination (TP-PA) and various EIAs and chemiluminescence immunoassays. Confirmation is important due to frequent false positive screening tests often ascribed to autoimmune disease, advanced age, injection drug use, pregnancy, and HIV infection (*CID* 1994;19:1040; *JID* 1992;165:1124; *JAIDS* 1994;7:1134; *Am J Med* 1995;99:55). In one review of 300,000 VDRLs, the rate of biologic false positives was 2.1% in persons with HIV compared to 0.24% in those without HIV (*Int J STD AIDS* 2005;16:722). Nontreponemal tests give antibody titers that correlate with disease activity. Many patients will have positive treponemal tests for life, but the VDRL and RPR usually become negative or persist at low titer. Some HIV-infected patients have "atypical serology" with unusually high, unusually low, or fluctuating titers, but "for most HIV-infected patients, serologic tests are accurate and reliable for the diagnosis of syphilis and for the response to therapy" (*MMWR* 2002;51[RR-6]:19). Some laboratories and blood banks now screen for syphilis with a treponemal test, usually EIA. These may also show false positives and need to be confirmed with a nontreponemal test with titer. If that test is negative, the lab should perform a different treponemal test that preferably uses different antigens than the initial test. If the second test is positive and the patient had prior treatment with no subsequent exposures, no further treatment is required. If there was no intervening treatment, the patient should be treated. If the second treponemal test is negative no further evaluation or treatment is needed (*MMWR* 2010;59:RR-12). The CDC prefers the traditional testing policy using the nontreponemal test first (Bolan, CDC letter to providers, 2/10/2011). For management guidelines and evaluation for neurosyphilis, see pg. 488.

Screening for Other Sexually Transmitted Infections (STIs):

- **Infections** with *N. gonorrhoeae* and/or *C. trachomatis* are common in HIV-infected patients (*AIDS* 2000;14:297) and are often asymptomatic in both men and women (*STD* 2001;28:33; *CID* 2002:35: 1010). Diagnosis of STIs is important because 1) they usually indicate ongoing high-risk behavior, 2) they may enhance transmission of HIV, and 3) detection and treatment can reduce likelihood of transmission (*Sex Transm Infect* 1999;75:3; *Lancet* 1995;346:530). Urine-based nucleic acid amplification tests (NAATs) are now generally available for *N. gonorrhoeae* and *C. trachomatis* for screening men and women with advantages of good sensitivity, good specificity and ease of specimen collection (*MMWR* 2010;59:RR-12). The usual cost is $40-100 per test. Rectal and pharyngeal *C. trachomatis* infections can be diagnosed by NAATs;

■ TABLE 2-17: **Routine Laboratory Tests**

Test	Cost*	Frequency and Comment
HIV Tests		
HIV confirmation	$100	HIV serology. Rapid HIV tests and EIA need confirmation by Western blot, IFA or HIV RNA. If confirmatory test is negative or indeterminant, repeat in 1 month. See pg. 9-20.
HIV viral load	$150-300	See pg. 20-27. Baseline and every 3-6 months.
CD4 count and CD4%	$100-150	See pg. 27-33. Baseline and every 3-6 months. Monitoring at 6-12 month intervals is appropriate in clinically stable patients with consistant HIV suppression.
HIV genotypic resistance test	$100-150	Baseline and with virologic failure.
HLA-B*5701	$100	Indicated if plan to treat with ABC.
Tropism test	$1960	Indicated if plan to use CCR5 antagonist (i.e., MVC) and with MVC failure.
Serologic Tests		
Hepatitis screen	$60-80	If acute hepatitis suspected, screen with anti-HAV IgM, anti-HCV and HBsAg ± anti-HBc IgM. For chronic hepatitis and immune status: anti-HAV, anti-HCV, HBsAg, anti-HBs and anti-HBc.
Total anti-HAV antibody[†]	$20-30	Screen at baseline for HAV immunity to determine need for vaccination.
anti-HBc or anti-HBs[†]	$10-15	HBV: Screen at baseline for immunity with anti-HBc, anti-HBs and HBsAg to determine need for vaccination. If prior HBV vaccination, then test anti-HBs. If anti-HBc present without anti-HBs or HBsAg, screen for chronic HBV with HBV DNA; if HBV DNA negative, give HBV vaccine. Repeat anti-HBs at 1-2 months after 3d vaccine dose to determine "take" (see pg. 57).
HBsAg[†]	$20-25	Screen for chronic hepatitis B. Consider HBV DNA in HBsAg negatives with abnormal transaminases.
anti-HCV[†]	$25 HCV EIA	Screen with anti-HCV; confirm positives with quantitative HCV RNA at $150. Consider HCV RNA in HCV-seronegatives at high risk, with abnormal transaminases, or with CD4 counts <200.
Syphilis: VDRL, RPR or treponema EIA[†]	$5-16	Confirm positives with FTA-ABS, MHA-TP or TP-PA. Repeat test annually in at-risk sexually active patients. Note concerns with EIA screening (pg 50).
anti-*Toxoplasma* IgG[†]	$12-15	Screen all patients at baseline, and repeat in sero-negatives if CD4 cell count is <100 cells/mm³ and patient does not take TMP-SMX for PCP prophylaxis or has symptoms suggestive of toxoplasmosis encephalitis. Agglutination assays for IgG are preferred. IgM is not useful.
Varicella IgG*	$10	If negative or unknown history for chickenpox or shingles to promote protection against exposure, varicella vaccination and/or post-exposure ZIG.

* Common charges are based on survey of five laboratories.
† Recommendations of Primary HIV Care Guidelines of IDSA (*CID* 2004;39:609).

(continued)

2 Laboratory Tests

Test	Cost*	Frequency and Comment
Chemistry		
Comprehensive Chemistry panel†	$10-15	Includes liver enzymes and renal function. Repeat every 6-12 months or more frequently in patients with abnormal results and with administration of hepatotoxic or nephrotoxic drugs, including most ART regimens. FBS at entry to care and repeat annually.
G6PD	$14-20	Timing and need for this test depends on the host demographics and use of high risk drugs (see pg. 61).
Lipid profile and blood glucose (fasting)	$20-40	Test at baseline and at 4-8 weeks after starting new ART regimen. Routine testing at 6-12 month intervals; more frequently based on initial results and risks.†
Hematology		
Complete blood count (CBC)†	$6-8	Repeat every 3 to 6 months, more frequently for low values and with marrow-toxic drugs.
Other		
Chest x-ray	$40-140	May be routine or restricted to those with past pulmonary disease, chronic pulmonary disease or a positive PPD or IFN gamma release assay.*
PAP smear†	$25-40	Repeat at 6 months and then annually if results are normal. Results reported as "inadequate" should be repeated. Refer to a gynecologist for results showing atypia or greater on the Bethesda scale (see pg. 55-56).
PPD test or interferon-gamma release assay	$10/PPD test $40/IFN gamma release assay	Test at baseline. Annual testing should be considered in previously PPD-negative patients who have risk for tuberculosis, and repeat testing should be considered if initial test was negative and the CD4 count has subsequently increased to >200 cells/mm^3 in response to ART.
Urine NAAT: *C. trachomatis* in sexually active females ≤25 years†	$40-100	Recommended by CDC HIV prevention guidelines for sexually active females <25 years (*MMWR* 2010; 59:RR12). Advocated as marker of high risk behavior with need for enhanced counseling and for treatment + contact tracing. Repeat annually in sexually active patients. and more often in high-risk patients (see pg. 19). The Primary Care HIV Guidelines recommend screening all men and women for gonorrhea and *C. trachomatis* (*CID* 2009;49:651).
Urinalysis	$10	Assessment is especially important in African-Americans, those on TDF, and with co-morbidities: diabetes, hypertension or hepatitis C. If ≥1 + proteinuria, measure hour urine protein/creatinine ratio.

* Common charges are based on survey of five laboratories.

† Recommendations of Primary HIV Care Guidelines of IDSA (*CID* 2004;39:609).

(continued)

Laboratory Tests

Test	Cost*	Frequency and Comment
General Health Screens		
Mammography	$100-350	Indicated annually in women >50 years.
Colonoscopy	$300-800	Indicated in patients >50 years and every 10 years thereafter.[†]
Prostate-specific antigen	$50-100	Men >50 years
Bone densitometry	$150-900	Patients with risk factors for osteoporosis (see pg. 554). MRI for patients with hip pain.

* Common charges are based on survey of five laboratories.

† Recommendations of Primary HIV Care Guidelines of IDSA (*CID* 2004;39:609).

these test are more sensitive than culture at these sites (*STD* 2008;35:435 and 637; *JCM* 2010;48:1827; *JCM* 2009;47:902), but they are FDA-cleared only for diagnostic testing for urethral or endocervical infection. Alternative less expensive tests include endocervical and urethral swabs to detect *N. gonorrhoeae* and/or *C. trachomatis* by culture, nucleic acid hybridization, DFA or EIA.

- **Screening (CDC Guidelines):** The CDC recommends annual screening for *C. trachomatis* in all females <25 years who are sexually active. For women who are >25 years this screening is recommended if there are specific risks such as a new sex partner or multiple sex partners. *C. trachomatis* screening of sexually active young men is recommended in settings of high *C. trachomatis* prevalence such as STD clinics and some MSM (*MMWR* 2010;59:RR-12). Routine screening of sexually active MSM is recommended at least annually for 1) HIV (if not known to be positive); 2) syphilis; 3) urinary NAAT testing for *N. gonorrhoeae* and *C. trachomatis*; 4) rectal infection with *N. gonorrhoeae* and *C. trachomatis* in men who have had insertive intercourse in the prior year, preferably with a rectal swab for NAAT testing; and 5) pharyngeal test for *N. gonorrhoeae* in men who have had receptive oral intercourse in the prior year, preferably using NAAT (testing for pharyngeal *C. trachomatis* is not recommended).

- **The HIV Primary Care Guidelines** (*CID* 2009;49:651) recommend screening all patients for syphilis (RPR or VDRL) and "consider" first voided urine NAAT tests for *N. gonorrhoeae* and *C. trachomatis*. Women should have vaginal secretions examined for *Trichomonas*, and women <26 years and others at increased risk should have a cervical specimen for NAAT for *Chlamydia* species. Patients reporting receptive anal sex should have rectal cultures for *N. gonorrhoeae* and *C. trachomatis*. The screening tests noted should be repeated annually in sexually active patients.

Laboratory Tests

2

Chest X-Ray: A routine baseline chest x-ray is sometimes recommended for detection of asymptomatic tuberculosis and as a baseline for patients who are at high risk for pulmonary disease. Nevertheless, in a longitudinal study of 1,065 patients at various stages of HIV infection, showed routine x-rays performed at 0, 3, 6, and 12 mos (*Arch Intern Med* 1996;156:191) detected an abnormality in only 123 (2%) of 5,263 x-rays. None of the asymptomatic PPD-negative patients had evidence of active tuberculosis, and only 1 of 82 with a positive PPD had an abnormality on x-ray. The authors concluded that routine chest x-rays in asymptomatic HIV-infected patients with negative PPD skin tests are not warranted.

Tuberculin Skin Test and IFN-Gamma Release Assays:
The CDC recommends the Mantoux method TST (tuberculin skin test or interferon-gamma release assays (IGRAs) for detection of latent TB (see pg. 69). The TST test uses the intradermal injection of 5TU of PPD, for HIV-infected patients who have not had a prior positive test. TST should be repeated annually if initial test(s) were negative if the patient belongs to a population with a high risk of tuberculosis (such as residents of prisons or jails, injection drug users, and homeless individuals). The PPD should also be repeated following immune reconstitution when the CD4 count increases to >200 cells/mm^3. Induration of ≥5 mm at 48-72 hrs constitutes a positive test. Anergy testing is not recommended.

IGRAs, FDA-approved tests that measure release of interferon-gamma, derived from *M. tuberculosis* include:

- *QuantiFERON-TB Gold* test
- *QuantiFERON-TB Gold In-Tube* test
- *T-SPOT.TB* test

All require fresh whole blood that is mixed with TB antigens and reported as positive, negative or indeterminate (*T-Spot.TB* also has a "borderline" result). Advantages compared to PPD testing include: 1) Better specificity (92-97% vs. 55-95%); 2) Single patient visit is required; 3) Results are available in 24 hrs; 4) It does not boost with subsequent tests; and 5) There are not false positive tests with BCG vaccination. Disadvantages include: 1) need to process blood sample within 8-16 hrs; 2) limited data on ability to predict who will get active TB; 3) limited data in selected populations: children <5 years, recent TB exposures, immunocompromised patients and results with serial testing; and 4) Cost (*Ann Intern Med* 2007;146:340; *PLoS One* 2008; 6:e2665; *MMWR* 2006;54 RR15:49; *Proc Am Thorac Soc* 2006;3:103).

Note: A meta-analysis of TST showed good performance characteristics except in patients with a prior BCG (*Ann Intern Med* 2007;16:340).

Pap Smear: The CDC recommends that a gynecological evaluation with pelvic exam and Pap smear be performed at baseline, repeated at 6 mos and annually in women with HIV infection. The cervical screening is performed with conventional or liquid based cytologic tests (Paps test) and can include HPV-DNA tests. Cytopathic findings are reported by the Bethesda classification: atypical squamous cells (ACS), low grade squamous epithelial lesions (LSIL), or high grade squamous epithelial lesions (HSIL). The ACS category is subclassified as atypical squamous cells of undetermined origin (ASC-US) and atypical squamous cells – cannot exclude HSIL (ACS-H). HIV-infected women with ASC-H, LSIL or HSIL should undergo colposcopy. With ASC-US (indicating some abnormal areas on the cervix) the recommendations include: 1) colposcopy; 2) repeat Pap test at 6- to 12-mo intervals until there are two consecutive negatives; or 3) test for high risk HPV DNA.

Recommendations for women with an abnormal Pap test are based on the 2006 Consensus Guidelines for Management of Abnormal Cervical Cytology (www.mmhiv.com/link/2006-ASCCP-Abnormal).

More aggressive testing in women with HIV is recommended because of prior reports indicating a several-fold increase in rates of squamous intraepithelial lesion (SIL) (33-45% HIV+ vs 7-14% HIV-negative) and a 0- to 9-fold increase in rates of cervical cancer in women with HIV (*Arch Pediatr Adolesc Med* 2000;154:127; *Obstet Gynecol Clin N Am* 1996;23,861; *JAIDS* 2003;32:527; *JAIDS* 2004;36:978). Severity and

■ TABLE 2-18: **Comparison of Cervical and Anal Cancer** (Adapted from Darragh and Winkler, *Cancer Cytopath* 2011;119:5)

Issue	Cervical Cancer Decreasing	Anal Cancer Increasing
Prevalence in general population	8.1/100,000	1.6/100,000
Prevalence in HIV population	5.6/100,000	34.6/100,000
Median CD4 at diagnosis (cells/mm³)	287	276
Duration of HIV (median)	8.2 years	12.4 years
HPV types	16-50%	16-66%
	18-20%	18-5%
National guidelines	Yes	No
Median age at diagnosis	48 years	60 years
Palpation useful	No	Yes
Cytology useful	Yes	Probably
HPV testing useful in screening	Yes	No
Management	Colposcopy	High resolution anoscopy
Availability of well trained cytologists	Extensive	Limited
Treatment: High grade lesions	Laser, LEEP	Infrared coagulation, excision

2 Laboratory Tests

frequency of cervical dysplasia increase with progressive immune compromise, but this association is weak and there is some evidence that cervical cancer rates are not decreasing in the HAART era (*Curr HIV Res* 2010;8:493; *JID* 2010;201:681; *JID* 2010;201:650). There is a strong association between HIV infection and detectable and persistent HPV infection by HPV types associated with cervical cancer (16, 18, 31, 33, and 35) (*CID* 1995;21[suppl 1]:S121; *NEJM* 1997; 337:1343; *JID* 2001;184:682). See pg 531.

Human Papilloma virus (HPV) testing:
There are over 100 HPV types and more are benign. High risk ongenic types (especially type 16 and 18) may cause cancer of the cervix, penis vulva, vagina, anus or oropharynx. Nononcogenic types (especially types 6 and 11) may cause genital warts or respiratory papillomatosis. The lifetime risk of HPV in sexually active persons is >50% and persistence of oncogenic type is the greatest risk for cancer. HPV tests that are FDA-cleared are HCII High-Risk HPV test (Qiagen), HCII Low-Risk HPV test (Qiagen), Cervista 16/18 test and Cervista HPV High-Risk test (Hologics) (2010 CDC Guidelines for Sexually Transmitted Diseases (*MMWR* 2010;59 RR-12:1).

Anal PAP smear for SIL and carcinoma in MSM:
Anal cancer is similar to cervical cancer in many ways: both are caused by infection with one of several oncogenic HPV subtypes, low-grade lesions often progress to high-grade lesions, and Pap smear may be an effective screening method (*Am J Med* 2000;108:674). The prevalence of HPV in MSM is 60-75% (*JID* 1998;177:361), and the frequency of anal carcinoma in MSM with HIV infection is 35/100,000, or about 80 times that of the general population (*Lancet* 1998;351:1833; *Cancer* 2010;116:5507; *Int J Cancer* 2010;127:875; *AIDS* 2010;24:535). The rate increases with CD4 counts <500 cells/mm^3 (*AIDS* 1998;12:495).

- **Method**: No preparation is required. Use a Dacron (not cotton) swab to obtain the specimen before rectal exam, (i.e. before lubrication is introduced). The patient should not have had an enema or anal sex in the prior 24 hrs. The swab is moistened with saline or non-sterile water, the anus is spread so the aroderm points out, the swab is inserted into the anal canal; it must be inserted at least 2 cm from the anal verge. It is then withdrawn gradually while rotating the swab with mild pressure to the anal wall. The swab is immersed in methanol-based solution, agitated and submitted to the lab.

- **Sensitivity and specificity:** A review of 7 reports on anal cytology showed sensitivities of 42-98% and specificities of 33-96% (*AIDS* 2010;24:463) and specificity of 32-59% for anal Pap smears (*CID* 2006;43:223).

- **High resolution anoscopy (HRA):** Patients with cytology results showing ASC-US, LSIL or HSIL should be referred for HRA, which is comparable to cervical colposcopy and is considered complementary

Laboratory Tests

to cytology in high risk patients (*Dis Colon Rectum* 2009;52:1854; *AIDS* 2010;24:373). The American Society for Colposcopy and Cervical Pathology offers an annual workshop on HRA (www.mmhiv.com/link/ASCCP-HRA-Workshop). A cost analysis concluded that direct use of HRA was more cost effective than cytology or HPV testing (*AIDS* 2011;25:635).

INDICATIONS are controversial and there is no consensus. Some authorities recommend anal Pap smears in all patients with histories of receptive anal intercourse at 1-3 year intervals, which is comparable to recommendations for cervical Pap smears (*Am J Med* 2000;108: 634). Others are more selective based on the large variation in reported sensitivity and specificity, and the uncertain relative value of Pap tests vs. HRA (*AIDS* 2010;24:463). The 2010 STD Guidelines (*MMWR* 2010;59 RR-12:1) state, "Because the increased incidence of anal cancer in HIV-infected men screening for anal intraepitelial neoplasia by cytology can be considered."

TREATMENT: Abnormal anal Pap smears should lead to referral for high-resolution anoscopy and biopsy (*CID* 2004;38:1490). A cost effective analysis (Canada) found that the best strategy was use of HRA without pre-sreening by anal Pap.

EVALUATION: A meta-analysis of 21 published studies from 1996 to 2005 (*CID* 2006;43:223) concluded that anal Pap smears are of "modest accuracy" that is similar cervical Pap smears. Limitations are: 1) lack of randomized trials; 2) limited treatment data; and 3) poorly-defined natural history.

Hepatitis A Serology:
HAV serology (total anti-HAV antibody) is performed to identify candidates for the HAV vaccine, which is indicated for susceptible persons with chronic HCV infection, injection drug use, MSM, persons with clotting disorders, persons with chronic liver disease, and travelers to HAV-endemic areas (*MMWR* 1996;45[RR-15]:1) (see pg. 75). Some authorities believe that all HIV-infected persons who are susceptible should be vaccinated. The prevalence of anti-HAV IgG is 40-70% in adults in the US and most European countries (*CID* 1997; 25:726; *MMWR* 1999;48:[RR-12]:1). To diagnose acute hepatitis the preferred test is anti-HAV IgM. The anti-HAV IgG becomes positive at 8-16 wks.

HBV Tests: See pg. 507.
- HBeAg: Indicates infection with high rate of infectivity and of viral replication.
- Anti-HBe (HBeAb): May be present with chronic infection or immunity. Main use is chronic infection in whom HBV DNA indicates low viral titer and low degree of infectivity.
- HBV DNA: Marker of viral replication.
- Anti-HBc IgM: Indicates recent infection (within 6 mos).

SCREENING TESTS: All HIV-infected patients should be screened with HBsAg and anti-HBs. Routine testing for HBcAb is optional.

BASELINE EVALUATION: See pg. 51, 507.

- Anti-HBs and HBsAg negative: vaccinate (see pg. 75)
- HBsAg positive: evaluate for chronic infection with HBeAg, HBV DNA, liver function tests
- Anti-HBc positive, anti-HBs/HBsAg-negative: rule out chronic HBV infection with HBV DNA, vaccinate if negative

■ TABLE 2-19: **Hepatitis B serology** (*MMWR* 2010;59 RR-12)

HBsAg	Total Anti-HBc	HBc IgM	Anti-HBs	Interpretation
–	–	–	–	Never infected
+	–	–	–	Acute HBV (< 18d)
+	+	+	–	Acute HBV
–	+	+	–	Acute – resolving
–	+	–	+	Past infection – Immune
+	+	–	–	Chronic HBV
–	+	–	–	False positive (susceptible)
–	+	–	+	Immune if > 10 IU/mL

HCV (*MMWR* 2004;53,[RR-15]:1; 2008 DHHS OI Guidelines): The seroprevalence of HCV is 1.8% in the general population, 4-6% in MSM, and 70-90% in IDUs and hemophilia patients (see pg. 513).

SCREENING: All HIV-infected persons should be tested for HCV infection using the sensitive third-generation EIA screening assay for anti-HCV antibodies (*Hepatology* 2002;36;S3). The third-generation EIAs have a sensitivity and specificity of >99% in immunocompetent patients, but there may be false-negatives with severe immunosuppression (e.g. CD4 counts <100 cells/mm^3) (*JAIDS* 2002;31:154) and some with acute HCV infections. A rapid point-of-care test from *OraQuick* is available using venous blood, finger stick blood, serum, plasma or oral fluid with sensitivities and specificities of 99.2-100% (*J Clin Virol* 2010;48:15; *J Virol Methods* 2011;172:27). Results are available in 10-20 minutes. A confirmatory test with HCV RNA is needed. Many authorities prefer the older more established screening tests using EIA, RIBA or PCR. Qualitative or quantitative HCV RNA assays should be ordered in patients with suspected false-negative results (e.g., seronegative injection drug users or patients with unexplained transaminase elevation) (*JID* 1994;170:433; *Blood* 1993; 82:1010).

CONFIRMATORY TEST: For patients with a positive EIA screening test or rapid test, qualitative HCV RNA assay is recommended for confirmation, although it may not be necessary with EIA screening in

Laboratory Tests

patients with risk factors for HCV infection and an abnormal ALT. Qualitative HCV RNA assays have a threshold of detection of 50-100 IU/mL. A negative test does not exclude HCV, because HCV RNA levels may periodically decline below limits of detection; repeat testing at 3-6 mos is recommended to rule out chronic HCV infection. Tests for quantification of HBsAg are also available and can be used to measure response to treatment (*J Clin Virol* 2011;50:292)

EVALUATION: 1) Quantitative HCV assay, 2) liver function tests and 3) HCV genotype. Quantitative HCV assays (bDNA or RNA PCR) are VL assays that have a threshold of detection of 500 IU/ mL and may be used in place of the qualitative RNA test to establish the diagnosis, because this test will be necessary for clinical management anyway.The HCV RNA does not correlate with disease severity or rate of progression; its principal use is to monitor response to therapy. Hepatic transaminases should be measured in patients with chronic HCV infection, although there may be significant liver disease with persistently normal AST and ALT levels. An HCV genotype should be measured, because the genotype is an important predictor of response to therapy. Genotype 1 accounts for about 75% of US cases and shows relatively poor response to interferon treatment. Patients who are non-immune should be vaccinated against HAV and HBV. Those who are considered candidates for HCV therapy should be evaluated as recommended (see pg. 516).

■ TABLE 2-20: **Tests for HCV**

Test	Cost	Comment
Anti-HCV EIA	$25-45	Indicates past or present HCV infection. Sensitivity of the third generation tests is >99%.
		EIA lacks specificity in low-prevalence populations – supplemental assay required for confirmation.
		RIBA – of little utility in HIV-infected patients.
Qualitative HCV RNA (HCV RT-PCR)	$160-200	RT-PCR technology to detect HCV RNA; may have false-positives and negatives.
		Threshold for detection is 50 IU/mL.
		Usual use is to confirm serology results.
Quantitative HCV PCR or bDNA	$160-225	Determines concentration using RT-PCR or bDNA technology. Less sensitive than qualitative RT-PCR. Threshold of detection is 500 IU/mL; most patients with chronic HCV infection have 10^5-10^7 c/mL.
		HCV RNA level is not useful for determining prognosis; it is used to monitor response to therapy. Magnitude of HCV RNA level may predict response. It has largely supplanted qualitative HCV RNA tests due to adequate sensitivity and comparable cost.
Genotype	$200-250	6 genotypes – genotype 1 predominates in U.S. (70%) and shows poorest response to therapy. Better response with genotypes 2 and 3.

2 Laboratory Tests

Toxoplasma Serology: _Toxoplasma_ serology (anti-_Toxoplasma_ IgG) is recommended to assist in the differential diagnosis of complications involving the CNS, to identify candidates for toxoplasmosis prophylaxis (_Ann Intern Med_ 1992;117:163), and to counsel patients on preventive measures if seronegative (see pg. 70). The preferred method is an agglutination assay for IgG; IgM assays are not useful, and the Sabin-Feldman dye test is less accurate. Toxoplasma IgG must be stipulated because most labs will do the IgM assay unless IgG is specified. Seroprevalence among adults in the US is 10-30%, and the seroconversion rate is up to 1% per year. The sensitivity of the test is 95-97%. Most infections in AIDS patients represent relapse of latent infection, which is noted in 20-47% of those with the combination of CD4 counts <100 cells/mm^3, positive _Toxoplasma_ serology, and no prophylaxis (_CID_ 1992;15:211; _CID_ 2002;34: 103).

A negative _Toxoplasma_ serology should be repeated after the CD4 cell count is ≤100 cells/mm^3 if the patient does not take atovaquone or TMP-SMX prophylaxis for PCP (2009 Guidelines for Prevention and Treatment of Opportunistic Infections in HIV-Infected Adults and Adolescents: www.mmhiv.com/link/2009-OI-NIH-CDC-IDSA) or whenever the diagnosis of toxoplasmosis encephalitis is being considered when prior tests were negative or not done (see pg. 486).

CMV Serology: See pg. 441. This test is not recommended for baseline screening in the 2009 Guidelines for Prevention and Treatment of Opportunistic Infections in HIV-Infected Adults and Adolescents (www.mmhiv.com/link/2009-OI-NIH-CDC-IDSA) due to limited clinical utility in most patients. However, it _is_ recommended in the IDSA HIV Primary Care Guidelines for persons defined as having low risk for CMV infection (_CID_ 2009;49:66). The major potential benefit is that a negative test usually excludes CMV disease (_Ann Intern Med_ 1993;118:12; _Lancet_ 2004; _Lancet_ 2004;363:2116). Other uses of serology: 1) identification of seronegative patients for counseling on CMV prevention (although the message is not different from the "safe sex message" for preventing HIV transmission); 2) assessment of the likelihood of CMV disease in late-stage HIV infection, although invasive CMV disease has become a rare complication in the HAART era; 3) identification of seronegative individuals who should receive CMV-antibody-negative blood or leukocyte-reduced blood products for nonemergent transfusions (_JAMA_ 2001;285:1592); and 4) CMV serology is the "C" in TORCH testing in neonates. Seroprevalence for adults in the United States is about 50%; in MSM and injection drug users it is >90% (_JID_ 1985;152:243; _Am J Med_ 1987;82:593). The 2009 Primary Care Guidelines for HIV Management from IDSA (_CID_ 2009;49:651) recommend a baseline anti-CMV IgG in low-prevalence populations, but this has never proven useful in preventing or predicting CMV disease in HIV-infected persons (_JCM_ 2000;38:563).

Glucose-6-Phosphate Dehydrogenase Levels (G6PD): G6PD deficiency is a genetic variation that predisposes to hemolytic anemia following exposure to oxidant drugs commonly such as dapsone, primaquine and TMP-SMX. Over 150 G6PD variants are inherited on the X chromosome, but the most frequent are GdA-, which is found in 10% of black men and in 1-2% of black women, and Gdmed, found predominantly in men from the Mediterranean area (Italians, Greeks, Sephardic Jews, Arabs), India, and Southeast Asia. The 2009 IDSA Guidelines for Primary HIV Care recommend qualitative screening for G6PD deficiency on entry to care in patients with a predisposing racial or ethnic background (*CID* 2009;49:651). A review of 1,110 tests in an HIV program in Texas found positive results in 75 (6.8%) including rates of 68/699 (9.7%) in African-Americans, 5/253 (2.0%) in Hispanics and 1/153 (0.7%) in Caucasians (*J Infect* 2010;61:399). With most defects, the hemolysis is mild and self-limited because only the older red cells are involved, and the bone marrow can compensate even with continued administration of the implicated drug. The limited hemolysis in patients may be significant in patients who have anemia from other causes. The severity of anemia also depends on the concentration of the drug in red cells and the oxidant potential of the inducing agent. In the series noted above with 75 HIV-infected patients, 40 received TMP-SMX and 5 (6.7%) developed acute hemolytic anemia (*J Infect* 2010;61:399). The most likely offending agents in patients with HIV infection are dapsone and primaquine. Sulfonamides cause hemolysis less commonly. A PubMed review (1950-2009) identified 7 drugs with evidence to support prohibiting in patients with G6PD-deficiency: dapsone, methylene blue, nitrofurantoin, phenazopyridine, primaqine, rasburicase, and toluidine blue (*Drug Saf* 2010;33:713). Typical findings with hemolysis include elevated indirect bilirubin, elevated LDH, decreased haptoglobin, methemoglobinemia, reticulocytosis, Coombs test negative, and a peripheral smear showing the characteristic bite cells. During hemolysis, G6PD levels are usually normal because the susceptible red cells are destroyed; testing must consequently be delayed until about 30 days after discontinuation of the offending agent. Results are reported as % normal G6PD enzyme activity classed as normal (60-150%), moderately severe (10-60%), and severe (<10%) deficiency. Laboratories report results as units/g Hgb, with these three categories of deficiency.

HLA-B*5701: It appears that possibly all true abacavir (ABC) hypersensitivity reactions (HSR) have a genetic basis attributed to carriage of the MHC class I allele HLA-B*5701 (*PNAS* 2004;101:4180; *AIDS* 2005;19:979). The large definitive trial was PREDICT, a prospective double-blind trial in which 1660 patients with intended ABC use were tested and randomized for prescribing physicians to know or not know results of the HLA-B*5701 screening test (*NEJM* 2008;358:568). ABC HSR was confirmed with a blinded independent

■ TABLE 2-21: **Results of PREDICT in 1,660 patients (*NEJM* 2008;358:568)**

	Clinically suspected HSR[†]		Immunologically confirmed HSR[†]	
	Pos	Neg	Pos	Neg
HSR	30	36	23	0
No HSR	19	792	25	794
PPV	62%	-	46%	-
NPV	-	96%	-	100%

Abbreviations:
HSR = hypersensitivity reaction;
PPV = Positive predictive value;
NPV = negative predictive value

† Prevalence of HLA-B* 5701 is highly variable by race:
US Caucasians 8%, US Asians 1%, US African-Americans 2%, US Hispanics 2%,
UK 8%, Western Europe -7%, China and Japan <1% S. American Caucasians 5-7%,
Australians 8%, Sub-Saharan Africa <1%, Mediterranean 1-2%, India 5-20%
(*HIV Ther* 2003; 8:36)

skin patch test that is not commercially available. The sensitivity of HLA B*5701 testing was 43% in patients with clinically suspected ABC HSR and 100% for immunologically confirmed reactions. Specificity was 97% and 98% respectively (Table 2-21). The conclusion was that a negative test for HLA-B*5701 had a 100% negative predictive value, meaning a that a negative test excluded the possibility of HSR within the limits imposed by the sample size. A subsequent review of 9,720 patients in 272 HIV centers in Europe found positive results in 5-6.9% of whites and 0.4% of blacks (*Pharmacogenet Genomics* 2010; 20:307). This report emphasized the 100% sensitivity of the test. The DART trial in Uganda found no positive tests in 247 participants and a 2-3% rate of "false positive HSRs" (*Trop Med Int Health* 2010;15:454). HLA-B*5701 testing is now recommended in any patient in whom first use of ABC is being considered. The investigator largely responsible for developing the test and the principle investigator of PREDICT is unaware of false negative tests (S. Mallol, personal communication 2/13/11). The need for screening in low prevalence populations in resource-limited setting is unclear. Quality assurance testing in 7 labs with 96 specimens showed 100% concordance (*Antivir Ther* 2007; 12:1027) (see pg. 179).

DXA (Dual-Emission X-ray Absorptiometry) scans for bone density measurement (*CID* 2010;51:937): See pg. 15, 19.

BACKGROUND: HIV infection and its treatment is associated with high rates of decreased bone density resulting in increased rates of osteoporosis (*AIDS* 2006;20:2165) and fragility fractures (*J Clin Endocrinol Metab* 2008;93:3499; *CID* 2010;52:1061).

TESTING: The **standard test** to evaluate BMD is dual-energy x-ray absorptiometry (DXA). Results are classified by WHO based on the decrease in standard deviations (SD) below a reference population of young healthy women. This is used for persons ≥50 years, and it is expressed as a "T score." Osteopenia is defined by a hip T score of -1- 2.49 and osteoporosis is defined by a T score >-2.5. For persons <50 years the standard metric is a "Z-score" based on SD below sex and ethnic matched controls, but osteoporosis in this low age group cannot be based exclusively on BMD.

INDICATIONS for DXA from four sources:

- **The National Osteoporosis Foundation:** a) women >65 years; b) men >70 years; c) persons with a fragility fracture at any age; and d) patients with an additional risk – decrease the age threshold to 50 years for men and women (HIV is not a recognized additional risk).

- **The 2009 IDSA/HIVMA Guidelines for HIV Primary Care:** These guidelines endorse the above recommendations (*CID* 2009;49:65)

- **An ad hoc group of experts in bone disease in HIV infection:** Their recommendation is for screening DXA scans in: a) all postmenopausal women, b) all men >50 years old and c) those of any age with a fragility fracture (*CID* 2009;51:937).

- **US Preventive Services Task Force (*Ann Intern Med* 2011;154:356):** The recommendation for risk assessment to predict low bone mineral density (BMD) and fractures is the Fracture Risk Assessment (FRAX) tool of WHO (www.mmhiv.com/link/FRAX) to estimate 10-year risk for fracture because the clinical data are easily obtained. The threshold recommended for screening is 10% for a fracture in 10 years. The most common screening tests are DXA of hip and lumbar spine and quantitative ultrasonography of the calcaneus (which predicts fractures of the hip and spine as well as DXA). Screening recommendations are for women >65 years and younger women with a 10% risk for fracture in 10 years. Data are considered inadequate for a recommendation in men.

Testosterone Levels:

INDICATIONS:

- **IDSA HIV Primary Care Guidelines (*CID* 2009:49:651):** Male patients who complain of fatigue, weight loss, loss of libido, erectile dysfunction, depressive symptoms or evidence of reduced bone mineral density.

- **An Endocrine Society Clinical Practice Guideline (*J Clin Endocrinol Metab* 2010;95:2536):** Male patients with signs and symptoms unequivocally associated with low serum testosterone: reduced libido, decreased spontaneous erections, breast discomfort, gynecomastia, loss of axillary or pubic hair, small testes, hot flashes or sweats.

TEST: Morning total serum testosterone. It should be noted that some authorities prefer screening with free testosterone levels (*CID* 2009; 49:651). Abnormal tests should be repeated by repeating the test. Free serum testosterone should be measured in some men who have levels at or near the lower limit of normal. Testing should not be done during an acute illness. Testing of LH and FSH will distinguish primary (testicular) and secondary (pituitary-hypothalamic) hypogonadism (*J Clin Endocrinol Metab* 2010; 95:2536).

MEDICAL MANAGEMENT: See pg. 394.

Screening for Cardiovascular Disease

MARKERS OF IMMUNE ACTIVATION: Patients with HIV infection have an increased risk of cardiovascular disease due to HIV *per se* and/or to its treatment (*JID* 2010;201:1788). Thus, cardiovascular disease is now recognized as a major cause of death in this population (*AIDS* 2010;24:1537). Factors that contribute to this risk include: 1) some antiretroviral agents (IDV, LPV, SQV, ABC, ddI) (*JID* 2010;201:318); and 2) immune activation, presumably due to HIV *per se* (*JAIDS* 2010;55:615; *PLoS Med* 2008;5:e203). Inflammatory markers thought to correlate with immune activation mediated risks include hsCRP, IL-6 and D-dimer (*PLoS Med* 2008;5:e203; *AIDS* 2009;23:929; *JAIDS* 2010;55:316). Viral suppression with ART reduces these markers but does not usually bring them down to normal levels (*JID* 2010;201:1788). These markers (hsCRP, IL-6 and D-dimer) are readily available in clinical laboratories and are relatively inexpensive. Nevertheless, none are accepted as useful for monitoring cardiovascular risk in patients with HIV infection in any guidelines including the 2011 DHHS Guidelines, the 2010 IAS-USA Guidelines or the 2009 HIV Primary Care Guidelines (*CID* 2009;49:651) (see pg. 85).

Vitamin D Deficiency

STANDARD TEST: Serum 25-hydroxyvitamin D (25OHD) level is the standard and reflects the total vitamin D from diet, sunlight, and adipose stores in the liver.

NORMAL LEVELS: The threshold to define insufficiency is arbitrary. The WHO defines insufficiency as a level <20 ng/mL, but many labs now define deficiency as levels <20 ng/mL and insufficiency at <30 ng/mL (*NEJM* 2011;364:248). Note that 50-80% of the general population have vitamin D levels <30 ng/mL (*Arch Intern Med* 2009;169:626). The 2011 IOM review of vitamin D concluded there is an exaggerated estimation of the frequency of Vitamin D deficiency due to the use of thresholds of 25OHD, which should be <12 ng/mL for deficiency, <20 ng/mL as inadequate, and ≥50 ng/mL for toxicity (www.mmhiv.com/link/IOM-Vitamin-D). The 2010 International Osteoporosis Foundation recommended a target of 30 ng/mL in elderly people (*Osteoporos Int* 2010;21:1151).

Laboratory Tests

HIV INFECTION: Vitamin D insufficiency is common in persons with HIV infection in three reports showing levels <30 ng/mL in 60-74% (*Antiviral Ther* 2006;11:L9; *AIDS Res Hum Retroviruses* 2009;25:9; *CID* 2011;52;396). It is possibly noteworthy that these figures are actually higher than those in NHANES, which is a CDC-based population survey of 5,000 randomly selected US citizens. Risk factors and odds-ratios for low levels in the SUN study were black race (OR = 4.5) and Hispanic ethnicity 2.8. Antiretroviral agents implicated include EFV (*CID* 2011;52:396; *Antivir Ther* 2010;15:425; *AIDS* 2010;24:1923), TDF (*JAIDS* 2010;54:496) and possibly PIs (*AIDS* 2003;17:513).

POSSIBLE CONSEQUENCES:

- Most important is impact on BMD with osteomalacia, osteoporosis and fragility fractures (*NEJM* 2007;357:266; *J Clin Endocrinol Metab* 2001;86:1212; *JCI* 2006;116:2062; *NEJM* 1197;337:670). Note that these are the only clearly established consequences.

- Muscle weakness (*Mayo Clin Proc* 2006;81:353)

- Cognitive dysfunction (*J Nat Med Assoc* 2009;101:349)

- Cardiovascular risks (*Eur Heart J* 2010;31:2253; *Mol Nutr Food Res* 2010;54:1103; *Cardiovasc Ther* 2010;28:e5)

- Diabetes (type 2) and metabolic syndrome (*AIDS* 2011;25:531; 2010;25:525)

- Immune function (*Curr Infect Dis Rep* 2011;13:83)

RECOMMENDATIONS:

- **The IOM report** is based on review of over 1,000 publications and makes the following conclusions (www.mmhiv.com/link/IOM-Vitamin-D); (*JAMA* 2011; 305:453):

  □ The 25OHD level to define vitamin D "deficiency" should be <12 ng/mL and "inadequate" at 12-20 ng/mL.

  □ The only clear consequence of low 25OHD levels is bone health.

  □ The estimated average dietary intake for adults 600 IU/d and 800 IU/d for persons >71years (assumes minimal sun exposure; the upper limit of intake is 4,000 IU/d to avoid toxicity.

- **International panel of experts** (2010 International Scientists to D* Action (www.mmhiv.com/link/2010-DAction): defines 25OHD deficiency as <40-60 ng/mL and recommends intake of 2000 IU/d.

- **European AIDS Clinical Society 2009 Guidelines** define vitamin D deficiency as 25 OHD level <10 ng/mL and insufficiency as <20 ng/mL; the recommendation for intake is 800-2,000 IU/d.

Laboratory Tests

3 | Disease Prevention: Prophylactic Antimicrobial Agents and Vaccines

Recommendations of the 2009 Guidelines for Prevention and Treatment of Opportunistic Infections in HIV-Infected Adults and Adolescents (www.mmhiv.com/link/2009-OI-NIH-CDC-IDSA; *MMWR* 2009;58(RR-11): 1-66)

ANTIMICROBIAL PROPHYLAXIS AND VACCINES

Pneumocystis jiroveci : See pg. 462.

INDICATION: CD4 <200 cells/mm^3, prior PCP, thrush, CD4% <14 or CD4 count 200-250 cells/mm^3 with monitoring 3-4 mo intervals.

PREFERRED REGIMEN: TMP-SMX 1 DS qd or 1 SS qd

ALTERNATIVE REGIMENS

- TMP-SMX 1 DS 3x/wk
- Dapsone 100 mg qd or 50 mg po bid
- Dapsone 50 mg qd + pyrimethamine 50 mg/wk + leucovorin 25 mg/wk
- Dapsone 200 mg/wk + pyrimethamine 75 mg/wk + leucovorin 25 mg/wk
- Aerosolized pentamidine 300 mg/mo by *Respirgard II* nebulizer using 6 mL diluent delivered at 6L/min from a 50 psi compressed air source until reservoir is dry (usually 45 min), with or without albuterol (2 whiffs) to reduce cough and bronchospasm
- Atovaquone 1500 mg po qd with meals (*NEJM* 1998;339:1889)
- Atovaquone 1500 mg po + pyrimethamine 25 mg + leucovorin 10 mg qd.
- Other considerations for unusual circumstances: intermittent parenteral pentamidine and oral clindamycin plus primaquine.

RISK: The risk of PCP without prophylaxis is 60-70% per year in those with prior PCP and 40-50% per year for those with a CD4 count <100 cells/mm^3. The mortality for patients hospitalized and treated for PCP in the HAART era is 10-20% (*PLoS One* 2009;4:e7022). PCP prophylaxis reduces the risk of PCP 9-fold, and patients who develop PCP despite prophylaxis have a lower mortality rate (*Am J Respir Crit Care Med* 1997;155:60). The major reasons for PCP prophylaxis failure are CD4 count <50 cells/mm^3 and non-adherence (*JAMA* 1995; 273:1197; *Arch Intern Med* 1996;156: 177). Provider error in prescribing accounts for about 20% of failures (*CID* 2007;44:879). A 2010 report found that the incidence of PCP among patients with viral suppression, CD4 counts of 100-200 cells/mm^3 and no PCP propylaxis

Disease Prevention: Prophylactic Antimicrobial Agents and Vaccines

3

was 0/1000 person-years follow-up, suggesting that PCP prophylaxis is unnecessary in these patients (*CID* 2010;51:611).

TMP-SMX has established efficacy for reducing the incidence of bacterial infections and toxoplasmosis. This drug is active against most *Salmonella, Nocardia, Legionella,* most methicillin-sensitive *S. aureus* (MRSA), community-acquired MRSA (USA 300 strains), many gram-negative bacilli, most *H. influenzae,* and about 70% of *S. pneumoniae.* No other PCP prophylaxis regimen has this spectrum of activity.

ADVERSE REACTIONS: Adverse reactions sufficiently severe to require discontinuation of the drug are noted in 25-50% with TMP-SMX, 25-40% with dapsone, and 2-4% with aerosolized pentamidine (*NEJM* 1995:332:693). Patients who have a non-life-threatening reaction to TMP-SMX should continue this drug if it can be tolerated. Those who have had such a reaction in the past could be rechallenged, possibly using desensitization (see pg. 411). Gradual initiation of TMP-SMX prophylaxis reduces the rate of rash and/or fever by about 50% (*JAIDS* 2000;24:337). This suggests that most reactions are not allergic or IgE mediated. Pyrimethamine/sulfadoxine (*Fansidar*) is effective, but rarely used due to the risk of severe hypersensitivity reactions.

DISCONTINUATION OF PRIMARY OR SECONDARY PROPHYLAXIS: CD4 count > 200 cells/mm^3 x 3 mos. An exception is patients who develop PCP with a CD4 >200 cells/mm^3; in such patients continuation of PCP prophylaxis for life "is probably prudent" (2008 NIH/CDC/IDSA Guidelines for Prevention and Treatment of Opportunistic Infections in Adults and Adolescents. (*MMWR* Early Release 2009;58). A meta-analysis of 14 controlled trials involving discontinuation of PCP prophylaxis (*CID* 2001;33: 1901) found no difference in risk of PCP between those who continued prophylaxis and those who discontinued with a CD4 count >200 cells/mm^3. The rates were 19.1 vs. 18.2 PCP episodes per 1000 patient-years for primary prophylaxis and 43.5 vs. 41.9 PCP cases per 1000 patient-years for secondary prophylaxis. The rate of adverse reactions was 34.5 vs. 8.6 cases per 1000 patient-years favoring discontinuation. For secondary prophylaxis, a review of 96 cases followed an average of 42 mos showed no risk of PCP (*AIDS* 2004;18:2047). A more recent review with follow-up averaging 40 mos in 78 patients showed no cases of PCP (*AIDS* 2004;18:2047). More recent studies suggest that the risk of PCP is markedly attenuated when the virus is suppressed regardless of the CD4 count (*CID* 2010;51:611; *JID* 2011;203:364).

RESTARTING PRIMARY PROPHYLAXIS: CD4 count decreases to <200 cells/mm^3

SECONDARY PROPYLAXIS: Indications, regimens, stopping rules and restarting rules are the same as for primary prophylaxis.

TRANSMISSION RISK: Some authorities recommend avoidance of "high intensity exposure," meaning that a patient with PCP should not be placed in a room with a vulnerable patient (*NEJM* 2000;342:1416; *Am J Respir Crit Care Med* 2000;162:167; *Emerg Infect Dis* 2004;10:1713). Other reports do not support this recommendation (*JAMA* 2001;286: 2450), but a 2010 report of 394 PCP patients analyzed for the DHPS mutations supported the concept of nosocomial transmission (*CID* 2010;51:e28).

Mycobacterium tuberculosis : See pg. 462.

TESTS TO DETECT LATENT AND ACTIVE TB: Any patient with HIV infection and no prior record of a positive test or TB treatment should undergo diagnostic testing for latent TB with a tuberculin skin test (TST or PPD), an IFN γ release assay (IGRA) or both. The relative merits of these test methods in HIV-infected patients is unknown except that IGRAs are preferred in those previously given BCG (see pg. 54). Patients with negative skin tests should be retested if the CD4 count increases to >200 cells/mm^3 if the baseline test was performed at a CD4 count below that level. The test should be repeated annually in patients with risk for TB based on regional TB rates or sociodemographic factors. Patients with fibrotic changes on chest x-ray that are consistent with TB should receive INH prophylaxis regardless of TST results. Patients with positive tests should be evaluated for active TB, which should include a chest x-ray.

INDICATIONS FOR PROPHYLAXIS

- Positive skin test (≥5 mm induration) or IGRA and no prior history of treatment for active or latent TB
- Exposure to close contact with pulmonary TB
- A history of untreated or inadequately treated TB
- Evidence of old fibrotic lesions on chest x-ray in patients without adequate prior treatment regardless of PPD/IGRA results after active TB is excluded.

RISK (*MMWR* 1998;47:RR-20): Positive test for latent TB (positive PPD with ≥5 mm induration or positive IGRA) without prior prophylaxis or treatment, recent TB contact, or history of inadequately treated TB that healed (*MMWR* 2000;49[RR-6]). The risk of active TB in those with latent TB infection is magnified 7- to 80-fold by HIV co-infection (*Lancet* 2000;356:470; *MMWR* 2000;49[RR-6]). It also appears that active TB accelerates the rate of HIV progression (*JAIDS* 1998;19:361; *BMJ* 1995;311:1468; *JID* 2004;190:869). HIV-infected persons who are close contacts of active TB cases should be evaluated to exclude active disease and should receive treatment for latent TB infection regardless of PPD/IGRA results.

EFFICACY OF PROPHYLAXIS: The Cochrane Library review for TB with INH prophylaxis vs. no prophylaxis prophylaxis in patients with AIDS found an odds ratio for active TB of 0.38 in those with a positive PPD based on 12 controlled trials that included 8,578 randomized patients. No significant change in mortality was detected. Efficacy was similar for different recommended drug regimens (*Cochrane Database Syst Rev* 2010;20:CD000171).

PREFERRED

- Isoniazid (INH) 300 mg po + pyridoxine 50 mg qd x 9 mo
- INH 900 mg po + pyridoxine 100 mg twice weekly with DOT x 9 mo
- Exposure to drug resistant TB: Consult expert
- Alternative to INH: rifampin 300 mg qd or rifabutin (dose adjusted, see pg. 362)
- Note that the 2-mo regimen of pyrazinamide (PZA) + rifampin regimen is no longer recommended due to reports of 40 cases of severe hepatotoxicity, including 7 deaths with the PZA + rifampin 2-mo regimen (*MMWR* 2002;51:998; *MMWR* 2002;51:998; *Am Rev Respir Crit Care Med* 2001;164:1319).

PREGNANCY: INH regimens

MONITORING: Laboratory monitoring includes baseline tests of liver function (bilirubin ALT, AST and alkaline phosphotase) for INH recipients and liver function tests (as above) plus a CBC for rifampin/rifabutin recipients (*MMWR* 2000;49 RR-6:1). Patients should be clinically monitored monthly to detect hepatotoxicity or neuropathy, and they should stop treatment and report any symptoms of hepatitis: jaundice, dark urine, nausea, vomiting, abdominal pain, and/or fever >3 days. INH should be discontinued with ALT elevations to >5x ULN without symptoms or ALT to >3x ULN with symptoms. Monitoring of LFTs is recommended for patients with abnormal baseline LFTs and those receiving ART (*Am J Respir Crit Care Med* 2006;174: 935). In a review of 1995 HIV infected patients given INH prophylaxis in Botswanta, 19 (1.1%) developed hepatitis and there was one death (*Am J Respir Crit Care Med* 2010;182:278).

Toxoplasma gondii : See pg. 486.

INDICATION: *Toxoplasma* IgG positive plus CD4 <100 cells/mm^3

NOTE: Seronegative patients on PCP prophylaxis that does not cover *Toxoplasma* should have the serologic test repeated if the CD4 count decreases to <100 cells/mm^3

RISK: CD4 count <100 cells/mm^3 plus positive anti-*Toxoplasma* IgG conferes a risk of toxoplasmosis encephalitis of 33%per year (*JID* 1996;173:91; *CID* 2001;33:1747).

PREFERRED: TMP-SMX 1 DS qd

ALTERNATIVES

- TMP-SMX 1 SS qd

- Dapsone 50 mg qd po + pyrimethamine 50 mg/wk + leucovorin 25 mg/wk

- Dapsone 200 mg/wk po + pyrimethamine 75 mg/wk po + leucovorin 25 mg/wk po

- Atovaquone 1500 mg qd ± pyrimethamine 25 mg qd + leucovorin 10 mg qd

IMMUNE RECONSTITUTION: The safety of discontinuing primary and secondary prophylaxis for toxoplasmosis has been confirmed in prospective studies (*JID;181:1635; CID 2006;41:79*) and multiple observational studies (*Lancet* 2000;355:2217; *JID* 2000;181: 1635; *AIDS* 1999;13: 1647; *AIDS* 2000;14:383; *Ann Intern Med* 2002; 137:239).

DISCONTINUATION OF PROPHYLAXIS

- **Primary prophylaxis:** Discontinue prophylaxis with CD4 count >200 cells/mm^3 for >3 mos; restart when CD4 count is <100-200 cells/mm^3.

- **Maintenance therapy:** Discontinue prophylaxis with CD4 count >200 cells/mm^3 for ≥6 mos providing initial therapy for ≥6 wks has been completed and the patient is asymptomatic with respect to toxoplasmosis. Some authorities would include MRI evaluation in this decision. Restart prophylaxis when CD4 count is <200 cells/mm^3.

Mycobacterium avium complex (MAC): See pg. 459.

INDICATION: CD4 count <50 cells/mm^3 after ruling out active MAC infection.

RISK: CD4 count <50 cells/mm^3. The incidence of MAC with a CD4 <50 cells/mm^3 and no ART or prophylaxis is 20-40% (*JID* 1997; 176:126; *CID* 1993;17:7). The incidence of MAC has decreased precipitously in the HAART era, presumably due to both ART and effective MAC prophylaxis (*AIDS* 2010;24:1549; *Med Care* 2009;43 Suppl 9:1123-30).

PREFERRED:

- Azithromycin 1200 mg po once weekly

- Clarithromycin 500 mg po bid

- Azithromycin 600 mg po twice weekly

ALTERNATIVE: Rifabutin 300 mg po daily with dose adjustment for concurrent ARV agents (pg 362).

IMMUNE RECONSTITUTION: It is safe to discontinue primary and secondary MAC prophylaxis with immune reconstitution (*NEJM* 1998;338:853; *NEJM* 2000;342:1085; *Ann Intern Med* 2000;133:493; *JID* 1998;178:1446; *HIV Med* 2004;5:278).

Disease Prevention: Prophylactic Antimicrobial Agents and Vaccines

3

- **Primary prophylaxis:** Discontinue prophylaxis with CD4 count >100 cells/mm³ for >3 mos. Restart when CD4 count is <100 cells/mm³. The study that followed the largest group (592 patients) for the longest time (mean, 2.5 years) found only one case of MAC bateremia after stopping primary prophylaxis (*CID* 2005; 41:549).

- **Maintenance therapy:** Discontinue when CD4 cell count is >100 cells/mm³ for >6 mos, 12 mos of therapy have been completed, and the patient is asymptomatic for MAC. Restart when CD4 count is <100 cells/mm³.

Herpes Simplex Virus

RISK: The risk is outbreaks of HSV and transmission of HSV from infected patients or without active lesions. See pg. 447.

RECOMMENDATION: (*MMWR* 2010;55-12)

1) Disclosure of HSV-2 (and HIV) serostatus

2) Abstinence from sex during outbreaks with active herpetic lesions

3) Prophylactic valacyclovir (1 gm/d) for the partner with HSV-2 reduces recurrences of HSV outbreaks by 70-80% (*JAMA* 1998;280:887) but does not appear to reduce risk of HIV acquisition (*Lancet* 2008;371:2109). There is possible benefit of anti-HSV prophylaxis to prevent HIV transmission by the partner with HIV/HSV co-infection.

4) Use of condoms reduces risk of transmitting both HIV and HSV.

5) Acyclovir has established efficacy in preventing transmission of HSV-2 and is indicated independent of HIV for the patient with multiple recurrences.

INDICATION FOR PROPHYLAXIS AND REGIMENS USED: HIV-infected patient with HSV-2 co-infection (see pg. 447).

Varicella zoster virus

Note: There are two live virus varicella vaccines - one to prevent chickenpox in immunologically-naïve patients and the herpes zoster vaccine for patients with prior varicella infection who are at risk for shingles.

- **RISK:** Patient with negative VZV serology: approximately 1-3% of the US population; much less common in those born before 1980 (*JID* 2008;197 Suppl 2:S147). Routine varicella zoster IgG serology is recommended in HIV-infected patients if above factors do not indicate prior infection. Serologic tests for varicella correlate well with a history of varicella but not with vaccination for varicella (*Infect Control Hosp Epidemiol* 2007;28:564).

- **Pre-exposure vaccine prophylaxis:** CD4 > 200 cells/mm³ + patient risk defined by: 1) previously unvaccinated; 2) no history of chicken pox or herpes zoster; 3) seronegative to VZV; and 4) born after 1980. Note that serologic evidence of immunity is recommended for persons born before 1980 who are immunocompromised (*MMWR* 2007;56:RR-4:1).

HERPES ZOSTER VACCINE: This vaccine is a live attenuated high dose VZV vaccine intended to prevent herpes zoster (shingles) in patients with history of primary varicella. This vaccine is recommended by the CDC for persons >60 years of age, but it is contraindicated in patients with HIV infection with CD4 counts <200 cells/mm^3 (*MMWR* 2008;57:RR-5:1). A large study of immunocompetent adults over 60 years showed vaccine efficacy in preventing zoster of 55% (*JAMA* 2010;305:160). Patients with HIV infection who are >60 years and have a CD4 count >200 cells/mm^3 are now included in the CDC recommendations. A review of this vaccine given to HIV-infected patients with a CD4 count >400 cells/mm^3 showed safety, but only a modest immune response (*Human Vaccine* 2010;6:318). If the vaccine causes infection, the patient should receive acyclovir.

POST-EXPOSURE PROPHYLAXIS:

- **Risk:** Close contact with person with varicella or herpes zoster plus susceptibility as defined above.

- **Prophylaxis:** Varicella-zoster immune globulin (*VariZIG*) 125 IU/10 kg (to 625 IU) IM given within 96 hrs of exposure. Alternatives are varicella vaccine if the CD4 count is >200 cells/mm^3 or a course of acyclovir.

Note: (*VariZIG*) available at 800-843-7477.

INFLUENZA VACCINE: Killed influenza vaccine is recommended for all HIV-infected persons. The vaccine is generally well tolerated, but the antigenic response is not as good as in adults without HIV (*Vaccine* 2011;29:1359; *CID* 2011;52:138). As expected, serologic response correlated with CD4 count; one study reported a good response with a second dose at 21 days after the first (*CID* 2011;52:122). Immunosuppressed persons are a CDC priority for the killed virus influenza vaccine (*MMWR* 2010;59:1147). Risk of infection in adults is based on baseline serology appears to be increased even at CD4 counts >350 cells/mm^3 (*AIDS* 2011;52:219). One report found HIV status did not influence severity (*HIV Med* 2011;12:236).

S. pneumoniae : See pg. 562.

RISK: All patients with HIV infection. Risk for invasive pneumococcal infection was 50- to 100-fold greater than in patients without HIV infection in the pre-HAART era (*Ann Intern Med* 2000;132:182; *JID* 1996;173: 857; *JAIDS* 2001;27:35; *Am J Respir Crit Care Med* 2000; 162:2063). The risk of invasive pneumococcal disease has decreased substantially in the US following introduction of *Prevnar 7* for children apparently due to the herd immunity effect (*AIDS* 2010;24:2253).

3 Disease Prevention: Prophylactic Antimicrobial Agents and Vaccines

VACCINE: Use the 23-valent pneumococcal polysaccharide vaccine *(Pneumovax)* 0.5 mL IM

INDICATION FOR VACCINATION:

- CD4 count >200 cells/mm³ unless vaccinated in the past 5 years.
- Consider revaccination if >5 years from the time of initial vaccination or if vaccine was given when the CD4 count was <200 cells/mm³ and has subseqently increased above that level (optional).

EFFICACY: Studies of efficacy of pneumococcal vaccine in HIV-infected persons have shown variable results. A CDC report indicated 49% efficacy (*Arch Intern Med* 2000;160:2633), but others found poor efficacy in immunosuppressed hosts (*NEJM* 1986;315:1318; *JAMA* 1993;270:1826). A controlled study in Uganda found increased rates of pneumonia in vaccine recipients (*Lancet* 2000;355:2106), but a subsequent report indicated that vaccine recipients had a reduction in all-cause mortality (*AIDS* 2004;18:1210). The most complete and recent analysis was a review of 16 studies and concluded there is "only moderate support" for vaccination (*HIV Med* 2010;10:1468). Patients with low CD4 counts have a poor antigenic response (*JID* 2004; 190:707), but those who respond to ART have a good serologic response (*Vaccine* 2006;24:2563).The best evidence for benefit of pneumococcal vaccination are data showing that it reduces the high rates of pneumococcal bacteremia in patients with HIV infection (*Vaccine* 2004;22:2006; *Arch Intern Med* 2005;165:1533). One case-control study found that the major factors in reducing risk were ART (OR-0.23) and pneumococcal vaccination (OR 0.44) (*CID* 2007;45:e82), but much of the decrease in invasive pneumococcal infections in adults, including those with HIV infection, is attributed to the herd effect of *Prevnar 7*, which is licensed only for children (*JAIDS* 2010; 55:128). A randomized trial of *Prevnar* given to HIV-infected adult patients with pneumococcal bacteremia was highly effective in preventing recurrent pneumococcal sepsis and death with a 74% efficacy rate (P=0.002) (*NEJM* 2010;362:812). However, subsequent studies have shown *Prevnar 7* to be only slightly more immunogenic than *Pneumovax* in adults with HIV infection (*JID* 2010;202;1114). Note that studies of *Prevnar 7* immunization and *Pneumovax* revaccination in adults with HIV do not lead to either robust or sustained antibody responses (*JID* 2010;202:114). The current recommendation is *Pneumovax* for adults and adolescents if the CD4 count is >200 cells/mL and there has been no prior PPV vaccination in the prior 5 years (*MMWR* 2009;58 RR-4). *Prevnar 13* is undergoing studies in HIV-infected patients (*AIDS* 2010;24:2253).

Hemophilus influenzae

The risk to adults with HIV infection is low for *H. influenzae* type B. Most infections are due to non-type B strains that are not covered by the vaccine. The Hib vaccine is not recommended.

Hepatitis A

RISK: 1) MSM, 2) drug users (injection and non-injection), and 3) persons with chronic liver disease, including chronic HBV and HCV (*MMWR* 2002;51[RR-6]:61). Susceptibility is defined by negative total HAV antibody, which is present in 30% of American adults. Some authorities recommend HAV vaccination for all non-immune patients as defined by negative total anti-HAV antibody.

INDICATION: 1) Chronic liver disease, travelers to countries where HAV is endemic or epidemic, IDU or MSM; plus 2) seronegative for HAV (optional test); plus 3) CD4 >200 cells/mm³.

VACCINE: HAV vaccine 0.5 mL IM x 2 separated by 6 mos.

Hepatitis B: See pg. 507

RISK: In the era of ART, liver disease, in large part due to HBV and HCV, has become a major cause of death (*Lancet* 2002;360:1921; *JID* 2003;188:571). The prevalence of chronic HBV in HIV infected persons is reported in 6-15% MSM, 10% IDU and 4-6% heterosexuals (*J Hepatol* 2006;44 Suppl 6). The prevalence of HBV antibody indicating prior infection is 24-76% (*J Hepatol* 2006;44 S6; *MMWR* 2008;57 RR-8:S1).

VACCINE: HBV vaccine is available as single antigen formulation (*Recombivax HB* and *Engerix B*) and in combination with HAV vaccine as *Twinrix*. The recommended doses for single antigen vaccine (*MMWR* 2006;55:RR 16) (Table 3-1).

■ TABLE 3-1: **Recommended HBV Vaccine Dosing**

Doses	Adults >20 yrs dose (ug)*	Immunosuppressed ≥20 yrs
Recombivax HB	10	40
Engerix B	20	40
Twinrix *	20	—

* HAV and HBV vaccine

The vaccine schedule: 0, 1 and 6 mos; 0, 1 and 4 mos; 0, 2 and 4 mos and 0, 1, 2 and 12 mos. The vaccine schedule for *Twinrix* (Hepatitis A and B) is 0,1 and 6 mos or 0, 1, 2 and 12 mos.

Alternative vaccine schedules: Response rates based on achieving HB_s titers of >10 mIU/mL with the standard CDC recommended vaccine regimen have been low (18-72%) compared to those without HIV (>90%) (see below). Higher response rates are noted with increased doses and with intradermal vaccination. A trial comparing standard vaccine with 4 IM doses of 40 ug (instead of 20 ug) at weeks 0, 4, 8, and 24 was 82% and 4 intradermal injections of low doses (4 ng) at weeks 0, 4, 8, and 24 showed responses in 77% (*JAMA* 2011;305:1432).

3 Disease Prevention: Prophylactic Antimicrobial Agents and Vaccines

INDICATION: CD4 count >350 cells/mm^3 and negative anti-HBs and negative HBs antigen screening tests. Note that most patients with isolated anti-HBc are not immune and should be vaccinated (*JAIDS* 2003;34:439).

RESPONSE: Response rates to standard HBV vaccine in patients with HIV are only 40-60% compared to >90% in other populations (*Ann Intern Med* 1988;109:101; *AIDS* 1992;6:509; *AIDS Resp Ther* 2006;3: 9; *AIDS Rev* 2009;11:157; *Vaccine* 2005;23:2902; *CID* 2005;41:1045; *CID* 2004;38:1478). The 2008 NIH/CDC/IDSA Guidelines on the Prevention and Treatment of Opportunistic Infections in HIV-Infected Adults and Adolescents (*MMWR* 2009;58 RR 11:1) recommend the standard 3 dose series, but some studies suggest a possibly better response with double-dose or 40 mcg doses IM at 0, 1 and 6 mos (*Vaccine* 2000;18:1161;*Vaccine* 2005;23:2902; *J Clin Gastro* 1992; 14:27). For example, a study of double dose vaccine given in 4 doses (0, 1, 2 and 6 mo) found a protective antibody response in 89% of HIV-infected patients with a median CD4 count of 401 cells/mm^3 (*Vaccine* 2010;28:1447). However, another study reported a response rate of 51% in patients given the double dose after failure to response to the standard dose series (*JID* 2008;197:292). The recommendation for patients with a low CD4 count to delay vaccination until immune reconstitution. Repeat anti-HBs at 1 mo after the 3rd dose (*Ann Intern Med* 1988;109:101). If anti-HBs is <10 IU/mL consider repeating the series or using the double dose regimen.

Twinrix: This product may be used to simultaneously immunize HIV-infected patients for HAV and HBV using a 0, 1 and 6 mos schedule (*MMWR* 2001;50:806). Studies in 2,165 healthy adults showed antigenic response to the HAV component in 99.9% and the HBV component in 98.5%.

Hepatitis C: See pg. 513

INDICATION: Acute HCV infection defined as ≤6 mos from time of HCV exposure. Goal is to prevent chronic HCV infection.

PROPHYLAXIS: Peg-IFN in standard dose x 24 wks (*Gastroenterology* 2006;130:632). The addition of ribavirin is arbitrary.

Influenza

INDICATION: All patients annually.

RISKS: See pg. 562.

Human Papilloma Virus (*MMWR* 2010;59:630)

RISKS: See pg. 56-57.

VACCINES: HPV vaccines licensed in the US are the bivalent *Cervarix* vaccine and the quadrivalent *Gardasil* vaccine. Both vaccines protect

■ TABLE 3-2: **Vaccine Recommendations for Patients with HIV (*MMWR* 2009;57:Q1)**

Vaccine	HIV
Hepatitis A	Recommended if at risk (non-immune with chronic liver disease, MSM, IDU, hemophilia, or travel to endemic areas). Also, can consider in all non-immune patients without above risks. Consider HAV vaccine, or combined HAV/HBV vaccine (*Twinrix*) given at 0, 1 and 6 mos (3 doses) or 0, 7, 21-30 days with booster at 12 mos.
Hepatitis B	Recommended if non-immune; given at 0, 1 & 6 mos. Consider double dose (40 ug/mL) (*Recombivax* in 3 dose schedule) or 20 ug/mL doses (*Engerix B*) given in 4 doses – 0, 1, 2 and 6 mos.
Influenza: *FluMist* *	Contraindicated
Influenza: IM vaccine	Recommended yearly; most effective if CD4 >100 cells/mm³
MMR*	Recommended with exposure or travel. Contraindicated with CD4 count <200 cells/mm³.
Meningococcal vaccine	Use if indicated
Pneumococcal vaccine	Recommended when CD4 >200 cells/mm³. One time revaccination at 5 years recommended for immunodeficient patients.
Tetanus-diphtheria (Pertussis)	Recommended; give booster every 10 yrs or with tetanus-prone injury
Varicella (Varivax)*	Indicated for non-immune patients (approx. 5% in U.S. are susceptible). Contraindicated with CD4 <200 cells/ mm³
Smallpox*	Contraindicated except with exposure
Human papilloma virus	Recommended for women and high risk men 11-26 years; 3 doses separated by 2 mos (1st and 2nd) and 6 mos (2nd and 3rd)
Herpes zoster (*Zostavax*)*	Adults > 60 years. Contraindicated with CD4 < 200 cells/mm³
Travel-related vaccines	
Polio and typhoid*	Use inactivated (killed vaccine)
MMR	If CD4 very low + travel to measles endemic, use immune globuli
Yellow fever*	Live virus vaccine; safety with HIV is uncertain, especially with CD4 count <200 cells/mm³; may need vaccine waiver letter. Many consider safe with CD4 >200 cells/mm³
Influenza	Southern hemisphere travel; flu season is April-Sep
Rabies	If indicated
Japanese encephalitis	If substantial risk
Cholera*	Use killed recombinant vaccine; not recommended

* Live attenuated vaccines – alternative non-live options are available for typhoid, influenza, polio and cholera

Disease Prevention: Prophylactic Antimicrobial Agents and Vaccines

3

against infections against HPV types 16 and 18 that account for 70% of cervical cancers. The quadrivalent vaccine also protects against HPV types 6 and 11 that cause 90% of genital warts. Both vaccines are given in three 0.5 mL doses IM at 0, 1-2 mos and 6 mos. Prevaccination screening for HPV is not recommended. These are not live vaccines. Pregnancy is a contraindication.

INDICATIONS: Either vaccine is recommended for females ages 11-12 years and can be given to females ages 13-26 years who have not started or completed the series. Benefit is greatest if HPV is given before sexual debut. The vaccines are available for eligible persons <19 years through Vaccines for Children (VFC) program (800-232-4636). The quadrivalent vaccine may also be given to males ages 9-26 years to prevent genital warts (*MMWR* 2010;59:630). Vaccine efficacy of the quadrivalent vaccine for preventing genital warts is 60% (*NEJM* 2011;364:401). Vaccine efficacy in women for preventing genital infection or lesions involving HPV types in the vaccine approach 100% with a 3-4 year follow-up (*NEJM* 2007;356:1928; *BMJ* 2010; 341:c4455; *Cancer Prev Res* 2009;2:868). One report showed a 78% reduction in anal intraepithelial neoplasia (a precursor of anal cancer) in vaccine recipients (Jessen H. 2010 IAS, Vienna:Abstr. THLBB101), and some have strongly advocated routine use of the quadrivalent vaccine MSM up to 26 years (*Vaccine* 2010;28:6858; *Lancet* 2010;10:815). A cost analysis of this strategy concluded it would be cost effective for MSM ages 12-26 years (*Lancet* 2010;10:845).

PREFERRED AGENT: HPV quadravalent vaccine 0.5 mL IM at 0, 2 and 6 mos.

■ TABLE 3-3: **Commonly Used Vaccines as Applied to Persons with HIV Infection***

Vaccine	Recommendation HIV	Cost AWP†	Series (doses)	Risk with HIV	Best Response‡
Tetanus diptheria	All persons	$5	1	Not different	CD4 >300
Influenza	All persons (killed virus)	$20	1	↑ Mortality	CD4 >100 VL <30,000
Hepatitis A	Risk MSM, IDU, Travel	$60	2	↑ Fulminant hepatitis	CD4 >500
Pneumovax	All persons	$20	1	↑↑ Pneumococcal bacteremia	CD4 >200
Hepatitis B	HBsAg and HBsAb negative	$60	3	↑ Progressive liver disease	CD4 >350 VL <10,000
Zoster	Age >60 CD4 >200	$200	1	↑↑ Rate zoster	CD4 >200

* Risk data are largely based on pre-HAART era data.

† AWP = Approximate average wholesale price (2010)

‡ Best response is for CD4 count in cells/mm³ +/- VL in c/mL.

Histoplasma capsulatum

RISK: For patients with a CD4 count <100 cells/mm^3 who live in the Midwest or Puerto Rico and are not taking ART, the risk is 2-5% (*CID* 2000;30:50).

INDICATION: CD4 count <150 cells/mm^3 and at high risk because of occupational exposure or residence in a community with a hyperendemic rate of histoplasmosis defined as >10 cases /100 person years.

RECOMMENDATION: Consider primary prophylaxis if CD4 <150 cells/mm^3 and residence in endemic area or occupational risk.

PREFERRED AGENTS: Itraconazole 200 mg qd po.

Coccidioides immitis

RISK: CD4 count <250 cells/mm^3 (*JID* 2000;181:1428) plus exposure in an endemic area (Southwest US, usually CA or AZ). The frequency in the endemic area was previously reported at about 4% per year in untreated AIDS patients, 0.2% per year for HIV without AIDS, and 0.015% per year in the general population (*JID* 2000;181:1428). A more recent review from the same endemic area shows a subtantial reduction in both risk and severity of this complication attributed to ART (*CID* 2010;50:1).

INDICATION: Consider annual serology for *C.immitis* for patients with CD4 counts <250 cells/mm^3 and residence in an endemic area. Indication for prophylaxis is positive serology (IgM or IgG).

RECOMMENDATION:

- Fluconazole 400 mg po qd
- Itraconazole 200 mg po bid

Pencillium marneffei

INDICATION: 1) CD4 count <100 cells/mm^3 for patients in highly endemic area (Southeast Asia)

PREFERRED AGENT: Itraconazole 200 mg po qd

Trypanosoma cruzi (Chagas disease)

INDICATION: 1) Antibody to *T. cruzi*, 2) no prior therapy and 3) infection likely to be <20 years' duration.

PREFERRED AGENT: Benznidazole* 5-8 mg/kg/d po x 30-60 days

ALTERNATIVE: Nifurtimox* 8-10 mg/kg/d po x 90-120 days

*Neither drug is available in US: obtain from CDC drug service

PREVENTION OF EXPOSURE

Enteric bacterial pathogenss

- The risk of infection with enteric bacterial pathogens is significantly increased with HIV infection and immunosuppression. The risk is most striking for *Salmonella* (*JID* 1987;156:998; *AIDS* 1992;6:1495; *CID* 1995;21:S84), but also noted with *Shigella* (*CID* 2007;44:327) and *Campylobacter* (*Ann Intern Med* 1984;101:187). These pathogens are generally transmitted by contaminated food or water and less commonly by fecal contact.

- **Recommendations for prevention:** 1) hand washing; 2) avoid undercooked eggs and other common food sources of *Salmonella*; 3) avoid undercooked meat; and 4) avoid cross-contamination with cutting boards, knives, hands, etc.

- **With travel to developing countries:** avoid undercooked meat, tap water or ice from tap water (unless water is boiled >1 minute or decontaminated with iodine or chlorine), unpasteurized milk and raw vegetables.

Toxoplasmosis

Major sources are contaminated stool from infected cats, soil contact and ingestion of uncooked meat. Seronegative patients with HIV infection should: 1) avoid undercooked pork, beef and venison; 2) wash hands after gardening, contact with raw meat or change of cat litter; 3) wash raw vegetables and avoid eating them raw; and 4) avoid changing cat litter, keep pet cats inside and feed cats commercial food or well cooked meat.

Cryptosporidiosis

Sources are stool from infected people and animals, and contaminated food and water. Prevention is most important with CD4 count <200 cells/mm^3. Patients with HIV should: 1) avoid contact with stool from patients with possible cryptosporidiosis and stool from pets, especially dogs and cats <6 mos of age; 2) avoid sex practices that involve oral contact with feces; 3) avoid drinking water from lakes or rivers; and 4) avoid eating raw oysters. During outbreaks involving drinking water: boil water for 3 minutes, put water through a 1 um micrometer, or use bottled water (see www.bottledwater.org or call 1-703-683-5213). Note that rifabutin and azithromycin may have a protective effect. Also note that bottled water is unregulated and many commercial supplies are not different from municipal water supplies which are regulated.

4 | Antiretroviral Therapy

■ TABLE 4-1: **Antiretroviral Drugs Approved by the FDA for Treatment of HIV Infection**

Generic Name (Abbreviation)	Brand Name	Manufacturer	FDA Approval Date
Zidovudine (AZT, ZDV)	Retrovir	GlaxoSmithKline (ViiV)	March 1987
Didanosine (ddl)	Videx	Bristol-Myers Squibb	October 1991
Zalcitabine (ddC)*	Hivid	Hoffmann-La Roche	June 1992
Stavudine (d4T)	Zerit	Bristol-Myers Squibb	June 1994
Lamivudine (3TC)	Epivir	GlaxoSmithKline (ViiV)	November 1995
Saquinavir (SQV hgc)	Invirase	Hoffmann-La Roche	December 1995
Ritonavir (RTV)	Norvir	Abbott Laboratories	March 1996
Indinavir (IDV)	Crixivan	Merck	March 1996
Nevirapine (NVP)	Viramune	Boehringer Ingelheim	June 1996
Nelfinavir (NFV)	Viracept	Pfizer (ViiV)	March 1997
Delavirdine (DLV)	Rescriptor	Pfizer (ViiV)	April 1997
Zidovudine/lamivudine (AZT/3TC)	Combivir	GlaxoSmithKline (ViiV)	September 1997
Saquinavir (SQV sgc)*	Fortovase	Hoffmann-La Roche	November 1997
Efavirenz (EFV)	Sustiva	DuPont Pharmaceuticals	September 1998
Abacavir (ABC)	Ziagen	GlaxoSmithKline (ViiV)	February 1999
Amprenavir (APV)*	Agenerase	GlaxoSmithKline (ViiV)	April 1999
Lopinavir/ritonavir (LPV/r)	Kaletra	Abbott Laboratories	September 2000
Zidovudine/lamivudine/abacavir (AZT/3TC/ABC)	Trizivir	GlaxoSmithKline (ViiV)	November 2000
Tenofovir DF (TDF)	Viread	Gilead Sciences	October 2001
Enfuvirtide (ENF)	Fuzeon	Hoffmann-La Roche	March 2003
Atazanavir (ATV)	Reyataz	Bristol-Myers Squibb	June 2003
Emtricitabine (FTC)	Emtriva	Gilead Sciences	July 2003
Fosamprenavir (FPV)	Lexiva	GlaxoSmithKline (ViiV)	November 2003
Lamivudine/abacavir (3TC/ABC)	Epzicom	GlaxoSmithKline (ViiV)	August 2004
Emtricitabine/tenofovir (FTC/TDF)	Truvada	Gilead Sciences	August 2004
Tipranavir (TPV)	Aptivus	Boehringer Ingelheim	June 2005
Darunavir (DRV)	Prezista	Tibotec (Janssen)	June 2006
Efavirenz/emtricitabine/tenofovir (EFV/FTC/TDF)	Atripla	Gilead Sciences / Bristol-Myers Squibb	July 2006
Maraviroc (MVC)	Selzentry	Pfizer (ViiV)	August 2007
Raltegravir (RAL)	Isentress	Merck	October 2007
Etravirine (ETR)	Intelence	Tibotec (Janssen)	January 2008
Rilpivirine (RPV)	Edurant	Tibotec (Janssen)	May 2011
Rilpivirine/emtricitabine/tenofovir (RPV/FTC/TDF)	Complera	Gilead Sciences	August 2011

* Withdrawn from the market.

4 Antiretroviral Therapy

Recommendations for Antiretroviral Therapy

Recommendations of the 2011 DHHS Guidelines, 2010 International AIDS Society USA, the 2008 British HIV Association Guidelines, the 2009 European AIDS Clinical Society and the 2010 WHO guidelines (see below).

Goals of Therapy (2011 DHHS Guidelines)

CLINICAL GOALS: Reduced morbidity and mortality associated with HIV infection and its treatment. Prolongation of life and improvement in quality of life.

VIROLOGIC GOALS: Greatest possible reduction in VL (preferably to <50 c/mL) for as long as possible to halt disease progression and prevent or delay resistance.

IMMUNOLOGIC GOALS: Immune reconstitution that is both quantitative (CD4 cell count in normal range) and qualitative (pathogen-specific immune response).

THERAPEUTIC GOALS: Rational sequencing of drugs in a fashion that achieves clinical, virologic, and immunologic goals while maintaining treatment options, limit drug toxicity and facilitate adherence.

EPIDEMIOLOGIC GOALS: Reduce HIV transmission

When to Start Therapy

The main determinants for initiating antiretroviral therapy in most patients are patient readiness and CD4 count. (Tables 4-2 through 4-6).

WHEN TO START ART: There are no large completed propective randomized trials to inform the decision of when to initiate ART. Contemporary guidelines from virtually all major global sources recommend initiating treatment in patients defined as "ready" for what may be lifelong treatment if there is an AIDS-defining diagnosis or a CD4 count <350 cells/mm^3. Current guidelines from Europe and WHO have retained the CD4 threshold of 350 cells/mm^3, with some exceptions based on co-morbidities such as AIDS-defining conditions, tuberculosis and pregnancy (Tables 4-4 – 4-6). Guidelines from the US (2011 DHHS and 2010 IAS-USA Guidelines) now recommend that ART for patients with CD4 counts <500 cells/mm^3 and that it be offered or considered optional for those who have CD4 counts >500 cells/mm^3. This assumes patient readiness and a patient who is not a "long-term non-progressor" (see pg. 2). It is important to emphasize that the urgency of ART, the strength of the recommendation and the quality of the evidence to support the recommendation correlate inversely with the CD4 count. Multiple other issues beyond "patient readiness" contribute to the urgency of ART, including co-morbidities, patient age, transmission risk, CD4 slope, VL and pregnancy. The following summarizes the rationale for the 2011 DHHS and 2010 IAS-USA Guidelines for initiating ART for virtually all patients with HIV infection:

DHHS GUIDELINES (2011)

- TABLE 4-2: **Indications to Start Antiretroviral Therapy (DHHS Guidelines, Jan. 11, 2011 revision)**

Indications to treat
■ CD4 count < 500 cells/mm³
■ CD4 count > 500 cells/mm³: Treatment should be offered or considered*
■ Any CD4 count: HIVAN, pregnancy, HBV co-infection with treatment, indication for HBV

* The Panel was divided with 50% favoring "treatment should be optional" and 50% favoring "treatment should be offered"

IAS-USA GUIDELINES (2010)

- TABLE 4-3: **Recommendations for Initiating Antiretroviral Therapy (2010 Recommendations of IAS-USA, *JAMA* 2010;304:32)**

Primary HIV	Symptoms
Chronic HIV with Symptoms	Treat
Asymptomatic	
CD4 <500 cells/mm³	Treat
CD4 >500 cells/mm³	Consider treatment
Factors or conditions favoring treatment at any CD4 count	■ CD4 slope >100 cells/mm³/yr ■ HIV VL >100,000 c/mL ■ High risk for CVD ■ Opportunistic infections including TB ■ High risk of transmission ■ HIVAN ■ Age >60 yrs. ■ Chronic HBV ■ Chronic HCV

BRITISH HIV ASSOCIATION GUIDELINES (2008)

- TABLE 4-4: **Recommendations of the British HIV Medical Association (*HIV Med* 2008;9:563)**

INDICATIONS TO TREAT
Primary HIV Infection
■ Clinical trial ■ Neurologic involvement, CD4 count > 200 cells/mm³ over 3 months or AIDS diagnosis
Established HIV infection
■ CD4 <200 cells/mm³ ■ CD4 201-350 cells/mm³ "when patient is ready" ■ CD4 >350 cells/mm³ + HIV co-morbidity, HBV co-infection requiring treatment, HCV co-infection ("some cases"), CD4% <14, CVD or high CVD risk (Framingham risk >20% in 10 years)
AIDS: (Except tuberculosis with CD4 >350 cells/mm³)

Antiretroviral Therapy

4

EUROPEAN AIDS CLINICAL SOCIETY GUIDELINES, VERSION 5 (2009)

■ TABLE 4-5: Recommendations for Initiating ART: European AIDS Clinical Society (EACS) ARV Guidelines 2009

Category	Indications
Primary HIV Infection	AIDS defining event, CD4 < 350 cells/mm³ at >3 months Consider if symptoms severe or prolonged, especially CNS Sx
Chronic HIV Infection Symptomatic	Treat
Asymptomatic	
CD4 < 350 cells/mm³	Treat
CD4 350-500 cells/mm³	Treat if HBV or HCV co-infection, HIV or "other organ deficiency" "Consider" if VL >100,000 c/mL, pregnancy, high, malignancy or cardiovascular risk or CD4 slope >50-100 cells/mm³/yr
CD4 > 500 cells/mm³	Can be offered if >1 condition listed in the CD4 strata 350-500
Any CD4 count	Can be offered on individual case basis

WHO GUIDELINES (2010)

■ TABLE 4-6: When to Start Antiretroviral Therapy – 2010 WHO Guidelines

Clinical setting	CD4 count
Any WHO stage	<350 cells/mm³
WHO stage 3-4	Any CD4 count
Tuberculosis (active)	Any CD4 count
Pregnancy	<350 cells/mm³ or WHO stage 3-4
Hepatitis B requiring treatment	Any CD4 count

* Clinical stages
- □ Clinical stage I: Asymptomatic or PGL, and/or normal activity
- □ Clinical stage II: Weight loss <10%, minor mucocutaneous conditions, zoster <5 years, recurrent URIs, and/or symptomatic plus normal activity
- □ Clinical stage III: Weight loss >10%, unexplained diarrhea >1 month, unexplained fever >1 month, thrush, oral hairy leukoplakia, pulmonary TB in past year, or severe bacterial infection, and/or bedridden <50% of days in the past month
- □ Clinical stage IV: CDC-defined AIDS and/or bedridden >50% of days in the past month

■ **Cohort Studies:** The NA-ACCORD cohort combines data for 22 cohorts in North America with >8000 patients and 61,798 patient-years of follow-up. This showed a significant survival advantage with ART initiated at a CD4 count of 350-500 vs. waiting until below that threshold (OR=1.7; p<0.001) and with a CD4 count of >500 vs. waiting until <500 (OR 1.94; p<0.001) (*NEJM* 2009;360:1815).

Other cohort reviews also show the survival advantage of ART initiated at high CD4 counts including the HIV-CASUAL Collaboration (*AIDS* 2010;24:123) which combined data from 12 cohorts with

Antiretroviral Therapy

62,760 HIV-infected patients. This showed an odds ratio for survival that correlated inversely with CD4 count relative to no therapy: <100 cells/mm³: 0.29; 200-350 cells/mm³: 0.55 and >500 cells/mm³: 0.77.

- **Immune Activation:** The health consequences of immune activation have been implicated as a cause of morbidity and mortality associated with HIV infection. These include most of the non-AIDS-defining conditions that are now the dominant complications associated with HIV infection, including cardiovascular disease, accelerated aging, liver, bone and metabolic disorders, non-AIDS associated cancers and possibly neurocognitive function (*NEJM* 2006;p355:2287; *Infect Dis Annu Rev Med* 2011;62:141; *BMJ* 2009; 338:3172). These complications are seen at all CD4 strata, and they correlate with elevations in biomarkers of immune dysfunction such as hsCRP, IL-6, and D-dimer (*Curr Opin HIV AIDS* 2010;5:498; *PLoS Med* 2008;5:e203). ART reduces the levels of these markers but not to normal (*AIDS* 2010;24:1657; *PLoS Med* 2008;5:e203; *CID* 2009;48:350; *PLoS Med* 2006;42:426).

- **Cost:** The cost of currently recommended ART regimens is about $12,000/year regardless of CD4 count (*AIDS* 2010;24:2705). Cost effectiveness of ART is well established in patients with low CD4 counts (*CID* 2006;42:1003) but is not available for therapy given at high CD4 thresholds. It is important to anticipate the impact of costs in the context of generic prices, which will include 3TC, EFV, SQV and NVP over the next several years. At least one analysis demonstrated that initiating ART at a CD4 count >500 cells/mm³ was even more cost effective than initiating ART with a CD4 count <350 cells/mm³ (*NEJM* 2001;344:824).

- **Transmission Risk:** There is a strong association between VL and probability of HIV transmission (*NEJM* 2000;342:921). These data are sufficiently robust to suggest that achieving an undetectable virus on ART might eliminate the possibility of sexual transmission (*Bulletin des Medicins Suisses* 2008;89:5) and a WHO mathematical model suggested that treatment of all infected people would end the epidemic (*Lancet* 2009;373:48). Although these issues are debated in terms of the practicality of application, there is no dispute that treatment of HIV-infected patients is a major prevention strategy (*CID* 2010;51:725). This has been confirmed by HPTN 052, a large multinational trial comparing early vs. deferred ART in HIV-infected patients with seronegative partners, which demonstrated a 96% reduction in sexual transmission to the uninfected partner (*NEJM* 2011, in press).

- **Reservations** about early therapy in the past were often based on concerns about potential long term complications of antiretroviral drugs and the prediction of increasing HIV resistance. However, the 25-year experience with 23 drugs has taught us that current regimens are generally well tolerated, and long term toxicity has become less concerning after 15 years of HAART, including reduced use of drugs with predictable long-term consequences such as d4T, ddI, ddC, and IDV. Concerns about increased rates of resistance have been quelled by sequential testing showing that rates of transmitted resistance are decreasing, presumably reflecting better and earlier ART treatment (*JAIDS* 2009;51:450).

COUNTER ARGUMENTS TO "EARLY ART"

- **CD4 Threshold:** There is good evidence to support ART at a CD4 threshold of 350 cells/mm^3 based on cohort data (*NEJM* 2010;363:257), but cohort data addressing the issue of benefit of ART in patients with CD4 counts >350 cells/mm^3 (*CID* 2003;37:951; *JID* 2006;194:612) are inconsistent (*JID* 2008;197:1133; *JID* 2008:197:1084).

- **Randomized Trial:** The optimal method to make important decisions in medicine is the randomized controlled trial. Such a trial has not been conducted using currently available ART agents, but the appropriate study (START) is now enrolling and may provide an answer based on high quality evidence with a randomized controlled trial.

- **Cost:** The current cost of ART is approximately $12,000/year with a CD4 count >500 cells/mm^3 (*AIDS* 2010;24:2705).

- **Long Term Toxicity:** The long term complications of treatment are largely unknown due to lack of data with long-term exposure. For example, there were some unexpected associations between antiretroviral agents and complications that emerged from the D:A:D study (*JID* 2010;201:318) and SMART (*NEJM* 2006;355:2283) with respect to cardiac, bone and renal disease that may be drug related.

SPECIAL CO-FACTOR CONSIDERATIONS

The following populations are identified in the 2011 DHHS Guidelines and/or the 2010 IAS-USA Guidelines as priorities for ART regardless of the CD4 count:

- Pregnant women: The purpose is to prevent perinatal transmission as well as to treat the mother (see pg. 152).

- HIV-associated nephropathy (HIVAN) since this may be seen at relatively high CD4 counts and the preventive benefit of ART is well established (see pg. 571).

- Hepatitis B co-infection to provide suppressive therapy for both HIV and HBV with drugs that are active against both viruses. Treating either infection alone risks resistance in the other virus, and often requires the use of suboptimal drugs (see pg. 507).

- Patients at risk of sexual transmission (e.g., patients with seronegative partners) based on the data cited above showing decreased risk of transmission in patients with treated HIV infection.

- Rapid CD4 decline is a suggested indication, although caution is advised due to the substantial variations in this measurement based on laboratory methods. It is suggested that loss of more than 100 cells/mm³/yr is "rapid" (see pg. 29).

- **A high viral load** (>100,000 c/mL) is associated with a more rapid CD4 decline, although this association is thought by some to be modest (*JAMA* 2006;296:498; *Lancet* 2007;370:407) and supporting data are not strong (Table 4-2).

- **Age** may also be a consideration, since it is associated with more rapid progression and poorer CD4 response to ART, presumably due to loss of thymic reserve (*Nature* 1998;396:690; *Ann Intern Med* 2008;148:178 and Table 4-2). The threshold suggested in the 2010 IAS-USA Guidelines is >60 yrs.

- **Acute HIV infection:** There is suggestive evidence that initiating ART during acute HIV infection has long-term benefit (*PloS Med* 2004;1:e36; *AIDS* 2004;18:709), including: 1) reduction in transmission at a time of great risk (*Ann Intern Med* 2007;46:591; *NEJM* 352:1873; *AIDS* 2011;25:941); 2) reduction in symptoms of acute infection and 3) possible reduction in the virologic set point and/or the rate of progression (*JID* 2007;195:1762; *JID* 2010;202: S2:S278). Treatment during acute or recent HIV infection is considered optional; participation in a clinical trial is recommended.

SURVIVAL PREDICTIONS

- Specific data for some of these risks are available from the "Risk Calculator" derived from a database of 40,000 patients and updated June 5, 2007 (Table 4.2; see www.art-cohort-collaboration.org). Options are for calculations at the start of ART or for 6 months after ART to account for response to treatment. The highest risk factors for poor outcome are low CD4 count (column 1), an AIDS diagnosis (column 2+3 vs. 4), injection drug use (column 2+3 vs. 5) and advanced age (column 6 vs. 7). VL had a very modest effect (columns 3 vs. 2). For example, an untreated person age 30-39 years with a CD4 count of 300 cells/mm³ and VL 50,000 c/mL has a 3.1% probability of death in 5 years, but this increases to 7.7% if the patient is over 50 years, is unchanged if the VL is >100,000 c/mL and increases to 9.1% if he/she is an injection drug user. The following table shows the variations in prognosis based on CD4 count (Column 1), VL (Column 2), a prior AIDS diagnosis (Column 3), IDU as a risk (Column 5), and age differences (Columns 6 and 7).

- The Veterans Aging Study Cohort Project (VACS) Index is a more recent version of the risk calculator that adds additional markers including anemia, liver injury, renal injury and hepatitis C co-infection – a total of 7 variables with 24 point allocations. This appears to provide a more accurate calculation of survival (*HIV Med* 2010;11:143). See www.vacohort.org.

4 Antiretroviral Therapy

■ TABLE 4-7: **Variables Associated with the Risk of an AIDS-defining Complication or Death in 5 Years for a Patient 30-39 Years**

CD4	VL (c/mL)		AIDS*	IDU*	Age* 16-29	Age* >50
	< 100,000	> 100,000				
1	2	3	4	5	6	7
<25	22%†	26%	46%	40%	23%	35%
25-49	19%	23%	42%	35%	21%	31%
50-99	18%	22%	39%	33%	19%	29%
100-199	12%	15%	28%	24%	13%	21%
200-349	8%	10%	10%	15%	8%	13%
>350	6%	8%	8%	13%	7%	11%

* VL at 100,000 c/mL
† Risk of AIDS defining diagnosis or death
Data from "Risk Calculator" of the ART Cohort Collaboration based on an analysis of 40,000 patients and last updated June 5, 2007 (*AIDS* 2007;21:1185)

What to Start

The Initial Regimen

Regimens that are most extensively used, best studied and recommended by virtually all guidelines are 2 NRTIs combined with a NNRTI, a ritonavir-boosted PI or RAL (Table 4-8 to 4-11).

FTC/TDF is the favored NRTI pair based on ease of administration, potency, experience, tolerability and toxicity. ABC/3TC is considered an alternative NRTI pair. Both are co-formulated and given as one pill daily.

- **3TC and FTC:** Virtually all regimens include 3TC or FTC, which are similar except for half-life; both are nearly completely free of side effects, both are active against HBV (with the potential for a severe flare of HBV if withdrawn or HBV resistance develops), and both select for the 184V mutation. Continued use of 3TC or FTC in the presence of the 184V mutation provides residual but reduced activity against HIV and does not risk additional NRTI resistance mutations.

- **TDF/FTC** is co-formulated as *Truvada*, with EFV (*Atripla*), and with RPV (*Complera*) to permit dosing with one pill daily. In a trial comparing AZT/3TC vs. TDF/FTC, each in combination with EFV, the TDF/FTC recipients had superior results at 144 weeks in terms of viral suppression to <50 c/mL (80% vs. 70%), CD4 count increases (mean of 312 vs. 271 cells/mm³), discontinuations for adverse reactions (9% vs. 4%), limb fat atrophy by DEXA scan, and number of M184V mutations (*NEJM* 2006;354:251; *JAIDS* 2006;43:535). A comparative trial (ACTG 5202) of TDF/FTC vs. ABC/3TC, each with either ATV/r or EFV, showed an increased rate of virologic failure in ABC/3TC recipients with a baseline VL >100,000 c/mL and greater safety events and NRTI modification (*NEJM* 2009;361:2230). No significant difference in virologic outcome was noted for patients

Antiretroviral Therapy

with a baseline VL <100,000 c/mL, although there were differences in safety endpoints favoring TDF/FTC (*Ann Intern Med* 2011; 154:445). No difference in outcome was noted for TDF/FTC vs. ABC/3TC in some other trials (*AIDS* 2009;23:1547). Disadvantages of TDF are poor CNS penetration (of uncertain significance), renal toxicity and greater loss of bone mineral density than with other agents. The potential for renal toxicity makes TDF a poor option if there is pre-existing renal disease with a creatinine clearance <50 mL/min and requires regular monitoring of renal function in all patients. Guidance on methods to monitor bone mineral density in TDF recipient are unclear but caution is advised in patients with osteoporesis or osteopennia. TDF and FTC are both active against HBV, making this a preferred dual NRTI in combination with a third antiretroviral agent in patients with HIV/HBV co-infection (*NEJM* 2007;356:1445; *Hepatology* 2006; 44:1110; *CID* 2010;51:1201).

- **ABC/3TC** is co-formulated as *Epzicom* for once-daily administration in combination with a third agent. ABC has been problematic due to a potentially serious hypersensitivity reaction (HSR), but this risk has been essentially eliminated by pre-treatment testing for HLA-B*5701 (*NEJM* 2008;358:568). ABC has the advantage over TDF of having no renal toxicity, but the disadvantages of possible reduced potency in patients with a baseline VL >100,000 c/mL (see ACTG 5202, pg. 181) and a possible increased risk of cardiovascular events. Both disadvantages are inconsistent across studies, making conclusions difficult, but, based on these concerns, 2011 DHHS Guidelines list ABC/3TC as an alternative to TDF/FTC, and there is a cautionary note for ABC use in patient with a high baseline VL or multiple risk factors for cardiovascular disease in the IAS-USA and European Guidelines. The main evidence for the risk of myocardial infarction (MI) comes from the D:A:D retrospective analysis of 33,347 patients, which found an OR for MI with ABC use was 1.9 (p<0.003) compared to other ART agents (*Lancet* 2008;371:1417). Similar associations were also shown in the SMART and STEAL studies (see pg. 183), but were not observed in several other trials. The greater risk for virologic failure is based on AGTC 5202, a large trial of treatment-naïve patients randomized to TDF/FTC vs. ABC/3TC. The study was unblinded in the subset of patients with a baseline VL >100,000 c/mL due to a significant difference in the number of virologic failures favoring TDF/FTC (*NEJM* 2009; 361:2230). This difference was not seen in the final analysis of the subset with a baseline VL <100,000 c/mL (*Ann Intern Med* 2011;154:445) and has been inconsistently seen in other reports (see pg. 183).

- **AZT/3TC** is coformulated as *Combivir* and has been used extensively since 1997. It is now generic and in the 2011 DHHS Guidelines classified as an acceptable dual-NRTI combination. It is acceptable due to decreased virologic and CD4 response compared to TDF/FTC, the need for twice-daily dosing, and a side effect profile

4 Antiretroviral Therapy

that includes GI intolerance, fatigue, bone marrow suppression, lipoatrophy and lactic acidosis (see pg. 416). The pivotal trial GS 934 comparing AZT/3TC with TDF/FTC, each with EFV, is summarized above (*NEJM* 2006;354:251).

■ **ddI + 3TC or ddI + FTC:** Toxicity of ddI includes pancreatitis, peripheral neuropathy, and lactic acidosis. There is also a possible association with non-cirrhotic portal hypertension. Clinical experience with this combination is limited, and most trials of ddI+3TC or ddI+FTC have either been non-comparative or have used non-standard comparators. One trial using ddI+FTC+EFV given once daily demonstrated good viral suppression (*Antivir Ther* 2003;8 Suppl 1:594).

■ **AZT, d4T and ddI:** Thymidine analogs and ddI are not generally recommended in US and European guidelines due primarily to mitochondrial toxicity (see pg. 165). These agents are commonly used in combination with 3TC in resource-limited countries for economic considerations and are considered generally safe if adequately monitored. AZT is considered an acceptable option in the 2011 DHHS Guidelines (Table 4-8), and AZT and ddI are in the 2010 Guidelines from the European AIDS Clinical Society (Table 4-10).

■ **NRTI pairings to avoid: 3TC + FTC** (redundant antiviral activity), **AZT + d4T** (antagonistic), **ddI + d4T** (toxicity), **TDF + ddI** (high rate of virologic failure, resistance, increased ddI toxicity and blunted CD4 response).

■ **AZT/3TC/ABC:** Inferior to AZT/3TC+EFV in treatment-naïve patients (*NEJM* 2004;350:1850). This "triple nucleoside regimen" was a "preferred regimen" for treatment-naïve patients until the announcement of results of ACTG 5095 in 2003 (see pg. 249). Nevertheless, this appears to be the best of the triple NRTI regimens.

■ **PI/r vs. NNRTI-based ART:** ACTG 5142 is an important study assessing the relative merits of NNRTI- vs. PI/r-based ART regimens. At 96 weeks, the combination of EFV+2 NRTIs was virologically superior (89% vs. 77% for VL <50 c/mL, p=0.006). However, recipients of LPV/r had a greater increase in median CD4 count (+285 cells/mm^3 vs. 240 cells/mm^3, p=0.01) and failure with LPV/r resulted in fewer major resistant mutations (16 vs. 0) (*NEJM* 2008;358:2095) (see pg. 249). This barrier to resistance seen with LPV/r applies to other PI/r-based ART regimens including DRV/r, ATV/r, FPV/r and SQV/r. The protection generally applies to the accompanying NRTIs as well. By contrast, virologic failure on EFV- or NVP-based ART commonly results in resistance to NFV and EFV as well as some of the co-administered NRTIs (see Table 4-18, pg. 114).

■ **EFV:** Efavirenz is a preferred 3rd drug in all guidelines for treatment-naïve patients largely because no other regimen has ever shown superior virologic efficacy in a major clinical trial. Other advantages

■ TABLE 4-8: Initial Regimen: DHHS Guidelines (October, 2011)

Category	Regimen
Preferred Regimens (alphabetical order)	ATV/r* + TDF/FTC† DRV/r + TDF/FTC† EFV‡/TDF/FTC† RAL + TDF/FTC†
Preferred Regimen (for pregnant women)	LPV/r (bid) + ZDV/3TC†(preferred for pregnant women)
Alternative Regimens (alphabetical order)	ATV/r* + ABC#/3TC† DRV/r + ABC#/3TC† EFV‡ + ABC#/3TC† FPV/r (qd or bid) + (ABC#/3TC† or TDF/FTC†) LPV/r (qd or bid) + (ABC#/3TC† or TDF/FTC†) RAL + ABC#/3TC† RPV§ + (TDF/FTC+ or ABC#/3TC†)

* ATV and ATV/r should not be used in patients on >20 mg omeprazole equivalent per day

† 3TC can substitute for FTC and vice versa

‡ EFV should not be used during the first trimester of pregnancy or in women of child-bearing potential trying to conceive or not using effective contraception

§ Use RPV with caution in patients with pre-treatment VL >100,000 copies/mL.. Use of proton pump inhibitors contraindicated

\# ABC should not be used in patients who test positive for HLA-B*5701. Use with caution in patients with high risk of cardiovascular disease or pretreatment VL >100,000 copies/mL

NOTE: See DHHS Guidelines for other regimen categories: 1) Acceptable regimens; 2) Regimens that may be acceptable but more definitive data are needed; and 3) Regimens that maybe acceptable but should be used with caution

■ TABLE 4-9: Initial Regimen: IAS-USA (*JAMA 2010;304:321*)

	NRTI pair	3rd drug
	Select one NRTI pair (second column) plus a third drug (third column)	
Preferred	TDF / FTC	EFV, ATV/r, DRV/r, RAL
Alternative	ABC / 3TC	LPV/r, FPV/r, MVC

■ TABLE 4-10: Initial regimen: European AIDS Clinical Society (EACS) 2009

	NRTI pair	3rd drug*
	Select one NRTI pair (second column) plus a third drug (third column)	
Preferred	ABC/3TC or TDF/FTC	ATV/r, DRV/r, LPV/r, SQV/r (1000/100 bid)
Alternative	AZT/3TC, ddl+3TC, ddl+FTC	FPV/r, SQV/r (2000/100 qd), RAL

* Doses in mg for 3rd drug: ATV/r 30o/100 qd; DRV/r 800/100 qd; LPV/r 400/100 bid or 800/200 qd; FPV/r 700/100 bid or 1400/200 qd; RAL 400 bid

■ TABLE 4-11: Initial Regimen for Resource-Poor Settings: WHO 2010

Criteria	Regimen
Standard	EFV + (AZT/3TC or TDF/FTC or TDF+3TC); or NVP + (AZT/3TC or TDF/FTC or TDF+3TC)
HBV Co-infection	(EFV or NVP) + (TDF/FTC or TDF+3TC)
Tuberculosis	EFV-based ART as soon as possible
Pregnancy	EFV* + (AZT/3TC or TDF/FTC); or NVP + (AZT/3TC or TDF/FTC)

* Do not start EFV in first trimester

4 Antiretroviral Therapy

are that it is available in a three drug combination for administration as a single pill for once daily administration. It has also been used extensively since FDA approval in 1998 giving the longest follow-up for any of the favored 3rd drug options for treatment-naïve patients. Major concerns with EFV are its low genetic barrier to resistance, the teratogenic effects that preclude use in the first trimester of pregnancy or in women who are vulnerable to pregnancy, and common early neuropsychiatric side effects, with the potential for more serious or prolonged psychiatric effects in a small proportion of patients. Other concerns with EFV are that the frequency of baseline resistance is comparatively high (see pg. 250), and there is a possibility of minor resistant variants that may predict failure but are missed with standard genotypic resistance testing at baseline (*JID* 2010;201:662). There is also uncertainty about long-term psychiatric complications (*Drug Saf* 2006;29:865; *JAIDS* 2006;29:865) and metabolic consequences with hyperlipidemia (*AIDS* 2009;23:1109; *JAIDS* 2010;55:39).

- **PIs:** Multiple ritonavir-boosted PIs appear comparably potent based on randomized clinical trials in treatment-naïve patients demonstrating similar virologic outcome (VL <50 c/mL by intent-to-treat analysis at ≥ 48 weeks). The flagship trials comparing PI/r vs. LPV/r are:

  - KLEAN (see pg. 282): FPV/r vs. LPV/r (*Lancet* 2006;368:476)
  - GEMINI (see pg. 374): SQV/r vs. LPV/r (*JAIDS* 2009;50:367)
  - CASTLE (see pg. 195): ATV/r vs. LPV/r (*Lancet* 2008;372:646)
  - ARTEMIS (see pg. 225): DRV vs. LPV/r (*AIDS* 2008;22:1389)

  The two PI-based regimens that are favored in US Guidelines for treatment-naïve patients are ATV/r and DRV/r, agents that have proven non-inferior or superior to LPV/r in viral suppression in CASTLE (see pg. 195) and ARTEMIS (see pg. 225), respectively, with better tolerability and fewer lipid effects. Again, neither ATV/r or DRV/r have proven inferior in viral suppression in a clinical trial of treatment-naïve patients.

- **ATV/r:** This drug was compared to EFV in ACTG 5202 (pg 100), which included 928 patients who were randomized to take either TDF/FTC or ABC/3TC with either EFV or ATV/r. Virologic outcome was similar for EFV vs. ATV/r at 96 weeks, with VL <50 c/mL in 13.5% of EFV recipients and 15% of ATV/r recipients (p=NS) (*Ann Intern Med* 2011;154:445). However, there were marked differences in the frequency of resistance mutations: the frequency of EFV resistance mutations in patients failing EFV was 68/126 (54%); with ATV/r, as with other RTV-boosted PIs, major PI resistance mutations were noted in only 7/38 (5%) of virologic failures. The companion NRTIs were also protected from NRTI resistance mutations among ATV/r recipients with virologic failures: NRTI resistance emerged in 12% vs. 37% (p=0.0003). Disadvantages of ATV/r are the potential for jaundice or scleral icterus, need to take a meal with dosing, the need for gastric acidity for adequate bioavailability, rare cases of nephrolithiasis and possible nephrotoxcity, drug interactions with concurrent use of TDF or EFV, the need for dose adjustment with hepatic insufficiency, and poor CNS penetration (uncertain significance). See pg. 193.

- **DRV/r:** This boosted PI is one of four ART combinations favored as preferred in both the 2011 DHHS Guidelines and 2010 IAS-USA Guidelines, but DRV/r-based ART has never been tested against the other three preferred regimens in both guidelines for treatment-naïve patients. Potency and tolerability were apparent from the ARTEMIS trial: 79% of 343 treatment-naïve patients given once-daily DRV/r had VL <50 c/mL at 96 weeks (*AIDS* 2009;23:1679). This included viral suppression in 76% of 141 participants with a baseline VL >100,000 c/mL and 79% of 269 with a baseline CD4 count <200 cells/mm^3. DRV/r was better tolerated from a gastrointestinal standpoint than LPV/r, and had less of an effect on lipids. Advantages over ATV/r include the lack of hyperbilirubinemia and potential for jaundice and the ability to combine the drug with PPIs. Disadvantages are the potential for rash, which can sometimes be treatment-limiting. See pg. 223.

- **Raltegravir (RAL):** STARTMRK (see pg. 354) compared EFV with RAL, each in combination with TDF/FTC, in 566 treatment-naïve patients (*Lancet* 2009;374:796). At 48 weeks VL was <50 c/mL in 86% of RAL recipients vs. 82% of EFV recipients (difference 4.2%; 95% CI=1.9-10.3) (see pg. 355). RAL recipients had a significantly shorter time to virologic suppression (of no clinical significance), significantly fewer adverse drug reactions leading to drug discontinuation, higher CD4 count responses, and less hyperlipidemia (*JID* 2011;203:1204). At 96 weeks (*JAIDS* 2010,55.39) VL was <50 c/mL in 84% of EFV recipients and 83% of RAL recipients. A subsequent non-comparative trial in 35 patients given RAL in combination with ABC/3TC found that 31 (91%) had a VL <50 c/mL (*HIV Clin Trials* 2010;11:260). Attempts to use RAL once daily have not been successful (*HIV Clin Trials* 2010;11:197; *JAC* 2010;44:145). RAL is a potent integrase inhibitor with few drug interactions, excellent tolerance, and advantages that it is taken bid and has a low barrier to resistance with cross resistance to the next generation agent eltegravir but not dolutegravir. See pg. 353.

- **Maraviroc (MVC):** The MERIT trial in both guidelines compared EFV vs. MVC in combination with AZT/3TC patients with R5 virus at screening (*JID* 2010;201:803) The once-daily MVC arm was stopped early due to excessive rates of virologic failure. At 48 weeks (n=721) MVC was inferior to EFV for suppression to <50 c/mL, but overall results were not significantly different when adjusted for erroneous baseline tropism screening using the more sensitive tropism assay, which is in current use. The main difference in outcome after the

4 Antiretroviral Therapy

tropism adjustment was the reason for failure. More MVC discontinuations were for viral failure (12% vs. 4%), and more EFV discontinuations were for adverse reactions (4% vs. 14%). The 96-week results of this trial showed similar results, with <50 c/mL in 59% of MVC recipients vs. 63% of EFV (*HIV Clin Trials* 2010;11:125). Other analyses of the MERIT data found that MVC recipients had greater CD4 cell increases at 96 weeks (median 212 vs. 171 cells/mm^3) (*HIV Clin Trials* 2010;11:125), better lipid profiles (*HIV Clin Trials* 2011;12:24) and slightly greater impact on markers of immune activation (*PLoS One* 2010;5:e13188) (see pg. 317).

INDIVIDUALIZED SELECTION OF THE INITIAL REGIMEN (TABLE 4-12):

The discussion above deals primarily with relative potency of available agents. Selection of an appropriate regimen requires consideration of patient-specific issues. These include the following:

- Prior resistance test results.
- Co-morbidities, including cardiovascular, renal, hepatic or metabolic disease, mental health disorders.
- Concurrent drugs (see Table 4-12).
- Pregnancy or pregnancy potential (see pg. 157).
- Patient preference, including issues of pill burden, number of doses and food/fasting requirements (see Table 4-15, pg. 103).
- Baseline test results, including CD4 count if NVP is being considered and HLA-B*5701 test results if ABC is being considered.
- Hepatitis B co-infection (see pg. 507).
- Acute HIV infection: If treatment is to be given before resistance test results are available, a PI/r-based regimen is commonly recommended, since patients are more likely to be infected with NNRTI-resistant virus than with PI-resistant virus.

Treatment of HIV-2 (*HIV-Med* 2010;11:611; *CID* 2011;52:1780):

BACKGROUND: See pg. 7.

- **Viral load:** There is one commercially available HIV-2 viral load assay (HIV- Type 2 RNA, quantitative, University of Washington Laboratory Medicine, CPT code 87539, 800-713-5198). There are no controlled trials of ART for HIV-2 infection or HIV-1/2 coinfection. Recommendations are largely based on anecdotal observations from clinical and *in vitro* reports.
- **NRTIs:** HIV-2 is generally sensitive to NRTIs but is relatively rersistant to AZT, has a low barrier to resistance to NRTIs and has high rates of K65R (*Leukemia* 1997;11 Suppl 3:120; *HIV Med* 2010;11:611).
- **NNRTIs:** HIV-2 is inherently resistant to this class due to Y188L polymorphisms (*Antiviral Ther* 2004;9:3) causing an altered binding

pocket resulting in high rates of failures reported with HIV-2 and HIV 1/2 infection (*AIDS* 2010;24:1043).

- **PIs:** PI-based ART is preferred but it is critical to select agents well and follow closely since options after failure are limited: NNRTIs are inactive and NRTIs have a low barrier to resistance. Most active are LPV, DRV and SQV (*AAC* 2008;52:1545); much less effective due to weaker binding are ATV, NFV and TPV (*AAC* 2008;52:1545; *JAC* 2002;46:731). Clinical experience with PI-based ART is somewhat worse with HIV-2 or HIV-1/2 compared to HIV-1 (*AIDS* 2010;24:1043; *Trop R Soc Med Hyg* 2010;104:151). The best and most extensive experience is with LPV/r (*AIDS* 2009;23:1171; *AIDS* 2006;20:127). A single proV47A mutation confers LPV resistance but hypersensitivity to SQV that may be useful for sequencing (*AAC* 2008;52:1545; *JAC* 2002;46:731).

- **RAL:** RAL is generally active against HIV-2, which shows the same resistance pathways as HIV-1. Published clinical experience in limited and variable (*Eur J Med Res* 2009;14 Suppl 3:47; *Antivir Res* 2010;86:224; *J Clin Virol* 2009;46:176; *AIDS* 2008;22:665; *AIDS* 2008;22:109; *JAC* 2008;62:941).

- **MVC:** HIV-2 appears capable of using other receptors, so MVC should not be used (*J Virol* 2005;79:1686; *J Virol* 1998;72:5425).

- **ENF:** HIV-2 is resistant to ENF *in vitro* (*Antiviral Ther* 2004;9:57).

RECOMMENDATIONS (2011 DHHS Guidelines; *CID* 2011;52:1334)

- **Patients with untreated HIV-2 moninfection** or **HIV1-2 dual infection** who require ART should be treated with 2 NRTIs and a boosted PI based on a limited experience (*BMC Infect Dis* 2008;8:21) including one series showing a good response in 17 of 29 (59%) HIV-2 monoinfected adults (*AIDS* 2009;23:1171; *HIV Med* 2010;11:611; *CID* 2011;52:1257). The largest published series includes 126 treated with LPV/r combined with 3TC plus either AZT or TDF) (*CID* 2011;52:1334). The mean CD4 counts in this group was + 12 cells/mm^3/month and the mean VL at one year was 2.2 log$_{10}$ c/mL.

- **Monitoring response:** Standard methods cannot be used due to inability to monitor VL response and unique resistance mutations (*JID* 2009;199:1323; *HIV Med* 2010;11:611). The recommendation is to follow CD4 count response with the understanding that it is a poor indicator of virologic response or failure (*AIDS* 2008;22:457).

Agents	Advantages	Disadvantages
2 NRTIs + 1 PI or RTV-boosted PI*		
ATV±RTV	■ Low pill burden ■ Once-daily dosing (ATV 400 mg qd or ATV/r 300/100 mg qd) ■ Minimal or no effect on lipids or insulin resistance ■ Fewer GI side effects than LPV/r in CASTLE ■ ATV may be given without RTV unless combined with TDF or EFV ■ Minimal resistance with initial failure of ATV/r ■ Major ATV-resistance mutation (I50L) has minimal PI cross resistance ■ Never beaten in a clinical trial	■ Food requirement ■ Side effects: Hyperbilirubinemia (clinically inconsequential unless it causes jaundice or icterus), possible nephrotoxicity, rash, nephrolithiasis (rare) and PR prolongation (inconsequential without 2nd QTc prolonging drug) ■ Reduced ATV AUC when combined with TDF or EFV (use ATV/r 300/100 qd with TDF and 400/100 mg qd with EFV). Cannot be combined with NVP. ■ More virologic failure and resistance with ATV than with ATV/r ■ Absorption dependent on food and acidic pH (PPIs, antacids and H2 blockers may decrease absorption)
DRV/r	■ Better GI tolerability and lipid effects compared to LPV/r in ARTEMIS ■ Minimal resistance with virologic failure ■ Once-daily dosing if no DRV resistance mutations ■ Potential for monotherapy after induction with 3 drugs (MONET trial, not currently recommended) ■ Never beaten in a clinical trial	■ Limited experience for long term durability and tolerability ■ Food requirement ■ RTV boosting required ■ Potential for rash and hepatotoxicity
FPV±RTV	■ Once daily regimen available (FDA-approved without prior PI failure), including FPV/r 1400/100 mg, with less RTV toxicity ■ No food effect ■ Minimal PI resistance with initial failure (FPV/r) ■ FPV/r comparable to LPV/r in KLEAN trial ■ FPV/r 1400/100 mg qd comparable to ATV/r for GI tolerability and lipid effects in (ALERT)	■ Rash, GI side effects ■ Hyperlipidemia ■ Less data with FPV/r 1400/100 mg/d compared to ATV/r or DRV/r; less data with FPV/r 700/100 mg bid compared to LPV/r ■ Use of unboosted FPV can cause DRV cross-resistance

IDV/r	■ Long term experience documenting sustained benefit in some pts.
	
	■ RTV boosting eliminates fasting requirement and q8h dosing requirement
	
	■ Potency 90% VL <500 c/mL at 24 wks (*NEJM* 1997;337:779)
		■ Nephrolithiasis and nephrotoxicity
		
		■ BID dosing required
		
		■ IDV/r combination issues
		  • 400/400 mg bid: poor GI tolerability
		  • 800/100 mg bid: risks nephrolithiasis
		
		■ Sicca syndrome, alopecia, paronychia
		
		■ Insulin resistance and hyperglycemia

continued on next page

Antiretroviral Therapy

Agents	Advantages	Disadvantages
2 NRTIs + 1 PI or RTV-boosted PI* (*continued*)		
LPV/r	■ Co-formulation (*Kaletra*) ■ Potency and long term durability documented ■ No food effect ■ Minimal PI resistance with initial failure ■ Once-daily therapy effective for treatment-naïve patients but not recommended with ≥3 LPV resistance mutations or in pregnancy ■ Preferred PI in pregnancy (DHHS guidelines)	■ Nausea, diarrhea ■ More virologic failures than EFV-based ART (ACTG 5142), DRV/r (ARTEMIS) and ATV/r (CASTLE) ■ GI side effects common ■ PI class metabolic toxicity ■ Requires RTV boosting at 200 mg/d (compared to 100 mg/d with ATV, DRV, FPV)
NFV	■ No PI cross-resistance with signature D30N mutation ■ Extensive experience	■ Diarrhea ■ PI class toxicity ■ Reduced potency compared with boosted PIs (main disadvantage) ■ Decreased efficacy with low CD4 and/or VL >100,000 c/mL ■ Fatty food requirement ■ PI cross-resistance with selection of L90M ■ The only "unboostable" PI ■ BID dosing required
SQV/r*	■ Non-inferior to LPV/r (GEMINI trial) ■ Less triglyceride elevation than LPV/r in GEMINI trial	■ Poor GI tolerability ■ PI class toxicity ■ RTV boosting required ■ Most published data are with *Fortovase* formulation, which is no longer available ■ Higher pill burden than other recommended PI/r combinations ■ FDA black box warning regarding QTc prolongation ■ Prolonged QTc with FDA recommendation for pre-treatment EKG (see pg. 376)
2 NRTIs + NNRTI		
EFV	■ Efficacy and durability well documented ■ Comparable potency with viral load >100,000 c/mL ■ Single tablet coformulation with TDF/FTC available ■ Long half-life helps prevent resistance with missed or delayed doses ■ May use with rifampin ■ Unbeaten in clinical trials for virologic efficacy and durability	■ Neuropsychiatric toxicity and rash ■ Teratogenicity: contraindicated in first trimester of pregnancy and with pregnancy potential ■ Low genetic barrier to resistance ■ Risk of resistance if all agents in regimen are stopped simultaneously ■ Reduced CD4 increase compared to PI, RAL and MVC-based regimens ■ Methadone interaction ■ Reduces PI levels ■ Metabolic side effects ■ High rate of transmitted resistance ■ Lower CD4 increase than with PIs, MVC or RAL

continued on next page

Antiretroviral Therapy

4

Agents	Advantages	Disadvantages
2 NRTIs + NNRTI *(continued)*		
NVP	■ Low pill burden ■ No food effect ■ Minimal lipid changes ■ Least expensive third agent ■ Pharmacologic barrier to resistance ■ Relatively few drug interactions ■ New extended dose once-daily formulation available	■ Hepatotoxicity, including potentially lethal hepatic necrosis ■ Restricted use based on CD4 count: women must have <250 cells/mm^3 and men <400 cells/mm^3 at initiation of therapy ■ High rate of rash, including life-threatening hypersensitivity reactions ■ Risk of resistance if all agents in regimen stopped at once ■ Low genetic barrier to resistance ■ Methadone interaction ■ Risk of resistance with single dose NVP for PMTCT (without NRTI "tail") ■ Reduces PI levels ■ Less clinical trial data than with EFV
RPV	■ Better tolerated than EFV (less rash, CNS side effects) ■ No known teratogenicity ■ Single tablet coformulation with TDF/FTC available	■ More virologic failure at VL >100,000 than EFV ■ May be less "forgiving" of non-adherence than EFV ■ More resistance with failure than EFV (NRTI, NNRTI) ■ Failure results in cross-resistance to ETR due to 138K mutation ■ Must be taken with meal for adequate absorption ■ Cannot be taken with PPIs; caution with H2 blockers, antacids
2 NRTIs + CCR5 antagonist		
MVC	■ Efficacy comparable to EFV (MERIT trial) ■ No food effect	■ Requires screening for tropism ■ Extensive drug interactions resulting in 3 different doses ■ Limited long-term experience ■ Requires BID dosing; QD dosing under study
2 NRTIs + Integrase Inhibitor		
RAL	■ Potency comparable to EFV (STARTMRK) ■ Well tolerated ■ No food effect ■ Few interactions	■ Lower barrier to resistance than PI/r ■ Requires BID dosing ■ Most data are with TDF/FTC
3 NRTIs		
AZT/3TC/ABC	■ Extensive experience ■ No food effect ■ May be given with rifampin ■ Low pill burden ■ Preserves PI and NNRTI options ■ Minimal drug interactions ■ Coformulated ■ Only triple NRTI regimen with good virologic results	■ Reduced potency at all baseline VL levels compared to EFV-based ART (ACTG 5095) ■ Side effects of AZT and ABC (see below) ■ Need for HLA-B*5701 screening ■ Requires bid dosing

continued on next page

Antiretroviral Therapy

■ TABLE 4-12: **Advantages and Disadvantages of Antiretroviral Agents and Combinations for Initial Therapy.***(Continued)*

Agents	Advantages	Disadvantages
2 NRTIs (as component of ART regimen)		
AZT/3TC (or AZT+FTC)	■ Extensive experience ■ Low pill burden ■ Co-formulated (AZT/3TC) ■ No food effect ■ M184V slows AZT resistance and increases AZT activity	■ AZT toxicity: anemia, neutropenia, GI intolerance and fatigue ■ TAMs and NRTI cross-resistance with prolonged failure ■ Mitochondrial toxicity (AZT) including lipoatrophy, lactic acidosis and hepatic steatosis ■ Requires bid dosing ■ Less effective than TDF/FTC (GS934) ■ Worse CD4 response than with ABC/3TC ■ More M184V mutations than with TDF/FTC
TDF/FTC or TDF+3TC	■ Once daily regimen ■ Both effective against HBV ■ Well tolerated ■ Low pill burden (1/d with FTC) ■ Avoids TAMs ■ Coformulated ■ Mitochondrial toxicity ■ Efficacy superior to AZT/3TC (*NEJM* 2006;354:251) and safer than d4T/3TC (*JAMA* 2004;292:191) ■ M184V increases TDF activity	■ Risk of ABC and ddI cross-resistance after failure with K65R (uncommon with TDF/FTC) ■ TDF decreases ATV levels (use ATV/r) and increases ddI levels and toxicity ■ Potential for TDF nephrotoxicity ■ Greater reduction in bone mineral density than with other ARVs
ABC/3TC or ABC+FTC	■ Once daily regimen ■ Low pill burden (1/d with 3TC) ■ Well tolerated ■ Avoids TAMs ■ Coformulated (ABC/3TC) ■ Low potential for mitochondrial toxicity	■ ABC hypersensitivity reaction (rare with HLA B*5701 screening) ■ Possible risk of ddI cross-resistance (L74V) or TDF and ddI cross-resistance (K65R) ■ Possible increased risk of cardiovascular disease during exposure
ddI+3TC or ddI+FTC	■ Once daily regimen ■ Avoids TAMs	■ Minimal data ■ ddI toxicity and food effect: neuropathy, pancreatitis, possible mitochondrial toxicity, possible non-cirrhotic portal hypertension ■ Risk of K65R with ABC and TDF cross-resistance ■ Increased toxicity when given with TDF, d4T or ribavirin
d4T+3TC or d4T+FTC (not recommended)	■ Good short-term tolerability ■ No food effect ■ M184V (3TC) slows d4T resistance	■ d4T toxicity: neuropathy, lactic acidosis, hepatic steatosis, lipoatrophy ■ TAMs and cross-resistance with prolonged failure ■ Requires bid dosing
ddI+d4T (not recommended)	■ Extensive experience in pre-HAART era	■ Contraindicated in pregnancy ■ Excessive mitochondrial toxicity and drug-specific toxicities (see above) ■ Food effect (ddI) and bid dosing ■ May increase risk of TAMs and multi-nucleoside resistance

continued on next page

Antiretroviral Therapy **4**

■ TABLE 4-12: **Advantages and Disadvantages of Antiretroviral Agents and Combinations for Initial Therapy.***(Continued)*

Agents	Advantages	Disadvantages
2 NRTIs (as component of ART regimen) *(continued)*		
AZT+ddI (not recommended)	▪ Extensive experience in pre-HAART era	▪ Side effects and toxicity of AZT and ddI (see above) ▪ May increase risk of TAMs and multi-nucleoside resistance mutations ▪ Complex dosing (AZT tolerability improved with food, ddI taken on empty stomach) ▪ Requires bid dosing
TDF+ddI (not recommended)	▪ Once daily regimen	▪ High rates of virologic failure with 3rd NRTI or with NNRTI ▪ Reduced CD4 response without dose adjustment ▪ Drug interaction requiring reduced dose of ddI ▪ Possible increased risk of ddI toxicity (see above)

*   Most PIs are associated with class adverse reactions (hyperlipidemia, insulin resistance, fat redistribution). ATV, DRV and FPV (1400/100) are exceptions.

All PIs, except nelfinavir, are boosted to give better pharmacokinetics.

Factors That Influence Probability of Prolonged Viral Suppression

REGIMEN POTENCY: The standard is to use 3 ARVs from at least 2 distinct classes. The January 2011 DHHS and 2010 IAS-USA Guidelines (pg 91) are identical with respect to the preferred regimens. They advocate TDF/FTC combined with EFV, DRV/r, ATV/r or RAL: all unbeaten for virologic efficacy in clinical trials for treatment-naïve patients, with acceptable side effect profile and adherence demands.

■ TABLE 4-13: **Efficacy of Antiviral Classes in Achieving an HIV Viral Load <50 c/mL at 48 Weeks (***AIDS* **2006;20:251)**

Class	VL <50	CD4 Increase
NNRTI	64%*	+173
PI/r	64%*	+200*
3 NRTIs	54%	+161
PI (unboosted)	43%	+179

*Significantly better than other categories (*P*<0.05)

ACTG 5142 AND ACTG 5202: These are the major trials comparing EFV with PI/r-based ART. ACTG 5142 demonstrated that EFV was superior to LPV/r in virologic suppression, but failure with EFV was associated with high rates of NNRTI resistance (48%), while there were no major PI mutations with LPV/r failure. Subsequently, ATV/r proved virologically superior to LPV/r (CASTLE), setting the stage for ACTG

5202, which compared EFV vs. ATV/r in 928 treatment-naïve patients (*Ann Intern Med* 2011;154:445). Virologic suppression was comparable, and is with other studies of ritonavir-boosted PIs, PI resistance mutations were infrequent in patients who failed therapy (see Table 4-14 below and Table 4-18, pg. 114).

■ TABLE 4-14: **ACTG 5202 – 96 Week Results for EFV + 2 NRTIs vs. ATV/r + 2 NRTIs (*Ann Intern Med* 2011;154:445)**

	ABC/3TC +		TDF/FTC +	
	ATV/r	EFV	ATV/r	EFV
Viral Failure				
Total	17%	15%	11%	10%
Baseline VL >100,000	12%	13%	10%	11%
Major resistance mutations				
NNRTI	1%	65%*	0	56%*
PI	1%	0	0	0
NRTI	14%	40%	9%	23%

* p<0.05

ADHERENCE: In a study by Paterson and colleagues (*Ann Intern Med* 2000;133:21) the adherence rate of >95% was required to achieve an 80% probability of virologic suppression to <400 c/mL at 24 weeks. With 90-95% adherence the probability of suppression dropped to 50%. However, while multiple studies have confirmed the importance of adherence (*AIDS* 2001;15:2109; *CID* 2001;33:386; *CID* 2002;34:115; *AIDS* 2004;35:S35), this early report is less relevant today, now that we are using boosted PIs and NNRTIs with long half-lives. More recent work has shown that adherence requirements vary depending on the regimen, which reflects regimen potency, pharmacokinetic properties, class- or agent-susceptibility, and within-class cross-resistance mutational patterns. Substantial experience shows that adherence to recommended regimens will achieve durable virologic suppression unless there is transmitted resistance. Some nuances of these conclusions:

- **Transmitted resistance** may be apparent with baseline testing, but resistant strains often have a competitive disadvantage over wild-type virus, but are in the latent pool and emerge only with antiviral pressure. Thus, relevant historical data include prior resistant tests, antiretroviral history and infecting source data.

- **Resistance mutations in the minority pool** or restricted to latently infected reservoirs and may cause virologic failure despite good adherence.

- The role of resistance mutations in reducing replication competence is poorly understood.

4 Antiretroviral Therapy

- PI/r-based regimens have a <u>genetic barrier to resistance</u> that is poorly understood; unlike NNRTI-based regimens, antiviral activity can often be achieved following virologic failure by simply improving adherence. This accounts for the relative safety of DRV/r, ATV/r or LPV/r monotherapy (*AIDS* 2008;22:385; *JAC* 2010;65:2436; *AIDS Rev* 2010;12:127; *Antivir Ther* 2011;16:59; *AIDS* 2010;24:2365; *AIDS* 2009;23:279).

- **Resistance testing** is commercially available for 5 of the 6 classes of antiviral agents for HIV-1. The exception is CCR5 antagonists (see pg. 48-49).

- **Analysis of minority strains** may become commercially available and could facilitate detection of minority strains (*JID* 2010;201:662).

- It is assumed that <u>resistant strains persist for the lifetime</u> of the patient, although this has been debated in the context of single-dose NVP to prevent perinatal transmission (*NEJM* 2010;363:1499).

- EFV has a **pharmacologic barrier** to resistance: the long half-life prevents resistance with missed doses, as demonstrated in the FOTO trial with Five (days) On and Two (days) Off (*HIV Clin Trials* 2007;8:19), which is not a recommended strategy based on the small size of the trial.

- **Genetic barrier:** EFV, NVP, ETR, 3TC, FTC, RAL, some unboosted PIs and ENF have a lower barrier to resistance compared to MVC and boosted PIs have a high barrier to resistance.

- **Cross-resistance** is agent-within-class specific. Thus, 103N causes resistance to EFV and NVP but not ETR or RPV; the 138K RT mutation, selected by RPV, causes cross-resistance to ETR. These patterns affect in-class sequencing decisions.

- The <u>184V RT mutation</u> is somewhat unique since it reduces activity of 3TC and FTC, but continued use does not risk additional resistance mutations (*JID* 2007;19:1537).

- The greatest challenge to patients for virologic control and prevention is <u>adherence to the initial regimen</u> since the level of HIV viremia is orders of magnitude higher. Thus, baseline VL often defines the risk of failure and resistance.

- **Adherence and resistance:** Poor adherence predicts virologic failure but not necessarily resistance. The highest risk of resistance to an unboosted PI-based regimen is virologic failure in the face of good adherence (*JAIDS* 2002;30:278; *AIDS* 2000;14:357; *AIDS* 2001;15:1701). In one study, 23% of patients with virologic failure ascribed to resistance had 92-100% adherence based on unannounced pill counts (*AIDS* 2003;17:1925). In another study, 88% of patients with resistance mutations had taken >70% of prescribed doses (*CID* 2003;37:1112). Both reports found virologic failure but virtually no resistance mutations with consumption of <60% of prescribed doses with unboosted or boosted PI-based ART. The assumption is that the drug level was inadequate to select resistant strains. More recent data suggest this association between adherence and resistance is related to drug class and to specific agents (*AIDS* 2006;20:223). As noted, virologic failure and resistance are less likely to occur with boosted PIs compared to unboosted PIs, due presumably to the pharmacologic barrier (*JAIDS* 2008;47:397; *CID* 2006;43:939).

  □ Details of resistance testing and mutational patterns associated with resistance are summarized on pgs 38-46.

- **Guidance for improved adherence:**

  1. **Common strategies and observations**
     □ Establish patient readiness before initiating treatment (but recognize relative urgency as noted on pg. 82).
     □ Use a standardized approach to assess adherence, but note that self-reported non-adherence is reliable.
     □ Use the entire health care team to reinforce adherence messages
     □ Realize that health care professionals are poor predictors of who will adhere.
     □ Adherence may decrease with time, becoming significantly worse at 6-12 mos than it is initially (*Topics HIV Med* 2003;11:185).
     □ Address obvious issues of convenience: pill burden, frequency of daily administrations, food or fasting requirements, tolerance, pill size. (Table 4-15)

- TABLE 4-15: **Convenience Factor**

Class	Once daily	Pill burden*		No food effect
NRTI*	ABC, ddI, TDF, FTC, 3TC	1/day: 2/day:	ABC/3TC TDF/FTC AZT/3TC	ABC, FTC. 3TC, TDF, d4T, AZT
NNRTI	EFV, NVP, ETR, RPV	1/day: 1 or 2/day: 2/day:	EFV, RPV NVP ETR	NVP
PI/r*	ATV/r, LPV/r DRV/r, FPV/r	2/day: 3/day: 4/day: 6/day: 8/day:	ATV/r DLV/r, FPV/r LPV/r, FPV/r SQV/r TPV/r	LPV/r
CCR5 antagonist	MVC	2/day	MVC	MVC
Itegrase inhibitors	RAL	2/day	RAL	RAL
NRTI pairs	ABC/3TC, TDF/FTC	1/day	ABC/3TC, TDF/FTC	ABC/3TC, TDF/FTC

* Data provided for NRTI is limited to combination formulations. The PI data are limited to boosted PIs and pill burden includes the ritonavir dose except LPV/r.

Antiretroviral Therapy

4

2. **Factors that predict reduced adherence:** Side effects, mental illness, active substance abuse, complex regimens, stigma, low level of literacy, comorbidities such as TB, asymptomatic status of patient when treatment begins, poverty issues (homelessness, transportation problems), poor understanding of regimen and inadequate pharmacy service (*Topics HIV Med* 2003;11:185; American Public Health Association, "Recommendations for Best Practices," www.mmhiv.com/link/APHA-Adherence).

3. **Adherence review and recommendations of the British HIV Association (www.mmhiv.com/link/BHIVA-Adherence)**

   □ Treatment simplification: A review of 53 clinical trials with 14,264 participants failed to show a significant correlation between pill count and viral suppression (*AIDS* 2006;20:2051). A review of the HIV literature on the benefit of fewer daily doses found only one study demonstrating a better outcome with once-daily ART (*JAMA* 2002;288:2868); however, it is generally preferred by patients (see pg. 123).

   □ Improvement in knowledge: Two reports found a benefit with educational sessions (*JAIDS* 2003;34:191; *Patient Educ Couns* 2003;50:187). Other reports found no benefit with individual counseling by a trained counselor or group support (*JAIDS* 2003;34:174; *J Assoc Nurses AIDS Care* 2003;14:52).

   □ Pagers, alarms, phones: One large randomized study found significantly more virologic failure in patients using a dose time alarm vs. controls (XV Int'l AIDS Conf 2004, Abstr. LbOrB15). (The presumed reason was because patients depended on the alarm, which sometimes failed).

   □ Practice with placebo: One controlled trial with a 5-wk training period found a benefit that was modest and transient (*AIDS* 2006;20:1295).

   □ Directly observed therapy: Several studies found improved virologic outcomes using DOT with methadone maintenance (*CID* 2004;38[suppl 5]:S409; *CID* 2004;38[suppl 5]:S414; *CID* 2006;42:1628; *CID* 2007;45:770; *Public Health Rep* 2007;122:472). However, a meta-analysis of 12 studies that satisfied methodological criteria and were published before July, 2001 showed no benefit (*Lancet* 2009;374:2064).

■ **Measuring adherence:** Physician estimate is notoriously unreliable (*Ann Intern Med* 2000;133:21). Patient self-report is most reliable when there is acknowledgement of poor adherence, when queries are non-judgemental of poor adherence, with simple standardized surveys for doses taken in past 3 days or one week taken at each clinic visit and when the queries are impersonal as with a form or computer program (*JAIDS* 2006;43 Suppl 1:S149). Pharmacy records can be very useful (*AIDS Behav* 2008;12:86) and have been shown to correlate with virologic outcome (*PLoS Med* 2008;5:el09).

- **Adherence recommendations:**
  1. Data do not support frequent, intensive or prolonged contact with adherence specialists; use of the entire HIV medicine team of health care providers appears more effective than an adherence specialist.
  2. Regimens should not be simplified if simplification reduces potency.
  3. Medication alarms may reduce adherence, because people may depend on them, and they often fail.
  4. Critical factors are patient understanding of the regimen, a good provider-patient relationship and a drug regimen that addresses patients needs as much as possible.
  5. Pharmacy records and pill counts are especially effective for documenting good or bad adherence.

Rapidity of VL Response: The trajectory of the VL response predicts the nadir plasma VL and consequently the durability of HIV response. There are exceptions: The VL response to RAL-based ART is substantially more rapid compared to EFV in the first 6 wks of treatment, although results at 24 and 48 weeks were similar. More recent work indicates that the dose response slope is class dependent and possibly dictated by the stage in the viral lifecycle at which the agent is active (*Nat Med* 2008;14:762). One large review found that the median time to a VL <50 c/mL in treatment-naïve patients was 13.5 wks (*Int J Sex Transm Dis AIDS* 2006;17:522) (see pg. 26). To achieve an optimal and durable virologic response, treatment-naïve patients treated with ART are expected to respond as follows:

- Decrease 0.7-1.0 $\log_{10}$ c/mL at 1 wk (*Lancet* 2001;358:1760; *JAIDS* 2002;30:167)
- Decrease 1.5-2.0 $\log_{10}$ c/mL to <5,000 c/mL at 4 wks (*AIDS* 1999;13:1873; *JAIDS* 2000;25:36). One review of 656 treatment-naïve patients given ART found that a VL reduction to <1000 c/mL by week 4 predicted an 82-95% probability of VL <50 c/mL at week 24 (*JAIDS* 2004;37:1155).
- Decrease to <500 c/mL at 8-16 wks and <50 c/mL at 16-24 wks (*Ann Intern Med* 2001;135:954; *JAIDS* 2000;24:433)

Failure to achieve these goals suggests lack of antiretroviral potency, non-adherence, resistance or inadequate drug levels due to drug interactions, poor absorption, etc.

When to Modify Therapy

- **Virologic failure:** The goal of therapy is a sustained VL <50 c/mL, according to 2010 IAS-USA Guidelines (*JAMA* 2008;300:555), the 2011 DHHS Guidelines, the 2008 British HIV Association, and the 2008 European AIDS Clinical Society Guidelines.

4 Antiretroviral Therapy

Test	Time	Comment
VL	Baseline, then at 2-4 wks, then at 4-8 wk intervals until <200 c/mL, then q3-6mos	• More frequently with treatment failure • Expectation: VL decrease by 0.7-1.0 $\log_{10}$ c/mL at 1-2 wks, 1.5-2.0 $\log_{10}$ c/mL at 4 wks, and <200 c/mL by 24-48 wks
CD4	Baseline and q3-12mos	• CD4 increase of 30-70 cells/mm³ expected by month 4, and 100-150 cells/mm³ by 1st yr • There are no clearly established methods to increase the CD4 response beyond HIV suppression. Interferon and steroids decrease the CD4 cell count substantially. • The risk of an OI is notably reduced if the VL is suppressed without a good CD4 cell count.

□ Rapidity of response: Response in treatment-naïve patients should be a decrease of 0.7-1.0 $\log_{10}$ c/mL at 1 wk, 1.5-2.0 $\log_{10}$ c/mL decrease at 4 wks and <50 c/mL at 16-24 wks (see pg. 26).

□ Sustained viral suppression: Viral suppression to <50 c/ml should be sustained and confirmed with VL measurements at 3- to 6-month intervals (Table 4-16). Note that the 2011 DHHS Guidelines changed this interval from 3-4 mos, noting that the frequency of testing can be decreased in patients with an established pattern of good adherence and consistent HIV suppression for at least 2-3 yrs.

□ Blips: A blip is defined as a transient VL >50 c/mL preceded and followed by measurements of <50 c/mL without a change in treatment. One study of patients with sustained levels <50 c/mL measured VL every 2-3 days for 3-4 mos. Blips were common (9/10 patients), low-level (median of 79 c/mL), transient (isolated events), unrelated to clinical events (illness, vaccination, etc.), inconsistent (noted in only one of duplicate samples), and appeared to represent a statistical variation around the mean VL below 50 c/mL, suggesting most that are unconfirmed with repeat testing are errors (*JAMA* 2005;293:817). The frequency of blips caused both the ACTG and the DHHS to change their definition of virologic failure to a confirmed VL >200 c/mL.

□ Frequency of virologic failure: In an analysis of 12 reports with 1,197 patients in the U.S., 62% failed to achieve the goal of VL <50 c/mL by 24 wks (*CID* 2004;38:614). A review of 14,264 treatment-naïve patients in clinical trials between 1994 and 2004 found that 45% failed to achieve a VL <50 c/mL at 48 wks, but this improved to 36% in 2003-04 (*AIDS* 2006;20:2051). More recent reports indicate further progress (Yazdanpanah Y. 17th Intern AIDS Conf. 2008; Abstr. THAB0406).

Antiretroviral Therapy

- Rationale for the 50-200 c/mL threshold: Sequence analysis of HIV clones from patients with sustained VL <50 c/mL shows no sequence evolution with emergence of resistance mutations (*JAMA* 2005;293:817; *JID* 2004;189:1444; *JID* 2004;189:1452; *J Virol* 2006;80:6441; *PloS Path* 2007;3:3122). Levels <200 c/mL are usually blips. A similar analysis in patients with persistent low-level viremia (50-400 c/mL) demonstrated acquisition of resistance mutations in 9/21 patients at a median follow-up of 11 mos (*CID* 2004;39:1030). Studies using "single copy" assays indicate that these patients maintain a viral steady-state with a median VL of 3 c/mL (*CID* 2008;47:102; *PloS Path* 2007;3:e46). These observations suggest that a VL <50 c/mL indicates an absence of viral replication; virus present below that cutoff appears to reflect release from the latent CD4 cell pool. It should be acknowledged that some authorities consider this to represent low level viral replication to be managed with ART intensification (*JID* 2011;203:906; *Curr Opin HIV AIDS* 2010;5:491).

- **Immunologic failure:** There is no consensus definition. The expected increase is about 100 cells/mm^3 at one year with baseline levels <350 cells/mm^3 and increases averaging about 50 cells/mm^3/year in the second and third year with median increases of 250-300 cells/mm^3 over 5 years (*Lancet* 2007;370:470; *CID* 2007;44:441). Initiation of treatment with CD4 counts <200 cells/mm^3 is associated with a reduced immunologic response (*CID* 2007;44:441; *JAIDS* 2004;36:702), with some studies showing a plateau of 350-500 cells/mm^3 at 4-6 years, indicating a limited immunologic reserve with late starts (*JAIDS* 2007;45:515). Other large cohort studies show continuing increases in the mean CD4 counts to levels of >600 cells/mm^3 even with late starts (*Lancet* 2007;370:407). Persistently low CD4 counts are infrequently complicated by AIDS-defining complications if there is good viral suppression. In most cases intensification or changes in the ART regimen in the face of viral suppression has not proven effective in restoring the CD4 count.

  - CD4 count increases despite virologic failure: Multiple studies have shown that suboptimal virologic response to ART is commonly associated with increases in CD4 counts. This has consistently been shown in the large "salvage" studies (RESIST, POWER, BENCHMRK, TORO), in which most of the patients in the control group given an optimized background regimen (OBR) without the investigational agent had increases in the median CD4 counts despite virologic failure. Nevertheless, the CD4 count increase was significantly less than that achieved with good viral suppression. (*NEJM* 2003;348:2175; *Lancet* 2006;368:406; *JAIDS* 2007;46:24; *JAIDS* 2007;46:125). Several large studies also show that OIs are uncommon with a VL <5,000 c/mL regardless of the CD4 count. See Table 4-19, pg. 115.

4 Antiretroviral Therapy

- Virologic failure and resistance: The VL also predicts the probability of resistance, since mutation rates are a function of replication rates and continued drug exposure drives strain selection with additional resistance mutations at rates that depend on the VL (replication rate). This means the rate of new resistance mutations will be orders of magnitude greater with a VL of 100,000 c/mL vs. 1,000 c/mL although both represent viral failure (*JAIDS* 2002;30: 154; *JAIDS* 2001;27:44; *AIDS* 1999;13:1035; *AIDS* 1999; 13:341).

- VL and CD4 slope: The CD4 response correlates inversely with viral suppression; the increase has a biphasic pattern, increasing by reported mean values of 50-120 cells/mm^3 during the first 3 mos, thereafter increasing by 2-7 cells/mo (*JID* 2006;94:29; *JAMA* 2002;288:222; *JID* 2002;185:471; *JAMA* 2004; 292:1911). Early studies suggested that the VL was the strongest predictor of the rate of CD4 decline in untreated patients (*Ann Intern Med* 1997;126:946), but more recent studies suggest that this association may have been overstated (*JAMA* 2006; 296:144918). These studies suggest that CD4 slope is primarily regulated by immune activation attributed to HIV viral replication, but possibly also influenced by co-morbidies (TB, HSV, CMV, etc.) and translocation of gut microbes and microbial products (*Nat Med* 2006; 12:1365; *Nat Rev Immunol* 2004;4:485). Nevertheless, it should be noted that the only therapeutic intervention with a major and sustained impact on outcome and CD4 increase is ART. This conclusion is supported by repeated studies showing that viral suppression is associated with a prompt increase in CD4 counts (without any apparent effect on co-pathogens or intestinal GALT); studies showing that there are no alternative interventions to increase CD4 response in patients with VL/CD4 discordance; and treatment interruption trials in which discontinuation of ART caused a prompt increase in VL and rapid CD4 count decline averaging 30-80 cells/mo during the first 2 months. There is no consensus, since some authorities have argued that the original data are correct, and re-analysis of the MACS data found that baseline VL strongly predicted long-term prognosis (*JAMA* 2007; 297:2349) (see pg. 29).

- Discordant CD4 count and VL results: Virologic suppression is associated with immune recovery, and the magnitude of the CD4 count increase correlates with viral suppression. However, there is substantial individual variation, and discordant changes in both directions are relatively common (*JID* 2001;183:1328; *CID* 2002;35: 1005). Most discordant results are enigmatic. An exception is treatment with the combination of TDF and full-dose ddI, which is associated with a blunted CD4 response and should not be used (*AIDS* 2004;18:2442). Some studies have shown superior CD4 count increases with RAL, MVC, or PI-based ART compared to NNRTI-based ART (*JAIDS* 2010;55:39; *PLoS One* 2010;5:e13188; *JID* 2010;201:

Antiretroviral Therapy

803; *Antivir Ther* 2009;14:771). Medications that most often cause reduced CD4 counts are interferon and corticosteroids (see pg. 31).

□ The approach to CD4/VL discordance: Decisions regarding antiviral agents are governed by VL: 1) Viral suppression appears to reduce the frequency of opportunistic infections independent of the CD4 count and 2) there are no interventions with ART known to confer benefit (other than avoidance of ddI+TDF and possibly AZT). It is possible that RAL, MVC, or PI-based ART would be superior for CD4 response compared to NNRTI-based therapy, but there are no clinical data supporting therapeutic switches. IL-2 increases the CD4 count but without apparent clinical benefit (*AIDS* 2005;19:279; *AIDS* 2006;20:405; *JAIDS* 2006;42:140).

- **Clinical failure:** This is defined as the occurrence or re-occurrence of an AIDS-defining opportunistic complication after 3 mos of ART. Immune reconstitution inflammatory syndrome (IRIS) (pg 525) should not be considered as evidence of treatment failure.

GUIDELINES FOR CHANGING ANTIRETROVIRAL REGIMENS

(Modified from 2011 DHHS Guidelines and 2008 IAS-USA Guidelines) Major reasons for changing the initial regimen are drug toxicity, virologic failure or because of miscellaneous issues such as cost, access or convenience.

- **Changes due to toxicity:** Single agent substitution can be made assuming there has been adequate virologic response and the substitution is rational on the basis of potency and prior resistance test results (Table 4-17).

■ TABLE 4-17: **Monitoring for Adverse Drug Reactions (ADRs) (***CID* 2006; 43:645 and 2008 DHHS Guidelines)

Test	Frequency	Comment
Chemistry	Entry to care and q6-12mos With ART: baseline, at 2-8 wks, then q3-6mos	■ Includes electrolytes, BUN, creatinine, estimated creatinine clearance, liver function tests ■ Some experts monitor serum phosphate with TDF
Fasting lipids: cholesterol (total, LDL, HDL), triglycerides	Entry to care and annually if normal With ART: baseline, at 4-8 wks, then q6mos if abnormal, q12mos if normal	■ Interpret in context of Framingham risks (pg 139) and ART agent-specific risks
CBC with differential	Baseline and q3-6mos	■ If given AZT, repeat at 2-8 wks and prn
Glucose (fasting)	Entry to care, then annual With ART: baseline, then q3-6mos	■ Test q3-6mos if last test abnormal, q6mos if normal
Urinalysis	Entry to care With ART: baseline, then q12mos	■ If on TDF repeat q6mos and prn

Antiretroviral Therapy

4

- **Changes due to convenience:** ART may be changed to improve convenience based on pill burden or dosing frequency (Table 4-15), drug interactions (such as the need for methadone or rifampin), or to eliminate side effects (such as substitution of RAL for ENF).

- **Changes due to virologic failure:** Virologic failure is defined by failure to achieve a decrease in VL by 1 log c/mL in the first 1-4 wks, a VL <500 c/mL at 24 wks, a VL <200 c/mL at 48 weeks and any sustained VL >200 c/mL after 48 weeks. Note that the ACTG and the 2011 DHHS Guidelines changed the VL threshold that defines virological failure as measured by standard laboratory testing from >50 c/mL to >200 c/mL. The reason is that most reports in the 50-200 c/mL range represent blips, but they cause concern, expense and inconvenience due to return visits and unnecessary resistance testing. Nevertheless, the therapeutic goal remains <50 c/mL, since this appears to indicate absence of viral replication based on studies showing lack of sequence evolution (*J Virol* 2006;80:6441; *J Virol* 2009;83: 8470), lack of virologic benefit with intensification (*PNAS* 2009;106:9403; *CID* 2010;50:912), and data suggeston that blips are not caused by replicating virus and are clinically inconsequential (*JAMA* 2005;293:817; *J Virol* 2004;78:968).

- **Risk factors for virologic failure:** 1) Suboptimal adherence: the most important factor in large studies (*AIDS* 2001;15:185); 2) date of initiation of ART: patients treated in the pre-HAART era often took sub-optimal regimens associated with high failure rates and high rates of resistance (*JID* 2008;197 Suppl 3:261); 3) agent-specific risks: NNRTIs, RAL, 3TC and FTC are more prone to resistance mutations than RTV-boosted PIs or MVC (Table 4 18); 4) high baseline VL (>100,000 c/ml): although most of the currently recommended regimens appear to be almost equally effective in patients with high or low baseline VL; 5) advanced HIV disease as indicated by low CD4 count or an AIDS defining illness; 6) failure of the drugs to reach the site of viral infection due to problems with adherence, drug interactions (methadone, rifampin, etc) and drug toxicity. Factors that affect drug pharmacology include renal disease, hepatic disease and the genetics of drug metabolism, especially as related to the P450 metabolic pathway; 7) comorbidities that substantially affect adherence such as depression, substance abuse, poverty and co-morbidity medical conditions; 8) lack of access to continuous therapy due to interruptions in pharmacy supply, drug payment issues and idiosyncracies of the health system; and 9) transmitted drug resistance that is in the latent pool and not detected with baseline testing (*JAMA* 2011;305:1327).

- **Evaluation of virologic failure should include:**
  - Comprehensive review of adherence-related issues, including detailed review of the regimen using pills or pill charts and timing of doses, assessment of food or drug interactions, review of drug

access and review of toxicities. Pharmacy records are valuable when available (*AIDS Care* 2010;10:1189).

□ Medical history review, including sequential CD4 counts, VLs, concurrent medications and co-morbidities.

□ Current and prior resistance tests. Most important in this assessment are the results of all current and prior resistance tests and prior antiretroviral exposure and response, including failure and toxicity. It must be emphasized that resistance mutations, once selected, are archived in the latent pool and will re-emerge under selective pressure (*JID* 2003;188:1433; *JAMA* 2011; 305:1327). Resistance mutations that are documented at any time are assumed to persist, and a history of virologic failure while on treatment with drugs with lower genetic barriers to resistance (3TC, FTC, NVP, EFV and RAL) should raise the possibility of resistance, which is still best documented with testing performed during treatment.

- **The most important principles for drug selection in the face of virologic failure are:**

  □ Use at least two and preferably three agents from ≥2 classes that are active based on a review of current and prior test results (see below) and treatment history.

  □ Address issues that prevented an adequate response to the prior or current regimen. The major concern is adherence; other issues are potency of the regimen, drug interactions and pharmacologic issues.

  □ The change in therapy due to virologic failure should occur rapidly to avoid the accumulation of additional resistance mutations that will further restrict future options (*AIDS* 2007;21:721). Exceptions are with 3TC and FTC.

  □ Do not stop therapy except for toxicity.

  □ Do not add a single drug to a failing regimen.

- **Resistance tests:** These tests are most accurate for evaluating resistance to drug classes being taken at the time the test is performed or within 4 wks of discontinuation of therapy. Transmitted mutations persist longer than acquired mutations; the duration of persistence depends somewhat on the effect of the mutation on replication capacity. For example, thymidine analog mutations (TAMs) and NNRTI mutations generally persist, whereas the strains with PI mutations or the M184V mutation are more quickly replaced by wild-type virus. Resistance assays do not reliably detect minority species (<20% of the viral population) (*JAMA* 2011;305:1327) and therefore are better at indicating what drug not to use and best for drugs that are currently being taken. Always consider prior resistance test results and treatment history, including duration of therapy in the presence of virologic failure and agent-specific genetic

4 Antiretroviral Therapy

barriers to resistance (high barrier with most boosted PIs and thymidine analogs; low barrier with 3TC, FTC, RAL and NNRTIs).

The sensitivity of resistance testing after ART is discontinued depends on the time off treatment and the drug being evaluated (*AAC* 2004;48:644). Wild-type virus may re-emerge as early as 4 wks after discontinuation, especially with respect to PI mutations, so 4 wks after drug discontinuation is the anticipated maximal duration of resistance test validity. Nevertheless, some mutations such as NNRTI or thymidine analog mutations, may persist for 9-12 mos or longer (*J Clin Lab Anal* 2002;16:76), possibly because they do not alter replication capacity (*J Med Virol* 2003;69:1). The M184V mutation more strongly influences replication capacity (*AAC* 2003;47:3377) and may become undetectable within 5-20 weeks after discontinuation (*AAC* 2002;46:2255; *AAC* 2004;48:644). With newer drugs used in highly treatment-experienced patients, the response rates are often dependent on the number of active drugs in the regimen and the number of resistance mutations affecting response to the newer agent(s) (see pg. 33-48).

STRATEGIES FOR VIROLOGIC FAILURE

In the first decade of HAART, the probability of success was greatest with the initial regimen and decreased with each successive regimen. This has changed with more recent drug development; in salvage trials, a large proportion of patients achieved full virologic suppression despite extensive drug resistance (*Lancet* 2007;370;29; *Lancet* 2007;369:1169; *Lancet* 2006;268:466; *NEJM* 2008;359:339). The goal of treatment remains full virologic suppression to <50 c/mL to prevent resistance, stop disease progression and preserve future treatment options. This goal is now achieved in most patients (*AIDS* 2010;24:2469; *NEJM* 2009;360:1815).

- **First regimen failure:** In most cases the usual regimen change after virologic failure of the initial regimen is to switch to an alternate regimen based on resistance tests, preferably performed on treatment or within 4 wks of changing or stopping treatment (2011 DHHS Guidelines; IAS-USA Guidelines). Lack of resistance despite failure typically indicates non-adherence. Resupression on PI/r-based ART can usually be achieved by improved adherence.

- **3TC and FTC resistance:** With virologic failure, an early NRTI resistance mutation to appear with most regimens containing 3TC or FTC is 184V, which reduces activity of 3TC and FTC. Some residual antiviral activity is retained, possibly due to decreased replication capacity associated with the 184V mutation. The mutation results in an increase in activity of AZT, d4T, and TDF without risk of further NRTI resistance mutations. For this reason it is sometimes recommended that 3TC or FTC be continued despite resistance, but in such cases these drugs should not be counted as active components of an antiviral regimen.

Antiretroviral Therapy

112

- **Virologic failure without resistance mutations:** If the test was performed on therapy, the usual cause is failure of the drug to reach the target due to inadequate adherence or, less often, due to drug interactions, noncompliance with food requirements, etc. This is most common with boosted-PI-based ART and usually means the regimen will be successful if properly taken.

- **PI-based regimen with virologic failure:** Patients failing PI-based regimens frequently have no PI resistance mutations, in which case the cause of failure is usually non-adherence. Options are: 1) correct errors in adherence, drug interactions or other pharmacologic issues that might account for suboptimal response; 2) add RTV boosting (applies only to FPV or ATV, if being given unboosted); 3) intensify with an additional agent; or 4) change regimen. Response should be monitored with VL testing at 2-4 wks after a new regimen. Multiple studies show that virologic failure on PI/r-based ART in patients without pre-existing PI mutations is not associated with primary PI resistance mutation (Table 4-18). The NRTIs given concurrently are also somewhat protected, although NRTI resistance can still occur, especially to 3TC or FTC (ACTG 5142; *NEJM* 2008;358:2059)

- **NNRTI-based regimen with failure:** Virologic failure with EFV usually results in a K103N mutation with cross-resistance to NVP, but retained susceptibility to ETR and RPV. Switch options usually include ETR as well as PI/r, RAL and MVC. The favored mutation with NVP resistance is the 181C, which substantially reduces activity of EFV and ETR. The favored mutation with RPV is 138K, which reduces ETR activity (*AAC* 2011;55:600). The switch to ETR for virologic failure or toxicity is generally straightforward (*AIDS* 2011;25:143). The switch from EFV to RPV is more complicated due to the long half-life of EFV and drug interations of RPV. Guidance in switching EFV → RPV is under investigation. It should be emphasized that there is no benefit and some potential harm to continuing EFV or NVP in the face of virologic failure with resistance. There is no benefit because once resistance has occurred there is no residual antiviral effect and no negative effect on viral fitness (*J Med Virol* 2003;69:1; *JID* 192:1537). The potential harm is the accumulation of NNRTI resistance mutations that will impair effectiveness of second generation NNRTIs such as ETR.

- **NRTI resistance with virologic failure:** A dual-NRTI combination is a standard component of the initial regimen. NRTI-containing regimens are usually superior to most available "NRTI-sparing" combinations (Tables 4-23A and 23B). 3TC or FTC are often continued even in the presence of the M184V mutation due to good tolerability, documented antiviral effect attributed to reduction in replication capacity and/or partial antiviral effect, and increased activity of AZT, TDF, and d4T (*JID* 2005; 192:1537; *J Virol* 2009;83:2036; *AIDS* 2006;20:795; *AAC* 2003; 47:3478). The

4 Antiretroviral Therapy

selection of the backbone is based on resistance testing, consideration of comorbid conditions (e.g., renal impairment, cardiovascular risk factors, HBV coinfection), and avoidance of incompatible or toxic combinations (e.g., AZT+d4T, ddI+d4T, ddI+TDF).

- **MVC**: This CCR5 antagonist offers a relatively new option for patients with extensive treatment experience and resistance. There are two caveats. First, the patient must be shown to have R5 virus using a tropism assay. Unfortunately, approximately 50-60% of patients with extensive treatment experience have dual/mixed (DM) or X4-tropic virus and are not candidates for MVC therapy (Table 2-16) (*CID* 2007;44:591-5). MVC has many drug interactions, so dose adjustments of MVC are commonly needed (Table 5-58A, pg. 321).

- **RAL:** The integrase inhibitor raltegravir offers another option, with advantages of potency, excellent tolerability, virtually assured susceptibility and minimal drug interactions. Results of these trials are summarized in Table 4-19 showing cross-study comparisons. Continued RAL with resistance mutations confers no therapeutic benefit (*JAC* 2009;64:1087).

■ TABLE 4-18: **Frequency of Resistance Mutations Associated with Virologic Failure**

Class	Agent	Trial	Resistance*
PI/r†	LPV/r	ACTG 5142 (1)	0/76
		ARTEMIS (2)	0/31
		CASTLE (3)	0/15
	ATV/r	ACTG 5202 (4)	0/140
		CASTLE (3)	1/15 (7%)
	DRV/r	ARTEMIS (2)	0/46
	FPV/r	SOLO (8)	0/32
Integrase Inhibitor	RAL	STARTMRK (6)	4/8 (50%)
		BENCHMRK (7)	64/94 (68%)
CCR5 Antagonist	MVC	MERIT (8)	13/29‡ (45%)
NRTI	EFV	ACTG 5142 (1)	11/46 (24%)
		ACTG 5202 (4)	49/154 (32%)
		MERIT (8)	9/13 (69%)

*   Resistance = Number of major resistance mutations to the agent noted / number of sensitivity tests done in virologic failures

†   Total for PI/r = 1/323 (0.3%)

‡   X4 virus 9/29 (31%); R5 resistance 4/29 (14%)

References: 1) *NEJM* 2008;358:2059; 2) *AIDS* 2009;23:1679; 3) *JAIDS* 2010;53:323; 4) *Ann Intern Med* 2011;154:445; 5) *AIDS* 2004;18:651; 6) *Lancet* 2009;374:796; 7) *NEJM* 2008;359:355; 8) *JID* 2010;201:803

Antiretroviral Therapy

- **Extensive drug resistance:** There are now 25 drugs and 6 classes, so nearly all patients have options (Table 4-1) as shown in the TRIO trials (*CID* 2009;49:1441; *Drugs* 2010;70:1629). This report showed that 90% of patients with "triple class resistance" had VL <200 c/mL at 24 weeks on a regimen of RAL+ETR+DRV/r. Nevertheless, there will always be patient situations in which no good options are available. In such patients, one option is participation in a clinical trial that targets multi-class failure patients, possibly with access to a new drug class or an alternative novel strategy. If virologic control cannot be achieved, the goal of therapy should be viral suppression to the greatest extent possible, with the goal of increasing or at least maintaining the CD4 count, since this ultimately determines the risk for most of the HIV-associated complications. It is noted that multiple studies have found CD4 counts tend to be stable or increase modestly despite VL indicating virologic failure (*AIDS* 1999;13:1035). In fact, a review of 6 seminal salvage trials (POWER, RESIST, TORO, DUET, MOTIVATE, BENCHMRK) in which patients in the control groups, who took only an optimized background regimen (OBR), experienced substantial increases in mean CD4 counts despite virologic failure rates of 60-80%. A review of RESIST, POWER, DUET and BENCHMRK trials demonstrated high failure rates in the OBR group (mean 54%), but the mean CD4 at one-year increased 38 cells/mm^3 vs. 103 cells/mm^3 in the group getting the test agent. Nevertheless, it must be emphasized that the goal of therapy is a VL <50 c/mL.

■ TABLE 4-19: **Flagship Salvage Trials: 48 Week Results**

Agent	Citation	Trial	No.	VL <50 OBR*	Mean CD4 count in OBR†
ENF	*JAIDS* 2005;40:404	TORO	661	8%	+90
TPV	*Lancet* 2006;368:466	RESIST	1,486	10%	+18
DRV	*Lancet* 2007;369:1169	POWER	255	10%	+19
RAL	*NEJM* 2008;359:1429	BENCHMRK	703	33%	+54
MVC	*NEJM* 2008;359:339/355	MOTIVATE	1,049	17%	+45
ETR	*Lancet* 2007;370:29/39	DUET	1,203	40%	+73

* OBR=Optimal background regimen
† Mean CD4 count increase (cells/mm^3) at 48 weeks in the OBR group with virologic failure rates of 60-92%

Continuing ART in the face of virologic failure has the benefit of reduced risk of clincial failure but at the cost of increasing resistance and decreasing future options. Prior studies show that continuing the same regimen with a VL >1000 c/mL results in an average loss of about one drug option per year (*Scand J Infect Dis* 2005;37:890; *CID*

4 Antiretroviral Therapy

2006;43:1329). These decisions are based on CD4 count and current options at the time the study was done. A concern with stopping ART is the rapid virologic rebound and CD4 decline as shown in the SMART trial (see Table 4-20, pg. 121).

- **Summary of recommendations for extensive resistance:**

1. The regimen should include <u>at least 2 and preferably 3 active drugs</u>.

2. <u>3TC or FTC</u> is often continued, despite resistance (but they do not count as active drugs). Use of other NRTIs to which the virus is resistant is arbitrary, but some studies show efficacy when options are limited (*JAIDS* 2011;57:24).

3. <u>First generation NNRTIs</u> (NVP or EFV) should be permanently stopped once resistance is observed. Second generation NNRTIs (RPV and ETR) may be options depending on resistance test results and ability to deal with RPV/EFV interactions.

4. Make optimal use of <u>current and historic resistance tests</u>.

5. With extensive resistance and limited options, consider <u>infrequently used agents</u> such as ENF or the TRIO combination (RAL+ETR+DRV/r) (*Drugs* 2010;70:1629). Recycling drugs with prior resistance has no established merit.

6. When necessary, seek access to <u>investigational drugs</u> through clinical trials or expanded access programs.

7. If at least <u>2 active agents are not available</u>, the goal of treatment is to: (a) reduce VL as much as possible and for long as possible; (b) maintain or increase the CD4 count; (c) reduce drug toxicity; and (d) limit use of drugs likely to lead to resistance mutations that may limit future treatment options. Note that patients with a VL <10,000 c/mL usually have a stable or increasing CD4 count on ART (*AIDS* 1999;13:1035).

8. The <u>urgency of decisions</u> in patients with limited options is usually driven by the risk of progression, which is largely reflected by the CD4 count.

9. <u>Mega-HAART, recycling, dual PIs and treatment interruption</u>, all historic tactics for managing patients with extensive drug resistance, are antiquated and should not be used.

Treatment Strategies
STOPPING HAART

- **Virologic failure:** Most patients with virologic failure that cannot be corrected with salvage regimens should not discontinue ART, since this results in a prompt increase in VL averaging 0.8-1.0 $\log_{10}$ c/mL (to pre-treatment baseline levels with a concurrent rapid decrease in CD4 count averaging 85-100 cells/mm^3 in 3 mos (*NEJM* 2003;349:

837; *JID* 2000;181:946). Thus, despite virologic failure as defined by the 200 c/mL threshold, the failing regimen often has significant activity. The attempt to determine the ARV agents that are responsible for this residual activity suggest a debated role for 3TC (and FTC by inference) and possibly other NRTIs and PIs, but not EFV or NVP (*JID* 2005;192: 1537). Nevertheless, continuation of antiviral agents in the face of ongoing viral replication has obvious risks based on cost, toxicity and resistance. With regard to resistance, the EuroSIDA study showed that continued use of a failing regimen resulted in an average of 2 new resistance mutations and loss of 1.25 active antiviral agents per 6 mos (*AIDS* 2007;21:721), which could have an important impact on future options (*JID* 2003;188:1001). The usual recommendation is not to discontinue ART, but to tailor the regimen to the individual patient based on critical need (CD4 count), the potential for selection of further resistance mutations that could affect future options, and the ability to achieve partial virologic control. Prior studies suggest clinical and immunologic benefit when the VL is maintained ≤10,000 c/mL (*Curr Opin Infect Dis* 2001; 14:23; *NEJM* 2001;344:472). With regard to agent selection, 3TC or FTC is usually for the reasons noted above. PI/r are often favored with selection based on the combination of genotype and phenotype sensitivity tests interpreted by an expert. RAL is preferably avoided unless there is likelihood of a fully-suppressive regimen; the concern is resistance to this and the next generation agents in this class. There is no evidence that EFV or NVP contribute to residual antiviral activity in the face of resistance, and continuation results in acquisition of new NNRTI mutations that could reduce susceptibility to ETR or RPV. Recommendations for the use of specific agents in non-suppressive regimens cannot be made based on available data.

STOPPING NVP AND EFV-BASED ART: These drugs have long half-lives. As a result, discontinuation of EFV- or NVP-containing regimens results in the equivalent of prolonged monotherapy drugs that have low barriers to resistance (*JID* 2006;42: 401). Methods to avoid resistance include staggered discontinuation with continuation of NRTIs for a period of time following discontinuation of the NNRTI, or substitution of a PI/r for the NNRTI for 2-4 weeks prior to discontinuation of the entire regimen.

- NVP: This drug auto-induces hepatic CYP3A4 metabolism over 2-4 wks to reduce half-life from 45 to 25 hrs (*JID* 1995;171:537). With single dose NVP used to prevent perinatal transmission, resistance mutations have been reported in 15-75% of treated women due to prolonged exposure to subtherapeutic levels of NVP (*JID* 2005;192:24). Resistance was significantly reduced with the use of AZT/3TC continued after administration of single-dose NVP for 3-7 days (*JID* 2006;193:482), although 5/39 (13%) developed primary resistance mutations despite use of AZT/3TC. On the basis of this observation, the 2008 Recommendations for Use of Antiretroviral Drugs in Pregnant HIV-Infected Women recommend that single-dose NVP be accompanied by a 7-day "tail" of AZT/3TC, and also acknowledges that this reduces but does not eliminate the risk of NVP resistance, since the right duration of the NRTI tail is unknown. The risk of developing NNRTI resistance after discontinuation of a suppressive NVP-based regimen may be lower than that seen with single-dose NVP, assuming the VL is suppressed at the time of discontinuation. Nevertheless, the concerns discussed below (EFV) also apply to NVP. Some have suggested that the "tail" should be up to 2 wks for NVP, particularly in the first 1-2 wks prior to autoinduction of metabolic pathways (*AIDS* 2007;21:1673). Another issue relating to this is reintroduction of NVP after discontinuation. The recommendation is to repeat the low-dose (200 mg qd) lead-in for 2 wks if the time off NVP exceeds 2 wks.

- EFV: The half-life of EFV ranges from 36 to 100 hrs, significantly longer than that of NVP. The major metabolic pathway is CYP2B6, and there are significant variations in half-life that are governed largely by polymorphisms at codon 516 of the CYP2B6 gene (*CID* 2006;42:401; *CID* 2007;45:1230; *JID* 2011;203:246). The result is that therapeutic levels can be detected for over 21 days after the drug is discontinued in some patients (*AIDS* 2005;19:716; *CID* 2006;42: 401). The risk of EFV resistance with discontinuation of all agents in EFV-based ART was 16% in SMART and anecdotally reported by others (*Lancet* 2006;368:459; *AIDS* 2007;21:1673, *CID* 2008;46: 1601). Recommendations to prevent resistance in this situation are to continue the two NRTs for 1-2 wks ("the NRTI tail" method) or substitution of a PI-based regimen for 3-4 wks (*AIDS* 2007;21:1673). Despite this recommendation it should be noted that the half-life of EFV is highly variable based on genetic variation in EFV metabolism, and the appropriate duration of this is not known, making the "NRTI tail" method unpredictable and the PI substitution method more attractive (2011 DHHS Guidelines).

INITIATING ART WITH AN HIV-ASSOCIATED COMPLICATION: Many patients present with an HIV-associated complication, and nearly all require ART as well as management of the complication, and this raises the question of timing of the initiation of ART. The issue is confounded by several interrelated variables, including: 1) the risk of the immune reconstitution syndrome (IRIS), 2) the urgency of starting ART based largely on the CD4 count, and 3) the complications incurred by treating the two conditions simultaneously in terms of drug interactions, drug toxicity and pill burden. The impression given in the early analyses was dominated by the philosophy that ART is rarely a therapeutic emergency, IRIS is a confusing and potentially serious complication, and these considerations justified a delay in starting ART. However, several studies have addressed this issue, and the emerging consensus is as follows:

Antiretroviral Therapy

- ART should be started immediately for conditions that represent important complications of advanced HIV and have no good therapeutic intervention other than ART (e.g., PML, microsporidiosis, cryptosporidiosis, HIV-associated nephropathy and HIV-associated dementia).

- For conditions for which there is effective therapy and a risk of IRIS such as MAC, PCP, cryptococcal meningitis and toxoplasmosis: ART should usually begin within 2 wks. This recommendation is based largely on results of ACTG 5164, a randomized trial of 283 treatment-naive HIV-infected patients with a median CD4 count of 29 cells/mm³ and a new AIDS-defining non-tuberculosis OI (*PLoS One* 2009;4:e5575). Participants were randomized to early ART (within 14 days) or delayed ART (after OI treatment completed). Results showed a significant benefit with early ART based on the study endpoint of AIDS progression or death (OR 0.51; 95 CI 0.27-0.94). The median time to initiate ART in this trial was 12 days in the early group and 45 days in the delayed group. A subsequent report on this study suggested that early ART did not increase the risk of IRIS with non-tuberculosis OIs (*PLoS One* 2010;5:e11416). Initiation of ART in patients with cryptococcal meningitis is debated based on a study from Zimbabwe that showed a mortality rate of 88% with ART given within 72 hours compared to 54% with ART delayed to 10 weeks (*CID* 2010;50:1532) The very high mortality rate in this trial makes it hard to interpret and generalize the findings, but many would avoid early initiation of ART in patients with cryptococcal meningitis, especially those with elevated intracranial pressures.

- Tuberculosis: See pg. 464-465.

IMMUNOLOGIC FAILURE: This refers to unexplained failure to achieve and maintain an adequate CD4 count despite virologic suppression. There is no consensus definition: some define it as failure to achieve an increase to selected thresholds that represent risks for HIV-related complications such as 50, 100 or 200 cells/mm³, some use a suboptimal CD4 cell response such as an increase of <50 cells/mm³/year, and some use thresholds of 350 or 500 cells/mm³ at 4-7 years. In a review of 53 therapeutic trials with 14,264 treatment-naïve patients, the median CD4 count increase at one year with good viral suppression was 180-200 cells/mm³ (*AIDS* 2006;20:2051). Immune recovery was significantly greater with boosted PIs than with NNRTI-based ART (+200 cells/mm³ vs. 179 cells/mm³).

- Factors contributing to poor CD4 response include interferon or prednisone therapy, advanced age, co-infection with HTLV-1, HTLV-2, HCV or HIV-2 and serious co-morbidities (see pg. 30-31).

- Antiretroviral drugs: The CD4 response: 1) is somewhat lower with EFV-based ART compared to alternative regimens including PI/r, MVC and RAL. The difference is often statistically significant in large

4 Antiretroviral Therapy

trials of treatment-naive patients, but there are no apparent medical consequences; 2) AZT-based regimens may have reduced response based on studies showing CD4 increase after switching to ABC or TDF (*NEJM* 2006; 354:251; and 3) the combination of TDF+ddI has been associated with a blunted CD4 response (*CID* 2005;19:569).

- Risk of an OI: The risk of an OI in patients with virologic suppression is substantially reduced despite a blunted CD4 response (*JID* 2005; 192:1407; *AIDS* 2006;20:371). The best documentation comes from the ClinSurv Study (*JID* 2011; 203:364), which analyzed data for 1,318 patients with VL <50 c/mL and CD4 counts <200 cells/mm³. There were only 42 new OI events with 5,038 patient-years follow-up or about 1/12 decades. Although PCP prophylaxis is still recommended in this group, the risk of PCP is very low. One study found showed zero cases of PCP per 1000 patient-years follow-up in patients with a CD4 count of 100-200 cells/mm³ (*CID* 2010;51:611).

- Interventions: Options to improve the CD4 response include changing the ART regimen. As noted, the CD4 response with EFV-based ART is somewhat less robust than with RAL-, DRV/r-, LPV/r- or MVC-based ART among those with viral suppression to <50 c/mL (see pg. 195, 248, 354). Nevertheless, this difference is of unclear clinical significance, and there has been no convincing benefit with drug switches. The usual approach is to ignore the issue based on the ClinSurv data. Another option is treatment intensification with additional antivirals despite effective viral suppression, but this approach has not succeeded in increasing the CD4 count (*PLoS One* 2011;6:e14764). There have also been attempts to supplement the regimen with an agent known to stimulate CD4 production. IL-2 increases CD4 count (*Arch Intern Med* 2007;167:597), but this was not associated with a clinical benefit in two large clinical trials (ESPRIT and SILCAAT) with 5706 randomized patients (*NEJM* 2009;361:1548). Some studies suggest a genetic basis for the blunted CD4 response in some patients (*JID* 2006;194:1098; *JAIDS* 2006:41:1). There are no management recommendations, and the highest priority remains virologic suppression with adequate attention to concurrent medications (steroids, etc) and co-morbidities that might be contributing.

INTERMITTENT TREATMENT INTERRUPTION: The rationale for intermittent treatment interruption had been to reduce drug cost, toxicity and inconvenience while maintaining viral suppression. However, the **SMART** trial demonstrated that CD4-based treatment interruption using a CD4 threshold of 350 cells/mm³ for interruption and 250 cells/mm³ for reinitiation was associated with a significantly higher risk of opportunistic infections and death than continuous ART (*JID* 2008;97:1145) (Table 4-20).

■ TABLE 4-20: **Results of SMART (*NEJM* 2006;355:2283)**

Drug	Interrupted ART n = 2720		Continuous ART n = 2752	
	N	Event rate (/100 p-y[†])	N	Event rate (/100 p-y[†])
Primary end point	120	3.3	47	1.3*
Death any cause	55	1.5	30	0.8*
Serious OI	13	0.4	2	0.1*
Major cardiovascular, hepatic, or renal disease	65	1.8	39	1.1*
Cardiovascular	46	1.3	31	0.8*
Renal	9	0.2	2	0.1*
Hepatic	10	0.3	7	0.2*
Grade 4 event	173	5.0	1480	4.2*

* P = <0.05

† p-y = person years

Scheduled interruptions: The **STACCATO** trial attempted the alternate-weeks strategy (also called **WOWO** for "week-on, week-off") with various regimens; virologic failure occurred in 53% in the experimental treatment group compared to 5% of controls treated with continuous ART (*Lancet* 2006;368:459). This study also showed a high rate of new resistance mutations in the WOWO group (*CID* 2005;40:728). A more recent trial with an 8 wks on, 8 wks off strategy was used in the **DART** study, but this was stopped early due to excessive HIV-related complications in the intermittent therapy arm (*Lancet* 2010;395:123). Another intermittent therapy study is called **FOTO**, "five [days] on, two off." With its long half-life, EFV presumably maintains its antiviral activity over the weekend. The initial experience with 20 participants in the FOTO trial has shown continued viral suppression in 19/20 taking NNRTI-based ART at 1 year (*HIV Clin Trials* 2007;8:256). This strategy should be reserved for patients in clinical trials until more data have accumulated. Treatment interruption is never recommended, especially if it results in virologic rebound.

MONOTHERAPY: The basic standard of at least two active drugs (and preferably three) was established in 1996 with the inception of the HAART era as shown in the Merck 035 trial (*NEJM* 1997;337:734). The combination of AZT/3TC+IDV achieved viral suppression (<50 c/mL) in 80% of patients compared to 43% given IDV alone and zero given AZT/3TC. Attempts to find exceptions have included several trials of monotherapy using boosted PIs. The goals are to reduce pill burden, cost and side effects. Results of 11 trials investigating this approach are summarized in Table 4-21, including 6 with LPV/r bid, 2 with DRV/r and 3 small trials with ATV/r. The format for 9 of the 11 was to achieve virologic suppression (VL <50 c/mL) on a standard 3-drug regimen, and then to discontinue NRTIs, leaving patients on boosted PI monotherapy, usually with continuation of the standard three-drug

4 Antiretroviral Therapy

regimen as the comparator. Monotherapy has been attempted only with PI/r based on the assumption that resistance would be unlikely and virologic control could be achieved by if necessary by restarting NRTIs.

Conclusions regarding these data based on the results in Table 4-21 and a review by I Perez-Valero and J. Arribas (*Curr Opin Infect Dis* 2011;24:7):

■ TABLE 4-21: **Monotherapy Trials with Boosted Protease Inhibitors**

Trial	Design*	Duration (wks)	Regimen	N	VL <50 c/mL
LPV/r					
MONARK [1]	Treatment-naive	48	LPV/r bid	83	67%
			LPV/r + AZT/3TC	53	75%
OK-04 [2]	Induction-maintenance	96	LPV/r bid	100	77%
			LPV/r + 2N	98	78%
KalMo [3]	Induction-maintenance	96	LPV/r bid	30	80%
			Current Rx	30	87%
SHCS [4]	Induction-maintenance	†	LPV/r bid	42	75%
			Current Rx	18	100%
STAR [5]	NRTI failure	48	LPV/r bid	100	64%
			LPV/r + TDF + 3TC	100	82%
Cameron [6]	Induction-maintenance	96	LPV/r bid	104	48%
			EFV + AZT/3TC	51	61%
DRV/r					
MONOI [7]	Induction-maintenance	48	DRV/r qd	113	94%
			DRV/r + 2 NRTIs	112	99%
MONET [8]	Induction-maintenance	48	DRV/r qd	127	86%
			DRV/r + 2 NRTIs	129	88%
ATV/r					
ATARITMO [9]	Induction-maintenance	24	ATV/r qd	27	93%
Karolinski [10]	Induction-maintenance	72	ATV/r qd	15	83%
ACTG5201 [11]	Induction-maintenance	28	ATV/r qd	34	85%

* Induction-maintenance consisted of randomization in patients with VL <50 c/mL

† Study discontinued due to excessive failure rates in the monotherapy arm (6 vs. 0) including 5 with high HIV levels in CSF [4]

References:
1) *AIDS* 2008;22:385, see pg. 312; 2) *JAIDS* 2009;51:147,see pg. 311; 3) *HIV Clin Trials* 2009;10:368, see pg. 311; 4) *AIDS* 2010;24:2347; 5) 2011 CROI;Abstr. 584, see pg. 312; 6) *AIDS* 2010;24L223; 7) *AIDS* 2010;24:2365, see pg. 228; 8) *JAIDS* 2010;47:223, see pg. 228; 9) *AIDS* 2007;21:1309; 10) *JAIDS* 2007;44:417; 11) *JID* 2009;199:866.

- **Relative merits:** 1) the best results have been with DRV/r given once daily in the MONET trial; 2) trials with ATV/r have been too small to allow for conclusions; and 3) the most extensive data are with LPV/r given twice daily.

- **Benefit:** a large proportion of patients can maintain suppression with DRV/r or LPV/r using an induction-maintenance approach.

- **Risks:** LPV/r monotherapy is associated with higher rates of low level viremia (50-500 c/mL) and higher rates of virologic failures than standard therapy, but most virologic failures can be "rescued" with reintroduction of 2 NRTIs, and resistance mutations are relatively rare. The SHCS trial (*AIDS* 2010;24:2347) suggests that LPV/r montherapy fails to protect the CNS. (This concern may apply to DRV/r also, but it has not been studied).

- **HIV guidelines** generally do not recommend PI/r monotherapy except for the European AIDS Clinical Society Guidelines, which state that it can be tried in adherent patients who have NRTI toxicity or other contraindications to standard ART.

NUCLEOSIDE-SPARING REGIMENS: Standard treatment of all treatment-naïve patients and most treatment-experienced patients consists of a "backbone" consisting of 2 NRTIs. However, there are multiple clinical settings in which use of these drugs are considered ill-advised, primarily due to safety concerns and sometimes resistance. Multiple NRTI-sparing regimens have been studied (Tables 4-22A and 4-22B). Most show limited benefit compared to standard treatment. It should be noted that 3TC and FTC are rarely contraindicated, since they have excellent tolerability, no well-characterized long-term metabolic complications and continued, although reduced, activity in the presence of the 184V resistance mutation. Continued use does not lead to additional resistance nor eliminate antiviral activity (*JAIDS* 2010; 54:51; *AIDS* 2006;20:795; *J Virol* 2008;80:201; *JID* 2005:192:1537.

REGIMEN SIMPLIFICATION: This term is defined in the 2011 DHHS Guidelines as a regimen change to achieve reduction in pill burden or frequency of administration, improve tolerability, improve potency or to respond to new data or treatment recommendations. The ultimate goal is to use a regimen that provides long-term viral suppression and to maintain a good quality of life with minimal risk. Data to support this approach come from studies demonstrating that long-term adherence to ART correlates with reduced adherence demands, reduced pill burden, and better patient satisfaction (*NEJM* 2006;354:251; *AIDS Res Hum Retroviruses* 2007;23:1505; *JAIDS* 2004;36:808). The best candidates for this type of regimen change are those without a history of treatment failure or with known susceptibility to the agents in the new regimen. See **SWITCHMRK** pg. 357.

4 Antiretroviral Therapy

■ TABLE 4-22A: NRTI-sparing Regimens - Treatment-naïve Patients

Trial	Regimen (dose in mg)	Duration	N	Comment
1	LPV/r 533/133 bid + NVP 200 bid vs. NVP/r and NVP + 2 NRTIs	96 wks	26	High rate ADRs – only 6/26 (23%) reached 96 wks. No benefit vs. controls.
ACTG 5142 [2]	LPV/r 533/133 bid + EFV 600 qd vs. (EFV or LPV) + 2 NTRIs	96 wks	250	Viral failure 26% (similar in all 3 groups). More resistance mutations in NRTI-free arm
Study 4001078 [3]	MVC 150 qd + ATV/r 300/100 qd vs. ATV/r + TDF/FTC	24 wks	60	More viral failures (20% vs. 11%; p = NS) and grade 4 hyperbilirubinemia (33%)
ACTG 5262 [4]	DRV/r 800/100 qd + RAL 100 bid	48 wks	112	DRV trough ↓ 57%. No comparator group. Increased failure rate and integrase resistance with baseline VL > 100,000 c/mL
ANRS-121 [5]	(EFV or NVP) + (LPV/r or IDV/r) vs. NRTI-containing regimen	24 wks	117	Viral failures greater with NRTI-sparing (28% vs. 12%) and more EFV resistance mutations; not recommended
ACTG A5110 [6]	LPV/r 533/133 bid + NVP 200 bid vs. LPV/r + (AZT or d4T) or LPV/r + ABC	48 wks	101	VL > 200 c/mL in 3-6% (all 3 groups). Significant increase in toxicity with LPV/r + NVP (p = 0.007)

References:
1) *JAIDS* 2009;50:335; 2) *NEJM* 2008;358:2095;
3) Mills A. 2010 IAC;Abstr THLBB203; 4) TAIWO B. 2011 CROI:Abstr. 551:5;
5) *AIDS* 2009;23:1605; 6) *JAC* 2009;63:998

■ **Within-class substitutions:** Examples include the desire to eliminate thymidine analogs (AZT, d4T) and ddI in favor of less toxic agents or more convenient pill combinations. Another example is the switch from LPV/r to an alternative boosted PI to simplify the regimen, reduce LPV/r-associated intolerance side effects, or improve potency (as with ATV/r or DRV/r).

■ **Out-of-class substitutions:** Examples include switches to lower pill burden combinations. More such switches will became available with the anticipated single tablet regimens.

■ **Toxicity:** ENF switches were common and usually successful in maintaining viral suppression when new agents such as RAL and ETR become available (*JAC* 2009;64:1341).

■ **Cost:** This has not been a major issue in the past but may become important in cases where the cost of ART is a critical issue and comparable agents become available in generic form.

Antiretroviral Therapy

Trial	Regimen (dose in mg)	Duration	N	Comment
SPARTAN [7]	ATV 400 bid + RAL 300 bid vs. ATV/r + TDF/FTC	24 wks	63	VL <50 c/mL: 84% vs. 76% in comparator; study halted for: RAL resistance, bid dosing and excessive jaundice Good virologic response, but RAL resistance mutations in 4 and grade 4 hyperbilirubinemia (21% vs. 0)
No Nuke ANRS-108 [8]	PI/r + NNRTI (primarily IDV/r or LPV/r + NVP or EFV) vs. NRTI-containing regimen	48 wks	45	Study goal was reversal of d4T or AZT lipodystrophy. Viral suppression retained and SC fat increased
ACTG 5110 [9]	LPV/r 533/133 bid + NVP 200 bid vs. LPV/r + NVP + ABC	48 wks	53	NRTI-sparing group: maintained viral control and ↓ lipodystrophy but had earlier ADRs (p <0.007)
MULTINEKA [10]	LPV/r 400/100 bid + NVP 200 bid vs. LPV/r + 2 NRTI	48 wks	34	VL <50 c/mL maintained with slight lipodystrophy improvement
ACTG A5116 [11]	LPV/r 533/133 bid + EFV 600 qd vs. EFV + 2NRTIs	2.1 yrs	226	LPV/r + EFV showed higher rates of viral failure (12% vs. 6%) and toxicity (17% vs. 4%)
PROGRESS [12]	LPV 400/100 + RAL 400 qd vs. LPV/r + TDF/FTC	48 wks	206	VL <50 in 83-85% in both groups; similar ADRs. Most participants had low baseline VL
Monotherapy Regimens	DRV/r, LPV/r			Table 4-21
TRIO	RAL + ETR + DRV/r			See TRIO pg. 228

* Induction-maintenance consisted of randomization in patients with VL <50 c/mL

† Study discontinued due to excessive failure rates in the monotherapy arm (6 vs. 0) including 5 with high HIV levels in CSF [4]

References:
7) Kozal M. 2010 IAS;Abstr. THLBB2004; 8) *HIV Med* 2008;9:625;
9) *JAC* 2009;63:998; 10) *CID* 2009;49:892; 11) *AIDS* 2007;21:325;
12) Reynes J. IAC;Abstr. MOAB0101

Dose Adjustments (ART Agents)

DOSE ADJUSTMENT FOR HEPATIC FAILURE: See 2011 DHHS Guidelines; for Child-Pugh Score (CPS), see Table 5-1, pg. 177.

- **NRTIs:** Minimal effect because these drugs have limited first-pass metabolism and low protein binding and are eliminated primarily by renal excretion. No dose adjustments with liver disease except for ABC. Avoid or consider 200 mg bid.

Antiretroviral Therapy

4

- **NNRTIs:** Liver dysfunction has minimal effect on trough levels of EFV, RPV, ETR and NVP. Avoid NVP with Child-Pugh Class B or C disease due to risk of hepatotoxicity. RPV has not been evaluated in patients with class C disease.
- **PIs:** These are extensively metabolized by cytochrome p450 enzymes; recommendations are:
  - **NFV, LPV/r:** Standard doses; use with caution.
  - **IDV:** Recommended dose is IDV 600 mg q8h. Limited clinical data.
  - **ATV:** Child-Pugh B – 300 mg qd without boosting; Child-Pugh C – Avoid.
  - **DRV/r:** Use with caution; not recommended with severe liver disease.
  - **FPV:** Treatment-naïve: C-P class A or B – 700 mg bid (unboosted), class C – 350 mg bid; treatment-experienced: C-P class A 700/100 bid, class B 450/100 qd; class C 300 mg bid + RTV 100 qd
- **Fusion inhibitor (ENF):** No dose change
- **CCR5 antagonist (MVC):** No recommendations; MVC levels likely to increase
- **Integrase inhibitor (RAL):** No dose adjustment for C-P class A & B; avoid with class C

DOSE ADJUSTMENT FOR RENAL FAILURE: See 2011 DHHS Guidelines and Table 4-35, pg. 148.

- **NRTI:** All require dose adjustment except ABC (see pg. 179).
- **NNRTIs: EFV, ETR, NVP, RPV:** No dose adjustment for mild renal disease; use with caution with moderate or severe renal disease
- **PIs:**
  - **DRV, FPV, IDV, LPV/r, RTV, SQV** and **TPV:** use standard dose
  - **ATV:** With hemodialysis use ATV/r 300/100 qd for treatment-naïve patients; avoid ATV and ATV/r in treatment-experienced patients
- **CCR5 antagonist (MVC):** 300 mg bid without potent CYP3A inducers or inhibitors; not recommended if postural hypotension or with potent CYP3A inducers or inhibitors.
- **Integrase inhibitor (RAL):** No dose adjustment

THERAPEUTIC DRUG MONITORING (TABLE 4-23): TDM is a potential method for determining appropriate drug dosing for HIV-infected patients with issues that are problematic, including adherence, drug interactions, pregnancy, concentration-dependent toxicities, interpatient variation and/or altered physiology due to hepatic, renal, or GI complications. TDM cannot be readily performed with NRTIs because the *in vivo* correlates are with intracellular concentrations rather than plasma concentrations, but plasma concentrations can be meaningful. There may also be interest in drug concentration in other compartments such as CNS, genital tract, etc. Nevertheless TDM for clinical care is not recommended by the 2011 DHHS Guidelines for several reasons:

- Lack of large prospective studies showing improved outcomes;
- Lack of consistent data indicating clinically significant levels that correlate with therapeutic response or toxicity;
- General unavailability of reliable laboratory resources to do this work;
- Requirement of fastidious technique for collecting and processing specimens;
- Substantial intrapatient variation.

Clinical trial data show that even with highly qualified labs and careful technique, results vary enormously. In one study with an average of 40 samplings per drug per patient, the coefficient of variation for drug levels was 44% for PIs and 25% for NNRTIs (*CID* 2006;42:1189). Nevertheless, there are exceptions and some high quality labs have shown clinical utility of TDM, including dose adjustment of EFV to prevent CNS toxicity (*Antivir Ther* 2011;16:189) or to monitor PI-based ART (*JAC* 2009;64:109).

■ TABLE 4-23: **Suggested Minimum Concentrations for Drug Susceptible HIV-1 Virus (2011 DHHS Guidelines)**

Drug	Conc. (ng/mL)	Drug	Conc. (ng/mL)
APV	400	LPV	1000
ATV	150	MVC	>50
DRV	3300	NFV	800
EFV	1000*	NVP	3000
ETR	275	RAL	72
FPV	400	SQV	100-250
IDV	100†	TPV	20,500

* C_{min} >4,000 ng/mL associated w/CNS toxicity
† C_{max} >10,000 ng/mL associated w/toxicity

Adverse Drug Reactions to Antiretroviral Agents:
2011 DHHS Guidelines; Consensus Panel (*CID* 2006;43:645)

For reviews from authoritative sources, see IAS-USA guidelines (*JAIDS* 2002;31:257); nutrition guidelines (*CID* 2003;31:Suppl 2); dyslipidemia guidelines (*CID* 2003; 31:216); review of cardiovascular risk and body fat abnormalities (*NEJM* 2005;352:48; *Circulation* 2008;118:198; *CID* 2006;43:645; *Top HIV Med* 2011;19:23).

4 Antiretroviral Therapy

Lipodystrophy

Lipodystrophy is a term that has been used to describe two distinct clinical entities: fat accumulation and lipoatrophy. **Fat accumulation** is seen within the abdominal cavity (visceral adipose tissue or VAT), the upper back (dorsocervical fat pad or "buffalo hump"), the breasts (gynecomastia), and in subcutaneous tissue (peripheral lipomatosis). Some patients have a combination of abdominal obesity, hypertension, dyslipidemia and insulin resistance resulting in the metabolic syndrome, which predisposes to cardiovascular disease (*Arteroscleroisis* 2010;208:222; *NEJM* 2003;349:1993; *JAIDS* 2002;31:363; *CID* 2007; 44:726). This is attributed to growth hormone deficiency that is most common in men with HIV and most frequently expressed as abdominal fat accumulation. The pathogenesis is complex, debated, and possibly multifactorial (*Curr Opin Infect Dis* 2011;24:43). Causal or contributing factors may be defective peripheral adipocytes (*Am J Clin Nutr* 2005;81:1405), adiponectin (*J Clin Endocrinol Metab* 2003;88:629), the hormone leptin (*CID* 2003;36:795), cortisol excess (*Diabetologia* 2004;47:1668) and/or a growth hormone related factor (*JAMA* 2008;300:509). HIV medication appears to play a role (*Top HIV Med* 2008;16:127; *Curr HIV Res* 2010;8:545). **Lipoatrophy** includes loss of subcutaneous fat in the face, extremities, and buttocks. Patients with peripheral lipoatrophy often have central fat accumulation as well (*JAIDS* 2005;40:121). Lipoatrophy is caused by NRTIs, especially d4T, and to a lesser extent to AZT and ddI (*Sex Trans Infect* 2001;77: 158; *NEJM* 2008;358:2095). The cause of lipoatrophy is mitochondrial toxicity, and a genetic predisposition has been defined (C/C at the HFE 187 locus) (*JID* 2008;197:858). The cause of fat accumulation is less clear as noted above, but some studies support the effect of these drugs on adipocyte cell physiology (*J Infect Chemother* 2011;17:183).

■ **Frequency and risk factors:** Lipodystrophy has been reported in 20-80% of patients receiving ART, a wide range reflecting a heterogeneous population and the lack of a standard case definition (*CID* 2006;43:645). The incidence based on perceived changes in body fat sufficiently severe to be detected by both the patient and physician in patients receiving 2 NRTIs plus a PI was 17%, with a median follow-up of 18 mos (*Lancet* 2001;357:592). In a meta-analysis of 5 series with 5435 ART recipients, fat accumulation was reported in 13-33% of patients and lipoatrophy in 13-34% of patients (*CID* 2003;36:S84). Reported rates of lipoatrophy reflected extensive use of thymidine analogs; rates are lower now due to decreased use of these agents. AZT, d4T and ddI are the only established causes of lipoatrophy. Risk factors include treatment with these agents, older age and nadir CD4 count <200 cells/mm^3 (*AIDS* 2010;24:353). Risk factors for fat accumulation are prior obesity, low CD4 count prior to treatment, treatment with PI or NNRTI and older age (*CID* 2006;43:645).

- **Antiretroviral Agents**

  □ Fat accumulation is often associated with PI-based ART (*AIDS* 2001;15:231; *AIDS* 1999;13:2493) with an odds-ratio in controlled trials of 2.6-3.4 (*CID* 2003;36[suppl 2]:S84), but it may be seen with HIV infection in the absence of PI exposure, with EFV treatment and without hyperlipidemia (*JAIDS* 2000;23:351; *Arch Intern Med* 2000;150: 2050; *JAIDS* 2007;45:508). Data suggest that unboosted ATV and RAL are unlikely causes compared to other agents (*J Infect Chemother* 2011;17:183). ACTG 5202 is the large 4-arm study comparing ATV/r vs. EFV and ABC/3TC vs. TDF/FTC. Trunk and VAT changes were greater for ATV/r than for EFV (37% vs. 21%), and the changes were similar for ABC/3TC vs. TDF/FTC (*Ann Intern Med* 2011;154:445).

  □ Lipoatrophy is more closely linked with NRTIs, especially d4T and less frequently ddI and AZT (*AIDS* 2000;14;F25; *AIDS* 1999;13: 1659; *CID* 2006;43:645; *NEJM* 206;354:251; *Curr Pharm Des* 2010;16:3339). The presumed mechanism is inhibition of DNA polymerase gamma resulting in depletion of mitochondrial DNA (*NEJM* 2002;346:81).

- **Evaluation** (*Lancet* 2000;356:1412; *Lancet* 2001;357:592; *AIDS* 1999;13:2493; *CID* 2003;36[suppl 2]:S63)

  □ Lipoatrophy: The major concern is cosmetic, so self-report and visual inspection are the best indicators. Anthropometric measurement of skin folds and limb diameter are sometimes used as well. Fat can be quantitated by CT scan, MRI, and DEXA (*JAIDS* 2002;31:2510; *AIDS* 2010; 24:1717), but these are expensive and not demonstrably better than self-report (*CID* 2006;43:645). They may be useful for study purposes.

  □ Fat accumulation: A waist-hip ratio >0.95 in men or >0.85 in women is useful. Some regard a waist circumference ≥102 cm (40 in) in men or >88 cm (35 in) in women as a better measure (*BMJ* 1995;311:158). CT scans or MRI are not clinically useful (*CID* 2006;43:645) and DEXA is not recommended except for research studies.

- **Treatment**

  □ **Low-fat diet and aerobic exercise** can be partly effective in treating fat accumulation (*AIDS* 1999;13:231; *Cochrane Database Syst Rev* 2005;18:CD001796), although this may exacerbate lipoatrophy.

  □ **Growth hormone:** The growth hormone deficiency noted with HIV infection is attributed to a reduced response to growth hormone releasing hormone (GHRH) noted in about 36% of men and 16%

of women (*JAMA* 2008;300:509). This is defined as a peak GH response following GHRH plus arginine testing of <7.5 ng/mL. In a placebo-controlled trial in men with HIV, abdominal fat accumulation and reduced GH response to GHRH, treatment with recombinant GH produced a significant reduction in abdominal and trunk fat, reduced diastolic blood pressure and reduced triglycerides (*JAMA* 2008;300:509). Side effects were rare except for an increase in the 2-hr post prandial blood glucose. Prior studies using high doses (up to 6 mg/d) have shown significant side effects including hyperglycemia, fluid retention, hypertension, carpal tunnel syndrome, further loss of subcutaneous fat, and the need for maintenance treatment (*JAIDS* 2002;35:240; *AIDS* 1999;13: 2099; *JAMA* 2008;300:509).

- **Thiazolidinediones:** There is conflicting evidence regarding the benefit of thiazolidinediones on lipoatrophy (*HIV Clin Trials* 2008; 9:254). An early report showed efficacy for lipoatrophy (*Ann Intern Med* 2000;133:263), but a placebo-controlled trial found no benefit with rosiglitazone (4 mg bid x 48 wks) in 108 patients with lipoatrophy (*Lancet* 2004;363:429). A subsequent trial with rosiglitazone (4 mg/d) for 48 wks found that it was superior to pravastatin (40 mg/d) or growth hormone (2 mg/d) for improving lipoatrophy (*HIV Clin Trials* 2008;9:254). Pioglitazone (30 mg/d) had a similar benefit in a controlled trial (*Antivir Ther* 2008;13:67). A meta-analysis of 7 studies of thiazolidinediones showed no change in visceral fat accumulation (*Top HIV Med* 2008;16:127); one study found a modest decrease with rosiglitazone (p<0.05) (*Ann Intern Med* 143;199: 253). These studies collectively suggest that these agents may have a modest effect on reversing HIV-associated lipoatrophy but no clear role in reducing visceral fat accumulation.

- **Tesamorelin** is an analog of growth hormone-releasing hormone (GHRH) that preserves the negative feedback inhibition. A trial comparing 2 mg/d vs. placebo showed a decrease in visceral adipose tissue (VAT) by 15% at 6 mos (*JAIDS* 2010;53:311). Another trial used tesamorelin in 265 patients for 6 mos followed by rerandomization to placebo or continued tesamorelin. At 12 months, the treatment group lost 18% VAT, while those on placebo developed reaccumulation (*JAIDS* 2010;53:311). Tesamorelin (*Egrifta*) was FDA approved November, 2010. It is given as a 2 mg dose daily for up to 6 months for lipodystrophy. The most common adverse reactions are arthralgias, skin rash at injection sites and increases in blood glucose. Concerns are the need for daily injections, the limited benefit with reversibility after discontinuation, the cost and the side effects (*J Clin Endocrinol Metab* 2010;95:4291).

- **Testosterone:** Testosterone gel in ART-treated men with low testosterone levels and abdominal fat accumulation may reduce abdominal fat but will also reduce limb fat (*CID* 2006;43:645) (see pg. 394).

- **Metformin** (500 mg bid) improves insulin sensitivity and results in weight loss and decreased fat accumulation (*JAMA* 2000;284:472; *AIDS* 1999;13:1000). It may also improve some markers of cardiovascular risk (*J Clin Endocrinol Metab* 2002;87:4611). A comparative trial of rosiglitazone (8 mg/d) or metformin (2 g/d) in patients with lipodystrophy found that metformin was superior for improving visceral fat and fasting lipids (*Ann Intern Med* 2005;143:337).

- **Restorative surgery** for fat accumulation includes removal of lipomas, breast fat tissue or dorsocervical fat pad by either surgery or liposuction (*Ann Plast Surg* 2007;58:255). A number of methods, including implants and injections, are being used for facial lipoatrophy. Controlled trials show minimal change in facial soft tissue by spiral CT scan, but adverse reactions are rare and patient satisfaction is generally good (*JAIDS* 2007;46:581; *AIDS* 2011;25:1; *AIDS* 2007;21:1147). Polylactic acid, for example, is FDA-approved for this indication, but it is expensive and usually requires multiple injections. Injections of fat or collagen are associated with rapid resorption, so the changes are short-lived. A review of 14 studies on various cosmetic surgery options with injectable fillers (poly-L-lactic acid, calcium hydroxylapatite, polyalkylimide gel, hyaluronic acid and silicone oil) for HIV-associated lipoatrophy found the cost for a single anatomical site ranged from $3,690 to $16,544, which is often not covered by payers. The procedures need to be repeated at 1-3 yrs (*AIDS Care* 2009;21:664).

- **Regimen changes** with a switch from PIs to an NNRTI are sometimes partially successful in reversing fat accumulation, although data are conflicting and changes are slow (*JID* 2001;184:914; *CID* 2000;31:1266). The SPIRAL study (see pg. 357) found that continuation of a PI/r-based regimen was associated with continued increases in visceral fat area by DEXA in patients, but no further increases were observed in the group switched to RAL (*AIDS* 2010;24:1697). Switching from d4T or AZT to ABC or TDF is associated with a measurable improvement in lipoatrophy, with increased limb-fat with ≥2 year follow-up. The more bothersome cosmetic change is buccal (cheek) lipoatrophy, which is stigmatizing and has proven difficult to measure and to reverse (*AIDS* 2006;20:2043;). The TARHEEL study showed that the switch from d4T to ABC or AZT was associated with significant increases in arm, leg, and trunk fat at 48 wks, but improvement was noted in <40% and was greater with DEXA than by self-report (*JAIDS* 2004;36:935; *CID* 2004;38:263). In patients not receiving AZT, ddI or d4T, there is no clear evidence or rationale for changing the ART regimen for lipoatrophy (*Curr Opinion Infect Dis* 2011;24:43).

4 Antiretroviral Therapy

Lactic Acidosis/Hepatic Steatosis

Lactic acidosis and hyperlactatemia is a potential side effect of d4T, and less commonly of AZT and ddl. It typically occurs after several months of treatment (median 9 mos) and may be asymptomatic (*CID* 2001;33:1931) or may present with symptoms that are usually vague, non-specific and progressive over weeks (*CID* 2007;45:261). A distinction is made between severe hyperlactatemia (2 consecutive lactate levels >5 mmol/L + HCO_3 <20 mmol/L and pH > 7.35) and lactic acidosis which is defined by the International Lactic Acidosis Group as an elevated lactate (>2 mmol/L) plus a pH <7.35 and HCO_3 <20 mmol/L (*AIDS* 2007;21:2455; *CID* 2007;45:254). Lactic acidosis is less common and potentially lethal. Many cases of hyperlactatemia without acidosis probably represent a laboratory artifact due to suboptimal collection of blood (*JAIDS* 2004;35:27; *CID* 2001;33:1931).

- **Cause:** The mechanism is NRTI inhibition of DNA polymerase gamma leading to anaerobic glycolysis with lactate production (*NEJM* 2002;346:811; *Nat Med* 1995;1:417; *J Clin Invest* 1995;96: 126; *Lancet* 1999;354:1112). *In vitro* assays of mitochondrial toxicity with inhibition of DNA polymerase gamma show that the rank order of NRTIs is ddC > d4T > ddl > AZT with minimal effect by 3TC, FTC, TDF and ABC (*CID* 2001;33:2072; *CID* 2002;34:838; *NEJM* 2006; 354:251; *CID* 2000;31:162; *AIDS* 2001;15:717).

■ TABLE 4-24: **Metabolic Impact of Antiretroviral Agents (Adapted from European AIDS Clinical Society: Guidelines on the Management of Metabolic Diseases of HIV, version 3, 2008)**

Less ──────────────────────────→ More

NNRTI	NRTI	PI
NVP	3TC, ABC, TDF FTC	FPV ATV
EFV	AZT, ABC	ATV/r SQV/r
	ddl	LPV/r, FPV/r* DRV/r*
	d4T	IDV/r, TPV/r RTV (full dose)

More ↓ (left side, pointing down)

* Authors disagree with placement since more recent data suggests minimal metabolic effect

- **Risk Factors:** The major risks are NRTI exposure (d4T > ddl > AZT), the duration of that exposure, female gender, pregnancy and obesity (*PLoS One* 2011;6:e18736). A review from Boston (2003-07) found an incidence of 3.2/100 pt-yrs in patients receiving ddl, d4T or AZT (*PLoS One* 2011;6:e18736). A review from South Africa found an

Antiretroviral Therapy

incidence in females of 16 cases/1000 pt-years compared to 1 case/1000 pt-years in men (*CID* 2007;45:261). In another review from South Africa, all cases were female, the median age was 36 years and the median patient weight was 81 kg (*S Afr Med J* 2006;96:722). Most cases in the early 1990s were attributed to AZT, but d4T and ddI account for nearly all cases reported in the first decade of HAART (*CID* 2002;34:838; *CID* 2007;45:254; *CID* 2007;45: 514; *CID* 2007;45:261; *S Afr Med J* 2006;96:722; *AIDS* 2007;21: 2455). In a case-control study of 110 cases, the greatest risks besides ddI or d4T exposures were female gender (OR=6), age > 40 yrs (OR=2.6) and CD4 count <200 cells/mm^3 (OR=7). (*AIDS* 2007;21:2455). Melformin is now one of the more common medication-associated causes in areas that have abandoned d4T and ddI (*Diabetologia* 2010;53:2546), but this risk is still extremely low (*Ann Intern Med* 2010;153:JC1).

- **Symptoms and diagnosis:** Patients with elevated serum lactate levels may be asymptomatic, chronically ill, or acutely ill. Symptoms are non-specific and vague, including non-intentional weight loss, GI complaints (anorexia, nausea, vomiting, abdominal pain) dyspnea and fatigue. Physical exam may show hepatomegaly, tachycardia, lipoatrophy and/or edema (*Ann Intern Med* 2000;133:192; *CID* 2002; 34:838; *AIDS* 2007;21:2455). Most patients have taken ddI or d4T for 6-12 mos, but cases occurring as early as 2 mohs or after 2 yrs have been reported. The diagnosis is confirmed by an elevated lactic acid level, which requires the use of a pre-chilled fluoride-oxalate tube and blood sampling without a tourniquet or clinched fist, with blood delivered rapidly to the lab on ice for processing within 4 hrs. The patient should not exercise for 24 hrs prior to sampling and should be well hydrated. Errors in quality control and overdiagnosis are common. The distinction between hyperlactatemia and lactic acidosis is based on measurement of pH and HCO_3 levels. Serious disease and mortality is are usually seen with lactic acidosis, and lactic acid levels obtained correctly correlate with prognosis: 0-2 mM is normal; 5-10 mM is associated with a 7% mortality; 10-15 mM with a >30% mortality, and >15 mM with a >60% mortality (*CID* 2002;34:838). Other common lab or radiographic abnormalities that suggest this diagnosis are elevated CPK, abnormal LFTs (prothrombin time, transaminase, bilirubin), LDH, anion gap >16; low serum albumin, pH and/or bicarbonate, and CT scan, ultrasound, or biopsy of liver showing hepatic steatosis.

- **Treatment:** Lactic acid levels <5 mM may not require treatment or may be managed with modification of NRTI therapy. Symptomatic patients usually have levels >5 mM and typically require discontinuation of NRTIs. In some cases, a switch from d4T, ddI, or AZT to ABC, 3TC, FTC, or TDF may be reasonable, provided the patient is not seriously ill and can be carefully observed. Lactic acid

 133

levels >10 mM, if properly obtained, should be viewed as a medical emergency because of the high mortality. Seriously ill patients require supportive care, which may include intravenous hydration, mechanical ventilation, and/or dialysis. Recovery is protracted. The half-life of mitochondrial DNA ranges from 4.5 to 8 wks, and the time required for clinical recovery is 4-28 wks (*AIDS* 2000;14:F25); *NEJM* 2002;346:811). Treatment with sodium bicarbonate is logical, but this has not been well supported in trials and may be detrimental (*Am J Physiol* 1982;242:F586; *J Hosp Med* 2010;5:E1; *Crit Care Med* 1991;19:1352). Other buffers have not been better. For NRTI-associated cases there are anecdotal case reports showing a possible benefit of thiamine (50 or 100 mg/d), riboflavin (50-200 mg/d), L-carnitine (990 mg tid), and co-enzyme Q10 (>50 mg/d) (*CID* 2006;43:645; *CID* 2002;34:838). The experience with riboflavin (50 mg/d) appears to be the most extensive and favorable. With regard to ART, switching to NRTIs unlikely to cause LA (3TC, FTC, ABC, TDF) can be considered, although some prefer to avoid all NRTIs until the lactate level measured monthly for at least 3 mos is normal. In one report 56 patients with hyperlactatemia or lactic acidosis attributed to d4T were given regimens containing AZT when ART was restarted and all tolerated it well (*CID* 2007;45:261). The preferred NRTIs in this setting are TDF, ABC, FTC and 3TC. The alternative is to use NRTI-sparing regimens (Table 4-22).

Insulin Resistance

Insulin resistance (impaired uptake of glucose by muscle and inhibition of hepatic glucogenesis) is common with PI-based ART, but diabetes (fasting blood sugar >126 mg/dL) is infrequent and rarely requires insulin, except in patients who are prone to diabetes (first-degree relative).

- **Definitions**
  - □ Insulin resistance: Tissues targeted by insulin fail to respond, leading to increased production of pancreatic insulin
  - □ Impaired glucose (prediabetes): A1C 5.7-6.4%, blood glucose of 140-199 mg/dL 2 hr after a 75-gm glucose loading dose, or fasting blood glucose of 100-125 mg/dL after an 8-hr fast.
  - □ Diabetes: Criteria of American Diabetes Association (*Diabetes Care* 2011;34 Suppl 1:S1): 1) A1C >6.5%; 2) blood glucose >200 mg/dL 2 hr after a 75-gm glucose loading dose; 3) fasting blood glucose ≥126 mg/dL after 8-hr fast; or 4) symptoms of diabetes and random blood glucose >200 mg/dL.

- **Frequency:** Insulin resistance is noted in 30-90% of patients treated with PIs, and overt diabetes occurs in 1-11%, with a mean of approximately 7% at 5 years (*AIDS* 1999;13: F63; *Lancet* 1999;353: 2s093; *Arch Intern Med* 2000;160:2050). In an analysis of the MACS database, the incidence of diabetes mellitus was 4.7/100 person-years for ART recipients, a 4.1-fold risk compared to untreated controls (*Arch Intern Med* 2005;165:1179). Insulin resistance has been demonstrated with administration of LPV/r, IDV, and RTV to uninfected individuals. No changes are seen with unboosted ATV (*AIDS* 2006;20:1813; *JID* 2004;182:209; *AIDS* 2004; 18:2137), but RTV increases insulin resistance with ATV/r. Less data are available for SQV, DRV, FPV, or NFV (*CID* 2006;43:645). The changes in blood glucose are usually apparent within 2-3 mos and can be detected with a fasting blood glucose test (*Lancet* 1999;353:2093). With IDV, insulin resistance can be detected after a single dose (*AIDS* 2002;16:F1).

- **Screening**: The 2011 DHHS Guidelines recommend fasting blood glucose levels at the initial evaluation and then annually if untreated. With ART, the recommendation is FBS at baseline and then every 6 mos if the previous test was normal, and every 3 mos if it was abnormal; more frequent testing is appropriate with prediabetes and specific risks (see below).

- **Risk:** Insulin resistance is important because it is a risk factor for atherosclerosis (*NEJM* 1996;334:952; *Am J Med* 1997;103: 152), especially when accompanied by dyslipidemia, hypertension, and visceral fat accumulation, the components of metabolic syndrome (*J Intern Med* 1994;736:13). Risk assessment should include review of risk factors for diabetes and including obesity, the use of PIs other than unboosted ATV, the use of NRTIs (especially d4T and ddI), advanced age, family history of diabetes, nonwhite race, and possibly HCV coinfection (*JAIDS* 2003;32:298; *AIDS* 2005;19:1375; *CID* 2007;45:111). Drugs other than HIV agents associated with greater risk include steroids, niacin, growth hormone, and some antipsychotics.

- **Prevention:** ADA recommendatons for prediabetics (A1C 5.7-6.4%): weight loss of 7% body weight and moderate exercise (e.g., walking) for >150 min/wk. Consider metformin if A1C is >6% despite lifestyle changes.

TREATMENT

- Standard guidelines are recommended for management of diabetes (*Diabetes Care* 2011;34 Suppl 1:11).

  □ The treatment goal is an FBS of 70-130 mg/dL or A1C of <7.0%. This goal is based on large controlled trials demonstrating that glycemic control correlates with reduced microvascular and neurologic complications (*Lancet* 1998;352:854; *Lancet* 1998; 352:837; *NEJM* 2000;342:381; *NEJM* 2008;359:1577; *NEJM* 2009;361:1024; *NEJM* 2009;361:1024).

  □ The daily diet should consist of 50-60% carbohydrate, 10-20% protein, and <30% fat, with <100 mg cholesterol per day and <10% of total calories from saturated fat

4 Antiretroviral Therapy

□ When drug therapy is necessary, agents that reduce insulin resistance are most commonly prescribed, including metformin and the thiazolidinediones, which reduce insulin resistance and visceral fat accumulation (*AIDS* 1999;13:100; *JAMA* 2000;284:472; *Ann Intern Med* 2005;143:337), with a possible reduction in cardiovascular risk. LFTs need to be monitored (ALT q2mos x 12 mos) with thiazolinediones; a baseline ALT >2.5x ULN contraindicates use. A baseline elevation of creatinine or lactic acid to ≥2x ULN contraindicates metformin.

□ Monitoring: The 2011 ADA recommendation is for A1C measurement in diabetic patients >2 x/year if stable and >4 x/yr if treatment is changed or the patient is unstable.

□ Insulin: Use when oral agents fail. Start with 10-15 units q3d until FBS <110 mg/dL. May combine with metformin. Sulfonylureas and other drugs in different classes reduce blood glucose but do not reverse insulin resistance. An alternative strategy is to change the ART regimen to a non-PI-based regimen or a PI-based regimen less likely to cause insulin resistance, such as ATV-based ART (*AIDS* 1999;13:805; *JAIDS* 2001;27:229; *CID* 2000;31:1266).

■ TABLE 4-25: **Recommendations of European AIDS Society for Treatment of Diabetes in Person Receiving ART (2007)**

Goal: HbA1c <6.5-7 without hypoglycemia and FBS 73-110 mg/dL

Intervention	Expected ↓ HbA1c	Comment
Lifestyle change	1-2	
Metformin 500-1500/d & ↑ to 2-3 g/d in 4-6 wks	1.5	GI intolerance, Contraindicated in renal failure Preferred for obese patients May worsen lipoatrophy
Thiazolidinedione* ■ Rosiglitazone 4-8 mg/d ■ Pioglitazone 15-45 mg/d	0.5-1.4	Fluid retention, heart failure and weight gain Preferred for patients with lipoatrophy
Insulin	unlimited	Hypoglycemia May require large doses (1-2 IU/kg)

* Subsequent to these guidelines in 2007, Rosiglitazone has been withdrawn from the market in Europe, and Pioglitazone is withdrawn in some countries.

Cardiovascular disease

Cardiovascular disease (CVD) is the major cause of death in the US and a major cause of death with HIV infection in the HAART era. According to the D:A:D analysis of 2,482 deaths with 180,176 person-years of follow-up, CVD, along with chronic hepatitis and non-AIDS malignancy, were the major non-AIDS causes of death, each accounting for 15-17% (*AIDS* 2010;24:1537). There are substantial data indicating that HIV infection increases the risk of an acute myocardial infarction (MI) by approximately 60% compared to age-matched controls (*J Clin Endocrin*

Metab 2007;92:2506). This risk is multifactorial, including some factors that are reversible and many that are HIV-related. The relative risk for an acute MI by the D:A:D analysis are summarized in Table 4-26.

■ TABLE 4-26: **Risk Factors for an Acute Myocardial Infarction (MI) in D:A:D***

Risk category	RR[†]
PI exposure (/yr)	1.1
Age (/5)	1.2
Male sex	2.1
BMI 30	1.3

Smoking
    Current
    Former
	
	2.9
	1.6

Prior CVD event	4.6
Diabetes	1.7
Hypertension	1.3
Total cholesterol (mmol/L)	1.3
Family history	1.4

   *   D:A:D data (*NEJM* 2007;356:1723)
   †   RR = Adjusted relative risk

An analysis of 6.517 patients in a Boston healthcare system from 1998-2008 found a significant risk associated with a VL >100,000 c/mL (OR 2.2; p=0.01) and a decreased risk with a VL <400 c/mL (OR 0.6; p=0.6). Similarly, a CD4 count <200 cells/mm^3 appeared to be a significant risk (OR 1.5; p=0.02) and increasing the CD4 count 50 cells/mm^3 correlated with a decreased risk (OR 0.95; p=0.001) (*JAIDS* 2010;55:615).

There are also substantial data suggesting HIV treatment may be an important risk factor (see below). The possible central role of immune-activation as indicated by elevated inflammatory markers is consistently shown but causally enigmatic (*PLoS Med* 2008;5:e203; *JID* 2010;201:1788; *Curr Infect Dis Rep* 2011;13:94). Large population based trials, including SMART, has shown that ART reduces markers of inflammation but does not normalize them (*AIDS* 2010;24:1657). Nevertheless, discontinuation of ART in the SMART trial was associated with a substantial in the risk of an AMI (OR 1.6; p=0.05) (*NEJM* 2006;355:2283).

■ **Hyperlipidemia:** Changes in blood lipids are an important concern in patients with HIV infection with and without ART. Studies in the pre-HAART era indicated that HIV-infection was associated with elevated triglyceride levels and decreased levels of LDL-C and HDL-C (*Am J Med* 1991;90:154; *JAMA* 2003;289:2978). The decrease in HDL-C and increase in triglyceride levels increased the risk of cardiovascular disease (CVD); studies comparing HIV-positive and -negative individuals demonstrate a 1.5- to 2.0-fold increase in CVD associated

4 Antiretroviral Therapy

with HIV infection (*Circulation* 2008;118:198). Although the rate of CVD is significantly higher, the absolute rate is low.

- **Agents:** D:A:D is a large cohort of HIV-infected patients designed to evaluate CVD. It is observational, but robust in numbers and methods that include review of all CVD events by blinded cardiologists. Early studies based on the analysis of 23,000 HIV-infected patients showed that the highest risk was patients with RTV-boosted PIs (*JID* 2004;189:1056). The presumed mechanism was drug-induced lipid elevation. RTV at a dose of 100 mg bid in seronegative patients increased TG levels 27%, LDL-C 16% and total cholesterol 17% (*HIV Med* 2005;6:421; *NEJM* 1995;333:1528). LPV/r did not increase TG or LDL-C levels more, but did increase the total cholesterol. FPV, DRV and TPV all show this effect with increases in TG and LDL-C with RTV boosting; the magnitude of the change is dependent on the dose of RTV (*Lancet* 2006;368;476; *Lancet* 2007;369:1169), and there is an independent effect of the PI on cholesterol. The exception is ATV, which has no apparent independent effect on lipids, but a very modest effect with RTV boosting at 100 mg/d (*AIDS* 2006;20:711). d4T and AZT are also associated with elevated triglyceride levels (*JAIDS* 2006;43:535; *JAMA* 2004;292:191). A more recent D:A:D analysis based on 178,835 person-years of follow-up and 580 MIs found a significant risk with only 4 ART agents: recent exposure to ABC or ddI and cumulative exposure to IDV/r or LPV/r (*JID* 2010;201:318). The data for ABC are particularly controversial due to conflicting results in both prospective and retrospective studies (see pg. 183). With regard to lipids and other ART agents: effects are less or nil with NVP and RPV compared to EFV (*AIDS* 2003;17:1195; *Curr Infect Dis Rep* 2011; 13:1). MVC caused less dyslipidemia than EFV in the MERIT trial (*Clin Trials* 2008;30:1228). RAL does not appear to alter blood lipids (*NEJM* 2008;359:339; *Lancet* 2010;375:396). ART-associated changes are usually apparent within 2-3 mos of initiating therapy.

- **Risk:** An increased risk of cardiovascular disease associated with ART was initially assumed based on serum lipid changes. The D:A:D data (summarized above) showed 126 MIs among 23,468 patients with a relative risk (RR) of 1.25; for smoking it was 2.2 (*NEJM* 2003;349:1993). With long-term follow-up (>4 yrs), the rate of MIs in patients receiving ART was about 26% above predicted rates (*HIV Med* 2006;7:218). A review of 9 studies indicated a significant risk of CVD in 7 reports (*Circulation* 2008;118:e29); other reports also show a modest increased odds ratio for coronary events with use of ART (*JAMA* 2003;289:2978; *AIDS* 2003;17:1179). These data collectively indicate that HIV infection is associated with an increased risk of CVD and MIs, and contributing factors include HIV infection *per se*, selected ART regimens and traditional risks such as smoking.

- **Risk assessment** should include a review of other CV risk factors as defined below based on guidelines from the AHA, the ACTG/IDSA and the Framingham 10-year risk calculator.

- □ **CVD risk assessment recommendations:**
  - Fasting lipid profile prior to starting ART and at 4-8 wks with new regimen; then every 6 mos if abnormal and every 12 mos if normal at previous visit.
  - Add the number of risks; if >2 calculate the 10-year risk (Framingham criteria)
  - Address non-lipid modifiable risk factors including smoking and diet
  - If lipid threshold is exceeded despite lifestyle changes, consider anti-lipid agent and modification of ART regimen

- □ **Framingham Risk Assessment:** The tool estimates the 10-year risk of developing an MI with death using 7 variables: 1) age in years; 2) sex; 3) total cholesterol (average of >2 measurements); 4) HDL cholesterol in mg/dL (average of >2 measurements; 5) smoking (positive if any cigarette smoking in the past month); 6) systolic blood pressure and 7) hypertension treatment (yes/no).

  The calculation is readily available from multiple sources including:
  - www.mmhiv.com/link/10-yr-risk-1
  - www.mmhiv.com/link/10-yr-risk-2

■ TABLE 4-27: **Cardiovascular Health Assessment (American Heart Association;** *Circulation* **2010;121:586)**

Metric	Ideal Cardiovascular Health
Current smoking	Never or quit >12 mos ago
Body mass index	BMI <25 kg/m²; waist circumference <88 cm (f) or 92 cm (m)
Physical activity	≥150 min/wk moderate intensity or ≥75 min/wk vigorous intensity
Diet	Low glycemic load on trans fat; high cereal fiber, folate marine omega-3 fatty acid, polyunsaturated:saturated fat ratio
Alcohol	Light or moderate
Total cholesterol	<200 mg/dL
Blood pressure	120/<80 mg Hg
Fasting blood glucose	≤100 mg/dL

■ **Biomarkers:** The markers most commonly used to measure immune activation in research studies have been hsCRP, IL-6 (and D-dimer) (*PLoS Med* 2008;5:e203). Studies in patients without HIV have found the best outcomes in those with a hsCRP <2 mg/L and LDL <70 mg/dL (*J Am Coll Cardiol* 2005;45:1644). IL-6 is another favored marker used in the SMART trial. These markers also predicted death

4 Antiretroviral Therapy

in participants in SMART when adjusted for CD4 count and viral load (*JAIDS* 2003;32:2010; JID 2010;201:1796). D-Dimer, a marker of thrombotic activity, has also been predictive of death in persons with and without HIV infection (*AIDS* 2009;23:929). The data show that these biomarkers predict CVD and death, and that levels are increased with HIV infection and decreased, but do not return to normal, with ART (*Curr Opin AIDS* 2010;5:511; JID 2010;201:1788). For more information on these biomarkers, see pg. 64.

SPECIFIC RECOMMENDATIONS

- **Management:** Recommendations are from the ACTG and IDSA (*CID* 2003;37:613), the academic consortium (*CID* 2006;43:645), IAS-USA Guidelines, the European AIDS Clinical Society Guidelines 2008, and the National Cholesterol Education Program guidelines III (*JAMA* 2001;285:2486) and the American Heart Association (*Circulation* 2010:121:586). Note that LDL-C guidelines were modified based on more recent data that now target LDL-C <70 mg/dL in the two highest risk groups (*J Am Coll Cardiol* 2004;44:720).

  There is also a shift in conclusions about HDL-cholesterol, "the good cholesterol." This is atheroprotective by promoting efflux of cholesterol from macrophages. HDL cholesterol can be converted to a dysfunctional form, so levels may be deceptive. Thus, it is the HDL efflux capacity that is most relevant (*NEJM* 2011;264:127). The American Heart Association has also redefined the interpretation of triglycerides as an important biomarker of CVD risk with optimal levels ≤150 mg/dL, borderline 150-200 mg/dL; high 200-499 mg/dL and very high ≥500 mg/dL. They note that lifestyle changes can reduce levels by 50%, and therapy is advocated for levels >500 mg/dL to prevent pancreatitis, but it is not known if this intervention prevents CVD (*Circulation* 2011;123:2292).

  □ **Baseline assessment:** Lipid panel, including cholesterol, LDL and HDL cholesterol, and triglycerides after fasting at least 8 hrs (preferably 12 hrs). Non-fasting lipid panels can also provide useful information about cholesterol subsets. Fasting is necessary for accurate measurement of triglycerides and the calculation of LDL cholesterol but has minimal effect on total cholesterol. LDL-C is calculated by the Friedewald equation: LDL-C=TC-(HDL-C)-TG/5 (*JAIDS* 2002;31:257). LDL cholesterol measurements are unreliable with triglyceride levels >400 mg/dL. In this situation, clinicians can subtract HDL cholesterol levels from total cholesterol to obtain a non-HDL cholesterol level (*JAMA* 2001; 285:2486) or can use direct LDL measurements. Interpretation must take into account secondary causes of dyslipidemia including nephrosis, alcoholism, thiazides, testosterone treatment, estrogen treatment, hypogonadism, uncontrolled diabetes, and cocaine abuse. Goals of therapy for LDL cholesterol levels are summarized in Table 4-28.

■ TABLE 4-28: **National Cholesterol Education Program Guidelines** (*Circulation* 2004;110:227)

Risk category	LDL goal (mg/dL)	Lifestyle change	Drug therapy
Atherosclerosis, diabetes, or multiple risk factors	<70	<100	>130 100-130 optional

≥2 risk factors:
smoking, HBP, HDL <40 mg/dL, hereditary factors*
    10-yr risk 10-20%
    10-yr risk <10%
	
	<100
	<130
		
		<130
		<130
			
			>130
			>160

0-1 risk factors*	<160	<190	160-190 optional >190

* Age: male >45 yrs, female >55 yrs; HDL-C <40 mg/dL; BP >140/90 or antihypertension drugs; smoking; coronary artery disease in a first-degree male relative <55 yrs or female relative <65 yrs

□ **Monitoring:** The lipid profile should be repeated at 6-mo intervals if abnormal, and at 12-mo intervals if normal (2011 DHHS Guidelines).

TREATMENT OF HYPERLIPIDEMIA: See *Circulation* 2011;123:243.

GUIDELINES FOR PREVENTION OF CVD*: (*Circulation* 2011;125:1245)

* **Class I-V:** I = Benefit >>> Risks; III = Benefit > Risk.
  Evidence level: Level A – strong evidence ; C – weak evidence

■ **Lifestyle** (Table 4-27, pg. 139)

□ Smoking: Do not smoke (IA) (see Table 7-28, pg. 567)

□ Exercise: Walking >150 min/wk or vigorous exercise >75 min/wk Note that more is better (IB)

□ Diet: Rich in fruits and vegetables, whole grain, high fiber, fish (especially oily fish >2 x/wk); reduce intake of saturated fat, cholesterol, alcohol, sodium and glucose; avoid trans-fatty acids (IB)

□ Weight: BMI <25 (IB)

□ Omega-3 fatty acids by fish eating or pills (EPA 1800 mg/d)

■ **Major Risks**

□ Blood pressure: <120/80 mm Hg;

medications for BP >140/90 mm Hg: thiazides, beta-blockers, ACE inhibitors

□ Lipids: LDL-C <100 mg/dL, HDL-C >50, TG <150 mg/dL; LDL-C <70 for high risk (see Table 4-28)

□ ASA: 75-325 mg/d with coronary artery disease, diabetes, age >65 (and no risk for GI bleed or hemorrhagic stroke)

4 Antiretroviral Therapy

- **Antiviral substitution:** The **D:A:D trial** with 178,835 person-years of observation and 580 patient deaths found a significant association with death from an acute MI with use of LPV/r, IDV/r, ABC and ddI. The association with LPV/r and IDV/r was with cumulative use; for ABC and ddI it was recent exposure. The association with PIs is usually thought to reflect their association with dyslipidemia; the mechanism with NRTIs is not well established. There are extensive data about the impact of various classes and agents from clinical trials that permit generalizations:

  - **NRTIs:** A review of the CNICS cohort with 2,267 treated patients found that TDF, 3TC an ABC had minimal impact compared to the thymidine analogs, ddI was associated with the highest LDL-C increases and d4T recipients had the highest triglyceride increases (*AIDS* 2011;25:185).

  - **PI/r regimens** often have the poorest atherogenic lipid profile – most marked with LPV/r (ATAZIP: *JAIDS* 2009;23:16) and RTV (CASTLE: *JAIDS* 2010;53:323) and a meta-analyis (*JAC* 2010;65:1878). ATV appears to be essentially "lipid neutral" without boosting (*JAIDS* 2009;57:153). RTV promotes an atherogenic lipid pattern in a dose dependent fashion as shown in the LESS trial (*HIV Clin Trials* 2010;11:239).

  - **NNRTIs:** EFV has a modest impact on LDL-C and TG levels as shown in the MERIT trial with comparison to MVC (*HIV Clin Trials* 2011;12:24) and compared to RAL in STARTMRK (*JAIDS* 2010; 55:39).

  - **MVC:** This agent appears to be "lipid neutral" as shown in MERIT (*HIV Clin Trials* 2011;12:24).

  - **RAL:** Appears to be lipid neutral according to the SWITCHMRK (*Lancet* 2010;375:396) and SPIRAL (*AIDS* 2010;24:1697). Substituting an NNRTI, ATV or ATV/r for another boosted PI has improved lipid profiles (*JAIDS* 2005;39:174); *AIDS* 2005;19:917). Switching to ABC or TDF from d4T may also be effective (*AIDS* 2004;18:1475). One report found that statin therapy was more effective than changing antiretroviral agents (*AIDS* 2005;19:1051).

- **Drug therapy (Tables 4-29 through 4-32)**

  - **Statins**: These are the most effective drugs for reducing LDL-C; they also decrease TG. The clinical benefit correlates with the LDL-C decrease. An analysis of 700 HIV-infected patients showed that lipid goals were achieved more frequently with atorvastatin or rosuvastatin compared to pravastatin (*CID* 2011; 52:387) A meta-analysis of 58 placebo-controlled trials found that all-cause mortality was reduced by 10% for every 1.0 mmol/L decrease in LDL cholesterol with no threshold (*Lancet* 2010; 376:1670). Once started, statins are usually continued for a lifetime. If stopped, lipid levels return to baseline within 2-3 wks.

Antiretroviral Therapy

Statins have beneficial anti-inflammatory effects that are not completely explained by lipid reduction. The JUPITER study with rosuvastatin showed that the cardiac event rate and the hsCRP results were significantly reduced even after adjusting for the change in LDL-cholesterol (*Am J Cardiovasc Drugs* 2010;10:383). Statin therapy has been noted to reduce hsCRP levels (*Arch Med Res* 2010;41:464). This has been noted in HIV-infected patients as well (*AIDS* 2011;25:1128). The latter report showed a median decrease of hsCRP of 3.0 to 2.4/L (p <0.001) that did not correlate with changes in lipids.

□ **PI interactions:** Most statins are metabolized using cytochrome P3A4; all PIs inhibit CYP3A4. The greatest effect is with lovastatin and simvastatin; atorvastatin is only partially metabolized by CYP3A4; pravastatin and rosuvastatin are not metabolized by this mechanism, except for the interaction of DRV/r and pravastatin (see Table 4-29). Inhibition of CYP3A4 causes significant toxicity potential when used with PIs but not NNRTIs.

■ TABLE 4-29: **Statins**

| Agent* | Form | Dose (FDA) | | Decrease LDL |
		Initial mg/day	Max mg/day	
Atorvastatin (*Lipitor*)	Tabs – 10, 20, 40, 80 mg	10	80	35-60%
Fluvastatin (*Lescol*)	Caps – 20, 40 mg; 80 mg XL	20-40	80	20-40%
Pravastatin (*Pravachol*)	Tabs – 10, 20, 40, 80 mg	20-40	80	30-40%
Rosuvastatin (*Crestor*)	Tabs – 5, 10, 20, 40 mg	10	40	45-60%

* Lovastatin (*Mevacor*) and simvastatin (*Zocor*) are not included due to major drug interactions with all PIs.

□ **Adverse effects:** In a review of 700 HIV-infected patients given statins, 6.4% discontinued treatment due to toxicity, and rates were nearly equal for pravastatin, atorvastatin and rosuvastatin (*CID* 2011;52:387). The most common was CPK elevation, and the most severe was rhabdomyolysis with renal failure. Obtain baseline CPK levels and repeat the test if myalgias develop; some recommend discontinuing statins or lowering the dose if the level is 3-5x ULN (Treatment Guidelines, *Med Letter* 2003;3:15). Other ADRs include gastrointestinal symptoms and increased transaminase levels in 1-2%, which are often corrected by use of an alternative statin. A rare polyneuropathy has been reported (*Neurology* 2002;58:1333).

4 Antiretroviral Therapy

■ TABLE 4-30: **Drug Interactions: Effect of ARV Agents on AUC of Statins**

Statin*	ATV	DRV/r	EFV	ETR	FPV/r	LPV/r	SQV/r	TPV
Atorvastatin	ND	↑4.0	ND	ND	1.5	↑4.9	↑0.8	↑8.0
Pravastatin	ND	↑1.8	↓0.4	–	ND	↑1.3	↓0.5	ND
Rosuvastatin	↑2.1	↑–	ND	–	–	↑2.0	↑–	↑1.2

ND = No data; "–" = no significant effect (Adapted from the 2011 DHHS Guidelines).

* For atorvastatin – concurrent DRV/r increases the atorvastatin 4-fold.
Lovastatin and simvastatin are not included – both are contraindicated for concurrent use with PIs. Both may be used with EFV and ETR with doses based on lipid response without exceeding the recommended dose.

□ **Fibrates:** These agents (fenofibrate and gemfibrozil) are used to treat triglyceride levels >400-500 mg/dL (Table 4-31). Levels <150 mg/dL are considered normal, and levels >400 mg/dL represent an independent risk for cardiovascular disease. These drugs can be used concurrently with statins as shown in ACTG5087, which found good results with the combination (*J Clin Lipidol* 2010;4:279).

   □ **Triglyceride levels >400 mg/dL:** Preferred treatment is with fibrates, either micronized fenofibrate 48-145 mg qd or gemfibrozil 100 mg bid. If triglyceride levels remain >500 mg/dL, consider fish oil 3-6 gm/d (*CID* 2005;41:1498).

■ TABLE 4-31: **Triglycerides: Preferred Fibrates**

Agent	Form	Regimen
Gemfibrozil (*Lopid* and generic)	Tabs – 600 mg	600 mg bid before meals
Fenofibrate (*TriCor* and generic)	Tabs: 48, 145 mg Caps: 67, 100, 200 mg	48-145 mg qd 200 mg qd

□ **Niacin:** Reduces LDL-C and triglycerides. Concerns are flushing, minimal published experience in HIV-infected patients with dyslipidemia, and possible insulin resistance (*Antivir Ther* 2006;11: 1081). One report showed favorable results with a mean decrease of 34% in TG with ER niacin, combined with ASA pretreatment to avoid flushing. Recently, the AIM-HIGH study, a large clinical trial in which niacin was used to increase HDL-C in patients with coronary heart disease, was halted when it became clear that elevations in HDL-C did not decrease cardiovascular risk.

□ **Fish oil:** Active components are omega-3 fatty acids, which are used to treat high TG. The usual dose in 3-6 gm/d, it is generally well tolerated, and data supporting efficacy in HIV-infected patients is modest but good (*CID* 2005;41:1498; *Antiviral Ther* 2006;11:1081). Use is generally reserved for patients who fail fibrates.

Antiretroviral Therapy

- Ezetimibe: This agent in a dose of 10 mg/d reduces absorption of cholesterol. A study in HIV-negative patients raised doubts about benefit (*NEJM* 2008;358:1507), but a subsequent report with 44 HIV-infect patients given ezetimbe and a statin showed good tolerance and good LDL response (*AIDS* 2009;23:2133).

■ TABLE 4-32: **Drug Treatment of Lipid Abnormalities**

Abnormality*	Preferred	Alternative	Comment
High LDL-C only	Statin	Fibrate	Pravastatin (20-80 mg/d) or atorvastatin (10-80 mg/d); 40 mg/d is maximum with PIs; avoid pravastatin with DRV/r
High TG only	Fibrate	Statin	Gemfibrozil or fenofibrate; fish oil (1-2 gm bid)
High LDL-C + TG 200-500	Statin	Fibrate	Pravastatin (20-80 mg/d) or atorvastatin (10-80 mg/d); 40 mg/d is maximum with PIs; avoid pravastatin with DRV/r Alternative: fluvastatin (20-80 mg/d) or fenofibrate (48-267 mg/d)
High LDL-C + TG >1000	Fibrate	Fish oil Niacin Statin	Gemfibrozil (900-1200 mg/d) or fenofibrate (67-267 mg/d) Fish oil (1-2 gm bid) Niacin 1.0-1.5 gm/d + statin

* TG=triglyceride, LDL-C=LDL cholesterol

Hepatotoxicity

Most ARV agents have been implicated as potential causes of hepatotoxicity, but frequency, severity, and mechanism are highly variable (Table 4-33 and 4-34). Many cases are confounded by the presence of pre-existing liver disease ascribed to HBV, HCV, or alcoholism. The most common manifestation is an asymptomatic increase in transaminase levels, which often resolves without discontinuation of the implicated agent.

■ TABLE 4-33: **Grading of Hepatotoxicty (ACTG)**

Grade	ALT/AST (x ULN)	AlkPhos x ULN	Bilirubin x ULN
1	1-2.5x	1-2.5x	1.0-1.5x
2	2.5-5x	2.5-5x	1.5-2.5x
3	5-10x	5-10x	2.5-5x
4	>10x	>10x	>5x

- HBV or HCV co-infection: Both are associated with increased mortality with HIV co-infection, although the mechanisms are unclear. HCV often represents a marker of injection drug use, which may account for the difference (*JAIDS* 2003;33:365; *CID* 2003;36: 363). HBV is immune-mediated, so immune restoration with ART may account for an increase in HBV progression.

4 Antiretroviral Therapy

- **NRTIs:** Three mechanisms of liver injury are described: 1) hepatic steatosis that accompanies lactic acidosis caused by thymidine analogs (d4T or AZT) or ddI; 2) ABC hypersensitivity; and 3) flares of chronic hepatitis due to the use of drugs active against HBV, including 3TC, FTC or TDF. The mechanism may be HBV resistance, IRIS, or discontinuation of these drugs. The frequency of resistance to 3TC and presumably FTC is 30-50% after 1 year of exposure; it is <2% with TDF (*AIDS* 2003;17:1649). The ABC HSR is a serious multisystem reaction that is seen in 4-5% of ABC recipients with >90% occurring in the first 6 wks of treatment. This reaction is prevented by screening for HLA-B*5701 (*NEJM* 2008;358:568)

- **NNRTIs:** All five NNRTIs may cause hepatotoxicity with elevated transaminases. Reported rates of grade 3-4 hepatotoxicity are 8-15%, and are highest with NVP (*HIV Clin Trials* 2003;4:115; *AIDS* 2003;17:2191; *J Hepatol* 2002;36:283). NVP appears to cause liver disease by two possibly distinct mechanisms. The serious form is symptomatic hepatitis, sometimes associated with hepatic necrosis, which usually occurs in the first 6 wks of treatment, is accompanied by a systemic response (fever, rash, GI symptoms), and resembles a hypersensitivity reaction (*AIDS* 2003;17:2209). This reaction is reported in 11% of women who start NVP as initial treatment with a CD4 count >250 cells/mm³; the risk is also increased in previously untreated men who initiate NVP with a CD4 count >400 cells/mm³. This reaction may not be reversible even when detected early. Frequent monitoring of transaminase levels is commonly advocated, but there is no evidence that this predicts the event. See pg. 335 for management guidelines. The second type of hepatotoxicity usually occurs later in the course of therapy, presents with elevated transaminase levels, and is similar for the transaminitis seen with PIs, NVP, and EFV, especially in patients with HBV or HCV co-infection. Most are asymptomatic. Current recommendations are to discontinue the NNRTI only when there are symptoms or the transaminase levels reach an arbitrary threshold of 5x ULN. Many will spontaneously resolve even when treatment is continued with ALT levels >10x ULN (*Clin Liver Dis* 2003;7:475; *AIDS* 2003;17:2209).

- **PIs:** Hepatotoxicity with PIs is usually characterized by asymptomatic elevations in transaminase levels caused by unknown mechanisms. Liver biopsies in such cases are usually nonspecific and do not show drug-induced injury. Most have resolution of the abnormal tests despite continuation of the implicated drug. Grade 3-4 toxicity (ALT to 5-10x ULN) is most common in patients with HBV or HCV co-infection; it appears to be most frequent with RTV (*JAMA* 2000;283:74) and is dose-related. The recommended intervention is to alter therapy if hepatitis is symptomatic or if the ALT increases above an arbitrary threshold of 5x-10x ULN in the absence of symptoms, especially if the high levels of ALT persist.

Antiretroviral Therapy

Class & Agents	Frequency Grade 3-4	Mechanism
NRTI		
d4T, AZT, ddl	6-13%	**Mitochondrial toxicity** with hepatic steatosis; d4T most common
FTC, TDF, 3TC	6% (?)	**HBV flare** with NRTI: withdrawal or resistance **HBV IRIS**
ABC	5%	**Hypersensitivity**; genetic predisposition; does not occur with negative HLA-B*5701 screen
PI		
All agents	3-10%	**Mechanism unknown**; consequences unknown; transaminase levels may return to normal while continuing PI. Greatest risk with HCV or HBV coninfection.
IDV and ATV	>50%	**Indirect hyperbilirubinemia:** no liver injury, but may cause scleral icterus or jaundice in 3-5% ATV/r > ATV > IDV
TPV	<1%	**Hepatotoxicity:** symptomatic hepatitis that may progress to hepatic failure and death. Most hepatotoxic PI.
NNRTI		
NVP	1-11%	**Hypersensitivity:** symptomatic hepatitis (usually with nausea, vomiting, rash and/or fever in the first 12-16 wks of treatment) (*JID* 2005; 191:825). Risks: baseline CD4 count >250 cells/mm^3 in women, >400 cells/mm^3 in men; rate is 11% in women initally treated with CD4 >250 cells/mm^3 and <2% with CD4 <250 cells/mm^3. **Delayed hepatotoxicity** can also occur: transaminase elevation. Greatest risk is with HBV or HCV co-infection.
EFV, DLV, ETR, RPV	8-15%	**Transaminase elevation**; mechanism unknown; analogous to hepatitis with PIs. Greatest risk with HBV or HCV co-infection.

† Adapted from Olgledigbe and Sulkowski, *Clin Liver Dis* 2003;7:475; Sanne, *JID* 2005;191:825; Price and Thio, *Clin Gastroenterol Hepatol* 2010;8:1002)

Nephrotoxicity:

There are only 3 antiretroviral drugs that are known to have potential for nephrotoxicity: TDF (see pg. 388), ATV (see pg. 193), and IDV (see pg. 294).

4 Antiretroviral Therapy

ART dose modification for liver or renal disease: See Table 4-35

■ TABLE 4-35: **Dosing of Antiretroviral Agents in Renal and Hepatic Failure (2011 DHHS Guidelines)**

Drug NRTIs	Standard Dose	Renal Insufficiency CrCl = mL/min			Hemodialysis[§]	Hepatic Failure
AZT**	300 mg bid	CrCl <15: 100 mg tid or 300 mg qd			100 mg tid or 300 mg qd[†]	Usual dose
ddl	**>60 kg** 400 mg qd **<60 kg** 250 mg qd	CrCl* 30-59 10-29 <10	>60 kg 200 mg/d 125 mg/d 125 mg/d	<60 kg 125 mg/d 100 mg/d 75 mg/d[†]	As with CrCl <10 mL/min[†]	Usual dose
d4T	**>60 kg** 30-40 mg bid **<60 kg** 30 mg bid	CrCl* 26-50 10-25	>60 kg 20 mg bid 20 mg qd	<60 kg 15 mg bid 15 mg qd	Dose after HD	Usual dose
TDF**	300 mg qd	CrCl 30-49 300 mg q48h 10-29: 300 mg 2x/wk <10: No recommendation			q7d (dose post HD)	Usual dose
TDF/ FTC	300/200 mg qd	CrCl 30-49: 300/200 q48h <30 (No recommendation)			Avoid	Usual dose
3TC**	300 mg qd or 150 mg bid	CrCl 30-49: 150 mg qd 15-29: 150 mg, then 100 mg qd 5-14: 150 mg, then 50 mg qd <5: 50 mg, then 25 mg qd			50 mg, then 25 mg qd Take post-dialysis	Usual dose
FTC**	200 mg qd	CrCl ≥50: 200 mg q24h 30-49: 200 mg q48h 15-29: 200 mg q72h <15: 200 mg q96h			200 mg q96h	Usual dose
ABC**	300 mg bid	Usual dose			Usual dose	C-P 5-6: 200 mg bid >6: Avoid

Drug NNRTIs	Standard Dose	CrCl < 10 - >60	Hemodialysis[§]	Hepatic Failure
EFV**	600 mg qd	Usual dose likely	Usual dose	Use with caution
EFV/ TDF/ FTC	1 tab qd	CrCl <50: Coformulation not recommended	Avoid	Use with caution
NVP	200 mg qd x 14 days then 200 mg bid	Usual dose	Usual dose	C-P >6: Avoid
ETR	200 mg bid	Usual dose	Usual dose	Caution with C-P C
RPV	25 mg qd	Usual dose	Caution	CP-C: No studies

continued on next page

Antiretroviral Therapy

148

Drug PIs	Standard Dose	CrCl* < 10 - > 50	Hemodialysis[§]	Hepatic Failure
SQV/r	1000/100 mg bid	Usual dose	Usual dose	Moderate: Caution Severe: Avoid
LPV/r	400/100 mg bid or 800/200 mg qd	Usual dose	Usual dose	Use with caution
ATV	400 mg qd ATV/r 300/100 qd	Usual dose	Usual dose	C-P 7-9: 300 mg qd CP >9: Avoid C-P >6: Avoid RTV
FPV	1400 mg bid FPV/r 700/100 bid FPV/r 1400/100-200 mg qd	Usual dose	Usual dose	PI-naïve (FPV) C-P 5-9 700 mg bid ≥10 350 mg bid PI-naïve or -experienced (FPV/r) C-P 5-6 700 bid/100 qd 7-9 450/bid/100 qd ≥10 300 bid/100 qd
DRV/r	600/100 mg bid	Usual dose	Usual dose	Avoid with severe liver disease
NFV	1250 mg bid	Usual	Usual	Severe liver disease: Avoid
TPV/r	500/200 mg bid	Usual	Usual	C-P 5-6: Caution C-P ≥7: Avoid
ENF	90 mg SC bid	Usual dose	Usual dose	Usual dose
RAL	400 mg bid	Usual dose	Usual dose	Usual dose
MVC	150-600 mg bid	CrCl <30 300 mg bid; 150 mg bid if postural hypotension With potent CYP3A inducers or inhibitors: Avoid	Use with caution	Use with caution

* CrCl = creatinine clearance in mL/min (Cockcroft-Gault equation). For men it is $\frac{(140 - \text{age in yrs}) \times \text{wt (kg)}}{72 \times \text{serum creatinine}}$; for women multiply the result x 0.85.

** Most co-formulated NRTI-containing products should not be used with CrCl <50 mL/min

† Oral solution.

§ Administer post-dialysis on dialysis days. Hemodialysis removes ddI; d4T; 3TC; TDF; and NFV (*AIDS* 2000;14:89). Hemodialysis removes little or none of the following: AZT; ABC; EFV; IDV and RTV. There are sparse data on dose adjustment for most antiretroviral agents based on removal with peritoneal dialysis. Removal is anticipated or established with d4T, which should be dosed post dialysis. Others are not removed or are not expected to be removed.

¶ C-P Score = Child-Pugh Score (see pg. 177).

Antiretroviral Therapy

4

Increased Bleeding in Patients with Hemophilia

Increased spontaneous bleeding episodes in patients with hemophilia A and B have been observed with the use of PIs (*Hemophilia* 2008; 14:140; *AIDS* 2003;17:2397). Most of the reported episodes involved joints and soft tissues. However, more serious bleeding episodes, including intracranial and GI bleeding, have also been reported. The bleeding episodes occurred a median of 22 days after initiation of PI therapy. Some patients received additional coagulation factor while continuing PI therapy (*Hemophilia* 2000;6:487). **TPV** has a black box warning for intracranial hemorrhage based on a report of 13 cases in 2006 (Health Care Provider Letter from Boehringer Ingelheim Pharmaceuticals, June 30, 2006). A predisposition to intracranial hemorrhage represents a relative contraindication to TPV.

Osteopenia/Osteoporosis and Osteonecrosis/Avascular Necrosis See pg. 62, 554.

Osteoporosis is characterized by reduced bone strength with predisposition to fragility fracture, defined as a fracture associated with trauma equivalent to less than a fall from the standing position. Osteoporosis can be diagnosed by measuring bone-mineral density (BMD) using dual-energy x-ray absorptiometry (DXA). The metric used for evaluation is the T score in persons >50 years. The metric used in persons <50 years is the Z score. See pg. 63 for the WHO standards and methods to define osteoporosis. **Osteomalacia** indicates reduced mineralization of bone usually caused by Vitamin D deficiency and may lead to reduced BMD, but is a different condition.

Reduced BMD appears to be promoted by HIV *per se* as noted in a meta-analysis that found osteoporosis to be at least 3 times more common with HIV infection compared to uninfected age-matched controls (*AIDS* 2006;20:2165; *AIDS* 2010;24:2827). A non-progressive loss of BMD is seen with all ART regimens studied. However, the magnitude of BMD loss is greater with TDF (*CID* 2010;51:937; *JID* 2011;203:179). This was demonstrated in the ASSERT trial (*CID* 2010;51:963), which compared ABC/3TC with TDF/FTC and found significantly greater differences in BMD with DXA scans of the hip (-3.6% vs. -1.9%; p=0.001) and lumbar spine (-3.6% vs. -1.6%; p=0.04). Other contributing factors to bone disease in HIV-infected persons are poor nutrition, wasting, smoking, alcohol use, male hypogonadism, reduced vitamin D levels and ART, regardless of regimen used. The mechanism responsible for ART-associated BMD reduction is unknown.

Recommendations for testing are from Bone Disease in HIV Infection: A Practical Review and Recommendation for HIV Care Providers (*CID* 2010;51:937) (see pg. 63; for management guidance, see pg. 555). Recommendations for testing are all post-menopausal women and men >50 years old, based on the fact that HIV infection is now considered to be a risk factor for decreased BMD.

Antiretroviral Therapy

Associated conditions that are most important include: hypogonadism (early menopause, low testosterone, premenopausal oligomenorrhea); adrenal insufficiency; malabsorption; hemophilia; emphysema; lifestyle issues (smoking, alcohol >3 drinks/d, methadone, opiates, sedentary); calcium deficiency; vitamin D deficiency; and selected medications (glitazones, steroids, PPIs).

Diagnostic evaluation: History and physical exam, CBC, chemistry profile, BUN, calcium, phosphate, albumin, alkaline phosphotase, serum 25-hydroxyvitamin level, TSH, parathyroid hormone, 24-hr urine calcium and creatinine, total and free testosterone. Estradiol, FSH, LH, prolactin levels should be ordered in amenorrheic women, and fractional excretion of phosphate should be measured in TDF recipients (simultaneous serum phosphate and creatinine, spot urine phosphate and creatinine) (see *Bone Disorders 3rd Edition*, Livingstone C, Phil PA, Elsevier 2008 and *CID* 2010;51:937; see also pg. 62).

Vitamin D deficiency (*BMJ* 2010;340:b5664)

- **Typical presentation:** musculoskeletal pain and weakness in adults; rickets in children
- **Risk factors:** skin pigmentation, inadequate sun exposure, malabsorption renal or liver disease
- **Sources of vitamin D:** sun (90% of supply) 20-30 min with face exposure at midday is equivalent to 2000 IU vitamin D. Food sources: oily fish, egg yolk, mushrooms, supplemented cereals, margarine and milk
- **Recommended vitamin D intake:** 600 IU (10 ug)/d for adult

What to tell patients about vitamin D and calcium (*J Clin Endocrinol Metab* 2011;96:69) based on the 2010 IOM report (see pg. 65).

- **Bone health** is the only benefit of calcium and vitamin D intake for which there is evidence of disease. (The panel was not convinced that vitamin D treatment played a role in cancer, diabetes, heart disease, autoimmune disease or other health concerns).
- **The recommended daily intake of calcium** is 1000 IU/d for women 19-50 years and for men 19-70 years. For vitamin D the RDA is 600 IU/d for persons 1-70 years and then increases to 800 IU/d for persons >70 years. The upper limit of tolerance is 2000 IU/d for calcium and 400 IU/d for vitamin D.
- **Treatment of osteoporosis:** Alendronate reduces the hip fracture risk by 51% and increases bone mineral density at 3 years by 4.7-6.1%. Bisphosphonates are more efficient, but calcium and vitamin D are inexpensive and should be part of the treatment.

Recommendations for ART in Pregnancy (Based on DHHS Guidelines Recommendations for Use of Antiretroviral Drugs in Pregnant HIV-1-Infected Women for Maternal Health and Interventions to Reduce Perinatal HIV-1 Transmission in the United States September 14, 2011)

MAJOR RESOURCES IN THE US

- 2011 DHHS Guidelines: Recommendations for Use of Antiretroviral Drugs in Pregnant HIV-Infected Women for Maternal Health and Interventions to reduce perinatal HIV transmission in the US (September 14, 2011) (www.mmhiv.com/link/DHHS-Perinatal

- Perinatal HIV Hotline: 888-448-8765; www.mmhiv.com/link/NCCC-Perinatal-Hotline

■ TABLE 4-36: **2011 DHHS Guidelines for Pregnant Women**

Recommendations
Those already receiving ART with viral suppression: Continue same regimen. Exception is to avoid EFV in the first trimester.
Previous ART: Treatment should be based on baseline resistance testing and any prior history of ART. Avoid EFV in the first trimester and NVP with a baseline CD4 count >250/mL.
See relevant sections of the book for guidance in drug selection with hepatitis B co-infection, hepatitis C co-infection or HIV-2 infection.
Altered dosing of some PIs may be required with pregnancy including LPV/r.

WHO RECOMMENDATIONS

- <u>Women who need treatment for their own health</u>
  - □ Indication: CD4 <350 cells/mm³ or WHO stage 3 or 4
  - □ When to start: as soon as feasible
  - □ Regimen: AZT/3TC plus EFV or NVP
  - □ Infant prophylaxis: NVP daily or AZT bid from birth to 4-6 mos

- <u>Women who do not need ART for their own health but need to prevent MTCT</u>
  - □ <u>Option A</u>: antepartum AZT bid plus single dose NVP at onset of labor plus AZT/3TC during labor and delivery until 7 days post partum. With no breast feeding: infant to receive AZT from birth to 4-6 wks.
  - □ <u>Option B</u>: AZT/3TC+NVP to delivery if not breast feeding; if breast feeding continue until one week after breast feeding stopped using AZT/3TC+LPV/r or AZT/3TC/ABC or TDF+3TC+EFV.

- Mechanisms of prophylaxis to prevent perinatal HIV transmission: all phases of pre- and post-exposure prophylaxis contribute.
  - □ Decrease maternal viral load to reduce infant exposure from maternal blood and genital secretions.
  - □ ART reduces transmission even when maternal HIV VL is <1000

c/mL (*JID* 2001;183:539). Thus, the maternal VL correlates with the probability of transmission, but there is no VL threshold that can be considered risk free (*NEJM* 1996;335:1621).

□ Maternal VL at delivery and receipt of antenatal ART independently correlate with risk of transmission (*NEJM* 1996;335:1621).

□ Drugs that cross the placenta to provide systemic levels in the infant; this is particularly important at delivery (see Table 4-37).

□ ART to the mother only at the time of labor and/or only post-partum to the infant reduces infant risk of infection (*Lancet* 2003;362:1171; *JAMA* 2004;292:202; *AIDS* 2005;19:1289).

■ TABLE 4-37: **Safety of Antiretroviral Agents in Pregnancy***

ARV	FDA Cate-gory[†]	Placental Passage Newborn:Maternal Drug Ratio	Long-term Animal Carcinogenicity Studies	Rodent Teratogen
ABC	C	Yes (rats)	Positive (multiple timors in rodents)	Positive (anasarca and skeletal malformations at 1,000 mg/kg, 35 x human exposure, during organogenesis)
ATV	B	Unknown	Positive (adenomas in female mice)	Negative
AZT	C	Yes (human) [0.85]	Positive (rodent, vaginal tumors)	Positive (near-lethal dose)
ddI	B	Yes (human) [0.5]	Negative (no tumors, lifetime rodent study)	Negative
d4T	C	Yes (rhesus) [0.76]	Positive (high doses only)	Negative (but sternal bone calcium decreases)
DLV	C	Unknown	Not completed	Ventricular septal defect
DRV	C	No studies	Negative in rodents	Negative in rodents
EFV	D	Yes (cynomolgus monkeys, rats, rabbits) [~1.0]	Positive (liver adenomas and cancer in female mice)	Anencephaly; anophthalmia; microphthalmia (cynomolgus monkeys)
ENV	B	Unknown	Not done	Negative
FPV	C	Unknown	Positive (liver tumors in rats)	Positive (thymic elongation; incomplete ossification of bones; low body weight)
FTC	B	Yes (rodents)	Negative for tumors	Negative
IDV	C	Minimal (human)	Positive (thyroid adenomas)	Negative (but extra ribs in rats)
LPV/r	C	Yes (human) [0.2]	Positive (liver adenomas and cancer in mice)	Negative (but delayed ossification and increase in skeletal variations in rats at maternally toxic doses)
MVC	B	Unknown	Not done	Negative
NFV	B	Minimal (human)	Not completed	Negative

(continued on next page)

Antiretroviral Therapy

4

153

ARV	FDA Category[†]	Placental Passage Newborn:Maternal Drug Ratio	Long-term Animal Carcinogenicity Studies	Rodent Teratogen
NVP	B	Yes (human) [~1.0]	Positive (hepatic adenomas and cancer)	Negative
TDF	B	Yes (rats and monkeys) [0.95]	Positive (liver adenomas in mice at high doses)	Negative
3TC	C	Yes (human) [~1.0]	Negative (no tumors, lifetime rodent study)	Negative
TPV	C	Unknown	Not completed	Negative, but decreased bone formation in mice
RAL	C	Yes – rodents	In progress	Negative
RTV	B	Minimal (human)	Positive (rodent liver adenomas and cancer in male mice)	Negative (but cryptorchidism in rats at maternally toxic doses)
SQV	B	Minimal (human)	Negative	Negative

* Adapted from 2010 Guidelines for Use of Antiretroviral Drugs in Pregnant HIV-1 Infected Women for Maternal Health and Interventions to Reduce Perinatal HIV-1 Transmission in the U.S., July 8, 2008

† See pg. 178 for pregnancy categories.

2010 DHHS RECOMMENDATIONS

Principles of treatment

- The National Perinatal HIV Hotline provides clinical consultation on all aspects of perinatal HIV care: 1-888-448-8765.

- All pregnant women should receive ART regardless of CD4 count or VL.

- AZT should be included in the regimen unless: 1) severe toxicity precludes use; 2) there is documented resistance; or 3) the woman is already fully suppressed.

- Resistance testing should be performed before starting or changing therapy if the VL exceeds 500-1,000 c/mL.

Currently receiving ART or prior ART

- VL <50 c/mL: Continue current therapy if effective but: 1) avoid EFV in first trimester; 2) continue NVP if VL suppressed even if CD4 count is >250 cells/mm³; 3) continue oral therapy during intrapartum period and give IV AZT by continuous infusion during labor; and 4) if VL remains at 38 weeks, give infant AZT for 6 weeks starting as soon as possible after birth.

- Virologic failure: Perform resistance test and select appropriate regimen on basis of resistance test results and pregnancy guidelines

(Table 4-38). Include AZT if tolerated and active by resistance testing and avoid EFV (1st trimester) and ddI/d4T.

Treatment-naïve

- ART is recommended for all pregnant women regardless of VL.

- Pregnant women who require ART for their own health: Start ART as soon as possible. Regimen is selected by resistance test plus: 1) avoid EFV in the first trimester; 2) avoid ddI/d4T; 3) preferential use of AZT (if active and tolerated); 4) preferential use according to guidance in Table 4-38; 5) use NVP only if CD4 count is <250 cells/mm^3 and then only if benefit exceeds risk of hepatotoxicity; and 6) if VL >1000 c/mL near the time of delivery, schedule C-section at 38 wks and give infant a 6-wk course of AZT starting as soon as possible after birth.

- Pregnant woman who is treated only to prevent perinatal transmission: As above (resistance test, >3 active drugs selected by Table 4-38, avoid EFV, preferential use of AZT, continue ART through delivery with AZT given IV during labor) but: 1) consider AZT monotherapy if VL <1000 c/mL; and 2) consider delay until after the first trimester. Following delivery, ART may be stopped but if regimen includes an NNRTI, the recommendation is to continue NRTIs until 7 days after the VL is <1000 c/mL, consider AZT monotherapy (see below).

- HIV infection untreated prior to labor: 3 options:

Mother (in labor)	Infant
1) AZT IV during labor*	AZT x6 weeks† starting 6-12 hours after birth
2) AZT IV during labor* + NVP PO* + 3TC x7 days postpartum	AZT x6 weeks plus single dose NVP
3) AZT IV during labor*	AZT x6 weeks plus other agent but specific regimens are not well defined

* Mother: AZT IV 2 mg/kg continuous infusion over 1 hour and then 1 mg/kg/hr until delivery plus NVP 200 mg po at onset of labor

† Infant <35 wks: 1.5 mg/kg/dose IV or 2.0 mg/kg/dose po q12h advancing to q8h at 2 wks of >30 wks gestation at birth if mother did not receive intrapartum NVP

- Infant born to HIV infected mother who has not received ART: AZT x 6 wks for the infant (see doses above) or AZT plus additional drugs that are not well defined.

Major obstacles in reducing perinatal HIV transmission in the US

- Transmission rates in the US are reduced to <2% and the number of HIV-infected infants is <200/year (*MMWR* 2006;55:592; *Am J Obstet Gynec* 2007;197 Suppl 3:S10). Major obstacles to further reductions:
  - □ Failure in antenatal testing

4 Antiretroviral Therapy

- Absent or delayed prenatal care
- Acute HIV infection in late pregnancy and breastfeeding
- Lack of full implementation of prevention methods

Special situations

- Hepatitis: Screen for HAV, HBV, HCV. Pregnant women who are HBsAg- and HBsAb-negative should receive HBV vaccine

- HBV/HIV co-infection: Interferon is not recommended in pregnancy. There are several scenarios, with management recommendations that are complicated by overlapping activities and resistance patterns:

  - Requires treatment for HIV and/or HBV: 3-drug regimen including TDF/FTC or TDF+3TC. TDF causes bone changes when used in large doses in animals and is not generally recommended in pregnancy, but the exception may be HIV/HBV coinfection.

  - Requires treatment for HBV only: Stop ART postpartum and treat HBV with interferon or continue 3 drug ART regimen that includes TDF/FTC. (Note: Many authorities now prefer continuing ART).

  - Requires treatment of HIV infection: Continue 3 drug regimen with 2 agents active against HBV.

  - Requires treatment of neither HIV or HBV: Discontinue ART postpartum and monitor carefully for HBV flare. Alternative would be to give NRTI regimen that does not have activity against HBV such as AZT/ddI which can be discontinued post-partum. (Note: Many authorities now prefer treatment of HIV and HBV).

  An infant born to a mother with HIV/HBV coinfection should receive HBIG and the 3 dose vaccine series.

- HCV/HIV co-infection: Interferon is not recommended in pregnancy, and ribavirin is contraindicated. Standard indications for HIV management apply, but obtain transaminase levels at two weeks after starting ART and then monthly after initiating ART. Infants born to mothers with HCV/HIV should have an HCV RNA test at 2-24 wks of age and/or HCV antibody after 15 mos.

Stopping ART during pregnancy

- For severe adverse drug reactions, patient requests, emergency surgery or hyperemesis – stop all drugs.

- With planned treatment interruption using NNRTI-based ART, the recommendation is to continue 2 NRTIs for one week after stopping NNRTI (but optimal time is unknown and may be longer) (*CID* 2006; 44:1123; *HIV Med* 2004;5:180) (see pg. 331).

- Restarting NVP after previous discontinuation reintroduce with 200 mg qd for 2 wks if >2 wks have elapsed since discontinuation.

Virologic failure near term

- C-section: Schedule elective C-section at 38 wks if VL >1000 c/mL

	Agent	Comment
NRTIs		
Recommended	AZT	Preferred based on experience and extensive studies.
	3TC	AZT/3TC is standard NRTI backbone for pregnant women.
Alternatives	ddI	Avoid use with d4T and AZT.
	FTC	Levels are slightly lower in 3rd trimester but standard doses are adequate.
	d4T	Do not use with AZT or ddI.
	ABC	Need HLA B*5701 test to avoid HSR (see pg. 61). Use triple NRTI regimen (AZT/3TC/ABC only when standard regimen cannot be used.
	TDF	Category B. An alternative NRTI and preferred in HBV co-infected pregnant patients. Concern for decreased bone growth is based on juvenile monkeys given 8X the equivalent dose for humans. The prevalence of birth defects in the APR was 2.4% compared to 2.7% in the US population and no such birth defects were observed. Studies for TDF-associated renal disease have shown no abnormal renal function including cystatin levels through 2 years of age (Linde R, et al. 2010 CROI).
NNRTIs		
Recommended	NVP	Avoid initiating NVP in women with baseline CD4 >250 cells/mm³, but women already receiving NVP can continue.
Use in special circumstances	EFV	FDA Pregnancy Class D. Neural tube defects in 3/20 primates and 5 retrospective case reports of women given EFV in first trimester. Consider use in second or third trimester if there are no other alternatives and if contraceptive use is assured after pregnancy.
Insufficient data	ETR	Inadequate safety and pharmacokinetic data in pregnant humans.
PIs		
Recommended	LPV/r	Limited studies in pregnant women are ongoing, but this is now the recommended PI in pregnancy. Based on studies with prior formulation, the recommended dose is 2 tablets bid or 3 tabs bid during third trimester based on PK studies.
Alternatives	NFV	Adequate levels with 1250 mg bid, except 3rd trimester when levels are variable. Alternative when prevention of perinatal transmission is only goal.
	IDV/r	Theoretical concern for hyperbilirubinemia. Considered alternative to LPV/r and SQV/r. Must be boosted.
	SQV/r	Most studies in human pregnancy were done with *Fortovase*, which is no longer available. Recommended dose is SQV/r 1000/100 mg bid.
	ATV/r	Two of three studies show reduced ATV levels with ATV/r treatment and further reduced with concurrent TDF. Theoretical concern is increased indirect bilirubin, but hyperbilirubinemia in the neonate has not been observed yet. ATV or ATV/r are considered alternative PI regimens in pregnancy. Unboosted ATV is an option if RTV is not tolerated, but boosting is required if TDF is given.

Antiretroviral Therapy

4

■ TABLE 4-38: **Recommended Antiretroviral Therapy in Pregnancy (2010 DHHS Guidelines)** (*continued*)

Recommendation	Agent	Comment
PIs (continued)		
Insufficient data	FPV/r	Inadequate safety and pharmacokinetic data in pregnant humans. Must be boosted.
	TPV/r	
	DRV/r	
CCR5 Antagonists		
Insufficient data	MVC	Inadequate data on safety and efficacy in pregnancy
Entry Inhibitors		
Insufficient data	ENF	Inadequate data on safety and efficacy in pregnancy
Integrase Inhibitors		
Insufficient data	RAL	Inadequate data on safety and efficacy in pregnancy

Monitoring HIV during pregnancy

- HIV VL: The risk of transmission correlates with maternal VL, so rapid suppression is important. The recommendation with initial or changed ART is VL testing at 2-4 wks, then monthly until it is <50 c/mL and then then at least every 3 mos. The expectation is a decrease by >1 log by week 4 and <400 c/mL by 24 wks. Failure to achieve these goals should result in an alternative regimen based on resistance tests and pregnancy caveats. The VL should be assessed at 34-36 wks gestation to inform the mode of delivery decision.

- CD4 count: Monitor every 3 mos.

- Ultrasound: Recommended to confirm gestional age in first trimester and for the timing of any planned C-section. Most experts also recommend US in second trimester due to limited experience with ART exposure.

- If amniocentesis is indicated it should be performed in women on ART, preferrably when the VL is undetectable.

- Adverse drug reactions: See pg. 127.

Intrapartum care

- Intrapartum IV AZT is recommended regardless of the prior ART regimen. The recommended regimen is: 2 mg/kg over 1 hr followed by 1mg/kg/hr until delivery. With C-section, IV AZT should be given starting 3 hrs before surgery. AZT is recommended unless there is documented resistance or severe toxicity.

- Discontinue d4T during labor (with IV AZT).

- Intrapartum NVP is not recommended as a single dose of 200 mg po at onset of labor in women receiving ART due to lack of efficacy and increased risk of resistance (*JAMA* 2002; 288:198).

Antiretroviral Therapy

- Patients with <u>VL >1000 c/mL</u> near delivery should undergo scheduled C-section at 38 wks.

- <u>Women who present in labor</u> without prior HIV testing should have a rapid HIV test; if positive, IV AZT should be given during labor and the infant should receive the 6-wk course of AZT as described above.

- <u>If single-dose NVP is given</u>, consider adding 3TC during delivery and give AZT/3TC for 7 days postpartum (to reduce NVP resistance).

Postpartum follow-up

- The <u>decision to continue or stop ART</u> depends on nadir CD4 count, diagnoses of HIV complications and patient preference.

- <u>Breastfeeding</u> is not recommended where affordable alternatives are available.

- <u>Contraceptive counseling</u> is critical.

Interventions for Preventing Perinatal Transmission

The largest U.S. report is the Women and Infants Transmission Study (WITS) Group (*MMWR* 2006;55:592).

HIV Testing and Counseling

HIV TESTING: Standard serologic test with signed, informed consent and/or pretest plus post test counseling is required in some states and opt-out testing is used in most others. All pregnant women should be tested, and the test should be repeated in high-risk patients in the third trimester at 28 wks by CDC recommendations. Patients with an indeterminate test should have an HIV VL test. The rapid test (see pg. 16) is recommended for previously untested women presenting in labor. Women with symptoms suggesting acute HIV infection in the third trimester should be tested using a VL assay. Legally mandated counseling and written consents are seen as barriers to case detection, so that "opt-out testing" is strongly recommended (see pg. 9) (*MMWR* 2006;55: RR14). 2008 DHHS Guidelines (July 6, 2008).

Factors that Reduce Perinatal Transmission

For women who do not breastfeed, intrauterine transmission previously accounted for 25-40% and delivery for 60-75% (*MMWR* 2001;50[RR-19]:63). It should be emphasized that all three components of the AZT regimen (pre-natal, perinatal, and post-natal) have merit. The main currently advocated interventions are ART for the mother plus AZT for the exposed infant and C-section in selected cases. In ACTG 367, a retrospective analysis of 2,756 women, the rates of transmission were 1.3% with ART, 0.8% with ART and a VL <1,000 c/mL and 0.5% with C-section (*NEJM* 2007; 356:135).

VL: There is a direct correlation between maternal VL and probability of perinatal transmission varying from 41% with a VL >100,000 c/mL to

4 Antiretroviral Therapy

0% with a VL <1000 c/mL (*NEJM* 1999;13:407; *JID* 2001;183:206; *JAIDS* 2002;29:484). Despite these findings, there is no VL that can be regarded as safe, because other factors also play a role (*AIDS* 1999;13:1377; *AIDS* 1999;13:407; *JID* 1999;179:590). In an analysis of seven prospective studies, there were 44 cases of HIV in babies born to 1,202 women with VL <1,000 c/mL (*JID* 2001;183:539).

AZT: This drug should be included when possible because it has the largest experience for safety and efficacy. This includes significant reduction in perinatal transmission that is independent of VL (*NEJM* 1996;335:1621; *Lancet* 1999;354:156) and possibly independent of AZT resistance (*JID* 1998;177:557). Analysis of ACTG 076 showed that AZT significantly reduces perinatal transmission even in women with baseline VL <1,000 c/mL (*JID* 2001;183:539). This provides the rationale for AZT monotherapy in untreated pregnant women with a baseline VL <1,000 c/mL, although most experts would recommend this treatment only if a standard ART regimen was refused.

NVP: NVP is the best studied drug other than AZT. Single-dose NVP is the regimen now used most frequently to prevent maternal-to-child transmission in resource-limited countries (*BJOG Int J Obstet Gynecol* 2005;112:1196). However, concerns with this approach include evidence of HIV resistance, even with a single dose at delivery (*NEJM* 2004;351:229). Efficacy in preventing perinatal transmission has been demonstrated in multiple studies, most performed in resource limited areas, with a single maternal dose of 200 mg PO at delivery and one infant dose of 2 mg/kg. This regimen proved easy to implement, cheap, and effective, and transmission rates fell to 7-12% (*JAIDS* 2005;39:121; *JID* 2003;187:725). Addition of AZT, with or without 3TC, at 28-32 wks to the single intrapartum dose of NVP further reduced transmission to 3–7% (*NEJM* 2004;351:217; *AIDS* 2005;19:309).

Single-dose NVP is slightly superior in preventing perinatal transmission compared to a 6-wk course of AZT (*AIDS* 2005;19:1289). However, an analysis of 229 participants given NVP at 6-8 wks postpartum showed NVP resistance mutations in 66 (32%), including the K103N mutation in 48 (21%) (*NEJM* 2004;351: 229). Subsequent reports using allele-specific PCR to detect genotypic resistance in minority species show that resistance mutations are present in 60-80% of patients after single-dose NVP (*JID* 2005;192:24; *AIDS* 2006;20:995). Furthermore, a study from Thailand showed that the women given single-dose NVP subsequently had a suboptimal response to this drug when it was used therapeutically (*NEJM* 2004; 351:229). More recent reports from the OCTANE A5208 trial showed that single-dose NVP at delivery was associated with high rates of virologic failure with NVP-based ART compared to LPV/r-based ART when these drugs were given at >6 mos after delivery (*NEJM* 2010;363:1499). The same high failure rate to NVP treatment of infants after NVP exposure at delivery was reported in the P1060 trial (*NEJM* 2010;363:1510). There have been two strategies to deal with this problem: one is to avoid the risks of NVP monotherapy by adding a 4- to 7-day tail with AZT/3TC or a dose of TDF/FTC, both of which substantially reduce the risk of NNRTI resistance mutations (*NEJM* 2007;356:135; *Lancet* 2007;370:1698). The second strategy is to delay subsequent NVP therapy until > 6 mos post-partum based on the belief that there will be a decrease in NNRTI resistance mutations over time (*AIDS* 2006;20:995). Although eradication of such strains from the latent pool appears to violate one of the basic concepts of HIV pathogenesis, one report found that NVP therapy started within 6 mos of single-dose NVP was associated with failure in 42%, while a delay to >6 mos resulted in failure in only 12%, which was comparable to rates seen with NVP given to treatment-naïve women (*NEJM* 2007;356:13). Long-term durability of NNRTI-based regimens in women who have received single-dose NVP has not been assessed.

CESAREAN SECTION: C-section has established efficacy in reducing perinatal transmission when maternal VL exceeds 1,000 c/mL. A meta-analysis of 15 studies with 8,533 mother-infant pairs showed a 2-fold reduction in perinatal transmission in women given AZT vs. no ART and a 4-fold reduction when AZT was combined with C-section. A study of the European Mode of Delivery Collaboration randomly assigned patients to vaginal delivery vs. C-section. The C-section group had a perinatal transmission rate of 3/170 (1.8%) compared with 21/200 (10.5%) in the vaginal delivery group. However, C-section confers far less benefit for pregnant women given ART due to the substantial reduction in perinatal transmission rates with effective viral suppression (*Br Med J* 2001;322:511). The C-section decision is based on the risk/benefit ratio. There appears to be a slightly increased risk of this surgery to both mother and infant (*Am J Obstet Gynecol* 2002;186: 784; *JAIDS* 2001;26:236; *Am J Obstet Gynecol* 2000;183: 100; *Am J Obstet Gynecol* 2001;184:1108).

The rate of reduction in perinatal transmission varies with ART regimen and maternal VL at delivery (*AIDS* 2000;14:263; *CID* 2001;33:3). The 2010 DHHS Guidelines recommend offering C-section to HIV-infected women with a VL >1000 c/mL at 38 wks. Table 4-39 shows the relative rates of perinatal transmission with and without C-section in the HAART era, as well as an unexplained large difference in the frequency of C-sections in Europe compared to the US (*CID* 2005;40:458). C-section performed at the time of labor or in a patient with ruptured membranes incurs a 5- to 7-fold increased risk of infectious complications and no benefit for reducing perinatal transmission. Other risks for adverse outcomes are non-elective C-section, malnutrition, obesity, smoking, genital infection, low socioeconomic status, prolonged labor, and membrane rupture. The major complications noted in these patients are wound infections, pneumonia, and endometritis. In the largest U.S. study (WITS), there were 2 deaths among 207 HIV-infected women who underwent C-section; both had PCP (*JAIDS* 2001;26:218).

4 Antiretroviral Therapy

	1996	2003
Major form of therapy	AZT or none	HAART ± C-section
Perinatal transmission rate	22.6%	1.2%

Elective C-section performed to prevent perinatal transmission should be done at 38 wks instead of the usual 39 wks. The decision to recommend the procedure at 38 vs. 39 wks has the advantage of reducing the risk of labor and premature rupture of membranes, but a slight increased risk of infant respiratory distress (*Acta Pediatr* 1999;88:1244).

■ TABLE 4-40: **Rates and Results of Cesarean Section to Prevent HIV-Infection in Europe and the U.S.**

	Europe* n = 1579	U.S.[†] n = 1398
Mode of Delivery		
Vaginal	369 (23%)	1098 (79%)
Elective C-section	971 (61%)	108 (8%)
HIV transmission		
Vaginal	24/369 (6.5%)	38/1398 (3.5%)
C-section (elective)	16/971 (1.7%)	1/108 (1%)

* *CID* 2005;40:458
† *JAIDS* 2005;38:87

BREASTFEEDING: The estimated exposure in the average patient without ART is >60,000 infected cells and 500,000 cell-free virions/d (*JID* 1998;177:34). The frequency of HIV transmission with breastfeeding is 10-16% (*JID* 1996;174:722; *JAMA* 2000;283:1167; *Lancet* 1992;340:385; *JAMA* 2000;283:1175). The risk appears to be greatest in the first 4-6 mos (*JAMA* 1999;282:744). The risk is increased 2-fold with mastitis and 50-fold with a breast abscess. Other risk factors include cracked nipples, infant with thrush, primary HIV infection during pregnancy or breast-feeding, prolonged breast-feeding, mixed breast-feeding and early abrupt cessation of breast-feeding (*AIDS* 2006;20:1539; *NEJM* 2008;359:130; *PLoS Med* 2008;5:e63; *NEJM* 2010;363:2271). Breastfeeding is consequently discouraged for HIV-infected women in the developed world, where there are readily available affordable alternatives. The issue is more complex in developing countries, where breastfeeding is critical for infant nutrition and survival (*JAMA* 2000;238:1167) and is advocated in conjunction with ART in the 2010 WHO Guidelines. It is estimated, for example, that 1.7 million babies develop HIV each year due to breastfeeding but that 1.5 million babies would die each year if not breastfed (*Br Med J* 2001;322:511; *Lancet* 2000;355:451).

Evolving data from multiple large trials in low resource countries show benefit for reducing HIV transmission during breast feeding by the following:

Antiretroviral Therapy

- Continued ART in mother during period of breastfeeding – Mma Bana study <1% transmission from breastfeeding mothers on ART (Shapiro R, et al. 5th IAS Cape Town, 2009:Abstr. WeLLB101).
- Exclusive breast-feeding vs. mixed feeding (*AIDS* 2008;22:883).
- Continued breast feeding vs. abrupt cessation (*NEJM* 2008;359:130; *PLoS Med* 2008;5:e63).
- Antibiotic treatment of subclinical mastitis (*J Trop Pediatr* 2006;52: 311).
- Provision of nutrition counseling, clean water and breast milk substitutes (*PLoS Med* 2007;4:e17).
- 3TC prophylaxis for the infant for 6 mos (*JAIDS* 2008;48: 315).
- NVP/AZT prophylaxis to the infant for 14 wks (*NEJM* 2008;359: 179). Note that shorter course NVP is less effective (*Lancet* 2008;372: 300).

■ TABLE 4-41: **Eligibility for ART or ARV Prophylaxis in HIV-infected Pregnant Women + Breastfeeding (WHO 2009)**

Indications for ART or ARV prophylaxis	
CD4 <350 cells/mm³: ART	
CD4 >350 cells/mm³: ARV prophylaxis	
WHO stage 3 & 4 (symptomatic): ART	
WHO stage 1 & 2: ARV prophylaxis	
ART regimens (Treatment)	
Preferred: AZT/3TC + (NVP or EFV)	
Alternative: NRTIs: TDF/3TC or TDF/FTC (+ NVP or EFV)	
ARV Prophylaxis	
Option A	**Option B**
Mother	**Mother**
Antepartum AZT as early as 14 weeks gestation	*Antepartum ARV as early as 14 weeks gestation*
SD-NVP onset of labor	AZT/3TC + LPV/r
AZT/3TC in labor & delivery	AZT/3TC/ABC
AZT/3TC x 7 days postpartum	AZT/3TC + EFV
	TDF + 3TC + EFV
Infant	**Infant**
Breastfeeding: Daily NVP birth to 1 wk	Breastfeeding: Daily NVP birth to 6 wks
Non breastfeeding: AZT or NVP x 6 wks	Non breastfeeding: NVP x 6 wks

Issues with Antiretroviral Agents: See Table 4-37.

SAFETY OF ANTIRETROVIRAL THERAPY: See pg. 153-154. Existing data support the safety of all commonly used antiretroviral agents in pregnancy except ddI + d4T and EFV (*JAIDS* 2000;25:306; *MMWR* 2002;51[RR-7]:1; *NEJM* 2002;346:1879). The combination of **ddI + d4T** (no longer recommended in non-pregnant patients) should be

4 Antiretroviral Therapy

avoided or used cautiously due to reports of 3 maternal deaths ascribed to lactic acidosis and/or hepatotoxicity. **EFV** should be avoided in the first trimester due to neural tube defects in 3/20 monkeys and neural tube defects in at least 3 infants born to women exposed in the first trimester of pregnancy (EFV package insert). Safety in the second and third trimesters is not established but is considered probable since the neural tube is formed by that time. EFV exposures should be reported to the Pregnancy Registry (see below). **NVP** appears safe when given at delivery (*JAIDS* 1999;354:795) but shows high rates of hepatotoxicity, including fatal hepatic necrosis and death when given to pregnant women with a CD4 count >250 cells/mm^3 (see Nevirapine, pg. 330). **TDF** given in high doses to gravid monkeys caused a reduction in body length and reduction in insulin-like growth factor (*JAIDS* 2002;29:207). A report from France suggested mitochondrial toxicity with neurologic sequelae in 8 of 1754 infants exposed to **AZT** alone or AZT/3TC *in utero* (*Lancet* 1999;354:1084). Evaluation of over 16,000 infants exposed to AZT *in utero* has not confirmed the report and showed no evidence of immunologic, cardiac, oncogenic, or neurologic consequences (*NEJM* 2000;3:805). The conclusion is that AZT exposure *in utero* causes mitochondrial toxicity in ≤0.3% (*NEJM* 2002;346:1879). Rodent studies show an increase in vaginal tumors but only at 30x the size-adjusted dose in humans (*J Nat Cancer Inst* 1997;89:1602). There are no supporting data in humans (*JAIDS* 1999;20:43). A 2006 study from the Pregnancy Registry suggested a relationship between AZT exposure in the first trimester and hypospadias (*JAIDS* 2007;44:299).

THE ANTIRETROVIRAL PREGNANCY REGISTRY

Antiretroviral Pregnancy Registry
Research Park, 1011 Ashes Drive
Wilmington, NC 28405
Toll-free from US and Canada (800) 258-4263
Fax (800) 800-1052
From other countries (910) 256-0238
www.apregistry.com

The purpose of the registry is to detect major teratogenic effects of antiretroviral agents. The summary from January 1, 1989 to July 31, 2010 showed 159 outcomes with birth defects among 5,348 (3.0%) live births (2.8/100), which is similar to 3.1/100 rate in the CDC population-base surveillance system. First trimester exposures compared to second- and third-trimester exposures also showed no significant difference (2.8/100 vs. 2.2/100 live births). The largest experience is with AZT (2.9%) and 3TC (3.2%). The sample size was large enough to have detected a 2-fold increase in birth defects, but none was noted (APR, accessed April 15, 2011). See updated data in Table 4-42.

Antiretroviral Therapy

■ TABLE 4-42: **Pregnancy Registry: Birth Defects with First Trimester Exposure January 1, 1989 – April 15, 2011**

Agent	Defect/live birth	Agent	Defect/live birth
3TC	113/3754 (3.0%)	FTC	17/641 (2.7%)
ABC	21/717 (2.9%)	IDV	6/284 (0.8%)
ATV	11/448 (1.2%)	LPV	14/676 (2.1%)
AZT	113/3534 (3.2%)	NFV	45/1182 (3.8%)
d4T	19/797 (2.5%)	NVP	25/970 (2.6%)
ddI	19/404 (4.7%)	RTV	30/1271 (2.4%)
EFV	17/604 (2.8%)	TDF	26/1092 (2.4%)

Intrapartum care: (Data from Registry based on 13,538 pregnancies): Live births 1%; still births 2%; spontaneous abortion 2%; and induced abortion 3%.

PHARMACOLOGY: All NRTIs and NNRTIs cross the placenta; PIs cross poorly (*AIDS* 2002;16:889) (see Table 4-37). Passage of ARVs into breast milk is assumed; it is established for AZT, 3TC, and NVP. LPV/r is the preferred PI for use in pregnancy, but ATV/r also shows favorable pharmacokinetic results in pregnancy (*HIV Clin Trials* 2001;2:460).

RESISTANCE TESTING: Resistance testing should be performed before therapy in all pregnant women (2010 DHHS Guidelines). If there is AZT resistance, this drug should still be given IV during labor and PO to the infant (ACTG 1087, intrapartum and postpartum components).

Adverse Effects of Antiretroviral Agents

GI INTOLERANCE: Nausea and vomiting associated with early pregnancy may complicate drug administration or exacerbate the GI side effects of ART regimens. Possible solutions are antiemetics or altered regimens.

HYPERGLYCEMIA: Some PIs are associated with insulin resistance, and gestational diabetes is a concern with pregnancy. Some authorities advocate a glucose tolerance test with a 50-gm glucose load in early pregnancy with retesting at 24-28 wks gestation.

MITOCHONDRIAL TOXICITY: Pregnancy is associated with increased susceptibility to mitochondrial toxicity with lactic acidosis (*NEJM* 1999;340:1723; *Semin Perinatol* 1999;23:100), so caution is advised when using d4T, ddI, and, to a lesser extent, AZT.

NVP: This drug has been widely advocated for pregnant women based on extensive experience in limited resource countries, but most support is for single-dose treatment to prevent perinatal transmission at delivery. NVP is associated with severe rashes and symptomatic hepatitis including death in at least 6 pregnant women (*JAIDS* 2004;36:772). Most severe rash reactions and liver toxicity occur in the

4 Antiretroviral Therapy

first 6-18 wks. The risk of symptomatic hepatitis is up to 11% in women who initiate NVP with a CD4 count >250 cells/mm³, so the drug should be avoided in this group. With lower CD4 counts the drug may be given with careful monitoring in the first 18 wks to detect hepatotoxicity (transaminase levels), rash, fever and GI symptoms. Women already receiving NVP should simply continue it.

ACTG 076 Protocol (*MMWR* 2002;51[RR-7]:1)

- **Antepartum:** AZT 300 mg bid or 200 mg tid from week 14 to delivery.

- **Intrapartum:** AZT IV 2 mg/kg first hour, then 1 mg/kg/hr until delivery

- **Postpartum:** AZT syrup, 2 mg/kg q6h (or 1.5 mg/kg q6h IV) x 6 wks for the infant

Postexposure Prophylaxis (PEP)

Occupational Exposure

BASICS

- **Resources**

  □ An important resource is the Post Exposure Prophylaxis Hotline (PEPline) from the <u>National HIV/AIDS Clinicians' Consultation Center</u> in San Francisco which provides a 24 hr/d consultation service for post-exposure propylaxis for HIV, HBV and HCV (1-888-448-4911).

  □ <u>CDC guidance</u> This document (www.mmhiv.com/link/2005-CDC-OccupationalExposure) is valuable in risk assessment, but many authorities consider it to be outdated for recommended ARV options.

- **Priority considerations** (*Top HIV Med* 2010;18:174)

  □ The <u>decision to treat</u> should not be delayed by the need for additional information or a lab test, etc. The "72 hour window" implies the "window" is closed at 72 hours, but time delays within that period are important and relative.

  □ <u>The recommendation for PEP</u> is made by the treating physician. The decision to receive PEP is made by the healthcare worker.

  □ <u>Risk assessment</u> for probability of HIV transmission is based on the type of exposure and the HIV status of the source (Tables 4-43 to 4-45). The risk of transmission with a needle stick injury (percutaneous inoculation from an HIV infected source is estimated at 0.3% (95% CI 0.2-0.5). Important variables that increase this risk are a device used in an artery or vein (OR=4.3), high viral load in the source (OR=5.6), visible blood on the sharp source (OR=6.2) and deep penetration (OR=15.0) (*NEJM* 1997;337:1485). The risk for HIV exposure by splashes to broken skin or mucous membranes is estimated at 0.09% (95 CI 0.006-0.5) (*Arch Intern Med* 1993;153:1451).

- **Regimens**
  - □ The 2005 CDC recommendations for a two-drug regimen (Tables 4-44 and 4-45) were for AZT/3TC based largely on passively collected data in patients and non-human primate studies showing efficacy (*JID* 1991;163:625; *J Virol* 2000;74:9775). However, experience has taught that newer NRTIs are better tolerated, equally potent, and also work in the primate model for PEP (*CID* 2004;39:395). Consequently, many authorities now advocate TDF/FTC as preferred (*NEJM* 2009;361:1767; *JAIDS* 2008;47:494; *PLoS Med* 2008;5:e29; *Top HIV Med* 2010;18:74). Preexisting renal disease with a CrCl <50 mL/min is a TDF contraindication. For the third drug in the 3-drug regimen (Tables 4-44 and 4-45), the drugs usually used include RAL, DRV/r or ATV/r based on tolerability and potency (*Top HIV Med* 2010;18:174; *NEJM* 2010;361:1768).
  - □ An additional factor in drug selection is information from the source such as a high VL despite exposure (suggesting resistance), host medical record or knowledge of prior resistance tests suggesting possible transmission of a resistant strain.
- Hepatitis B and C
  - □ Healthcare workers with sharps injuries also have the risk for HBV and HCV transmission. See recommendations for management of HBV exposure (see pg. 172) and HCV exposure (see pg. 173).

RISK OF TRANSMISSION (*MMWR* 2005;54:RR-9)

- A total of 23 studies of needle sticks among health care workers (HCWs) in the pre-HAART era found HIV transmission in 20 of 6,135 (0.33%) exposed to an HIV-infected source (*Ann Intern Med* 1990;113:740). With mucosal surface exposure, there was one transmission among 1,143 exposures (0.09%), and there were no transmissions among 2,712 intact skin exposures. As of June 2005, there were a total of 57 HCWs in the United States who had occupationally acquired HIV infection as indicated by seroconversion in the context of an exposure to an HIV-infected source. This group includes 6 HCWs who received PEP using recommended regimens initiated within 2 hrs after exposure. An additional 136 HCWs who had possible occupationally acquired HIV did not have documented seroconversion in the context of an exposure (*NEJM* 2003;348:826). Occupations among 56 confirmed cases: nurses (23), laboratory technicians (20), and physicians (6). All transmissions involved blood or bloody body fluid except for three involving laboratory workers exposed to HIV viral cultures. Exposures were percutaneous in 48, mucocutaneous in 5, and both in 2 cases. To date, there are no confirmed seroconversions in surgeons and no seroconversions with exposures to a suture needle. Data since 2005 are incomplete.

Antiretroviral Therapy

4

- A retrospective case-control study of needle stick injuries from an HIV-infected source by the CDC included 33 cases who sero-converted and 739 controls (*MMWR* 1996;45:468; *NEJM* 1997;337: 1485). The risks for seroconversion included: 1) deep injury; 2) visible blood on the device; 3) needle placement in a vein or artery; and 4) a source with late-stage HIV infection (presumably reflecting high VL). There was also evidence that AZT prophylaxis was associated with a 79% reduction in transmission rates. Nevertheless, there are at least 21 cases of failures with PEP prophylaxis (*NEJM* 2003;348: 826).

■ TABLE 4-43: **Risk of Viral Transmission with Sharps Injury from Infected Source**

Source		Prevalence (U.S. general population)	Risk/exposure with sharps injury
HIV		0.3%	0.3%
HBV	HBsAg +	0.1-0.3%	1-6%*
	HBeAg +	0.05-0.1%	22-31%*
HCV		1.8%	1.9%

* Unvaccinated HCW

PEP RECOMMENDATIONS AND CHOICE OF REGIMEN: Recommendations are based on the type of exposure, HIV status of the source, or, if the status is unknown, the risk status of the source.

MANAGEMENT RESOURCES

- National Clinicians' Postexposure Prophylaxis Hotline (AETC, CDC): 888-448-4911 or www.mmhiv.com/link/NCCC-PEPline
- Hepatitis information line: 888-443-7232 or www.mmhiv.com/link/CDC-Hepatitis
- CDC Guidelines for occupational exposure (*MMWR* 2005;54:RR-9).
- CDC Reporting (occupationally acquired HIV and PEP failure): 800-893-0485 or www.mmhiv.com/link/CDC-HIV-Hepatitis-PEP
- HIV/AIDS treatment information: www.aidsinfo.nih.gov

TESTING IN THE SOURCE PATIENT: If there is no recent positive or negative serology, a rapid test (see pg. 16) is preferred. Results should be available in <1 h. Rapid tests are as reliable as standard serology for excluding HIV infection (false negatives in "window" period), and testing is highly cost effective in preventing unnecessary empiric short-term courses of antiretroviral agents (*Infect Control Hosp Epidemiol* 2001;22:289). Standard serologic tests may take 3-7 days, but a negative EIA screening assay is usually available in 24-48 hrs and is adequate for the decision to discontinue PEP if the rapid test is not available. The CDC recommends opt-out HIV testing, which should facilitate testing the source, although few states have laws that still require counseling and signed informed consent (*MMWR* 2006;44:RR14). If the source has had an illness compatible with acute HIV syndrome, testing should include plasma HIV RNA levels.

Antiretroviral Therapy

■ TABLE 4-44: **HIV Postexposure Prophylaxis for Percutaneous Injuries**

Exposure	Status of Source		
	HIV + and Low Risk*	HIV + and High Risk*	Unknown
Not severe: Solid needle, superficial	2-drug PEP[†]	3-drug PEP[†]	Usually none; consider 2-drug PEP[‡]
Severe: Large bore, deep injury, visible blood in device, needle in patient artery/vein	3-drug PEP[†]	3-drug PEP[†]	Usually none; consider 2-drug PEP[‡]

* Low risk: Asymptomatic HIV or VL <1,500 c/mL. High risk: Symptomatic HIV, AIDS, acute seroconversion, and/or high VL.

† Concern for drug resistance: Initiate prophylaxis without delay and consult an expert.

‡ Consider 2-drug PEP if source is high risk for HIV or exposure is from an unknown source with HIV infection likely.

■ TABLE 4-45: **HIV Postexposure Prophylaxis for Mucous Membranes and Non-intact Skin Exposures***

Exposure	Status of Source		
	HIV + and Low Risk[†]	HIV + and High Risk[†]	Unknown
Small volume (drops)	Consider 2-drug PEP	2-drug PEP	Usually no PEP; consider 2-drug PEP[‡]
Large volume (major blood splash)	2-drug PEP	3-drug PEP	Usually no PEP; consider 2-drug PEP[‡]

ˣ Non-intact skin: Dermatitis, abrasion, wound

† Low risk: Asymptomatic or VL <1500 c/mL. High risk: Acute seroconversion or high VL.

‡ Consider if source has HIV risk factors or exposure from unknown source where HIV-infected source is likely.

MONITORING AND COUNSELING THE HCW

- **Testing the HCW:** HIV serology should be performed at the time of injury, and repeated at 6 wks, 3 mos, and 6 mos. It should be repeated at 12 mos in HCW who acquired HCV with the injury, since this may delay HIV seroconversion (*NEJM* 2003;348:826; *Am J Infect Control* 2003;31:168).

- **VL:** VL testing is sometimes done because HIV viremia precedes positive serology, but caution is need in the interpretation due to high rates of false positives with VL levels <10,000 c/mL (*JID* 2004;190:598). Confine VL testing to patients with a febrile illness consistent with the acute retroviral syndrome since these patients may be in the window that precedes seroconversion.

- **Precautions to prevent sexual transmission:** The HCW should be advised to practice safe sex or abstain until serology is negative at 6 mos postexposure. The greatest risk is the first 6-12 wks, and many authorities recommend these precautions only to the 3-mo test.

4 Antiretroviral Therapy

Agent	Comment
Nucleoside Analogs	
AZT	Only drug with established efficacy; high rates of GI intolerance, fatigue and headache; monitor CBC
3TC	3TC or FTC included in most regimens due to good tolerability, potency, and qd dosing – High rates of resistance if source has virologic failure
d4T	Potent; good short-term tolerability; better tolerated than AZT, but rarely used for ART or PEP - Avoid ["Avoid" in bold as below]
ABC	Need for immediate PEP doesn't allow for HLA B*5701 prescreening; potential for hypersensitivity reaction (reported in 5-9%) – **Avoid**
ddI	Fasting requirement, GI intolerance. **Avoid**
TDF	Well tolerated, effective for PEP in primate model, benefit of qd dosing
FTC	Similar to 3TC and coformulated with TDF
Non-nucleoside RTIs	
EFV	Potent, but concern for short-term CNS toxicity in HCW – Not attractive in this setting
NVP	**Avoid:** FDA has reports of 22 PEP recipients with serious reactions to NVP, including 12 hepatotoxicity cases (one requiring a liver transplant) and 14 skin reactions, including 3 with Stevens Johnson syndrome
ETR	Active against some NVP and EFV resistant strains. Often combined with DRV/r – attractive when resistance in transmitted strain is a concern
RPV	Limited experience but probably similar to ETR for resistance advantages
Protease Inhibitors	
LPV/r	Potent and often favored among PIs.
ATV ± RTV	Potent, well tolerated, qd dosing, boosted well with RTV; food requirement, risk of jaundice, boosting requirement with concurrent TDF, gastric acid required - avoid with PPIs
NFV	Alternative options are better
FPV ± RTV	Potent, option of once-daily therapy; no food effect
IDV/r	Alternative options are better
SQV/r	Potent, option for once daily therapy
DRV/r	Potent and well tolerated. Attractive for PEP, especially if resistance is suspected in the source
Entry Inhibitors	
ENF	Some theoretical advantages with blocking entry, but no experience in PEP and requirement for time-consuming reconstitution and SC injection
Integrase Inhibitors	
RAL	Potent and well tolerated. Attractive option, especially if transmitted resistance is a concern
CCR5 Antagonist	
MVC	Transmitted HIV is almost exclusively R5 – so this should be effective

Antiretroviral Therapy

- **Time:** PEP should be initiated as quickly as possible, preferably within 1-2 hrs of exposure and up to 36 hrs postexposure. The median time from exposure to treatment in 432 HCWs with HIV exposure from October 1996 to December 1998 was 1.8 hrs (*Infect Control Hosp Epidemiol* 2000;21:780).

- **Side effects:** For HCWs who receive PEP, about 74% experience side effects, primarily nausea (58%), fatigue (37%), headache (16%), vomiting (16%), or diarrhea (14%). About 50% discontinue treatment before completion of the 4-wk course due to multiple factors including side effects of drugs (*Infect Control Hosp Epidemiol* 2000;21:780). The side effects largely reflect the drugs advocated in the 2005 CDC guidance, especially AZT.

- **Pregnancy:** EFV, TDF, and the combination of ddI + d4T should be avoided in pregnancy. Favored agents for HCWs who are pregnant are summarized on Table 4-41, pg. 163. CDC guidelines state that pregnancy should not preclude ART. Counseling non-pregnant HCWs with childbearing capacity should include a discussion of these risks including the extensive safety data of most drugs in the Pregnancy Registry (Table 4-45). The same applies to breast feeding.

- **Breastfeeding:** Consider temporary discontinuation of breastfeeding during antiretroviral therapy.

- **Resistance testing:** Guidance for drug selection may be available from the source in terms of: 1) VL to assess risk; and 2) treatment, response, and results of resistance to inform drug selection. This testing may also be done in the source at the time of injury if precludes rapid institution of PEP. Most authorities recommend that decisions be based on the drug history and VL of the source. In a review of 52 patients who were the source of occupational exposures, 39% involved stains with major mutations conferring resistance (*NEJM* 2003;348:826). This is another issue for which assistance from an HIV expert is appropriate.

HEALTH CARE WORKER-TO-PATIENT TRANSMISSION

- **History:** This became a topical issue in 1990 a Florida dentist was identified as the source of HIV infection for 6 dental patients (*Ann Intern Med* 1992;116:798; *Ann Intern Med* 1994;121:886). The source of the virus was established by genetic sequencing (*J Virol* 1998;72:4537), but the mechanism of transmission was never established. This disclosure led to a series of "look-backs" in which serologic tests were performed on >22,000 patients who received care from 59 health providers with known HIV infection. No transmissions were identified (*Ann Intern Med* 1995;122:653). Since that time, there have been 2 additional cases in France, one traced to a total hip procedure and two others with C-sections (*AIDS* 2006;20:285; *Ann Intern Med* 1999;130:1). As of 2002, totals for known transmissions from infected surgeon to patient are 375 for HBV, 7 for HCV, and 2 for HIV (*Hosp Infect Control* 2003;7:88).

4 Antiretroviral Therapy

- **Management of HIV-infected HCW**
  - □ Concern about the incident with the Florida dentist led to a federal law in 1991 requiring states to establish guidelines for HIV-positive HCWs. Most states adopted CDC recommendations that required persons who perform "exposure-prone invasive procedures" (surgery in a blind body cavity) to 1) advise the patient of the HCW's serostatus and 2) obtain written informed consent from the patient. This applies to surgeons, nurses, and other members of the operating team.
  - □ A review by Dr. Julie Gerberding, an expert in this topic and Director of the CDC at that time, emphasized that patients who have exposures analogous to what would be defined as a potential risk for occupational exposure to a HCW should be managed by standard guidelines with respect to counseling, serologic testing, and antiretroviral therapy.

OCCUPATIONAL EXPOSURE TO HEPATITIS B VIRUS (HBV)

- **Efficiency of transmission:** Highly dependent on vaccine status of HCW and the HBeAg status of the source.

- **HBV postexposure prophylaxis:** Recommendations are based on the vaccine status of the healthcare worker, evidence of serologic response (anti-HBs levels >10 mIU/mL), and the HBsAg status of the source. Responder status of the HCW is best assessed with serology at 1-6 mos after completion of the 3-dose series. Response is age-related: 95% for persons 20-30 years of age, 86% at 40-50 years of age, and 45% at ≥65 years of age. Titers decrease an average of 10%/yr, but prior responders with antibody titers >10 mIU/mL are probably protective. Non-responders have a 55% probability of response to re-vaccination.

■ TABLE 4-47: **HBV Postexposure Prophylaxis**

Vaccination Status of HCW	HBsAg Status of Source	
	HBsAg Positive	Source Unknown
Unvaccinated	HBIG* + vaccine series (3 doses)	HBV vaccine (3 doses)
Vaccinated		
Responder[†]	No Rx	No Rx
Non responder	HBIG x 1 + vaccine series or HBIG x 2 [‡]	Rx as source positive if high risk
Antibody status unknown	Test for anti-HBs ■ Anti-HBs >10 mIU/mL – no Rx ■ Anti-HBs <10 mIU/mL – HBIG x 1 + vaccine booster	Test for anti-HBs ■ Anti-HBs >10 mIU/mL – no Rx ■ Anti-HBs <10 mIU/mL – HBV vaccine series with titer at 1-2 mo

* HBIG = Hepatitis B immune globulin; dose is 0.06 mL/kg IM. Should be given as soon as possible and within 7 days.
† Responder defined by antibody to HBsAg of >10 mIU/mL.
‡ HBIG + the vaccine series is preferred for non-responders who did not complete the 3-dose series; HBIG x 2 doses is preferred if there were 2 vaccine series and no response.

Antiretroviral Therapy

- **Vaccine efficacy:** 80-95% when considering all vaccine recipients; 99% for responders.

OCCUPATIONAL EXPOSURE TO HEPATITIS C VIRUS (HCV)

- **Efficiency of transmission:** A review of 25 studies published from 1991 to 2002 found that the rate of HCV transmission following a sharps injury from an HCV-infected source was 44/2357 (1.9%) (*Clin Microbiol Rev* 2003;16:546). Cutaneous exposure to contaminated blood with intact skin does not appear to confer risk.

- **Seroprevalence of HCV (U.S.):** General population 1.8%; HCW 0.5-2%; gay men 2-6%; hemophilia patients 60-90%; injection drug users 60-90%.

- **HCV postexposure management**

  □ Source testing: Anti-HCV; confirm positives with qualitative PCR

  □ HCW: Anti-HCV and ALT at baseline and at 3-6 mos. Confirm positive serology with qualitative PCR.

  □ HCV RNA may be tested at 4-6 wks to detect acute HCV prior to seroconversion. Persons with documented acute HCV infection should have positive quantitative HCV PCR at 2-4 wks, usually accompanied by asymptomatic elevation of ALT. This precedes anti-HCV seroconversion.

  □ No prophylaxis with immune globulin (*CID* 1993;16:335) or with antiviral agents (interferon + ribavirin) is recommended (*CID* 1993;16:335; *JID* 1996;173:822; *Clin Microbiol Rev* 2003;16:546).

- **Management of patients with occupationally acquired HCV:** Postexposure monitoring with HCV PCR will detect early seroconversion. One report showed a high rate of HCV cure with treatment of acute HCV (*NEJM* 2001;345:1452) and others have had a similar experience in HCWs with occupationally acquired HIV (*Infection* 2005;33:30). Nevertheless, this approach has received varying degrees of endorsement (*Infect Control Hosp Epidemiol* 2001;22:53). The major concerns are the drug-associated toxicity for treatment of an infection that has a 20-40% probability of spontaneous clearance (*Hepatology* 2001;34:341; *Hepatology* 2002; S195; *Hepatology* 2001;34:341; *Hepatology* 2002;36:1020), the relatively benign long-term prognosis in persons without additional risk factors (*Hepatology* 1999;29:908), and the lack of data to show treatment at this stage is superior to standard guidelines for management of chronic infection (*Clin Microbiol Rev* 2003;16:546). Treatment in the acute phase should therefore be considered experimental. This strategy is also endorsed by the European guidelines (*Euro Surveill* 2005;10:260).

4 Antiretroviral Therapy

Non-occupational HIV Exposure
(Sexual Contact or Needle Sharing)

RISK OF TRANSMISSION

Follow-up: a more recent report indicated that the risk was greatest with acute HIV infection when the VL was highest (0.008/coital act in 5 mos after conversion compared to 0.0007/coital act in 8 year with chronic infection; *JID* 2005;191:1403).

■ TABLE 4-48: **Risk of HIV Transmission with Single Exposure from an HIV-infected Source**

Exposure	Source	Risk/10,000 exposures
Blood transfusion	Donegan E, *Ann Int Med* 1990;113:733	9,000
Needle-sharing IDU	*JAIDS* 1995;10:175	67
Receptive anal intercourse	*Br Med J* 1992;304:809	50
Needle stick injury	*Am J Med* 1997;102:9	30
Receptive vaginal intercourse	*Br Med J* 1992;304:809 *Sex Transm Dis* 2002;29:38 *Am J Epid* 1998;148:88	10
Insertive anal intercourse	*Br Med J* 1992;304:809 *Sex Transm Dis* 2002;29:38	6-7
Insertive vaginal intercourse	*Br Med J* 1992;304:809 *Sex Transm Dis* 2002;29:38	5

■ TABLE 4-49: **Risk of HIV Transmission in 415 Untreated Discordant Couples (*NEJM* 2000;342:921)**

Viral Load	Transmissions/100 Person-ys
<400 c/mL	0
400-3,500 c/mL	4.8
3,500-50,000 c/mL	14.0
>50,000 c/mL	23.0

■ TABLE 4-50: **Recommended Tests on Exposed Person and Source**

Exposed Person	Baseline	During PEP	4-6 wks	3 mo	6 mo
HIV serology	+		+	+	+
CBC, LFTs, BUN, creatinine	+	+			
STD (GC, chlamydia, syphilis)	+	+*	+*	–	–
HBV	+	–	+*	+*	–
HCV	+	–	–	+	+
Pregnancy	+	+*	+*		
If HIV seroconversion					
HIV VL			+	+	+
Resistance test			+	+	+
CD4 count			+	+	+

*　As clinically indicated
　For source, tests at baseline: HIV serology, STD screen (GC, *C. trachomatis*, and syphilis), HBVsAg, HCV Ab

Antiretroviral Therapy

CDC RECOMMENDATIONS FOR NON-OCCUPATIONAL EXPOSURE TO HIV, HBV AND/OR HCV (*MMWR* 2004;54[RR-2:1])

Recommendations are based to a large extent on probability of HIV infection in the source, the ability to deliver PEP within 72 hrs of exposure and the type of exposure. The recommendations are summarized in the following table.

■ TABLE 4-51: **CDC Recommendations for HIV Prophylaxis After Non-occupational Exposure (nPEP)**

nPEP is recommended if there is substantial risk of exposure within 72 hours and:
1. Exposure of vagina, rectum, eye, mouth, other mucosal surface, nonintact skin or subcutaneous **and**
2. Exposure with: Blood, semen, vaginal secretions, rectal secretions, breast milk, bloody fluid **and**
3. From: Source likely to be infected **and**
4. Time from exposure: <72 hours

nPEP is not recommended if there is:
1. Delay >72 hours from time of exposure **or**
2. Negligible risk based on exposure with: urine, nasal secretions, saliva, sweat or tears if not visibly contaminated with blood (regardless of HIV status of source)

nPEP recommended on case-by-case basis if:
1. Substantial risk exposure (defined above)
2. Within 72 hours of exposure **and**
3. Source patient HIV status unknown

Recommended regimens:
The recommendations follow the 10/29/04 recommendations of DHHS guidelines for initial treatment of HIV infection, with the exception that NVP has been removed from the list.

Preferred regimens
■ EFV* + (3TC or FTC) + (AZT or TDF)
■ LPV/r + (3TC or FTC) + AZT

Alternative regimens
■ EFV* + (3TC or FTC) + (ABC, ddI, or d4T)
■ ATV (or ATV/r) + (3TC or FTC) + (TDF, AZT d4T, ABC, or ddI)
■ FPV + (3TC or FTC) + (AZT or d4T) or (ABC, TDF, or ddI)
■ FPV/r + (3TC or FTC) + (AZT d4T, ABC,TDF, or ddI)
■ IDV/r + (3TC or FTC) + (AZT d4T, ABC,TDF, or ddI)
■ LPV/r + (3TC or FTC) + (d4T, ABC, TDF, or ddI)
■ NFV + (3TC or FTC) + (AZT, d4T, ABC, TDF, or ddI)
■ SQV/r + (3TC or FTC) + (AZT, d4T, ABC, TDF, or ddI)
*Avoid in pregnancy

4 Antiretroviral Therapy

5 | Drug Information

DRUG PROFILES are listed alphabetically by generic drug names.

TRADE NAME and pharmaceutical company source are provided unless there are multiple providers. Trade names are for United States brands.

COST is based on average wholesale price (AWP) according to www.mckesson.com (2010). Prices are generally given for generic products when generics are available.

PHARMACOLOGY, SIDE EFFECTS, AND DRUG INTERACTIONS: Data are from Drug Information 2010, American Hospital Formulary Service, Bethesda, MD; *PDR* 2010; published conference abstracts (CROI, IAC, ICAAC, IAS, HIV Pharm Workshop 2009-10).

CREATININE CLEARANCE (COCKCROFT-GAULT EQUATION)

- **Males:** $\dfrac{\text{Weight (kg) x (140 - age)}}{72 \text{ x serum creatinine (mg/dL)}}$

- **Females:** Determination for males x 0.85

- **Obese patients:** Use lean body weight.

- **Formula assumes stable renal function.** Assume creatinine clearance (CrCl) of 5-8 mL/min for patients with anuria or oliguria.

- **Pregnancy and volume expansion:** GFR may be increased in third trimester of pregnancy and with massive parenteral fluids.

Note: <u>MDRD equation</u>: 186 x serum creatinine $(\text{mg/dL})^{-1.154}$ x Age $^{-0.203}$ x (1.212 if Black) x (0.742 if female). This has not been validated in HIV-infected patients.

■ TABLE 5-1: **Child-Pugh Calculation**

Points	1	2	3
Bilirubin (mg/dL)	< 2	2-3	> 3
Albumin (g/dL)	> 3.5	3.5-2.8	< 2.8
PT (seconds)	< 4	4-6	> 6
Ascites	Absent	Mild-mod	Severe
Encephalopathy*	Absent	Mild (1-2)	Severe (3-4)
INR	< 1.7	1.7-2.3	> 2.3
Child-Pugh A = 5-6 points, B = 7-9 points, C = 10-15 points			

* 1 Personality change, ↓attention span, mild asterixis; uncoordinated; EEG slowing

  2 Lethargic; asterixis; EEG slowing, triphasic

  3 Asleep; asterixis; EEG slowing, triphasic

  4 Comatose, decerebrate, EEG-Severe slowing

5 Drug Information

PATIENT ASSISTANCE PROGRAMS: Most pharmaceutical companies that provide this service require all of the following:

- Income eligibility criteria such as an annual income <$12,000 for an individual or <$15,000 for a family
- Non-availability of prescription drug payment from public or private third party sources
- A prescription and a letter of verification

Note: Most will provide a 3-mo supply subject to rereview after that time (see www.needymeds.com).

CLASSIFICATION FOR DRUG USE IN PREGNANCY BASED ON FDA CATEGORIES: Ratings range from "A" for drugs that have been tested for teratogenicity under controlled conditions without showing evidence of damage to the fetus to "D" and "X" for drugs that are definitely teratogenic. The "D" rating is generally reserved for drugs with no safer alternatives. The "X" rating means there is absolutely no reason to risk using the drug in pregnancy.

■ TABLE 5-2: **FDA Pregnancy Classification**

Category	Interpretation
A	**Controlled studies show no risk.** Adequate, well-controlled studies in pregnant women have failed to demonstrate risk to the fetus.
B	**No evidence of risk in humans.** Either animal findings show risk, but human findings do not, or, if no adequate human studies have been performed, animal findings are negative.
C	**Risk cannot be ruled out.** Human studies are lacking, and animal studies are either positive for fetal risk, or lacking as well. However, potential benefits may justify the potential risk.
D	**Positive evidence of risk.** Investigational or postmarketing data show risk to the fetus. Nevertheless, potential benefits may outweigh the potential risk.
X	**Contraindicated in pregnancy.** Studies in animals or humans, or investigational or postmarketing reports, have shown fetal risk that clearly outweighs any possible benefit to the patient.

PREGNANCY REGISTRY FOR ANTIRETROVIRAL DRUGS: This is a joint project sponsored by pharmaceutical companies and an advisory panel with representatives from the CDC, NIH, obstetrical practsitioners, and pediatricians. The registry allows anonymity of patients and birth outcome follow-up is obtained by registry staff. Healthcare professionals should report prenatal exposures to antiretroviral agents to: Antiretroviral Pregnancy Registry, Research Park, 1011 Ashes Drive, Wilmington, NC 28405; 800-258-4263; fax 800-800-1052; (www.apregistry.com). For interpretation of rates it should be noted that the rate quoted for infants without exposure to antiretroviral agents is 2.7/100 live births and 2.09/100 live births for the first 7 days. Data are provided for antiretroviral agents with >200 first trimester exposed live births.

■ TABLE 5-3: **Classification of Controlled Substances**

Category	Interpretation
I	**High potential for abuse and no current accepted medical use.** Examples are heroin and LSD.
II	**High potential for abuse.** Use may lead to severe physical or psychological dependence. Examples are opioids, amphetamines, short-acting barbiturates, and preparations containing codeine. Prescriptions must be written in ink or typewritten and signed by the practitioner. Verbal prescriptions must be confirmed in writing within 72 hours and may be given only in a genuine emergency. No renewals are permitted.
III	**Some potential for abuse.** Use may lead to low-to-moderate physical dependence or high psychological dependence. Examples are barbiturates and preparations containing small quantities of codeine. Prescriptions may be oral or written. Up to five renewals are permitted within 6 months.
IV	**Low potential for abuse.** Examples include chloral hydrate, phenobarbital, and benzodiazepines. Use may lead to limited physical or psychological dependence. Prescriptions may be oral or written. Up to five renewals are permitted within 6 months.
V	**Subject to state and local regulation.** Abuse potential is low; a prescription may not be required. Examples are antitussive and antidiarrheal medications containing limited quantities of opioids.

ABACAVIR (ABC)

TRADE NAME: *Ziagen* (GlaxoSmithKline)

CLASS: Nucleoside analog

FORMULATIONS, REGIMEN AND COST:

- ***Ziagen***
  - Formulations: 300 mg tab; 20 mg/mL oral soln.
  - Regimen: 300 mg bid or 600 mg qd
  - AWP: $615/mo
- ***Trizivir:*** AZT/ABC/3TC (300/300/150 mg tab)
  - Regimen: 1 tab bid
  - AWP: $1,608/mo
- ***Epzicom* (or *Kivexa*):** ABC/3TC (600/300 mg tab)
  - Regimen: 600 mg qd (1 tab)
  - AWP: $1,073/mo

PATIENT ASSISTANCE: 866-728-4368

FOOD: Take without regard for meals

RENAL FAILURE: ABC – no dose adjustment; *Trizivir,* and *Epzicom* – not recommended with CrCl <50 mL/min; use separate components with dose adjustment.

HEPATIC FAILURE: Based on limited clinical data, 200 mg bid may be used for Child-Pugh class A (CP score 5-6). Some use the standard dose. Some use standard dose. Contraindicated for classes B and C (CP score 7-12). No data in moderate to severe hepatic impairment.

Drug Information

5

ADVANTAGES: Well tolerated, once-daily therapy, no food effect and excellent CNS penetration.

DISADVANTAGES: Hypersensitivity reaction in 5-8% of patients. Screening for HLA-B*5701 nearly eliminates the risk of this reaction and should be performed prior to administration (see pg. 61). Reports from D:A:D and SMART studies suggest that ABC may be associated with an increased risk of cardiovascular disease (this is debated), and ACTG 5202 suggests that ABC/3TC may be inferior to TDF/FTC in treatment of patients with a baseline VL >100,000 c/mL (see below).

POTENCY: With monotherapy, ABC reduced viral load 1.5-2.0 logs – significantly more than AZT, ddI, 3TC, and d4T. Most trials have shown good potency when combined with an NNRTI or PI/r (Table 5-4). ACTG 5202 is a randomized trial comparing ABC/3TC vs. TDF/FTC combined with EFV or ATV/r. After enrollment of >1800 participants, the study was stopped by the DSMB due to excessive rates of virologic failure in ABC/3TC recipients with a baseline VL >100,000 c/mL (*NEJM* 2009;361:2230). The difference was highly significant (p=0.003) and was independent of the third drug (EFV or ATV/r). Suboptimal response with ABC/3TC treatment of patients with baseline VL >100,000 c/mL has not been seen in other trials, but these have smaller sample sizes or trial designs that are less optimal. Results of ACTG 5202 for patients with a baseline VL <100,000 c/mL showed no difference between these two NRTI pairs, which was surprising, although meta-analysis of 12 trials with 5,168 patients found TDF/FTC was superior in virologic outcome with baseline VL >100,000 c/mL (p<0.002) and <100,000 c/mL (p=0.02) (*HIV Med* 2009;10:527).

CLINICAL TRIALS OF ABC/3TC AS INITIAL THERAPY

Comparison of NRTIs and NRTI combinations:

- **CNA 30024** compared AZT/3TC and ABC/3TC, each with EFV, in 699 treatment-naïve patients. At 48 weeks VL was <50 c/mL in 69% and 70%, respectively, by ITT analysis (*CID* 2004;39:1038). ABC/3TC was associated with less anemia, nausea, and vomiting, but more hypersensitivity reactions. This paved the way to coformulation (*Epzicom*).

- **Comparison of ABC/3TC once- vs. twice-daily: ESS 3008** compared twice-daily vs. once-daily ABC/3TC combined with a PI or NNRTI. Viral suppression was sustained at 48 weeks in 81% in the once-daily group vs. 82% in the twice-daily group. Adherence was better in the once-daily group. (*JAIDS* 2005;40:422). (Note: The intracellular half-life is 12-21 hr, justifying once-daily dosing.)

- **BICOMBO:** Comparison of ABC/3TC vs. TDF/FTC: 333 patients with virologic control while receiving a 3TC-containing regimen were randomized to TDF/FTC vs. ABC/3TC as the NRTI backbone (*JAIDS* 2009;51:290). Results at 48 weeks showed virologic failure in 4 (2%) in the ABC/3TC group vs. none in the TDF/FTC group.

■ TABLE 5-4: **Major Clinical Trials of ABC in Initial Therapy**

Study	Regimen	N	Dur (wks)	VL <50	VL <400
CNA 3014 *Curr Med Res Opin* 2004;20:1103	AZT/3TC/ABC	164	48	60%	66%*
	AZT/3TC+IDV	165		50%	50%
CNA 3005 *JAMA* 2001;285:1155	AZT/3TC/ABC	262	48	31%	51%
	AZT/3TC+IDV	265		45%*	51%
ACTG 5095 *NEJM* 2004;350:1850	AZT/3TC/ABC	382	48	61%	74%[†]
	AZT/3TC+EFV±ABC	765		83%*	89%[†]
CNA 30024 *CID* 2004;39:1038	ABC/3TC+EFV	324	48	70%	
	AZT/3TC+EFV	325		69%	
CNA 30021 (ZODIAC) *JAIDS* 2005;38:417	ABC (qd)+3TC+EFV	384	48	66%	—
	ABC (bid)+3TC+EFV	386		68%	—
ESS 30009 *JID* 2005;192:1921	ABC/3TC+TDF	102	12‡		51%‡
	ABC/3TC+EFV	169	48	71%	75%*
ESS 30008 *JAIDS* 2005;40:422	ABC/3TC (qd) + 3rd agent	130	48	82%	
	ABC/3TC (bid) + 3rd agent	130		81%	
HEAT (Smith KY, et al. 17th Intern. AIDS Conf. 2008:Abstr. LBPE1138)	ABC/3TC+LPV/r	343	96	60%	
	TDF/FTC+LPV/r	345		58%	
ALTAIR *CID* 2010;51:855	EFV/TDF/FTC	114	48		95%*
	ATV/r+TDF/FTC	105			96%*
	AZT+ABC+TDF/FTC	103			82%
ACTG 5202 *Ann Intern Med* 2011;154:445	ABC/3TC + EFV or ATV/r	719	96		82%
	TDF/FTC + EFV or ATV/r	767			89%*

* Superior to comparitor (*P*<0.05)

[†] VL <200 c./mL

‡ Study terminated due to high failure rate; VL <50 c/mL at 12 wks was 17% (TDF) vs. 50% (EFV). The triple NRTI arm had high rates of K65R and 184V resistance mutations.

- **HEAT:** Comparison of ABC/3TC+LPV/r vs. TDF/FTC+LPV/r in 688 treatment-naïve patients (*AIDS* 2009;23:1547). Virologic suppression at 48 weeks was comparable (Table 5-5), and rates of treatment limiting side effects and changes in lipid profile were similar. CD4 count recovery among ABC/3TC recipients (median increase 250/mm³ vs. 247/mm³) by week 96.

- **ACTG 5202:** This was a 4 arm trial of 1,858 treatment-naïve patients randomized to receive blinded ABC/3TC vs. TDF/FTC and open label EFV vs. ATV/r. The DSMB recommended early unblinding in the subset with a baseline VL >100,000 c/mL due to excessive virologic

Drug Information

5

■ TABLE 5-5: **Results of HEAT (ABC/3TC+LPV/r vs. TDF/FTC+LPV/r) at 48 weeks (AIDS 2009;361:2230)**

	ABC/3TC+LPV/r n=343	TDF/FTC+LPV/r n=345
VL <50 c/mL	68%	67%
Response w/baseline VL >100K c/mL	63%	65%
CD4 count (cells/mm³)	+201	+173
Virologic failure (VL > 50 c/mL)	12%	11%
GFR decreased	5%	5%
Suspected ABC HSR*	4%	1%

* HSR=hypersensitivity reactions

(Note that the patients were not prescreened for HLA-B*5701)

failures in the ABC/3TC vs. TDF/FTC recipients (15% vs. 7%; p <0.003) (*NEJM* 2009;361:2230). A more recent analysis showed a significantly lower virologic response rate in patients given ABC/3TC (*Ann Intern Med* 2011;154:445) (see Table 5-4).

■ **ASSERT:** Open-label trial in 385 treatment-naïve, HLA-B*5701 negative patients randomized to ABC/3TC+EFV vs. TDF/FTC/EFV. At 96 weeks ABC/3TC recipients had lower rates of viral suppression (VL <50 c/mL in 59% vs. 71%; p<0.05), a non-significant trend toward better renal function (change in GFR of +1.48 vs. -1.15 mL/min/1.73 M² (p=NS) and less decrease in bone mineral density at hip and lumbar spine (hip: -2.17% vs. -3.55%) (*JAIDS* 2010;55:49; *CID* 2010;51:973).

■ **ACTG 372A: ABC Intensification:** The addition of ABC to patients who had stable HIV suppression failed to confer clinical or virologic benefit (*HIV Clin Trials* 2010;11:312).

RESISTANCE: ABC selects primarily for 74V and, to a lesser extent, K65R. The 184V mutation by itself does not reduce *in vitro* or clinical activity, but when combined with 2 or 3 TAMs there is reduced activity, and with ≥4 TAMs there is no activity (*Topics HIV Med* 2006;14:125; *Antiviral Ther* 2004;9:37). Mutations at RT codons 65R and 74V lead to cross-resistance to ddI, and K65R leads to loss of susceptibility to TDF, especially when not accompanied by M184V. Each of these mutations results in a 2- to 4-fold decrease in susceptibility to ABC. Significant resistance requires multiple mutations, usually in addition to the 184V mutation (*JAC* 2010;65:307). In combination with TDF there is selection for 65R (*AAC* 2004;48:1413). The initial use of d4T or AZT drives TAMs, which reduce activity of all NRTIs. In contrast K65R protects against TAMs and enhances activity of AZT and d4T (*AIDS* 2007;21:405; *JID* 2004;189:837; *JAIDS* 2010;61:346). This is an additional reason for starting with ABC/3TC or TDF/FTC. However, such sequencing considerations have become less important in developed countries because of the declining use of d4T and AZT. They remain relevant in resource-limited settings.

Drug Information

RISK OF CARDIOVASCULAR DISEASE: This is a controversial association with no consensus. A retrospective review of the D:A:D observational cohort for cardiovascular disease risks associated with NRTI use included 33,347 patients and 157,912 patient-years of follow-up. There were 517 myocardial infarctions, including 192 in patients receiving ABC-containing regimens. The relative risk for recent ABC use was 1.9 (95% CI 1.5-2.5) (*Lancet* 2008;371:1417). More recent analysis of the D:A:D database continues to show this association (*JID* 2010;201:318). Analysis of SMART data for 1019 patients who received continuous ABC and 2882 patients treated with alternative NRTIs found that the relative risk for acute myocardial infarction with ABC use was 4.3 (*JID* 2008;197:1133). Switching from ABC to TDF has also been noted to decrease augmentation index, a measure of arterial stiffness, and Framingham risk score by 2% (*AIDS* 2010;24:2403). **Arguing against this association** are the following: 1) The risk was observed only with use in the prior 6 mos, indicating that the risk resolves when ABC is stopped; 2) No likely pathophysiological mechanism is apparent; 3) Markers of inflammation and coagulation do not correlate with ABC use (*AIDS Res Ther* 2010;7:9; *AIDS* 2010;24:f1; *AIDS* 2010;24:1657); 4) Other studies including a pooled analysis of 14,683 treated patients (9,639 ABC recipients) have not shown this risk (*Lancet* 2008;371: 1413); 5) An FDA review of 26 controlled clinical trials with 9,832 patients found no association between ABC use with AMIs (OR = 1.06) (Ding X. 2011 CROI, Abstr. 808; 6) ACTG 5001/ALLRT, a retrospective analysis of 6 ACTG trials in 3,205 treatment-naïve patients followed 17,404 patient years with 36 MI events, failed to show an ABC risk (*CID* 2011;52:429); and 7) It has also been argued that the association, if real, may reflect preferenial use of ABC in patients with the metabolic syndrome or renal failure (*JID* 2010;201:315).

PHARMACOLOGY

- **Bioavailability:** 83%; alcohol increases ABC levels by 41% (clinical significance unknown). CNS penetration (see pg. 550t).

- **T½:** 1.5 h (serum); intracellular T½: 12-21 h. The active metabolite, carbovir triphosphate, has an intracellular half-life of >20 hrs (*AIDS* 2002;16:1196). CSF levels: Ranks class 3 in the 4 class CNS penetration classification (*Neurology* 2011;76:693) (see pg. 550).

- **Elimination:** 81% metabolized by alcohol dehydrogenase and glucuronyl transferase with renal excretion of metabolites; 16% recovered in stool, and 1% unchanged in urine. Metabolism does not involve the cytochrome P450 pathway. Plasma clearance correlates with body weight, suggesting the possibility of suboptimal levels in patients with greater body weight (*Br J Clin Pharmacol* 2005;59:183).

- **Dose modification in renal failure:** None (*Nephron* 2000;87:186). *Trizivir* and *Epzicom* should not be used when CrCl <50 mL/min because of the need to reduce dosages of the AZT and 3TC components.

Drug Information

5

SIDE EFFECTS

■ **Hypersensitivity reaction (Black box FDA warning):** In an analysis of 30,595 participants in clinical trials and expanded access programs prior to screening for HLA-B*5701, 1302 (4.2%) had definite or probable hypersensitivity reactions (HSR), and 19 were fatal, for a mortality rate of 0.03% (3/10,000) (*Clin Ther* 2001;23:1603). Of the 19 deaths, 6 occurred with re-challenge. The median time of onset was 9 days, and 90% occurred in the first 6 wks. Clinical features include fever (usually 39-40°C), skin rash (maculopapular or urticarial), fatigue, malaise, GI symptoms (nausea, vomiting, diarrhea, abdominal pain), arthralgias, cough, and/or dyspnea. The rash occurs in 70% who have HSR (*CID* 2002;34:1137). Laboratory changes may include increased CPK, elevated liver function tests, and lymphopenia. Nearly all true HSRs have symptoms involving ≥2 organs (*Drug Saf* 2006;29: 811).

Susceptibility to this reaction has been associated with the MHC class I allele HLA-B*5701 haplotype (*Lancet* 2002; 359:727; *Lancet* 2002;359:1121). The flagship study of HLA-B*5701 screening was the PREDICT trial in which 1956 patients were tested prior to use of ABC, with results communicated to physicians based on randomization. Patients who had suspected HSR had confirmatory patch tests for verification of this mechanism. Results are summarized in Table 5-6.

All patch test-confirmed cases had the HLA-B*5701 allele, giving a negative predictive value of 100% (*NEJM* 2008;358:568). Specificity was 30-55%. This suggests that a negative test provides near absolute assurance that the ABC HSR will not occur. There are no well confirmed published cases of ABC HSR in patients with negative tests for HLA-B*5701 (S. Mallal, personal communication, Feb, 2011). The current recommendation for resource-rich countries are: 1) All patients who are to receive ABC should have this screening test, 2) Those with positive tests should never receive ABC and 3) Those with negative tests who are given ABC should still be warned about ABC HSR, even though the risk is extremely low.

There are substantial geographic and ethnic differences in rates of HLA-B*5701, as shown below (*J HIV Ther* 2003;8:36; *CID* 2006; 43:103):

U.S.: White 8%, Asian 1%, African-American 2.5%, Hispanic 2%; South America: 5-7%; Western Europe: 5-7%; UK: 8%; Middle East

■ TABLE 5-6: **Results of PREDICT (*NEJM* 2008;358:9)**

	HLA-B*5701 Results	
	Known	Not known
Clinically suspected HSR	3.4%	7.8%
Patch test confirmed	0	2.7%

1-2%; India: 5-20%; China: 0; Japan: 0; Thailand: 4-10%; Australia: 8%; Africa: <1%. A review of tests of 9,720 patients in 272 European centers found a rate of 5%: 6.5% in whites and 0.4 in blacks (*Pharmacogenet Geonomics* 2010;5:307).

Testing for HLA-B*5701 is offered by commercial labs at a cost of about $90-130, or it can be done in some local facilities, especially those with transplant programs. The test results usually require 3-10 days for reporting, the results are definitive (yes/no) and it never needs to be repeated (since it is a genetic test). Patients who have poorly confirmed HSR and a negative test can usually be rechallenged safely (*Antivir Ther* 2008;13:1019).

Rechallenge with ABC in a patient with true hypersensitivity virtually always results in a reaction within hours and may resemble anaphylaxis in 20% with hypotension, bronchoconstriction, and/or renal failure (*AIDS* 1999:13:999). Treatment of rechallenge reactions is supportive with IV fluids, ventilator support, dialysis, etc. Steroids and antihistamines are not effective. Rechallenge has been associated with death, but this is rare. HSR should be reported to the Abacavir Hypersensitivity Registry at 800-270-0425. For more information call 800-334-0089.

Patients prescribed ABC, including those with negative screening tests, should be warned to consult their provider immediately if they note two or more of the hallmark symptoms, including fever, skin rash, typical GI symptoms, cough, dyspnea, and/or constitutional symptoms, especially during the first month of therapy. A warning sheet is usually provided to the patient by the pharmacist. A possible solution in unclear cases with negative screening for HLA-B*5701 is adminis-tration under observation, because patients experiencing true ABC HSR will predictably experience worsening symptoms with continued dosing. The patch test used in the PREDICT study is not commercially available.

- **Other side effects** include nausea, vomiting, malaise, headache, diarrhea, or anorexia.
- **Lactic acidosis**. Patients taking ABC can presumably develop lactic acidosis, although this is rare because ABC, like 3TC, FTC and TDF, has low affinity for mitochondrial DNA (*J Biol Chem* 2001; 276:40847).

BLACK BOX WARNINGS: 1) ABC HSR; 2) lactic acidosis

DRUG INTERACTIONS: Alcohol increases ABC levels by 41%; ABC has no effect on alcohol levels (*AAC* 2000; 283:1811). ABC AUC ↓40% with TPV/r co-administration; clinical significance unknown. Ribavirin – potential antagonism; lower rate of early virologic response in the treatment of HCV (Avoid or use with caution). Methadone clearance increased 22%; not clinically significant. Use standard dose.

5 Drug Information

PREGNANCY: Category C. The 2010 DHHS Guidelines for Antiretroviral Drugs in Pregnant HIV-Infected Women (www.mmhiv.com/link/2010-DHHS-Perinatal) recommend ABC as an alternative to AZT/3TC for the NRTI backbone. The Pregnancy Registry shows birth defects in 21/717 (2.9%) of first trimester exposures (www.apregistry.com; accessed 1/1/2011). Rodent teratogen test showed skeletal malformations and anasarca at 35x the comparable human dose. Placental passage positive in rats. Studies in pregnant women show the ABC AUC is not altered, so the standard dose is appropriate (*AIDS* 2006;28: 553).

ACYCLOVIR (also includes famciclovir and valacyclovir)

TRADE NAMES: *Zovirax* (GlaxoSmithKline, acyclovir), *Famvir* (Novartis, famciclovir), *Valtrex* (GlaxoSmithKline, valacyclovir). All three are also available as generics.

FORMS AND COST:

- **Acyclovir (*Zovirax*):** Caps: 200 mg at $.97. Tabs: 400 mg at $2.17, 800 mg at $4.21. Suspension: 200 mg/5 cc at $138/480 mL. IV vials: 1 gm at $19.20. 5% ointment: 15 g at $200.00 (Brand only) (utility limited); 5% cream: (5 g) $173.00;

- **Famciclovir (*Famvir*):** Tabs: 125, 250, 500 mg; $5.80, $6.30, $12.70;

- **Valacyclovir (*Valtrex*):** Tabs: 500 mg at $8.21, 1000 mg at $14.05

CLASS: Synthetic nucleoside analogs derived from guanine

PATIENT ASSISTANCE PROGRAM: 866-728-4368 (acyclovir and valacyclovir)

INDICATIONS AND DOSES: For oral therapy, acyclovir, famciclovir, or valacyclovir are advocated by the CDC for treatment and prevention of HSV (*MMWR* 2010;59:RR-12). They are generally considered equivalent, although some authorities prefer valacyclovir and famciclovir for the immuno-suppressed host (*Lancet* 2001;353:1513). Acyclovir is the only available IV formulation in this class. Recommendations based on 2010 CDC guidelines for treating HSV in patients with HIV co-infection (*MMWR* 2010;59 [RR12]:30-35) and the CDC-IDSA recommendations for treating VZV with HIV co-infection (*MMWR* 2004;53 [RR-15]:42-44) and *in vitro* activity of various antivirals against herpes viruses are summarized below.

HERPES SIMPLEX: (*MMWR* 2010;59 [RR12]:30-35) See pg. 447-449.

Initial Infection: All patients should be treated even if the infection is mild.

- Acyclovir 400 mg po tid or 200 mg 5 x/d x 7-10d
- Famcyclovir 250 mg po tid x 7-10d
- Valacyclovir 1 gm po bid x 7-10d

Suppressive Therapy (with HIV co-infection):

- Acyclovir 400-800 mg po 2-3 x d
- Famciclovir 500 mg po bid
- Valacyclovir 500 mg po bid

Episodic HSV Infection (with HIV co-infection):

- Acyclovir 400 mg po tid x 5-10d
- Famciclovir 500 mg po bid x 5-10d
- Valacyclovir 1 gm bid x 5-10d

Severe or Resistant Infection: Acyclovir 5-10 mg/kg IV q8h might be necessary. If lesions persist, test HSV for resistance (*Arch Intern Med* 2003;163:76). HSV strains resistant to acyclovir are usually sensitive to foscarnet, which can be given at 40 mg/kg IV q8h until lesions resolve. An infrequently used alternative is cidofovir 5 mg/kg/wk. Topical alternatives include imiquimod or 1% cidofovir gel (must be compounded by pharmacy). Topical treatment should be given once daily x 5/d.

Genital HSV in Pregnancy: Most neonatal HSV infections are aquired from women without a history of genital HSV (*NEJM* 1997;337:509). The greatest recognized risk is HSV acquired near delivery (30-50%); the risk is low in women who have a history of recurrent HSV or who aquire HSV in the first half of pregnancy (*JAMA* 2003;289:203).

Pregnant women should be asked if they have a history of genital HSV, and some authorities routinely test pregnant women for type-specific HSV. The safety of acyclovir, famciclovir and valacyclovir in pregnancy is not definitely established, but available data suggest that acyclovir is safe during the first trimester (*Birth Defects Res A Clin Mol Teratol* 2004;270:201). Recommendations based on these observations are:

- Acyclovir po can be given to pregnant women with initial genital HSV or severe recurrent infection; IV acyclovir should be given for severe HSV.
- Acyclovir po can be given to women who have a history of recurrent HSV to prevent recurrence in late pregnancy (*Obstet Gynecol* 2002;10:71; *Am J Obstet Gynecol* 2003;188:836; *Obstet Gynecol* 2003;102:1396).
- Women without signs or symptoms of genital HSV or prodromal symptoms can deliver vaginally. C-section should be performed if there is evidence of genital HSV at onset of labor.

HERPES ZOSTER

Recommendations of the 2009 Guidelines from NIH, CDC and IDSA (www.mmhiv.com/link/2009-OI-NIH-CDC-IDSA) (see pg. 449-451) for VZV in patients with HIV infection:

- **Dermatomal zoster:** Valacyclovir 1 gm po tid or famciclovir 500 mg po tid or acyclovir 800 mg po 5/d x 7-10d; may require longer duration. Extensive cutaneous lesions or visceral VZV: Acyclovir 10-

5 Drug Information

■ TABLE 5-7: **Activity of Antivirals Against Herpesviruses**

	HSV	VZV	EBV	CMV	HHV 6-8
Acyclovir	++	+	+	—	—
Famciclovir	++	+	+	—	—
Valacyclovir	++	+	+	—	—
Ganciclovir	++	+	++	++[*]	+
Foscarnet	+	+	++	++[*]	+
Cidofovir	+	+	++	++[*]	++

[*] Performed well in clinical studies

15 mg/kg IV q8h; change to po therapy when lesions start to regress using valacyclovir (1000 mg tid), famciclovir (500 mg tid) or acyclovir (800 mg 5 x/d) to complete 10-14 day course.

- **Progressive Outer Retinal Necrosis (PORN):** Ganciclovir 5 mg/kg IV q12h + foscarnet 90 mg/kg IV q12h + ganciclovir 2 mg/0.05 mL given by intravitreal injection 2 x/wk and/or foscarnet 1.2 mg/0.05 mL intravitreal injection 2 x/wk (plus ART).

- **Acute Retinal necrosis (ARN):** Acyclovir 10 mg/kg IV q8h x 10-14d, then valacyclovir 1000 mg po tid x 6wk.

- **VZV Resistant to Acyclovir:** Foscarnet 90 mg/kg IV q8h.

- **Oral Hairy Leukoplakia (EBV):** Indications to treat are unclear, but treatment is requested by some patients, usually for cosmetic reasons. One study of 18 patients given valacyclovir 1 gm q8h x 28 days showed clinical and virologic response in 16 (89%) and virologic response in 16 (89%). Recurrence after 1 mo off treatment occurred in 2 of 12 patients (17%) (*JID* 2003;188:883). An alternative is topical 1% penciclovir cream (*Oral Surg Oral Med, Oral Pathol, Oral Radid Endod* 2010;110:611).

- **HIV:** Acyclovir is reported to have a modest impact on the viral load with a decrease of about 0.5 $\log_{10}$ c/mL in some reports (*Lancet Infect Dis* 2010;10:455; *JAIDS* 2008;59:77)

PHARMACOLOGY

- **Bioavailability:** Acyclovir, 15-20% with oral administration

- **T½:** Acyclovir, 2.5-3.3 h, CSF levels: 50% serum levels

- **Elimination:** Renal. See Table 5-8 for dose adjustment in renal failure

- **Famciclovir:** CrCl 40-59 mL/min = 500 mg q12h; 20-39 = 500 mg q24h; <20 = 250 mg q24h (after HD on HD days)

- **Valacyclovir:** CrCl 30-49 = 1 gm q12h; 10-29 = 1 gm q24h; <10 = 500 mg q24h (post-HD on HD days)

SIDE EFFECTS: Acyclovir, famciclovir and valacyclovir are generally well tolerated.

- **IV Acyclovir:** Irritation and phlebitis at infusion site, rash, nausea and

Drug Information

■ TABLE 5-8: **Acyclovir Dose Modification in Renal Failure**

Usual Dose	Creatinine Clearance	Adjusted Dose
200 mg 5x/day	>10 mL/min	200 mg 5x/day
	≤10 mL/min	200 mg q12h
800 mg 5x/day	10-50 mL/min	800 mg q8h
	<10 mL/min	800 mg q12h
5-10 mg/kg IV q8h	25-50 mL/min	5-10 mg/kg q 12 h
	10-25 mL/min	5-10 mg/kg q 24 h
	<10 mL/min/HD	5 mg/kg q24h

vomiting, diarrhea, renal toxicity and crystalluria (especially with rapid IV infusion, prior renal disease, and concurrent nephrotoxic drugs), dizziness, dehydration, abnormal liver function tests, itching, and headache

- **High doses especially with renal failure:** CNS toxicity-agitation, confusion, hallucination, seizure, coma
- **Rare:** Nausea, vomiting, anemia, neutropenia, thrombocytopenia, and hypotension

DRUG INTERACTIONS

- Increased meperidine and theophylline levels
- Probenecid prolongs half-life of acyclovir. No dose adjustment.

PREGNANCY: Acyclovir, famciclovir, and valacyclovir are category B. Acyclovir is not teratogenic, but has potential to cause chromosomal damage at high doses. The CDC Registry shows no increased incidence of fetal abnormalities among >700 women for whom pregnancy outcome data were available (*MMWR* 1993;42:806). As noted above (see pg. 187), the CDC recommends use of acyclovir during pregnancy for selected cases of HSV and for varicella. This is the preferred agent for HSV in pregnancy because of substantial experience showing safety and efficacy (*Obstet Gynecol* 2005; 106:1341; *Obstet Gynecol* 2003;102:1396). Use for prophylaxis in pregnancy is being investigated.

ALBENDAZOLE

TRADE NAME: *Albenza* (GlaxoSmithKline)

FORM AND COST: 200 mg tablets at $2.96

INDICATION AND DOSE: Microsporidiosis other than infections caused by *Enterocytozoon bieneusi* and *Vittaforma corneae*; 400 mg po bid with fatty meal until CD4 count >200/mm³ for >6 mos (2009 Guidelines for Prevention and Treatment of Opportunistic Infections in HIV-Infected Adults and Adolescents; www.mmhiv.com/link/2009-OI-NIH-CDC-IDSA).

Drug Information

5

CLINICAL TRIALS: See pg. 457-458. Albendazole (400 mg bid until CD4 >200/ mm³) is highly effective with microsporidiosis involving *Encephalitozoon (Septata) intestinalis* (*Parasitol Res* 2003;90 Suppl 1:S14; *Gastroenterol Clin Biol* 2010;34:450) but is not effective against *E. bieneusi*, which account for about 80% of cases of microsporidiosis in AIDS patients. These species can be distinguished by special stain (Uvitex-2B) EM or PCR that is also used for species identification in disseminated microsporidiosis and intraocular infection with *E. cuniculi* (*Int J Med Microbiol* 2005;294:529; *Ethiop Med J* 2005;43:97). Some reports suggest fumigillin may be useful with *E. bieneusi* infection (*Transpl Infect Dis* 2009;11:83).

PHARMACOLOGY

- **Bioavailability:** Low (<5%), but absorption is increased 5-fold if taken with a fatty meal vs. in a fasting state. Should be taken with fatty meal.

- **T1/2:** 8 hrs

- **Elimination:** Metabolized in liver to albendazole sulfoxide, then excreted by enterohepatic circulation

- **Dose modification in renal failure:** None

SIDE EFFECTS: Adverse reactions are infrequent and include reversible hepatotoxicity, GI intolerance (abdominal pain, diarrhea, nausea, vomiting), reversible hair loss, hypersensitivity reactions (rash, pruritus, fever), reversible neutropenia, and CNS toxicity (dizziness, headache). Some recommend monitoring liver function tests every 2 wks. Fatal pancytopenia has been reported (*Am J Trop Med Hyg* 2005;72: 291).

PREGNANCY: Category C. Albendazole is teratogenic and embryotoxic in rodents at doses of 30 mg/kg. Not recommended for use in pregnancy; ART is preferred for microsporidiosis.

AMPHOTERICIN B

TRADE NAME: Parenteral form, generic; oral form is no longer available from commercial sources but can be prepared by a pharmacy.

FORMS AND COST: *Fungizone* at $17.00/d/50 mg vial; *Abelcet* $720/d/100 mg; *Amphotec* $160/100 mg; *AmBisome* $393/100 mg

CLASS: Amphoteric polyene macrolide with activity against nearly all pathogenic and opportunistic fungi.

INDICATION: (Table 5-9) Sharply reduced general usage in recent years due to concerns about nephrotoxicity and availability of alternatives such as posaconazole, voriconazole, caspofungin, and lipid amphotericin formulations (*CID* 2006;42:1289). Conventional amphotericin is still first line therapy for cryptococcal meningitis.

ADMINISTRATION – ORAL: Oral suspension for thrush is no longer available commercially, but it can be prepared by a pharmacist to a

Drug Information

strength of 5-10 mg/mL of amphotericin B. Dose: 1-5 mL qid; swish as long as possible, then swallow.

ADMINISTRATION – IV: Usual dose is 0.3-1.5 mg/kg/d given by slow IV infusion over ≥2-4 hrs (*BMJ* 2000;332:579). Some authorities advocate a test dose (1 mg in 50 mL DSW given over 30 minutes with cardiovascular monitoring for 4 hrs) as a test for hypersensitivity. The usual dose for cryptococcal meningitis is 0.7 mg/kg/d combined with flucytosine. Higher doses (1 mg/kg/d) of amphotericin appear to be more rapidly fungicidal (*CID* 2008;47:131). For infusion-related side effects, premedicate with NSAID +/- diphenhydramine or hydrocortisone 50-100 mg. Give meperidine for rigors.

PHARMACOLOGY

- **Bioavailability:** Peak serum levels with standard IV doses are 0.5-2 μg/mL. There is no significant absorption with oral administration; CSF levels – 3% of serum concentrations.

- **T/:** 24 h with IV administration, detected in blood and urine up to 4 wks after discontinuation.

- **Elimination:** Serum levels in urine; metabolic pathways are unknown.

- **Dose adjustment in renal failure:** None, but consider lipid amphotericin.

■ TABLE 5-9: **Amphotericin for Fungal Infections Associated with HIV Infection (2008 IDSA/NIH/CDC Guidelines for Prevention and Treament of Opportunistic Infections in HIV-infected Adults and Adolescents**

Fungus	Preferred	Amphotericin B regimens
Aspergillosis (pg. 421)	Voriconazole	Ampho B 1 mg/kg/d IV or Lipid ampho B 5 mg/kg/d IV
Candidiasis • Thrush (pg. 425)	Azoles Echinocandins	Ampho B 0.3 mg/kg/d IV or Ampho B suspension 100 mg/mL with 1 mL gargled 4x/d
• Esophagitis (pg. 427)		Ampho B 0.3-0.7 mg/kg/d IV Lipid ampho B 3-5 mg/kg/d IV
Coccidiodomycosis • Mild/moderate • Severe (non-meningeal • Meningitis (pg. 432)	Azole Ampho B Fluconazole	Ampho B 0.7-1.0 mg/kg/d IV Lipid ampho B 4-6 mg/kg/d IV until improved – then azole Ampho B intrathecal if azoles fail
Cryptococcosis • Meningitis (pg. 433)	Ampho B + 5FC	Ampho B 0.7 mg/kg/d IV Lipid ampho B 4-6 mg/kg/d IV Induction phase: a minimum of 2 wks
Histoplasmosis (pg. 451) • Mild/moderate • Moderate/severe (non-meningeal)	Itraconazole Ampho B	Liposomal ampho B 3 mg/kg/d IV Alternate: Ampho B 0.7 mg/kg/d IV *or* ampho B lipid 5 mg/kg/d IV Duration: 2 weeks or when clinically improved
• Meningitis	Ampho B	Liposomal ampho B 5 mg/kg/d IV x 4-6 wks
Penicilliosis (pg. 475) • Mild • Acute	Itraconazole Ampho B	Ampho B 0.6 mg/kg/d IV x 2 wks

Drug Information

5

SIDE EFFECTS: Oral form: Rash, GI intolerance, and allergic reactions. Toxicity with IV form is dose-related and less severe with slow administration.

- Fever and chills, usually 1-3 hrs post infusion and lasting for up to 4 hrs post infusion. Reduce with hydrocortisone (10-50 mg added to infusion, but only if necessary due to immunosuppression); alternatives that are now often preferred are meperidine, ibuprofen, or naproxen prior to infusion.

- Hypotension, nausea, vomiting, usually 1-3 hrs post infusion; may be reduced with compazine.

- Nephrotoxicity in up to 80% ± nephrocalcinosis, potassium wasting, renal tubular acidosis. Reduce with gradual increase in dose, adequate hydration, avoidance of concurrent nephrotoxic drugs, and possibly sodium loading. Discontinue or reduce dose with BUN >40 mg/dL and creatinine >3 mg/dL. Lipid amphotericin preparations are less nephrotoxic, are often preferred and could be substituted.

- Hypokalemia, hypomagnesemia, and hypocalcemia corrected with supplemental potassium, magnesium, and calcium.

- Normocytic normochromic anemia with average decrease of 9% in hematocrit.

- Phlebitis and pain at infusion sites: add 1200-1600 units of heparin to infusate.

DRUG INTERACTIONS: Increased nephrotoxicity with concurrent use of nephrotoxic drugs – aminoglycosides, cisplatin, cyclosporine, possibly tenofovir, foscarnet, cidofovir, methoxyflurane, vancomycin; increased hypokalemia with corticosteroids and diuretics. Potential for digoxin toxicity secondary to hypokalemia.

PREGNANCY: Category B. Not teratogenic in animals or humans. Preferred over azoles in first trimester if equally effective.

■ TABLE 5-10: **Relative Merits of Amphotericin B Formulations** (*CID* 2003;37:415; *NEJM* 1999;340:764; *CID* 2002;35:359)

Preparation:	Amphotericin B†	Amphotec ABCD†	Abelcet (ABLC)‡	AmBisome (LAmB)‡
Dose	0.5-1.2 mg/kg/d	3-4 mg/kg/d	2.5-5 mg/kg/d	3-6 mg/kg/d
C$_{max}$ (ug/mL)	0.5-2	3.1	1.7	83
Usual cost (AWP)†	$17/d	$280-300/d	$800-850/d	$950-$1300/d
Adverse reactions*			18%	
Chills	30%	53%	15-20%	18%
Fever >38^{50}C	16%	27%	10-20%	7%
Creatinine >2x base	30-50%	10-25%	15-20%	19%

† AWP based on 0.7 mg/kg for Amphotericin; 5 mg/kg for lipid amphotericin
* Comparison of ADR is based on *AmBisome* vs. Ampho, *Amphotec* vs. Ampho
‡ Amphotericin B formulation is recommended for cryptococcal meningitis

Drug Information

ALTERNATIVE PREPARATIONS: (*CID* 2009;49:1721; *CID* 2003;37:415; *Medicine* 2010;89:236; *CID* 2001;32:686; *CID* 2005;41:1448; *CID* 2010; 50:291).

Lipid preparations of amphotericin B include (Table 5-10):

- ***Abelcet* (ABLC) (Enzon, Inc.):** Amphotericin B complexed with 2 phospholipids – DMPC and DMPG

- ***Amphotec* (ABCD) (Three Rivers Pharmaceuticals, Inc.):** Amphotericin B colloidal dispersion with cholesterol sulfate

- ***AmBisome* (LAmB) (Astellas Pharma US, Inc.):** Liposomal amphotericin B is a true liposomal delivery system

ADVANTAGES: Compared with amphotericin B, these formulations cause less nephrotoxicity and infusion-related reactions (*NEJM* 1999;340:764). Comparative trials vs. amphotericin B consistently show that the lipid preparations are therapeutically equivalent and sometimes superior, especially *AmBisome*. The only reason these drugs are not generally preferred over amphotericin B is cost, which is $17/d for amphotericin B vs. $300-700/d for lipid formulations (AWP) at standard doses. With many infections the lipid formulations may be more cost-effective due to reduced rates of renal failure and dialysis (*CID* 2001;32:686; *CID* 2003;37:415; *CID* 2009;49:1721; *Medicine* 2010;89:236). Relative merits are summarized in Table 5-10.

AMPRENAVIR (APV) – see Fosamprenavir (pg. 281)

Amprenavir is no longer available.

ANCOBON – see Flucytosine (pg. 279)

ANDROGEL – see Testosterone (pg. 394)

ATAZANAVIR (ATV)

TRADE NAME: *Reyataz* (ViiV Healthcare)

CLASS: Azapeptide protease inhibitor (*CID* 2004;38:1599)

FORMULATIONS, REGIMEN AND COST:

- **Forms:** ATV – caps, 100, 150 and 200, and 300 mg
- **Regimen:** ATV – 400 mg qd (PI-naïve only); ATV/r – 300/100 mg qd (preferred). Must use ATV/r 300/100 mg (boosted) with TDF. ATV/r 400/100 mg with EFV. ATV/r 400/100 mg with TDF + H2 blockers.
- **AWP:** $1131/mo
- **Food:** Take with a meal

5 Drug Information

- **Interactions:** Requires gastric acidity; Avoid proton-pump inhibitors (omeprazole, etc). Dosing separation required with antacids, H2 blockers, etc.; see warnings
- **Renal failure:** Standard doses except in patients on hemodialysis, who should receive only boosted ATV since levels are significantly lower (Agarwala S. 8th Internat Clin Pharm HIV Ther 2007;Abstr. 2)
- **Hepatic failure:** With Child-Pugh score 7-9, dose is 300 mg qd (limited clinical data); avoid with Child-Pugh score >9.
- **Storage:** Room temperature, 15-30°C

PATIENT ASSISTANCE: 800-861-0048 (8 am-5 pm CST, Mon.-Fri.)

WARNINGS

- Avoid unboosted ATV with TDF, EFV, ETR and NVP (*JAC* 2005; 56:380); avoid buffered ddI (use ddI-EC)
- Caution with drugs that prolong QTc with clarithromycin, use half-dose clarithromycin or alternative such as azithromycin.
- Proton pump inhibitors (PPIs): Avoid if coadministration is needed. Give PPI (maximum dose omeprazole is 20 mg) 12 h before ATV/r (treatment-naïve patients) or avoid PPI (treatment experienced patients) with ATV/r and/or give ATV/r >10 h after H2 blocker (*HIV Med* 2007;8:335).
- H2 blockers: take H2 blocker 2 h after ATV/r
- Antacids: give ATV/r 2 h before or ≥1 h after
- Food requirement: increases ATV AUC 70%.
- Hepatic disease: see dose modification below (Pharmacology)

ADVANTAGES: 1) Potency, especially with RTV boosting; 2) lowest pill burden among PIs and once-daily regimen; 3) negligible effect on insulin resistance and lipids, even with RTV boosting; 4) unique major resistance mutation (I50L) that does not cause PI cross-resistance; 5) generally well tolerated (few GI side effects); and 6) therapeutically equivalent or superior to all other regimens when combined with 2 NRTIs in treatment-naïve patients.

DISADVANTAGES: 1) Indirect hyperbilirubinemia – medically inconsequential but may cause jaundice or scleral icterus (<5-7%); 2) drug interactions – see warnings; 3) requirement for a meal and gastric acid; and 4) need for RTV boosting when combined with TDF (or an NNRTI).

MAJOR TRIALS

Treatment-naïve patients: Table 5-11

- **Switch studies: ATAZIP** trial consisted of 248 patients with viral suppression on LPV/r-based ART who were randomized to continue the same regimen or switch to ATV/r-based ART. Results at 48 weeks showed higher rates of treatment failure with LPV/r (20% vs. 17%) (P=0.002) and significant reductions in triglyceride and total cholesterol levels with ATV/r (*JAIDS* 2009;51:29).

Drug Information

- **Induction-maintenance: ACTG 5201** was a single-arm open label pilot study to determine efficacy of ATV/r monotherapy (300/100 mg qd) in patients who had achieved viral suppression to <50 c/mL for ≥48 wks on a regimen of PI-based ART (*JAMA* 2006;296:806). At 24 weeks, 31/34 (91%) had a sustained virologic response. Resistance testing in the 3 patients with virologic failure showed no PI resistance mutations (see pg 122t).

- The **ARIES** trial randomized patients who had VL <50 c/mL on ATV/r+ABC/3TC to continued ATV/r (300/100 mg qd) or unboosted ATV (400 mg qd). At 84 weeks (48 weeks post randomization) the rates of continued viral suppression (VL <50 c/mL) were 181/220 (86%) in the unboosted ATV group and 169/209 (81%) in the ATV/r group. The overall rate of virologic failure was 2%, and there were no PI resistance mutations in those 8 patients. CD4 count increases and adverse reactions were similar in the two groups, but lipid profiles were better in the unboosted ATV group (*AIDS* 2010;24:2019).

- **ATV vs. ATV/r: BMS 089** compared ATV (400 mg vs. ATV/r (300/100 mg qd in treatment-naïve patients. There was a clear pharmacologic advantage to boosting, though lipid levels were also higher. The study was underpowered to detect differences in virologic outcome (*JAIDS* 2008;47:161) (Table 5-12). The conclusion was that boosted ATV is preferred over unboosted ATV, and they are equivalent in terms of viral suppression and CD4 count recovery, but it also produced higher lipid changes and more jaundice. These changes were correlated with the sustained trough level achieved with RTV boosting.

- **CASTLE: ATV/r vs. LPV/r in treatment-naïve patients:** This trial compared ATV/r (300/100 mg once daily) vs. LPV/r (400/100 mg twice daily) in 883 treatment naïve patients (*Lancet* 2008;372:646). All patients also received TDF/FTC. Virologic suppression was comparable at 48 weeks (78% vs. 76%), and ATV/r performed better with respect to lipid changes, diarrhea and quality of life (*Lancet* 2008;373:646). Efficacy was similar across baseline CD4 strata, but LPV/r performed numerically worse (63% vs. 78% w/ baseline CD4 <50 cells/mm^3). The 96-week data (*JAIDS* 2010;53:323) are summarized in Table 5-13. Another analysis of CASTLE data concluded that ATV/r-based ART was more cost-effective than LPV/r-based ART (*Scand J Infect Dis* 2011;43:304).

- **ATV/r vs. EFV:** ACTG5202 was an open-label trial in which 1400 participants were randomized to receive ATV/r vs. EFV, each combined with separately randomized TDF/FTC or ABC/3TC. Randomization was stratified by baseline VL less or greater than 100,000 c/mL. Participants with baseline VL >100,000 c/mL were unblinded after it was found that virologic suppression was greater in the TDF/FTC arm compared to the ABC/3TC arm (see Abacavir). Overall results at 96 weeks showed similar rates of viral suppression

Drug Information

5

Trial	Regimen	No	Dur (wks)	VL <50	VL <200 -400
BMS 034: Treatment-naïve (*JAIDS* 2004;36:1011)	ATV 400 mg/d+AZT/3TC	286	48	32%*	70%
	EFV+AZT/3TC	280		37%	64%
BMS AI 424-008: Treatment-naïve (Package label)	ATV+AZT/3TC	181	48	33%	67%
	NFV+AZT/3TC	91		38%	59%
BMS AI 424-007: Treatment-naïve (*JAIDS* 2003;32:18)	ATV+ddl+d4T	103	48	36%	64%
	NFV+ddl+d4T	103		39%	56%
CASTLE: Treatment-naïve (*Lancet* 2008;372:646; *JAIDS* 2010;53:323)	ATV/r (300/100 mg qd) + TDF/FTC	440	96	74%‡	—
	LPV/r (400/100 mg bid) +TDF/FTC	443		68%	—
BMS 089: Treatment-naïve (*JAIDS* 2008;47:161)	ATV+d4T+3TC	105	96	55%	70%
	ATV/r+d4T+3TC	95		65%	75%
ALERT: Treatment-naïve (*AIDS Res Ther* 2008;5:5)	ATV/r+TDF/FTC	53	48	75%	79%
	FPV/r 1400/100 mg +TDF/FTC	53		83%	87%
BMS 043: Failed one PI regimen (*CID* 2004; 38:1599)	ATV 400 mg/d + 2 NRTIs	144	24	59%	—
	LPV/r + 2 NRTIs	146		77%‡	—
BMS 045:† Failed ≥2 HAART regimens containing ≥1 PI (*AIDS* 2006;20:711)	ATV/r 300/100 mg/d + 2 NRTIs	120	96‡	56%	—
	LPV/r + 2 NRTIs	123		58%	—
	SQV/ATV 1200/400 mg qd + 2 NRTIs	115		38%‡	—
AI 424-009: Failed therapy (*AIDS* 2003;17:1339)	SQV/ATV 1200/400 mg qd + 2 NRTIs	34	48	—	41%
	SQV/ATV 600/1200 mg qd + 2 NRTIs	28		—	29%
	SQV/r 400/400 mg bid + 2 NRTIs	23		—	35%
ARIES: ATV vs. ATV/r after 36 wks on ATV/r (*AIDS* 2010;24:2019)	ATV/r 300/100 qd + ABC/3TC	209	48	81%	86%
	ATV 400 qd + ABC/3TC	210		86%	92%
ACTG 5202: (*Ann Intern Med* 2011;154:445)	ATV/r + TDF/FTC or ATV/r + ABC/3TC	702	96	—	90% 85%
	EFV + TDF/FTC or EFV + ABC/3TC	698		—	91% 91%

* Low frequency of VL <50 c/mL is attributed to use of inappropriate collection tube for VL testing (*J Clin Virol 2006*;35:420).

‡ The SQV/ATV group did poorly and this arm was stopped.

† Results for >1 $\log_{10}$ c/mL decrease or <400 c/mL.

Drug Information

■ TABLE 5-12: **BMS 089-ATV vs. ATV/r** (*JAIDS* 2008;47:161)

	ATV n = 94	ATV/r n = 103
Outcome at 48 wks		
VL <50/mL	70%	75%
CD4 count (median increase)	+189	+224
Pharmacokinetic substudy		
C trough (geometric mean ng/mL)	127	670
Inhibitory quotient	9	53
Lipid changes		
Total cholesterol (mg/dL)	+8%	+16%
Triglycerides (mg/dL)	+10%	+45%

to <200 c/mL between the ATV/r and EFV arms: 83% vs. 85%, respectively, and there was no significant difference when combining ATV/r with TDF/FTC (89%) vs. ABC/3TC (3%) (*Ann Intern Med* 2011;154:445). ATV/r was associated with less increase in LDL cholesterol and fewer major resistance mutations in failures: EFV 41/71 (65%) vs. ATV/r 12/83 (16%); the 12 resistance mutations included 11 184V mutations occurring in ATV/r-treated participants and one PI mutation (88N/S) (see Table 4-14, pg. 101).

NUC-sparing regimens: See pg. 122-123.

■ **ATV + RAL:** In the **SPARTAN** trial, patients receiving ART with virologic failure or intolerance were randomized to ATV 300 mg bid (unboosted) + RAL 400 bid (N=63) vs. standard therapy with

■ TABLE 5 13: **CASTLE Trial: ATV/r vs. LPV/r in Treatment-naïve Patients 96-week Results** (*JAIDS* 2010;53:323)

	ATV/r n = 440	LPV/r n = 443
VL < 50 c/mL	74%	68%
■ Baseline CD4 < 50/mm^3	78%	58%*
■ Baseline VL >100,000 c/mL	74%	66%
■ CD4 count (median)[†]	+219	+219
Lipids (% increase)		
■ Cholesterol	+16%	+29%
■ LDL cholesterol	+32%	+40%
■ Triglyceride	+23%	+49%
Discontinued for adverse reaction	3%	5%
Resistance mutations with failure		
■ Major PI	1/28	0/29
■ 184V	5	7

* P=<0.05

† 48-week data

5 Drug Information

TDF/FTC + ATV/r (n=31). Participants included were RAL-naïve, had no PI mutations and no proton pump inhibitor requirement. The study was stopped prematurely because of high rates of resistance among those failing therapy, and high rates of jaundice. Results in 22 patients showed good pharmacologic data for both antivirals, but substantial individual variation in tolerance (*Drug Monit* 2010;32:782).

- **ATV/r + MVC:** See pg. 124, 320.
- **SPARTAN-ATV + RAL:** See pg. 125, 358.
- **ATV + RAL + 3TC:** A pharmacokinetic study of ATV+RAL+3TC in 17 patients showed therapeutic levels of RAL and virologic control was achieved with a regimen of ATV (600 mg)+RAL (800 mg) and 3TC or FTC (Jansen A. 2011 CROI;Abstr. 634).

Multiple HAART failures

- **BMS 045:** Patients with ≥2 HAART failures with ≥1 PI, NRTI, or NNRTI were randomized to TDF/NRTI plus either LPV/r 400/100 mg bid, SQV/ATV 1200/400 mg qd, or ATV/r 300/100 mg qd with 2 NRTIs in each group. Results at 24 weeks showed the SQV/ATV group did poorly, and these patients were given the option to change (*AIDS* 2006; 20:711). Efficacy at 96 weeks for the remaining two groups was similar, and patients taking ATV/r had less hyperlipidemia and grade 2-4 diarrhea than those on LPV/r (3% vs. 13%) with ATV/r. Results are summarized in Table 5-11.

RESISTANCE: ATV/r selects for 13 mutations: **10F/I/V, 16E, 33F/I/V, 46I/L,** 54L/V/M/T, **I50L, 60E,** 62V, 71I/T/L, 82A/T, **84V, 85V,** 90M, and 93L. The mutations in bold are used in the ATV score. Virologic response with boosted ATV-based ART was noted in 100% of patients with 0 or 1 of these mutations, 80% of those with 2, 42% with 3, and none with ≥4 mutations (*AIDS* 2006;20:35). Another scoring system consists of 16E, 32I, 20I/M/R/T/V, 53L/Y, 64L/M/V, 71I/T/V, 85V and 93L/M. One, two, or three mutations were associated with response rates of 67%, 6%, and 0% respectively. The more recent IAS-USA resistance profiles (12/2010) lists just 3 major ATV resistance mutations: 50L, 84V and 88S with the notation that "often numerous mutations are necessary to substantially impact virologic response" (*Top HIV Med* 2010;18:158). The signature mutation is I50L in treatment-naïve patients treated with unboosted ATV, which does not cause cross-resistance with other PIs, including FPV, which has the signature mutation I50V. The I50L mutation reduces ATV activity by a median of 10-fold, reduces replication capacity to 0.3-42%, and increases susceptibility to other PIs (*AAC* 2005; 49:3825), although the clinical significance of this is unknown. Among 78 virologic failures in clinical trials, 23 had both phenotypic resistance and the I50L mutation (*JID* 2004;189:1802). The I50L mutation is often associated with 71V, which increases susceptibility to other PIs *in vitro* (*AAC* 2005;49:3825).

PHARMACOLOGY

Drug Information

- **Absorption:** Requires food and gastric acid for optimal absorption, which is highly variable. Food increases AUC 70%. ATV trough levels >150 ng/mL correlate with virologic response (*AIDS Patient Care STDS* 2008;22:7). RTV boosting (300/100 mg) increases ATV AUC 3- to 4-fold and C_{min} by 10-fold (*Clin Pharmacokin* 2005;44:1035).

- **Distribution:** Protein-binding 86%, CSF/plasma levels ratio is 0.002-0.02. Penetration into seminal fluid is poor, with a seminal/blood plasma ratio of 0.1 (*AAC* 2007;51:335). Ranks class 2 in the 4 class scoring system for CNS penetration (*Neurology* 2011;76:693) (see pg. 550t).

- **Serum half-life:** 7 hrs

- **Elimination:** Inhibitor and substrate for P450 3A4 and inhibitor of glucuronidation. Metabolized by the liver, and metabolites are excreted by the biliary tract; only 13% of unmetabolized drug is excreted in urine.

SIDE EFFECTS: Generally well tolerated with only 2% discontinuation rate for adverse events in one large trial (BMS 008).

- **Common:** Reversible increase in **indirect bilirubinemia** due to UGT 1A1 inhibition in 22-47%; this is medically inconsequential but may cause jaundice (reported in 7%). The levels of unconjugated bilirubin correlate with ATV trough levels (*HIV Clin Trials* 2008;9:213). An increase in bilirubin of ≥0.3 serves as a surrogate marker for ATV adherence (*AIDS* 2005;19:1700). ATV/r appears safe in patients with advanced liver disease (*AIDS* 2011;25:1006). Nevertheless, there is a strong association between the genetic variants of ATV metabolism and ATV/r discontinuation (*CID* 2011;203:246). Analysis of CASTLE data at 96 weeks found significantly more women than men discontinued ATV/r (22% vs. 15%) (*JAC* 2011;66:383).

- **Occasional:** GI intolerance with nausea, vomiting, abdominal pain; rash (reported in 1-6% and occasionally severe (*Can J Infect Dis Med Microbiol* 2009;20:e10); increase in transaminase levels.

- **Prolongation of QTc and PR interval**, including asymptomatic first-degree AV block. Studies with ATV/r 300/100 mg qd showed slight but not significant increases in PR interval averaging 3 msec and no change at 1 mo (*HIV Med* 2006;7:317). PR interval monitoring should be performed in patients with conduction defects or with concurrent use with other drugs that alter cardiac conduction, e.g., diltiazem, verapamil, saquinavir, clarithromycin (use half dose of clarithromycin and diltiazem with slow titration or consider alternative: azithromycin.

- **Metabolic complications and lipodystrophy:** ATV and, to a lesser extent ATV/r, appear to be "heart friendly" based on: 1) little or no effect on lipid levels (*AIDS* 2006;20:711; *JAIDS* 2005;39:174); 2) minimal or no effect on insulin resistance (*AIDS* 2006;20:1813); 3) not associated with increased levels of biomarkers of CVD (*AIDS* 2010;24:2657); and 4) an observational study showing decrease in

5 Drug Information

carotid intima-media thickness in patients on ATV/r (*AIDS* 2010;24:2797). ACTG 5224 compared rates of visceral fat accumulation in ACTG 5202 participants (MCComsey C. 2011 CROI:Abstr. 77). ATV/r was associated with significantly more trunk fat than EFV.

- **ATV-associated renal disease - Urolithiasis:** ATV occasionally causes urolithiasis that is presumably due to precipitation of the drug resulting in crystaluria in a fashion analogous to indinavir (*NEJM* 2006;355:2158; *AIDS* 2006;20:2131; *AIDS* 2007;12:1060; *AIDS* 2007;21:1215;*CID* 2007;45:e105). About 7% of ATV is excreted in the kidney, and ATV is poorly soluble. Spectrophotometry analysis of the stones shows crystals of ATV and no metabolites. The stones are yellow, friable and radiolucent. The frequency in one report was 11/1134 patients or 1/100 patients; continued use of ATV in 6 patients with symptomatic stones was complicated by a recurrence in only one (*CID* 2007;45:e105). A EuroSIDA review of 6,843 HIV-infected patients for evidence of renal disease showed the risk of decrease in baseline CrCL > 25% with ATV-based ART was an incidence risk ratio of 1.2/years (p <0.0003) (*AIDS* 2010;24:1667) after adjustment of factor associated with CKD. This risk actually exceeded the rate of chronic kidney disease associated with TDF use incidence risk ratio 1.16/yr (*AIDS* 2010;24:1667).

- **Interstitial nephritis:** with acute renal failure has been reported (*Am J Kidney Dis* 2004;44:e81; *Virchows Arch* 2007;450:665; *Antivir Ther* 2011;16:119). A review from EuroSIDA based on sequential data for 6,842 patients found 225 receiving ATV/r (3.3%) progressed to chronic renal disease for a relative risk of 1.21 (95% CI 1.09-1.34; p=0.0003) (*AIDS* 2010;24:1667).

BLACK BOX WARNINGS: None

DRUG INTERACTIONS

- **Avoid concurrent use with ATV/r: Astemizole, alfuzosin, bepridil, cisapride, ergotamine, fluticasone, indinavir, quinidine, irinotecan, lovastatin, midazolam*, nevirapine, pimozide, pitavastatin (do not co-administer with ATV/r), proton pump inhibitors, propafenone, flecainide, amiodarone, rifampin, simvastatin, triazolam, ranolazine, terfenadine, and St. John's wort.**

  * Contraindicated with oral **midazolam**; IV may be used with close monitoring.

- **Dose modification:** (ATV standard unless specified): **Rifabutin:** 150 mg q24-48h. Consider rifabutin TDM. **Clarithromycin:** ↑ clarithromycin AUC 94% and may cause QTc prolongation; use half dose clarithromycin or use azithromycin. **Oral contraceptive:** Estradiol AUC ↑48% and norethindrone AUC ↑110%; consider alternative contraception with ATV (do not exceed 30 mcg) or ATV/r (use at least 35 mcg). **Statins: Rosuvastatin** AUC ↑213%. Start with 5 mg. Pravastatin or atorvastatin may be preferred. **Anticonvulsants:** carbamapezine, phenobarbital and phenytoin may ↓ levels of ATV substantially; avoid or use ATV/r with caution. **Sildenafil:** Maximum of 25 mg q48h. **Vardenafil:** No data; use ≤2.5 mg/24 hrs, and ≤2.5 mg/72 hrs with ATV/r. **Voriconazole** has not been studied, but it is anticipated that co-administration may increase ATV levels and decrease voriconazole levels; avoid if possible (consider voriconazole TDM with co-administration). **Atovaquone/Proguanil:** ATV/r ↓atovaquone AUC 46%; ↓proguanil 41%. Consider alternative malaria prophylaxis. **Diltiazem:** ↑AUC 125%; use half dose and monitor EKG. **Calcium channel blocker:** Monitor EKG. **H2 receptor antagonists** (e.g., ranitidine, famotidine, cimetidine)**:** Separate doses by as much time as possible, preferably; give ATV 2 h before or 10 h after H2 blockers. **Posaconazole:** ATV AUC ↑ 2.5-fold. Posaconazole AUC ↑3.7-fold. Monitor for potential ↑adverse drug reaction. **Antacids and buffered medications:** Give ATV 2 h before or >1 h after antacid. **Proton pump inhibitors** such as omeprazole should be avoided. Co-administration of 40 mg omeprazole with ATV/r 300/100 mg resulted in a 75% reduction in ATV AUC. This restriction applies to all PPIs. With **omeprazole** 20 mg should be separated by 12 hrs, ATV (ATV/r 300/100) AUC decreased by 42%. Manufacturer states that it may be considered in PI-naïve patients, but it is best to avoid. This admonition does not apply to other PIs, except NFV.

■ TABLE 5-14: **Dose Adjustments for ATV/r with Other ARVs**

Drug	Effect on co-administered drug (AUC)	Effect on ATV (AUC)	Recommendation
ddI EC	↓ 34%	No change	ddI EC – must take on empty stomach and ATV with meal. Standard doses
TDF	↑ 37% (w/ATV/r) ↑ 24% (w/ATV)	↓ 25%	Use ATV/r 300/100 qd + TDF 300 mg qd
EFV	No change	↓ 74%	Use ATV/r 400/100 mg qd with food +EFV 600 mg qd Avoid co-administration in PI-experienced patient
NVP	↑ C_{min} 46%	↓ C_{min} 41%	Avoid co-administration due to potential toxicity
ETR	↑ 30-50%	↓ 14%	Avoid; clinical significance unclear
MVC	↑ 3.6x	----	Use MVC 150 mg bid + ATV or ATV/r standard dose
DRV	No change	No change	ATV 300 qd+DRV/r standard dose
FPV	↑ 78%	↓ 33%	Insufficient data
LPV/r	No change	↑ 45%	LPV/r 400/100 bid+ATV 300 qd
SQV	↑ 449%	Not measured	Insufficient data; poor clinical response
IDV	---	---	Avoid hyperbilirubinemia
RAL	↑ 41-72%	----	Use standard dose RAL + ATV/r 300/100 mg qd
TPV/r	↑ 11%	↓ 39%	Avoid

Drug Information

5

Methadone: No interaction with unboosted ATV. With ATV/r, monitor for withdrawal. **Bupenorphine:** AUC ↑93% and 66% with ATV and ATR/r, respectively. ATV may ↓ if unboosted. Use ATV/r with bupenorphine. Monitor for sedation. **Paclitaxel, Repaglinide:** may be increased with ATV. Use with close monitoring. **Bosentan:** avoid with unboosted ATV. With ATV/r ↓ bosentan to 62.5 mg qd or qod after ATV/r has reach a steady state (>10 days).

- **ART agents:** See Table 5-14.

PREGNANCY: Category B: The pharmacokinetics of ATV/r with standard dosing (300/100 mg/d) was reported in four studies: One showed the ATV AUC was not altered by pregnancy (*AIDS* 2007;21:2409) and three studies showed significant pregnancy-associated decreases of about 25% (Eley, 15th CROI, 2008; Mirochnick M. 16th CROI, 2009; Mirochnick M. *JAIDS* 2012;Epub Ahead: PMID21283017). Concurrent use of TDF is an important variable due to the effect of this agent on ATV levels. Perhaps the most relevant report is IMPAACT10426, designed to measure pharmacokinetics of ART agents in pregnancy. The authors of this report recommend a dose adjustment of ATV/r to 400/100 mg for pregnant women (Mirochnick M. *JAIDS* 2012;Epub Ahead: PMID 21283017). The dose adjustment becomes more critical in ART-experienced pregnant patients if ATV/r is combined with TDF. It is not known whether the increase in bilirubin levels noted with ATV will increase rates of hyperbilirubinemia in the neonate to clinically important levels. Transplacental passage is low (10-16%), and this has not been seen in clinical trials. The FDA approved ATV/r for use in pregnant women based on a trial of 41 HIV-infected pregnant women given ATV/r (300/100 or 400/100 mg qd in combination with AZT/3TC). The approval was supported by pharmacology data showing adequate levels in the second and third trimesters. The 2011 DHHS Guidelines for Antiretroviral Drugs in Pregnant Women recommend ATV/r as an alternative to the preferred LPV/r. Unboosted ATV "may be considered" if RTV is not tolerated, the patient is treatment-naïve, and TDF is not in the regimen. The Pregnancy Registry reports 11 birth defects in 448 (2.5%) ATV exposures which compares to the 2.7% rate without ART exposure (reports through 7/20/2010).

ATORVASTATIN

TRADE NAME: *Lipitor* (Pfizer)

FORMS AND COST: Tabs: 10 mg at $3.34, 20 mg at $4.77, 40 mg at $4.77, and 80 mg at $4.77

CLASS: Statin (HMG-CoA reductase inhibitor)

INDICATIONS AND DOSES: See pg. 142. Elevated total and LDL cholesterol and/or triglycerides. Recommended statin for hyperlipidemia with PI-based ART by IAS-USA (*JAIDS* 2002;31:257) and HIVMA/ACTG (*CID* 2003;37:613). Atorvastatin use in a double blind study in HIV infected

Drug Information

patients reduced markers of immune activation (*JID* 2011;203:756). A review of statin use and efficacy by HIV-infected patients also showed the favored agents in terms of use and efficacy in achieving NCEP goal were atorvastatin and rosurvastatin (*CID* 2011;52:387). With atorvastatin, the initial dose is 10 mg qd with increases at 2-4 wk intervals to maintenance doses of 10-80 mg qd or 10-40 mg qd for patients on PIs. Should be taken with or without food, preferably in the evening. See pg 143.

MONITORING: Blood lipids at ≤4-wk intervals until desired results are achieved, then periodically. Obtain transaminase levels at baseline, at 12 wks, and then at 6-mo intervals. Patients should be warned to report muscle pain, tenderness, or weakness promptly, especially if accompanied by fever or malaise. Obtain CPK for suspected myopathy.

PRECAUTIONS: Atorvastatin (and other statins) are contraindicated with pregnancy, breastfeeding, concurrent conditions that predispose to renal failure (e.g., sepsis, hypotension), and active hepatic disease. Alcoholism is a relative contraindication.

PHARMACOLOGY

- **Bioavailability:** 14%

- **T½:** 14 h

- **Elimination:** Fecal (biliary and unabsorbed) – 98%; renal – <2%

- **Renal failure:** No dose adjustment

- **Hepatic failure:** Levels of atorvastatin are markedly elevated.

SIDE EFFECTS

- **Musculoskeletal:** Myopathy with elevated CPK plus muscle pain, weakness or tenderness ± fever and malaise. Rhabdomyolysis with renal failure reported.

- **Hepatic:** Use with caution. Elevated transaminases in 1-2%; discontinue if ALT and/or AST shows unexplained increase >3x upper limit of normal (ULN) x 2.

- **Miscellaneous:** Diarrhea, constipation, nausea, heartburn, stomach pain, dizziness, headache, skin rash, impotence (rare), insomnia

DRUG INTERACTIONS

- **PIs:** Potential for large increase in statin AUC with most PIs: Increase with NFV, 74%; LPV/r, 5.8x; SQV/r, 4.5x; TPV/r, 9x; FPV, 1.3x; DRV/r, 4x. Start with 10 mg qd and monitor clinically for myopathy or consider pravastatin; avoid doses >40 mg/d with PIs. EFV decreases atorvastatin AUC 43%. ETR decreases atorvastatin AUC 37%. NVP – no data.

- **Others: Grapefruit juice** increases atorvastatin levels up to 24%; avoid large amounts before or after administration. **Erythromycin:** Atorvastatin levels increased by 40%. **Antacids:** Atorvastatin levels decreased by 35%. **Other interactions with increased risk of myopathy: Azoles** (ketoconazole, itraconazole), cyclosporine, fibric

5 Drug Information

acid derivatives, niacin, macrolide antibiotics, nefazodone. **Niacin and gemfibrozil:** Increased risk of myopathy; rhabdomyolysis reported only with lovastatin + niacin, but could occur with other statins.

PREGNANCY: Category X – contraindicated

ATOVAQUONE

TRADE NAME: *Mepron* (GlaxoSmithKline)

FORM AND COST: 750 mg/5 mL: $1,133 per 210-mL bottle (21-days)

PATIENT ASSISTANCE PROGRAM: 866-728-4368

INDICATIONS AND DOSE: PCP: Oral treatment of mild to moderate PCP (A-a O_2 gradient <45 mm Hg and P_AO_2 >60 mm Hg; less effective than TMP/SMX) and PCP prophylaxis in patients who are intolerant of TMP-SMX and dapsone; toxoplasmosis treatment (third line) and prophylaxis (third line). Note drug interaction with EFV and some boosted PIs (see Drug Interactions).

- **PCP treatment:** 750 mg (5 mL) twice daily with meals x 21 days
- **PCP prophylaxis:** 1500 mg qd or 750 mg bid with meals
- **Toxoplasmosis treatment (alternative):** 1500 mg po bid with meals alone or combined with either pyrimethamine 200 mg x 1, then 50-75 mg qd or sulfadiazine 1.5 g qid (*CID* 2002;34:1243).

PHARMACOLOGY

- **Bioavailability:** Absorption of suspension averages 47% in fed state (with meals). Concurrent administration of fatty food increases absorption by 2-fold. There is significant individual variation in absorption. Administration with fatty food needs emphasis.
- **T½:** 2.2-2.9 days
- **Elimination:** Enterohepatic circulation with fecal elimination; <1% in urine
- **CSF/plasma ratio:** <1%
- **Effect of hepatic or renal disease:** No data

SIDE EFFECTS: Rash (20%), GI intolerance (20%), diarrhea (20%). Possibly related headache, fever, insomnia. Life-threatening side effects: none. Percent requiring discontinuation due to side effects: 7-9% (rash, 4%).

DRUG INTERACTIONS

- **Rifampin:** ↓ atovaquone by 54%, ↑ rifampin by 30%; avoid co-administration
- **Tetracycline:** ↓ atovaquone by 40%. Avoid or use with caution
- **AZT** AUC increased 31% due to atovaquone inhibition of AZT gluconuridation (clinical significance unknown).
- Atovaquone AUC is reduced by 75% with concurrent **EFV**, and

LPV/r, and by 50% with **ATV/r** (*AIDS* 2010;24:1223). Levels of **proguanil** (relevant for the use of atovaquone/proguanil for malaria) were reduced by 38-43%. Consider as an alternative to ETV, LPV/r and ATV/r.

- **Warfarin** Possible increase in INR (*Ann Pharmacother* 2011;45:e3).

PREGNANCY: Category C. Not teratogenic in animals; limited experience in humans.

ATRIPLA – see Efavirenz (pg. 244), Emtricitabine (pg. 255), and Tenofovir (pg. 388)

AZITHROMYCIN

TRADE NAME: *Zithromax* (Pfizer)

FORMS AND COST: Tabs: 250 mg tab at $7.16; 600 mg at $18.66; 1 g packet at $24.15. *Z-Pak* (generic) with 6 tabs (500 mg, then 250 mg qd x 4 days) at $13.99 (generic); *Zmax* (single-dose therapy), 2 gm/60 mL at $77.44; *Tri-Pak* with 3 tabs (500 mg x 3 days) for exacerbations of bronchitis at $71.66; IV formulation as 500 mg vial at $10.00, suspension 200 mg/5 mL (30 mL) $32.93.

CLASS: Macrolide antibiotic

INDICATIONS AND DOSES: See Table 5-15 below.

ACTIVITY: <u>S. pneumoniae</u> (about 20-30% of *S. pneumoniae* strains are resistant to azithromycin and other macrolides in the U.S.), streptococci (not *Enterococcus*), erythromycin-sensitive *S. aureus, H. influenzae, Legionella, C. pneumoniae, M. pneumoniae, C. trachomatis, M. avium* complex (MAC), *N. gonorrhoeae, T. pallidum* (resistance increasing), and *T. gondii* are generally sensitive. There is concern about increasing macrolide resistance by *S. pneumoniae* (*AAC* 2002;297:1016; *JID* 2000;182: 1417; *AAC* 2002;46:265; *AAC* 2001;45: 2147). However, multiple clinical trials show that *in vivo* activity with pneumococcal pneumonia is much better than *in vitro* results. For <u>MAC bacteremia</u>, one study found that azithromycin 600 mg qd was equivalent to clarithromycin 500 mg bid (*CID* 2000; 31:1245) when used in combination with ethambutol. The VA trial found clarithromycin to be superior (*CID* 2000;31;1245). For <u>syphilis</u>, preliminary studies in patients without HIV infection showed that azithromycin (2 g po x 1) was equivalent to benzathine penicillin (2.4 mil units IM x 1) for treatment of early syphilis (*NEJM* 2005;353:1236*).* More recent studies have shown an explosive rise in *T. pallidum* resistance to azithromycin in San Francisco, from 0 to 56% in 2004 (*CID* 2006;42:337). <u>N. gonorrhoeae</u> has developed resistance to multiple antibiotics making cephalosporins the only recommended class in the US 2010 CDC Guidelines (*MMWR* 210;59:RR-12). For pharyngeal GC the recommendation is ceftriaxone 250 mg IM plus azithromycin 1 gm po x 1 (or plus doxycycline 100 mg qd x 7d).

5 Drug Information

PHARMACOLOGY

- **Bioavailability:** Absorption is ~30-40%. The 600 mg tabs and the 1 g powder packet may be taken without regard to food, but food improves tolerability.

- **T½:** 68 hrs; detectable levels in urine at 7-14 days; with the 1200 mg weekly dose, the azithromycin levels in peripheral leukocytes remain above 32 µg/mL for 60 hrs.

- **Distribution:** High tissue levels; low CSF levels (<0.01 µg/mL)

- **Excretion:** Primarily biliary; 6% in urine

- **Dose modification in renal or hepatic failure:** Use with caution.

SIDE EFFECTS: GI intolerance (nausea, vomiting, pain); diarrhea – 14%. With 1200 mg weekly dose, major side effects are diarrhea, abdominal pain, and/or nausea in 10-15%; reversible dose-dependent hearing loss is reported in 5% at mean day of onset at 96 days and mean exposure of 59,000 mg (package insert). Frequency of discontinuation in AIDS patients receiving high doses – 6%, primarily GI intolerance and reversible ototoxicity – 2%; rare – erythema multiforme, increased transaminases.

CONTRAINDICATIONS: Hypersensitivity to erythromycin

DRUG INTERACTIONS: Preferred macrolide for PI and NNRTI co-administration because it avoids the drug interactions of clarithromycin.

■ TABLE 5-15: **Azithromycin Regimens by Condition**

Indication	Dose[†]
M. avium complex (MAC) prophylaxis*	1200 mg po per week or 600 mg po twice weekly (2008 IDSA/NIH/CDC Guidelines for Treatment and Prevention of Opportunistic Infections)
MAC treatment*	500-600 mg po qd + EMB ± rifabutin (*CID* 2000; 31:1245; 2008 IDSA/NIH/CDC OI Guidelines (Alternative)
Pneumonia*	500 mg IV qd x ≥2 days (hospitalized patients), then 500 mg po qd x 3 to 10 days; outpatient: 1.5-2 gm po over 1, 3 or 5 days
Sinusitis*	500 mg po x 1, then 250 mg po qd x 4 (*Z-pak*) or 500 mg po qd x 3 days (*Tri-pak*)
*C. trachomatis** (nongonococcal urethritis or cervicitis)	1 g po x 1 or doxycycline 100 mg po bid x 7 days
Gonococcal urethritis or cervicitis	Ceftriaxone 250 mg IM x1 or cefixime 400 mg po x 1 or azithromycin 1 gm po + ceftriaxone 250 mg IM (2010 CDC Guidelines for STDs)
Toxoplasmosis	900-1200 mg po qd + pyrimethamine 200 mg po x1, then 50-75 mg qd + leukovorin 10-20 mg qd x ≥ 6 wks, then half dose of each

* FDA-approved indications.

† Caps must be taken ≥1 hr before or >2 hrs after a meal; food improves absorption and tolerance of tabs and powder.

Drug Information

Azithromycin increases levels of **theophylline** and **coumadin**. Concurrent use with antiretroviral agents, rifampin, and rifabutin is safe. Concurrent use with pimozide may cause fatal arrythmias and must be avoided.

PREGNANCY: Category B (safe in animal studies; no data in humans). Preferred macrolide for MAC prophylaxis and treatment in pregnancy.

AZOLES – see Table 5-16 (pg. 208)

AZT – see Zidovudine (pg. 416)

BACTRIM – see Trimethoprim-Sulfamethoxazole (pg. 409)

BENZODIAZEPINES

Benzodiazepines are commonly used for anxiety and insomnia. They are also commonly misused and abused, with some studies showing that up to 25% of AIDS patients take these drugs. The decision to use these drugs requires careful consideration of side effects along with a discussion of the following issues with the patient:

- **EFV** may cause false positive urine tests for benzodiazepine. This is due to 8 hydroxy-EFV (*CID* 2009;48:1787).

- **Dependency:** Larger than usual doses or prolonged daily use of therapeutic doses.

- **Abuse potential:** Most common in those with abuse of alcohol and other psychiatric drugs.

- **Tolerance:** Primarily to sedation and ataxia; minimal to antianxiety effects.

- **Withdrawal symptoms:** Related to duration of use, dose, rate of tapering, and drug half-life. Features include: 1) recurrence of pretreatment symptoms developing over days or weeks; 2) rebound with symptoms that are similar to but more severe than pretreatment symptoms occurring within hours or days (self-limited); and 3) the "benzodiazepine withdrawal syndrome" with autonomic symptoms, disturbances in equilibrium, sensory disturbances, etc.

- **Daytime sedation, dizziness, incoordination, ataxia, and hangover:** Use small doses initially and gradually increase. Patient must be warned that activities requiring mental alertness, judgment, and coordination require special caution; concomitant use with alcohol or other sedating drugs is hazardous. Patients often experience amnesia for events during the drug's time of action.

- **Drug interactions:** Sedative effects are antagonized by caffeine and theophylline. Erythromycin, clarithromycin, fluoroquinolones, all PIs

5 Drug Information

■ TABLE 5-16: Azoles and Antiretroviral Agents: Drug Interactions

Antifungal	ART	Effect AUC	Recommendation
	NNRTI		
Fluconazole (see pg. 276)	EFV	No effect	Standard doses
	ETR	ETR ↑86%	Caution
	NVP	NVP ↑110%	Risk hepatotoxicity – monitor*
Posaconazole	EFV	Posa ↓50%	Alternative or monitor*
	ETR	ETR ↑?	Standard doses
Itraconazole (see pg. 301)	EFV	Itra ↓40%	May need ↑ itra dose
	ETR	Itra ↓?, ETR ↑?	Monitor*
	NVP	Itra ↓?, NVP ↑?	Monitor*
Voriconazole (see pg. 413)	EFV	Vori ↓77%, EFV ↑44%	Vori 400 mg bid, EFV 300 mg qd
	ETR	ETR ↑36%	Standard doses and caution
	PI		
Fluconazole (see pg. 276)	ATV/r	No effect	Standard doses
	SQV	SQV ↑	No data for SQV/r
	TPV/r	TPV ↑50%	Flucon dose ≤200 mg/d
Posaconazole	ATV/r	ATV ↑146%	Monitor for ATV ADR
	ATV	ATV ↑268%	Monitor for ATV ADR
Itraconazole (see pg. 301)	LPV/r	Itra ↑	Itra dose ≤200/d or monitor*
	SQV/r	Itra ↑, SQV ↑	Itra dose ↓ or monitor
	Other	Itra ↑, PI ↑?	ATV/r, DRV/r, FPV/r, TPV/r Dose itra ≤200 mg/d and/or monitor
Itraconazole/ Voriconazole	MVC	MVC ↑	MVC 150 mg bid
Azoles	RAL	No interactions	Standard doses

* Indicates monitoring azole blood levels

cimetidine, omeprazole, and INH may reduce hepatic metabolism and prolong half-life. Midazolam and triazolam are thus contraindicated for co-administration. Lorazepam, temazepam, and oxazepam are safer alternatives. Rifampin and oral contraceptives increase hepatic clearance and reduce half-life.

- **Miscellaneous side effects:** Blurred vision, diplopia, confusion, memory disturbance, amnesia, fatigue, incontinence, constipation, hypotension, disinhibition, bizarre behavior

- **Antiretroviral agents:** Concurrent use of triazolam or midazolam with PIs or DLV is contraindicated.

SELECTION OF AGENT AND REGIMEN: Drug selection is based largely on indication and pharmacokinetic properties (Table 5-17). Drugs with rapid

Drug Information

onset are desired when temporary relief of anxiety is needed. The smallest dose for the shortest time is recommended, and patients need frequent re-evaluation for continued use. Long-term use should be avoided, especially in patients with a history of abuse of alcohol or other sedative-hypnotic drugs. Dose adjustments are usually required to achieve the desired effect with acceptable side effects. Long-term use (more than several weeks) may require an extended tapering schedule over 6-8 wks (20-30% dose reduction weekly) adjusted by symptoms and sometimes facilitated by antidepressants or hypnotics.

■ TABLE 5-17: **Comparison of Benzodiazepines**

Agent	Trade Name	Anxiety	Insomnia	Tmax (hrs)	Mean Half-life (hrs)	Dose Forms	Regimens
Chlordiazepoxide	Librium	+	–	0.5-4.0	10	5, 10, 25 mg tabs	15-100 mg/day hs or 3 to 4 doses
Clorazepate	Tranxene	+	–	1 2	73	3.75, 7.5, 15, 11.25, 22.5 mg tabs	15-60 mg/day hs or 2 to 4 doses
Diazepam	Valium	+	+	1.5-2.0	73	2, 4, 5, 10 mg tabs	15-60 mg/day hs or 2 to 4 doses
Flurazepam	Dalmane	–	+	0.5-2.0	74	15, 30 mg caps	15-30 mg/day, hs
Quazepam	Doral	–	+	2	74	7.5, 15 mg tabs	7.5-30 mg hs
Alprazolam	Xanax	+	–	1-2	11	0.25, 0.5, 1, 2 mg tabs 0.5, 1, 2, 3 mg SR tabs	0.75-1.5 mg/day in 3 divided doses
Lorazepam	Ativan	+	+	2	14	0.5, 1, and 2 mg tabs	0.25-0.5 mg tid up to 4 mg/day
Oxazepam	Serax	+	+	1-4	7	10, 15, 30 mg caps	15-30 mg tid-qid
Temazepam	Restoril	–	+	1.0-1.5	13	15, 30 mg caps	15-30 mg qhs
Triazolam*	Halcion	–	+	1-2	3	0.125, 0.25 mg tabs	0.25 mg hs
Midazolam*	Versed	+	+	2 min	1-5	IV vial	0.03-0.06 mg/kg

* Concurrent use of midazolam or triazolam and all PIs or DLV is contraindicated. Single dose IV midazolam may be considered with ATV, TPV/r, and LPV/r. Monitor closely.

BIAXIN – see Clarithromycin (pg. 217)

BUPROPION

TRADE NAME: *Wellbutrin, Wellbutrin SR, Wellbutrin XL, Zyban* (GlaxoSmithKline) and generic

FORMS AND COST: Tabs: 75 mg at $0.73, 100 mg at $1.85, 150 mg sustained-release at $2.51. *Wellbutrin* comes in 75 and 100 mg tabs; *Wellbutrin SR* comes in 100, 150, and 200 mg tabs; and *Wellbutrin XL* comes in 150 and 300 mg tabs.

CLASS: Atypical antidepressant

INDICATIONS AND DOSES: Depression: 150 mg qd x 4 days, then 300 mg qd (XL formulation) or 150 mg bid (SR formulation); antidepressant effect may require 4 wks. *Zyban* for smoking cessation. Dose same as SR formulation x 7-12 wks.

PHARMACOLOGY

- **Bioavailability:** 5-20%
- **T½:** 8-24 hrs
- **Elimination:** Extensive hepatic metabolism to ≥6 metabolites, two with antidepressant activity; metabolites excreted in urine.
- **Dose modification in renal or hepatic failure:** Not known, but dose reduction may be required.

SIDE EFFECTS: Seizures, which are dose dependent and minimized by gradual increase in dose; dose not to exceed 450 mg/d. Use with caution in seizure-prone patients and with concurrent use of alcohol and other antidepressants.

OTHER SIDE EFFECTS: Agitation, insomnia, restlessness; GI – anorexia, nausea, vomiting; weight loss – noted in up to 25%; rare cases of psychosis, paranoia, depersonalization.

DRUG INTERACTIONS: LPV/r decreases buproprion AUC 57% (*Hogeland et al. CPT* 2007;81:69); no seizures reported with PI co-administration.

BUSPAR – see Buspirone (below)

BUSPIRONE

TRADE NAME: *BuSpar* (Bristol-Myers Squibb) and generics

FORMS AND COST: Tabs: 5 mg tab at $0.77, 10 mg tab at $1.35, 15 mg tab at $2.00

CLASS: Nonbenzodiazepine-nonbarbiturate antianxiety agent; not a controlled substance

INDICATIONS AND DOSES: Anxiety: 5 mg po tid; increase by 5 mg/d every 2-4 days. Usual effective dose is 15-30 mg/d in 2-3 divided doses. Onset of response requires 1 week, and full effect requires 4 wks. Total daily dose should not exceed 60 mg/d.

PHARMACOLOGY

- **Bioavailability:** >90% absorbed when taken with food.
- **T½:** 2.5 hrs

Drug Information

- **Elimination:** Rapid hepatic metabolism to partially active metabolites; <0.1% of parent compound excreted in urine
- **Dose adjustment in renal disease:** Dose reduction of 25-50% in patients with anuria
- **Hepatic disease:** May decrease clearance and must use with caution.

SIDE EFFECTS: Sleep disturbance, nervousness, headache, nausea, diarrhea, paresthesias, depression, increased or decreased libido, dizziness, and excitement. Compared with benzodiazepines, there is no risk of dependency, it does not potentiate CNS depressants including alcohol, it is usually well tolerated by elderly, and there is no hypnotic effect, no muscle relaxant effect, less fatigue, less confusion, and less decreased libido but nearly comparable efficacy for prevention of anxiety (not effective for acute anxiety attacks). Nevertheless, the CNS effects are somewhat unpredictable, and there is substantial individual variation; patients should be warned that buspirone may impair ability to perform activities requiring mental alertness and physical coordination such as driving.

DRUG INTERACTIONS: Rifampin decreases buspirone AUC 90%; NNRTIs may also decrease buspirone (Lamberg TS et al. *Br J Clin Pharmacol* 1998;45:381; *Drugs* 2011;71:11).

PREGNANCY: Category B

CASPOFUNGIN

TRADE NAME: *Cancidas* (Merck)

FORMS AND COST: 50 mg vial $405; 70 mg vial $421

CLASS: Polypeptide antifungal; Echinocandin glucan synthesis inhibitor.

ACTIVITY: Active against nearly all *Candida* spp, although somewhat higher concentrations are needed for *C. parapsilosis* and *C. guilliermondii*. Most fluconazole-resistant strains are sensitive (*Am J Med* 2006;119:993). Active against most *Aspergillus* spp; the combination of caspofungin with voriconazole or amphotericin is synergistic or additive against *Aspergillus* spp (*CID* 2003;36:1445; *Cancer* 2006; 107:2888; *Med Mycol* 2006;44(Suppl):373). No activity against *C. neoformans*.

INDICATIONS: (1) Invasive aspergillosis, in patients intolerant of voriconazole or amphotericin B, caspofungin plus posaconazole has been used for invasive aspergillus refractory to standard treatment (*Mycosis* 2011;54 Suppl 1:1439); (2) Candidemia and other serious *Candida* infections, including *Candida* esophagitis refractory and resistant to azoles. FDA-approved for oropharyngeal, esophageal, and disseminated candidiasis and for invasive aspergillosis. The 2008 IDSA/FDA/CDC Guidelines for Opportunistic Infections list caspofungin and other echinocandins) as alternative options in fluconazole – refractory oral or esophageal candidiasis. A major concern is expense.

5 Drug Information

DOSE: 70 mg IV on day 1, then 50 mg qd

- Dose with renal failure: standard; Dose in obese patients: 70 mg qd
- Dose with hepatic failure: With Child-Pugh score of 7-9, give standard loading dose of 70 mg, then 35 mg qd. Use with caution with Child-Pugh score >9

PHARMACOLOGY

- **Absorption:** IV only
- **T½:** 9-11 h
- **Distribution:** Poor CNS, eye and urinary penetration
- **Elimination:** Metabolized by hydrolysis and acetylating; <2% excreted unchanged in urine

ADVERSE REACTIONS: Excellent safety profile; rare side effects are rash, facial swelling, nausea, vomiting, headache, fever, phlebitis, hypokalemia, increased alkaline phosphatase. Rare patients have histamine release symptoms with rash, fever, pruritis, and sensation of warmth that accompanies infusion.

DRUG INTERACTIONS: Cyclosporin increases caspofungin AUC 35%; co-administration is not recommended due to increase in liver enzymes. **Tacrolimus** levels reduced 20% with caspofungin; monitor tacrolimus levels. **Phenytoin, carbamazepine, phenobarbital, dexamethasone, EFV**, and **NVP** may decrease caspofungin; consider increasing dose to 70 mg/d with invasive disease. **Rifampin** decreases caspofungin by 30%; increase caspofungin dose to 70 mg/d or consider micafungin.

PREGNANCY: Class C: Embryotoxic with skeletal abnormalities in rats and rabbits; limited experience in humans. Amphotericin B is preferred.

CIDOFOVIR

TRADE NAME: *Vistide* (Gilead Sciences)

FORM AND COST: 1% gel (not commercially available but can be compounded by pharmacy); 375 mg in 5 mL vial at $888

PATIENT ASSISTANCE PROGRAM AND REIMBURSEMENT HOTLINE: 800-226-2056

ACTIVITY: Active *in vitro* against CMV, VZV, EBV, HHV-6, HPV, pox viruses (molluscum, vaccinia, smallpox), and HHV-8; less active against HSV (*Exp Med Biol* 1996;394:105). CMV strains resistant to ganciclovir with UL97 mutation are usually sensitive to cidofovir. Cidofovir-resistant strains are usually resistant to ganciclovir and sensitive to foscarnet. HSV that is resistant to acyclovir is often sensitive to cidofovir.

INDICATIONS AND DOSE: CMV retinitis (*Clin Opthalmol* 2010;4:285); efficacy in other forms of CMV disease has not been established but is expected (*Arch Intern Med* 1998;158:957). Topical use for **acyclovir-**

resistant HSV (*J Eur Acad Dermatol Venereol* 2006;20:887). Cidofovir applied topically has been used to treat disfiguring **HPV** lesions (*J Am Acad Dermatol* 2006;55:533). A trial in 185 patients with HIV-associated **PML** failed (*AIDS* 2008;22:1759). There is a suggested but unproven role in HHV-8 associated primary effusion lymphoma (*Clin Adv Hematol Oncol* 2010;8:372; *Clin Adv Hematol Oncol* 2010;8:367)

- **Topical Administration:** Withdraw contents of IV vial (375 mg/5 mL) and mix with 33 gm of *Orabase* gel with benzocaine.
- **Induction dose:** 5 mg/kg IV over 1 hr* weekly x 2 wks
- **Maintenance dose:** 5 mg/kg IV over 1 hr every 2 wks*

---

* Probenecid 2 g given 3 hrs prior to cidofovir and 1 g given at 2 and 8 hrs after infusion (total of 4 g). Patients must receive >1 L 0.95 N (normal) saline infused over 1-2 hrs immediately before cidofovir infusion.

CLINICAL TRIALS: Studies of the Ocular Complications of AIDS (SOCA) comparing cidofovir vs. deferred treatment of patients with CMV retinitis in the pre-HAART era demonstrated a median time to progression of 120 days in the treated group compared with 22 days in the deferred group (*Ann Intern Med* 1997;126:257). Dose-limiting nephrotoxicity was noted in 24%, and dose-limiting toxicity to probenecid was noted in 7%.

NOTES ON ADMINISTRATION

- Cidofovir is diluted in 100 mL 0.9% saline.
- Renal failure: Cidofovir is contraindicated in patients with preexisting renal failure (serum creatinine >1.5 mg/dL, creatinine clearance ≤55 mL/min or urine protein >100 mg/dL or 2+ proteinuria).
- Co-administration of nephrotoxic drugs is contraindicated. There should be a 7-day "washout" following use of these drugs.
- Dose adjustment for renal failure during cidofovir treatment:
  - Serum creatinine increase 0.3-0.4 mg/dL: Reduce dose to 3 mg/kg.
  - Serum creatinine increase ≥0.5 mg/dL or ≥3 + proteinuria: Discontinue therapy.
- Gastrointestinal tolerability of probenecid may be improved with ingestion of food or an antiemetic prior to administration. Anti-histamines or acetaminophen may be used for probenecid hypersensitivity reactions.
- Cases of nephrotoxicity should be reported to Gilead Sciences, Inc. 800-GILEAD-5, or to the FDA's Medwatch 800-FDA-1088.

PHARMACOLOGY

- **Bioavailability:** Requires IV administration; probenecid increases AUC by 40-60%, presumably by blocking tubular secretion. CSF levels are undetectable.
- **T½:** 17-65 h
- **Excretion:** 70-85% excreted in urine.

Drug Information

5

SIDE EFFECTS: The major side effect is **dose-dependent nephrotoxicity** including Fanconi syndrome (*JAC* 2007;60:193). Proteinuria is an early indicator. IV saline and probenecid must be used to reduce nephrotoxicity. Monitor renal function with serum creatinine and urine protein within 48 hrs prior to each dose. About 25% will develop ≥2 + proteinuria or a serum creatinine >2-3 mg/dL, and these changes are reversible if treatment is discontinued (*Ann Intern Med* 1997;126: 257,264).

OTHER SIDE EFFECTS: Neutropenia in about 15% (monitor neutrophil count), Fanconi's syndrome with proteinuria, normoglycemic glycosuria, hypophosphatemia, hypouracemia and decreased serum bicarbonate indicating renal tubule damage, ocular hypotony, anterior uveitis or iritis, and aesthenia.

Probenecid causes side effects in about 50% of patients including fever, chills, headache, rash, or nausea, usually after 3-4 treatments. Side effects usually resolve within 12 hrs. Dose-limiting side effect is usually GI intolerance. Side effects may be reduced with antiemetics, antipyretics, antihistamines, or by eating before taking probenecid (*Ann Intern Med* 1997;126:257).

DRUG INTERACTIONS: Avoid concurrent use of potentially **nephrotoxic drugs**. Patients receiving these drugs should have a ≥7 day "washout" prior to treatment with cidofovir. Probenecid prolongs the half-life of **acetaminophen, acyclovir, aminosalicylic acid, barbiturates, beta-lactams, benzodiazepines, bumetadine, clofibrate, methotrexate, famotidine, furosemide, NSAIDs, theophylline**, **TDF** and **AZT**.

PREGNANCY: Category C. Embryotoxic and teratotoxic in rats and rabbits. Not recommended for humans.

CIPROFLOXACIN – see Table 5-18, pg. 216

TRADE NAME: *Cipro* (Bayer) and generic

FORMS AND COST: Tabs: 250 mg, 500 mg at $5.36, 750 mg at $5.62; 500 mg XR at $10.90; 1000 mg XR at $11.10. Vials for IV use: 400 mg at $3.60.

CLASS: Fluoroquinolone antibiotic

INDICATIONS AND DOSES

- **Respiratory infections:** 500-750 mg po bid x 7-14 days. *P. aeruginosa*: use 750 mg po bid or 400 mg IV q8 hx ≥14 days.

- **Gonorrhea:** Fluoroquinolones are no longer recommended (2010 CDC Guidelines for STDs).

- ***M. avium:*** 500-750 mg po bid (alternative or 3rd or 4th drug with serious disease)

- **Tuberculosis:** 500-750 mg po bid (multidrug-resistant *M. tuberculosis* or liver disease). Preferred agent is moxifloxacin.

Drug Information

214

- **Salmonellosis:** 500-750 mg po or 400 mg IV bid x 7-14 d for mild disease or 4-6 wks for CD4 <200 and/or bacteremia (preferred).
- **UTI:** 250-500 mg po bid x 3-7 d (first line); uncomplicated UTI: ciprofloxacin XR 500 mg qd x 3 d.
- **Traveler's diarrhea:** 500 mg po bid x 3 d (first line).

ACTIVITY: Active against most strains of *Enterobacteriaceae, P. aeruginosa, H. influenzae, Legionella, C. pneumoniae, M. pneumoniae, M. tuberculosis, M. avium complex*, most **bacterial enteric pathogens** other than *C. jejuni* and *C. difficile*. Somewhat less active against *S. pneumoniae* than levofloxacin, and moxifloxacin. There is increasing and substantial resistance by *S. aureus* (primarily MRSA) (*CID* 2000;32:S114), *P. aeruginosa* (*CID* 2000;32:S146), *E. coli* and *C. jejuni* (*CID* 2001;32: 1201). There is also escalating concern about fluoroquinolone-resistant *S. pneumoniae, N. gonorrhoeae* and *Salmonella*. Fluoroquinolines are no longer recommended for **gonococcal infections** due to resistance (2010 CDC Guidelines STD recommendations) (*MMWR* 2010;59:RR-12; *Ann Intern Med* 2007; 147:81). Most strains of *Salmonella* are fluoroquinolone-sensitive in HIV-infected patients (*Trop Med Int Health* 2010;15:697). For **tuberculosis** there is considerable enthusiasm for fluoroquinolone use for resistant strains which are now in phase III testing at the FDA (*Lancet* 2010;10:621).

PHARMACOLOGY

- **Bioavailability:** 60-70%
- **T½:** 3.3 hrs
- **Excretion:** Metabolized and excreted (parent compound and metabolites) in urine
- **Dose reduction in renal failure:** CrCl>50 mL/min – 250-750 mg q12h; CrCl 10-50 mL/min – 250-500 mg q12h; CrCl<10 mL/min – 500 mg q24h

SIDE EFFECTS: Usually well tolerated; most common include:

- Fluoroquinolones are now a major cause of *C. difficile*-**associated colitis** (*Ann Intern Med* 2006;145:758; *NEJM* 2005;353:2433; *CID* 2008;47:818; *Infect Control Hosp Epidemiol* 2009;30:264). All agents in the class are implicated; relative rates are unclear.
- **GI intolerance** with nausea – 1.2%; diarrhea – 1.2%
- **CNS toxicity:** Malaise, drowsiness, insomnia, headache, dizziness, agitation, psychosis (rare), seizures (rare), hallucinations (rare)
- **Tendon rupture:** About 100 cases reported involving fluoroquinolones, with ciprofloxacin accounting for 25% (*CID* 2003;36:1404). The incidence in a review of 46,776 courses was 0.1% with increased rates in older age and steroids as confounding risks (*BMJ* 2002;324:1306).

5 Drug Information

- **Torsades de pointes:** Rates/10 million are: moxifloxacin – 0, ciprofloxacin – 0.3, levofloxacin – 5.4 (*Pharmacother* 2001;21:1468).

- *Candida* **vaginitis**

CAUTION: Fluoroquinolones are relatively contraindicated in persons <18 years due to concern for arthropathy, which has been seen in beagles, but application to human disease is debated (*Curr Opin Pediatr* 2006; 18:64). Some fluoroquinolones may cause false positive urine screening tests for opiates (*JAMA* 2001;286:3115).

DRUG INTERACTIONS (TABLE 5-19B): Increased levels of **theophylline, methotrexate**, and caffeine; reduced absorption with **cations (Al, Mg, Ca)** in antacids, sucralfate, milk and dairy products, **buffered ddl**. Take fluoroquinolone 2 h before cations.

PREGNANCY: Category C. Arthropathy in immature animals with erosions in joint cartilages; relevance to patients is not known, but fluoroquinolones are not FDA-approved for use in pregnancy or in

■ TABLE 5-18: **Fluoroquinolone Summary**

	Ciprofloxacin *Cipro*	Levofloxacin *Levaquin*	Moxifloxacin *Avelox*
Oral form	+	+	+
IV form	+	+	+
Price (AWP) oral formulation	$6.42 (500 mg), $12.84/d	$12.28 (500 mg tab)	$12.25 (400 mg tab)
T½	3.3 hrs	6.3 hrs	12 hrs
T½ renal failure	8 hrs	35 hrs	12 hrs
Oral bioavailability	65%	99%	90%

Activity *in vitro**
  P. aeruginosa
  S. pneumoniae
  Mycobacteria
  Anaerobes
	
	+++(60-80%)
	+
	++
	—
		
		++
		++
		++
		+
			
			+
			++
			+++
			++

Regimens (oral)	250-750 mg bid	500-750 mg qd	400 mg qd

* All fluoroquinolones are active against most *Enterobacteriaceae*, enteric bacterial pathogens (except *C. jejuni* and *C. difficile*), methicillin-sensitive *S. aureus*, *Neisseria* spp., and pulmonary pathogens including *S. pneumoniae, H. influenzae, C. pneumoniae, Legionella,* and *M. pneumoniae.*

Major advantages of newer fluoroquinolones are once-daily dosing, good tolerability, and activity against *S. pneumoniae,* including >98% of penicillin-resistant strains (*AAC* 2002;46:265). The major newly recognized class side effect is *Clostridium difficile*-associated diarrhea or colitis (*NEJM* 2005;353:2433; *NEJM* 2005;353:2442, *NEJM* 2005;353:2503). Other class side effects include prolongation of QT interval when given to persons predisposed primarily by concurrent medications (macrolides, class IA and III anti-arrhythmics), tendon rupture (risk with age and steroids), and CNS toxicity including seizures. All are contraindicated in persons <18 years and in pregnant women. Divalent and trivalent cations reduce absorption – avoid concurrent antacids with Mg^{++} or Al^{+++}, sucralfate, Fe^{++}, Zn^{++}, and buffered ddl; administer fluoronoquinolones 2 hrs before cations. The major concern is abuse and resistance, with particular concern for *P. aeruginosa, Enterobacteraceae, S. pneumoniae, S. aureus, C. jejuni, N. gonorrhoeae, C. difficile* and *Salmonella.*

children <18 years. Review of >400 first trimester exposures showed no anomalies. Use is justified in severe MAC or multi-drug-resistant tuberculosis.

CLARITHROMYCIN

TRADE NAME: *Biaxin* (Abbott Laboratories) and generic

FORMS AND COST: Tabs: 250 mg at $4.51, 500 mg at $4.94, 500 mg XL at $7.55 (for qd dosing). Suspension: 250 mg/5 mL at $110 per 100 mL.

PATIENT ASSISTANCE PROGRAM: 800-659-9050

CLASS: Macrolide antibiotic

CLINICAL TRIALS: See Table 19A. Clarithromycin is highly effective in the treatment and prevention of **Mycobacterium avium complex** (MAC) disease (*NEJM* 1996;335:385; *CID* 1998;27:1278). Clarithromycin was superior to azithromycin in the treatment of MAC bacteremia in terms of median time to negative blood cultures 4.4 wks vs. >16 wks (*CID* 1998;27:1278). However, this point is debated and may be a dose issue (*CID* 2000;31:1254). There is no evidence that it is superior to azithromycin for MAC prophylaxis. Clarithromycin and rifabutin should be given together with caution due to decreased levels of clarithromycin (*NEJM* 1996;335:428). This is the presumed explanation for the lack of superior outcome with rifabutin plus clarithromycin vs. clarithromycin alone for prevention of MAC (*JID* 2000;181:1289).

■ TABLE 5-19A: **Clarithromycin Indications and Doses**

Indication	Dose Regimen*
Pharyngitis, sinusitis, otitis, pneumonitis, skin and soft tissue infection[†]	250-500 mg po bid or 1 g (2XL tabs) qd
M. avium complex (MAC) prophylaxis[†]	500 mg po bid (2008 IDSA/NIH/CDC Guidelines)
MAC treatment[†] (plus EMB ± moxifloxacin or rifabutin)	500 mg po bid (+ ethambutol 15 mg/kg po/d + rifabutin 300 mg po/d) (2008 IDSA/NIH/CDC OI Guidelines)
Bartonella	500 mg po bid x ≥3 mos

* Doses of ≥2 gm/d are associated with excessive mortality (*CID* 1999;29:125).

† FDA-approved for this indication.

ACTIVITY: *S. pneumoniae* (20-30% of strains and 40% of penicillin-resistant strains are resistant in most areas of the United States), good activity vs. most **erythromycin-sensitive *S. pyogenes*, *M. catarrhalis*, *H. influenzae*, *M. pneumoniae*, *C. pneumoniae*, *Legionella*, *M. avium*, *T. gondii*, *C. trachomatis*, and *U. urealyticum***. Activity against *H. influenzae* is often debated, although a metabolite shows better *in vitro* activity than the parent compound, and the FDA has approved

Drug Information

5

clarithromycin for pneumonia caused by *H. influenzae*. There is concern about increasing rates of macrolide resistance by **S. pneumoniae** (*JID* 2000;182:1417; *AAC* 2001;45:2147; *AAC* 2002; 46:265). Clinical trials show *in vivo* results are superior to *in vitro* activity, but excessive rates of breakthrough pneumococcal bacteremia has been reported when clarithromycin is used alone. Many authorities now prefer a beta-lactam combined with a macrolide for serious pneumococcal infections, presumably due to the anti-inflammatory effect of the macrolide effect of the macrolide (*Drugs* 2011;7:131; *CID* 2002;35:556).

■ TABLE 5-19B: **Clarithromycin Interactions with Antiretroviral Agents**

Agent	Clarithromycin	ART Agent	Regimen
IDV	↑ 53%	↑ 29%	Standard – Reduce clarithromycin w/renal failure
RTV	↑ 77%	No data	Reduce clarithromycin dose by 50% if CrCl 30-60 mL/min, and by 75% if CrCl <30 mL/min
SQV	↑ 45%	↑ 177%	CrCl 30-60 mL/min: ↓50%; CrCl < 30 mL/min: ↓75%. May ↑ risk of QTc prolongation. Consider azithromycin.
NFV	No data	No data	Reduce clarithromycin with renal failure
LPV/r	↑ 77%	↑	Reduce clarithromycin dose by 50% if CrCl 30-60 mL/min, and by 75% if CrCl <30 mL/min
NVP	↓ 30%	↑ 26%	Standard; monitor for efficacy or use azithromycin
EFV	↓ 39%	↑	Avoid if possible; consider azithromycin
DLV	↑ 100%	↑ 44%	Dose reduction for renal failure Consider ↓ 50%
ATV	↑ 94%	↑ 28%	Use half dose clarithromycin and monitor for arrhythmia (QTc prolongation) or use azithromycin w/ESRD
DRV	↑ 57%	No change	Use half dose clarithromycin if CrCl 30-60 mL/min and reduce 75% if CrCl <30 mL/min
TPV	↑ 19%	↑ 66%	Use half dose clarithromycin if CrCl 30-60 mL/min and reduce 75% if CrCl <30 mL/min
FPV	No Change	↑ 18%	Standard doses w/FPV, but consider ↓ dose in renal failure w/boosted FPV
MVC	No change likely	Possible ↑	MVC dose is 150 mg bid
ETR	↓ 39%	↑ 42%	Consider azithromycin for MAC

PHARMACOLOGY

- **Bioavailability:** 50-55%
- **T½:** 4-7 hrs
- **Elimination:** Rapid first-pass hepatic metabolism plus renal clearance to 14-hydroxyclarithromycin
- **Dose modification in renal failure:** CrCl <30 mL/min half usual dose or double interval

SIDE EFFECTS (TABLE 19B): GI intolerance – 4% (vs. 17% with erythromycin); transaminase elevation – 1%, headache – 2%, PMC – rare. There are 38 cases of neurotoxicity reported (*J Clin Neurosci* 2011;18:313).

DRUG INTERACTIONS: Clarithromycin is a substrate and inhibitor of CYP3A4. It increases levels of **rifabutin** 56%, and levels of **clarithromycin** are decreased 50%. Consider using **azithromycin**. Clarithromycin should not be combined with **rifampin, ergot alkaloid, carbamazepine** (*Tegretol*), **cisapride** (*Propulsid*), **pimozide** (*Orap*), increased levels of pimozide and cisapride may cause fatal arrhythmias. The same concern for QTc prolongation applies to concurrent use with **atazanavir** and **saquinavir**. (Use 50% clarithromycin dose or use azithromycin, which has no substantial interaction with these drugs.) May increase serum level CYP3A4 substrates. See Table 5-18B for interactions and dose adjustments for clarithromycin use with NNRTIs and PIs.

PREGNANCY: Category C; teratogenic rats and mice, but not rabbits or monkeys. experience with >100 first trimester exposures in women showed no defects. Okay to use for MAC if no alternatives.

CLINDAMYCIN

TRADE NAME: *Cleocin* (Pharmacia) and generic

FORMS AND COST:

- **Clindamycin HCl caps:** 75 mg – $2.28 (*Cleocin*), 150 mg – $0.63 (generic), 300 mg at $3.75
- **Clindamycin PO₄ with 150 mg/mL in 2, 4, and 6 mL vials:** 600 mg vial at $2.56; 900 mg at $5.04

INDICATIONS AND DOSES

- **PCP:** Clindamycin 600-900 mg q6-8h IV or 300-450 mg q6-8h po + primaquine 15-30 mg (base)
- **Toxoplasmosis:** Clindamycin 600 mg IV or po q6h + pyrimethamine 200 loading dose, then 50 mg (<60 kg) or 75 mg po (>60 kg) qd + leucovorin 10-20 mg qd (may be increased to 50 mg qd).
- **Other infections:** 600 mg IV q8h or 300-450 mg po q6-8h

ACTIVITY: Most Gram-positive cocci are susceptible except *Entero-*

Drug Information

5

coccus and some community-acquired MRSA. Most anaerobic bacteria are susceptible, but IDSA guidelines for intra-abdominal sepsis (*CID* 2010;50:133) do not include clindamycin due to increasing resistance by *B. fragilis* (20-30%).

SIDE EFFECTS: GI – diarrhea in 10-30%. Up to 6% of patients develop *C. difficile*-associated diarrhea; may be severe (*Ann Intern Med* 2006;145:758); most respond well to discontinuation of the implicated antibiotic ± metronidazole (500 mg tid x 10 days) or oral vancomycin (125 mg qid x 10114/d) (*Infect Control Hosp Epidemiol* 2010;31:431). Other GI side effects include nausea, vomiting, and anorexia. Rash – generalized morbilliform rash is most common; less common is urticaria, pruritus, Stevens-Johnson syndrome.

DRUG INTERACTIONS: Loperamide (*Imodium*) or **diphenoxylate/atropine** (*Lomotil* and other antiperistaltic drugs such as narcotics) may increase risk of *C. difficile*-associated colitis and should not be used for therapy.

PREGNANCY: Category B

CLOTRIMAZOLE

TRADE NAMES: *Lotrimin* (Schering-Plough), *Mycelex* (Bayer), *Gyne-Lotrimin* (Schering-Plough), *FemCare* (Schering), and generic

FORMS AND COST:

- Troche 10 mg at $1.61
- Topical cream (1%) 15 g at $5.29; 30 g at $8.29
- Topical solution/lotion (1%) 10 mL at $6.00; 30 mL at $15.52
- Vaginal cream (1%) 45 g at $7.20

CLASS: Imidazole (related to miconazole)

INDICATIONS AND DOSES

- **Thrush:** 10 mg troche 5x/d; must be dissolved in the mouth. Clotrimazole troches are only slightly less effective than fluconazole for thrush but are sometimes preferred to avoid azole resistance (*HIV Clin Trials* 2000;1:47). The problem is the need for 5 doses/d, although treatment with lower doses is often successful. Recommended duration in 2008 IDSA/NIH/CDC Guidelines is 7-14 days.

- **Dermatophytic infections and cutaneous candidiasis:** Topical application of 1% cream, lotion, or solution to affected area bid x 2-8 wks; if no improvement, reevaluate diagnosis. Recommended duration in 2008 IDSA/NIH/CDC Guidelines is 3-7 days and daily use for suppressive therapy in women with severe recurrent disease.

- **Candidal vaginitis:** Intravaginal – Vaginal cream: One applicator (about 5 g) intravaginally hs x 7-14 days.

Drug Information

ACTIVITY: Active against *Candida* species and dermatophytes.

PHARMACOLOGY

- **Bioavailability:** Lozenge (troche) dissolves in 15-30 minutes; administration at 3-hr intervals maintains constant salivary concentrations above MIC of most *Candida* strains. Small amounts of drug are absorbed with oral, vaginal, or skin applications.

SIDE EFFECTS: Generally well tolerated. Topical to skin (rare) – erythema, blistering, pruritis, pain, peeling, urticaria; topical to vagina (rare) – rash, pruritis, dyspareunia, dysuria, burning, erythema; lozenges – elevated AST (up to 15% – monitor LFTs); nausea and vomiting (5%)

PREGNANCY: Category C. May be used for oral or vaginal candidiasis.

COMBIVIR – see Lamivudine (pg. 304); Zidovudine (pg. 416)

COMPLERA – see Rilpivirine (pg. 366); Emtricitabine (pg. 255) and Tenofovir (pg. 388)

CRIXIVAN – see Indinavir (pg. 294)

CYTOVENE – see Ganciclovir (pg. 288)

DAPSONE

TRADE NAME: Generic

FORMS AND COST: Tabs: 25 mg at $1.06, 100 mg at $1.30

- **Comparison prices for PCP prophylaxis:**
  - Dapsone (100 mg/d): $6.00/mo
  - TMP-SMX (1 DS/d): $5.40/mo
  - Aerosolized pentamidine: $98.75/mo (plus administration costs)
  - Atovaquone (1500 mg/d): $1256/mo

CLASS: Synthetic sulfone that inhibits folic acid synthesis.

■ TABLE 5-20: **Dapsone Indications and Dose Regimens**

Indication	Dose Regimen
PCP prophylaxis	100 mg po qd
PCP treatment (mild to moderately severe)	100 mg po qd (plus trimethoprim 15 mg/kg/d po, in 3 doses) x 3 weeks
PCP + toxoplasmosis prophylaxis	50 mg po qd (plus pyrimethamine 50 mg/week plus folinic acid 25 mg/week) or dapsone 200 mg (+ pyrimethamine 75 mg + leucovorin 25 mg) once weekly

Drug Information

5

EFFICACY: A review of 40 published studies found dapsone (100 mg qd) to be slightly less effective than TMP-SMX for PCP prophylaxis, but comparable with aerosolized pentamidine and highly cost-effective (*CID* 1998;27:191). For PCP treatment, dapsone/trimethoprim is as effective as TMP-SMX for patients with mild or moderately severe disease (*Ann Intern Med* 1996;124:792).

PHARMACOLOGY

- **Bioavailability:** Nearly completely absorbed except with gastric achlorhydria (dapsone is insoluble at neutral pH).

- **T½:** 10-56 hrs (average 28 hrs)

- **Elimination:** Hepatic concentration, enterohepatic circulation, maintains tissue levels 3 wks after treatment is discontinued.

- **Dose modification in renal failure:** None

SIDE EFFECTS

- **Most common in AIDS patients:** Rash, pruritis, hepatitis, hemolytic anemia, and/or neutropenia in 20-40% receiving dapsone prophylaxis for PCP at a dose of 100 mg qd.

- **Most serious reaction:**

  □ Dose-dependent <u>hemolytic anemia</u>, with or without glucose-6 phosphate dehydrogenase (G6PD) deficiency, and methemoglobinemia; rare cases of agranulocytosis (0.2-0.4%) and aplastic anemia. Suggested monitoring includes screening for G6PD deficiency prior to treatment, in high-risk patients. The defect is not always a contraindication to high risk drugs since most patients with positive tests tolerate these drugs (see below). An exception is patients with the high risk variant of G6PD deficiency. A review of G6PD deficiency prevalence in 1172 HIV-infected patients in Houston showed deficiency in 75 (6.8%): Blacks 66/699 (9.7%); Hispanics 5/253 (2.0% and whites 1/153 (0.7%) (*J Infect* 2010;61:399). During follow-up, 40 patients with deficiency given TMP-SMX or dapsone; 5 (7%) developed hemolytic anemia (the trigger was TMP/SMX in 4 cases). This study did not define the degree of G6PD deficiency. Other studies have shown hemolysis, and Heinz body formation are exaggerated in patients with G6PD deficiency, methemoglobin reductase deficiency, or hemoglobin M.

  □ <u>Asymptomatic methemoglobinemia</u> independent of G6PD deficiency has been found in up to two thirds of patients receiving dapsone 100 mg qd plus trimethoprim (*NEJM* 1990;373:776). <u>Acute methemoglobinemia</u> is uncommon, but the usual features are dyspnea, fatigue, cyanosis, deceptively high pulse oximetry, and chocolate-colored blood (*JAIDS* 1996;12:477). Methemoglobin levels are related to the dose and duration of dapsone therapy; TMP increases dapsone levels, so TMP may precipitate methemoglobinemia. Methemoglobin levels are usually <25%,

Drug Information

which is generally tolerated except in patients with lung disease. Patients with glutathione or G6PD deficiency are at increased risk. The usual laboratory findings are increased indirect bilirubin, haptoglobin <25 mg/dL, elevated LDH, and a smear showing spherocytes and fragmented RBCs. Treatment for severe hemolysis consists of oxygen supplementation, transfusion for anemia, and discontinuation of the implicated drug. This is usually adequate if the methemoglobin level is <30%. Activated charcoal (20 gm qid) may be given to reduce dapsone levels. Treatment for severe cases in the absence of G6PD deficiency is IV methylene blue (1-2 mg/kg by slow IV infusion). In less emergent situations methylene blue may be given orally (3-5 mg/kg q4-6h); methylene blue should not be given with G6PD deficiency because methylene blue reduction requires G6PD; hemodialysis also enhances elimination.

- **GI intolerance:** Common; may reduce by taking with meals.
- **Infrequent ADRs:** Headache, dizziness, peripheral neuropathy. Rare side effect is "sulfone syndrome" after 1-4 wks of treatment, consisting of fever, malaise, exfoliative dermatitis, hepatic necrosis, lymphadenopathy, and anemia with methemoglobinemia (*Arch Dermatol* 1981;117:38).

DRUG INTERACTIONS: Decreased dapsone absorption – **H$_2$ blockers, antacids, omeprazole, and other proton pump inhibitors**. Dapsone levels decreased 7- to 10-fold by rifampin; use alternative. **Coumadin** – increased hypoprothrombinemia; pyrimethamine – increased marrow toxicity (monitor CBC); **probenecid** – increases dapsone levels; **primaquine** – hemolysis due to G6PD deficiency. **Trimethoprim** – increases levels of both drugs; monitor for methemoglobinemia.

RELATIVE CONTRAINDICATIONS: G6PD deficiency – monitor hematocrit and methemoglobin levels if anemia develops.

PREGNANCY: Category C. No data in animals; limited experience in pregnant patients with Hansen's disease shows no toxicity. Can be used for PCP prophylaxis in pregnant women. Hemolytic anemia with passage in breast milk reported (*CID* 1995;21[suppl 1]:S24).

DARAPRIM – see Pyrimethamine (pg. 351)

DARUNAVIR (DRV)

TRADE NAME: *Prezista* (Tibotec)
CLASS: Protease inhibitor
PATIENT ASSISTANCE AND INFORMATION: 866-836-0114 (toll-free in US)
FORMULATION, REGIMEN, COST:

5 Drug Information

- **FORM:** 75 mg ($2.41/tab), 150 mg ($4.82/tab), 400 mg and 600 mg ($19.27/tab)
- **REGIMEN** (FDA revised label 12/13/2010):
  - Treatment-naïve: DRV/r 800/100 mg qd.
  - Treatment-experienced with no DRV-associated resistance mutations (11I, 32I, 33F, 47V, 50V, 54M, 74P, 84V, 89V): DRV/r 800/100 mg qd with food.
  - Treatment-experienced with >1 DRV resistance mutation (listed above): DRV/r 600/100 mg twice daily with food.
- **FOOD:** Take with food
- **RENAL FAILURE:** No dose adjustment
- **HEPATIC FAILURE:** No data; use with caution
- **STORAGE:** 15-30°C (59-86°F)

ACTIVITY: Median EC_{50} against clinical and lab strains range 0.7-5 ng/mL activity includes group M (A-G), O, and HIV-2.

ADVANTAGES: Potent anti-HIV activity; excellent activity against HIV strains that are resistant to other PIs; relatively good tolerability and less lipid effects than LPV/r; as effective or more effective than LPV/r for treatment-naïve patients; once daily dosing in treatment-naïve patients and treatment-experienced patients with no DRV resistance mutations; good CNS penetration; resistance relatively rare with DRV/r-based ART.

- TABLE 5-21A: **ARTEMIS Trial – DRV/r vs. LPV/r in Treatment-naïve Patients. 96 week Results (*AIDS* 2009;23:1679)**

	DRV/r* 800/100 qd n = 343	LPV/r* 400/100 bid or 800/200 qd n = 346
Baseline		
Viral load (median) (c/mL)	70,800	62,100
CD4 count (median) (cells/mm³)	228	218
VL >100,000 c/mL	36%	36%
Results (96 wk)		
VL <50 c/mL	79%	71%[†]
Baseline >100,000	76%	63%[†]
CD4 change (cells/mm³)	+171	+188
Adverse drug reactions (ADR)		
Discontinuations for ADRs	4%	9%[†]
Diarrhea	4%	11%[†]
Gr 2-4 ↑ Total cholesterol	18%	28%[†]
Triglyceride (median) (mg/dL)	+18	+56[†]

* All patients received TDF/FTC
† p <0.05

Drug Information

DISADVANTAGES: Food requirement, RTV requirement, relatively high rate of rash reactions; good CNS penetration.

CLINICAL TRIALS

TREATMENT NAÏVE

- **ARTEMIS Trial (Table 5-21A):** DRV/r vs. LPV/r in treatment-naïve patients with a VL >5000 c/mL and any CD4 count. Participants were randomized to DRV/r (800/100 mg qd) or LPV/r (400/100 mg bid or 800/200 mg qd in combination with TDF/FTC). All patients received TDF/FTC (*AIDS* 2008;22:1389). Results at 96 weeks are summarized in Table 5-20. DRV/r was equivalent to LPV/r in virologic response, showed better tolerability and had a better lipid profile (*AIDS* 2009;23:1679). A post-hoc analysis found suboptimal adherence had minimal effect on virologic outcome with DRV/r but a much greater effect on LPV/r (76% vs. 53%; p <0.01) (*JAC* 2010;65:1505). Only 6 of the 31 virologic failures were associated with PI resistance mutations (*AIDS* 2009;23:1829).

TREATMENT EXPERIENCED

- **TITAN Trial (Early virologic failure) Table 5-21B:** DRV/r (600/100 mg bid) + optimized background regimen (OBR) vs. LPV/r (400/100 mg bid) + OBR in patients who had failed prior therapy and were naïve to LPV/r (*Lancet* 2007;370:49). At 48 weeks, DRV/r was superior to LPV/r in virologic outcome, although statistically significant superiority was not maintained when patients with baseline LPV resistance were excluded (Table 5-21) (*AIDS* 2009;23:1829). At 96 weeks, VL was <50 c/mL in 60% of DRV/r recipients compared with 55% of LPV/r recipients. The frequency of diarrhea was significantly greater in LPV/r recipients (15% vs. 8%,

■ TABLE 5-21B: **TITAN Trial Comparing DRV/r- and LPV/r-based ART in Patient with Virologic Failure on PI-based ART at 48 Weeks (*AIDS* 2009;23:1829)**

	DRV/r n = 286	LPV/r n = 293
Baseline		
Viral load ($\log_{10}$ median)	4.3	4.3
CD4 count (median) (cells/mm³)	235	230
Prior PI therapy ≥ 2 agents	32%	30%
Outcome at 48 weeks		
Virologic failure (VL > 400 c/mL)	10%	22%*
No. with primary PI resistance mutations	6	20
No. with NRTI resistance mutations	4	15
CD4 count (median) (cells/mm³)	+97	+102
Discontinuations due to adverse reactions	7%	7%

*P=<0.05

Drug Information

5

p=0.01); lipid changes were similar in the two groups, and more of the virologic failures in the LPV/r arm had PI resistance mutations (*AIDS* 2009;23:1829).

- **DUET-1 and -2:** These two trials examined the potential benefit of ETR in patients starting DRV/r as part of a salvage regimen. Criteria for enrollment were virologic failure with ≥ 1 NNRTI mutations, ≥ 3 primary PI mutations and a VL >5000 c/mL. All patients received DRV/r + an optimized background regimen (OBR). The 24-week results were reported for DUET-1 (*Lancet* 2007;370:29) and DUET-2 (*Lancet* 2007;370:39). Table 5-22 presents pooled 48-week results of the two trials (*AIDS* 2009;23:2289; *Expert Opin Pharmacother* 2010;11:1433). Viral suppression to < 50 c/mL was achieved in 57% of the ETR recipients vs. 36% of the controls, the mean CD4 count increases were 128 vs. 86/mm³, respectively, and rash was more common in the ETR group (21% vs. 12%) (*Antiviral Ther* 2010;15:1045). At 96 weeks, viral suppression to < 50 c/mL was maintained in all but 3% of those who had viral suppression at 48 weeks (57% vs. 60%) (*Antivir Ther* 2010;15:1045).

- TABLE 5-22: **DUET-1 and -2: DRV/r+ETR+OBR vs. DRV/r+OBR: 48 week Results with Pooled Data for Both Trials (*AIDS* 2009;23:2289)**

	DRV/r + ETR + OBR n = 599	DRV/r + Placebo + OBR n = 604
Baseline (median)		
HIV VL $\log_{10}$ c/mL	4.8	4.9
CD4 count (cells/mm³)	99	109
Results (48 wks)		
VL <50 c/mL	61%	40%*
CD4 count ↑ (cells/mm³)	+98	+73[†]
Active OBR agents with DRV FC <10		
1	46%	6%
2	63%	32%
3	78%	67%
Resistance mutations with failure		
Major PI	1/28	0/29
184V	5	7
ADR - rash	19%	11%[†]

* P=<0.0001
† P=0.0006

Drug Information

- **POWER-1 and -2** (*Lancet* 2007; 369:1169) were Phase IIb trials that compared DRV/r plus an OBR (≥2 NRTIs ± ENF) to comparator PI (CPI) + OBR in patients with VL >1000 c/mL, prior treatment with PI-based ART, and at least one primary PI resistance mutation (30N, 46I/L, 48V, 50L/V, 82A/F/S/T, I84V, or 90M). The OBR included LPV/r (36%), FPV (34%), SQV (35%) and ATV (17%); 47% received ENF. DRV was superior to alternative regimens available at that time (Table 5-23). Combined 96-week data for POWER-1 and -2 (n=467) showed virologic suppression to <50 of 39% for DRV/r vs. 9% for CPI (*Antiviral Ther* 2009;14:859). See Tables 5-23, 5-24 & 5-25.

- TABLE 5-23: **POWER-1 and -2: DRV/r + OBR vs. OBR: Results at 48 Weeks (*Lancet* 2007; 369:1169)**

	DRV/r + OBR n = 131	Comparator PI + OBR n = 124
Baseline		
VL (log$_{10}$ c/mL median)	4.6	4.5
CD4 count (mean) (cells/mm³)	153	163
≥3 primary PI mutations	54%	62%
Outcome at 48 weeks		
VL <50 c/mL	67 (45%)*	12 (10%)
CD4 count (median) (cells/mm³)	+102*	+19
Discontinue for ADR	7%	5%
Resistance correlates		
1 active drug in OBR	17/34 (50%)	1/40 (5%)
≥2 active drugs	27/48 (56%)	10/60 (17%)

* P=<0.05

- TABLE 5-24: **DRV Mutation Score and Outcome: POWER and DUET Trials**

No. mutations	POWER (24 wks)		DUET (24 wks)	
	N	VL <50 c/mL	N	VL <50 c/mL
0	76	62%	67	64%
1	115	57%	94	50%
2	134	46%	113	42%
3	65	25%	58	22%
4	58	16%	41	10%

- TABLE 5-25: **Correlation Between Baseline Phenotypic DRV Resistance Test Results and Virologic Response (POWER)**

Phenotype -fold change	N	VL <50 c/mL at 24 weeks
0-2	136	60%
2-7	85	47%
7-30	63	24%
>30	56	18%

5 Drug Information

- **ODIN:** A phase III open-labeled trial in which treatment-experienced patients with no DRV resistance mutations were randomized to DRV/r (600/100 mg bid) vs. DRV/r (800/100 mg qd). The 48-week results with 490 participants showed nearly identical results for VL <50 c/mL (72.1% for once-daily dosing vs. 70.9% for twice-daily dosing) (Lathouwers E. ICAAC 2010;Abstr. H1811). The analysis also showed no difference based on baseline viral load, number of PI resistance mutations at baseline, the number of active NRTIs in the OBR, TLOVR results, number who developed DRV resistance (1 among 102 treatment failures) or the number who developed PI resistance mutations (12% vs. 10%).

- **TRIO:** This is a Phase II, non-comparative multicenter trial involving 103 patients with multidrug resistant HIV defined as: 1) >3 NRTI resistance mutations; 2) >3 PI resistance mutations with <3 primary DRV mutations (11I, 32I, 33F, 47V, 50V, 54 L/M, 73S, 76V, 84V, 89V); 3) Virologic failure on an NNRTI with <3 ETR mutations and 4) VL >1000 c/mL. Treatment consisted of RAL, ETR and DRV/r with or without ENF and NRTIs. Participants had baseline resistance patterns showing a median of 4 primary PI mutations, one NNRTI mutation and 6 NRTI mutations. At 48 weeks, 89 (86%) had VL <50 c/mL (*CID* 2009;49:1441). At 96 weeks, all patients with VL <50 c/mL at 48 weeks had VL <400 c/mL on the TRIO regimen (Fagard C. 2011 CROI:Abstr. 549). Pharmacology studies demonstrated that ETR increased trough levels of DRV and RAL, but the PK was variable (*AIDS* 2010;24:2581).

MONOTHERAPY: See pg. 122t.

- **MONET:** 256 patients who had viral suppression (<50 c/mL) for >24 wks with PI-based ART (57%) or NNRTI-based ART (43%) and a median baseline CD4 of 574/mm^3 were randomized to DRV/r monotherapy (800/100 mg qd) or DRV/r once daily plus two NRTIs (*AIDS* 2010;24:223). At 48 weeks, DRV/r monotherapy was non-inferior to standard therapy (*AIDS* 2010;24:223) (Table 5-26). One PI resistance mutation emerged in each group (*Antivir Ther* 2011; 16:59).

- TABLE 5-26: **MONET Trial: DRV/r vs. DRV/r + 2 NRTIs (48-week Results) (*AIDS* 2010;24:223)**

	DRV/r n = 127	DRV/r + 2 NRTIs n = 127
HIV VL <50 c/mL	86.2%	87.8%
Intent-to-treat*	84.3%	85.3%

* Intent-to-treat with switch = failure

- **MONOI:** This is another study of DRV/r monotherapy (600/100 mg bid) after viral suppression, which enrolled treatment-experienced patients with no prior history of PI failure. Virologic suppression was comparable at 48 weeks (92% vs. 88%) (*AIDS* 2010;24:2365). At 96

Drug Information

weeks, VL was <50 c/mL in 91/97 (94%) of the DRV/r (monotherapy) arm and 87/96 (90%) of the DRV/r+2NRTI arm (Marc-Antoine V. 2011 CROI:Abstr. 534).

NRTI-SPARING: See pg. 122-123.

- **A5262: DRV/r+RAL:** The trial was a single arm study with 112 treatment-naïve patients given DRV/r (800/100 mg qd) + RAL (400 mg bid). At week 48 there were 28 virologic failures including 11 who rebounded. Of the 28 failures, 13 (46%) had VL 50-200 c/mL. Higher failure rates correlated with low baseline CD4 count and VL >100,000 c/mL. Resistance testing showed 4 with RAL resistance mutations and no PI resistance mutations (Taiwo. 2011 CROI:Abstr. 551).

- **DRV/r+EFV:** In a pharmacologic study, DRV/r 900/100 mg qd was given for 10 days, followed by addition of EFV 600 mg qd (*AAC* 2010;54:2775). There was a 57% decrease in DRV trough levels and an increase in EFV AUC, but the results suggested adequate drug levels for treatment-naïve patients.

- **DRV/r+MVC:** A pharmacokinetic trial of MVC 300 mg qd + DRV/r 800/100 qd demonstrated therapeutic MVC levels suggesting potential for futher study (Taylor A. 2011 CROI:Abstr. 636).

RESISTANCE: No single PI mutation results in complete loss of DRV activity. Resistance is best determined by the cumulative number of resistance mutations ("DRV score") or by phenotypic resistance testing. Reduced *in vitro* and *in vivo* activity seen with the following protease gene mutations: 11I, 32I, 33F, 47V, 50V, 54L/M, 73S, 74P, 76V, 84V and 89V. The most common DRV resistance mutations are 33F, 32I and 54L (*AAC* 2010;54:3018). Correlation between the mutation score and virologic outcome in POWER and DUET trials is shown in Table 5-24 and for baseline phenotype resistance test in Table 5-25. Genotypic Interpretation Systems (GIS) performed well for predicting resistance phenotype in an analysis of 100 resistant HIV strains (*AAC* 2010;54:2473). As with other PI/r-based regimens, most virologic failures on DRV/r were not associated with PI or NRTI mutations (*AIDS* 2004;23:1829). SeeTables 5-24 and 5-25.

PHARMACOLOGY: See Tables 5-24 and 5-25.

- **Renal failure:** Pharmacology is not changed in persons with CrCl 30-60 mL/min; there are no data for patients CrCl <30 mL/min, but drug levels are unlikely to be affected.

- **Hepatic disease:** Pharmacokinetics are not significantly altered by mild or moderate liver disease (*Clin Pharmacokinet* 2010;49:343) There are no data for severe hepatic failure; use with caution or avoid.

- **Bioavailability:** 37% without RTV, 82% with RTV. RTV increases DRV exposure 14-fold. Food increases C_{max} and AUC 30%. DRV should always be given with RTV and food.

5 Drug Information

- **Single daily dose:** A PK substudy from ARTEMIS showed a median DRV trough level at 24 hrs post dose (800/100 mg) of >1000 ng/mL (median 3,300 ng/mL) – well above the EC_{50} of HIV, which is 55ng/mL for wild-type. A randomized trial with 590 treatment-naïve patients compared once-daily DRV/r (800/100 mg qd) to twice-daily DRV/r (600/100 mg bid), each combined with 2 NRTIs. Results at 48 weeks showed 72% (qd) and 70% (bid) had VL <50 c/mL (*AIDS* 2011;25:929).
- **T½:** 15 hrs when given with RTV
- **CNS Penetration:** 9.4%. Exceeded the CI_{50} of wild-type by 20-fold and scored highest in CNS penetration among PIs (*JAIDS* 2009;52:56). On the 4 category CNS penetration scoring system, DRV ranks in category 3 (*Neurology* 2011;76:693) (see pg. 550t).
- **Excretion:** Metabolized extensively by CYP3A; 80% recovered in stool, 4% in urine

SIDE EFFECTS

- **Hepatotoxicity:** Drug-induced hepatitis is reported in 0.5% of patients given DRV/r; this includes serious fatal cases which are more common in patients with pre-exisiting liver disease.
- **Rash:** Tibotec issued a warning on skin reactions to DRV in August, 2009. Phase 3 studies showed Grade ≥2 rashes in 9%, Grade 3-4 in 1.3%; the drug was discontinued in 2%. Severe rashes including Stevens Johnson syndrome and erythema multiforme have been reported (*JAIDS* 2010;53:614) but occurred in <0.1%. Rashes usually occur in the second week and resolve in 1-2 wks with continued treatment. Rash reactions are unusual after 4 wks of treatment. DRV should be stopped immediately if the rash is severe or accompanied by fever, malaise, fatigue, muscle or joint aches, blisters, oral lesions, facial edema, conjunctivitis, hepatitis or eosinophilia. LFTs should be monitored. DRV contains a sulfonamide moiety and should be avoided in patients with severe sulfonamide allergy.
- **Metabolic effects:** Glucose intolerance, fat redistribution, and lipodystrophy. Hyperglycemia (blood glucose ≥161 mg/dL) in 2-6%, triglycerides >400 mg/dL in 25%.
- **Transaminase elevations:** >2.5 ULN in 10%
- **GI intolerance:** Diarrhea, vomiting, and/or abdominal pain in 2-3%
- **Headache:** 1-4%

DRUG INTERACTIONS

- **Drugs contraindicated for concurrent use: astemizole, cisapride, ergot derivative, midazolam, pimozide, terfenadine, triazolam, alfuzosin, bepridil, flecainide, propafenone, amiodarone, quinidine, simvastatin, lovastatin and rifampin, fluticasone, lidocaine, rifampin, carbamazepine, phenobarbital, phenytoin, St. John's wort, simvastatin, pitavastatin, and lovastatin.**

Drug Information

- **Other cautions**

  Antifungals (see azoles, pg. 208) **Ketoconazole and itraconazole:** increased levels of both azoles and DRV. **Voriconazole** AUC decreased 40% by RTV 200 mg/d; use with caution or avoid and monitor voriconazole trough (see pg. 413). **Rifabutin:** Use rifabutin 150 mg q24-48h. Consider rifabutin TDM. **Calcium channel blockers** (felodipine, nifedipine, amlodipine, diltiazem and nicardipine): concentrations increased; monitor. **Steroids** (dexamethasone, fluticasone): Dexamethasone may decrease levels of DRV; systemic steroid levels increased with inhaled fluticasone; consider alternatives, especially for long-term use. **Statins:** Atorvastatin: AUC increased 4-fold; start with 10-20 mg and titrate up (max. 40 mg/d). Pravastatin AUC level increased by a mean of 81%, but 5-fold in some patients. Use lowest doses and monitor. **Immunosuppressants** (cyclosporine, tacrolimus, sirolimus): levels increased; monitor immunosuppressant levels closely. **Methadone:** DRV/r decreases R-methadone 16%; monitor for withdrawal. **Oral contraceptives:** Ethinyl estradiol levels decreased 44%; use alternative or additional birth control method. **PDE5 inhibitors** (sildenafil, vardenafil, tadalafil): Do not exceed 25 mg sildenafil q48h, 2.5 mg vardenafil q72h, or 10 mg tadalafil q72h. **SSRIs** (sertraline, paroxentine), AUC decreased 49% and 39%, respectively; monitor antidepressant response. **Clarithromycin:** Levels of clarithromycin increased 59%; reduce dose 50% if CrCl 30-60 mL/min, 75% if CrCl <30 mL/min. **Warfarin:** S-warfarin AUC decreased 21%. Monitor INR. **Trazodone:** Levels and side effects (nausea, dizziness, hypotension) of trazadone may increase. Use lower dose or use with caution. **ddI** should be taken 1 hr before or 2 hrs after DRV. **Anti-arrhythmics:** bepridil, lidocaine, quinidine, amiodarone may increase levels; avoid. **Buprenorphine:** Nor-buprenorphine AUC increased 46%; no dose adjustment but monitor for sedation. **Carbamazepine:** DRV serum concentration unchanged, carbamazepine serum concentrations increased 45%. Monitor carbamazepine concentrations with co-administration. **Colchicine:** DRV/r increases colchicine level.

- **Concurrent use with other ARVs** (Table 5-27). The combination of DRV/r and EFV is of interest as a potential NRTI-sparing regimen. A pharmacokinetic study showed that EFV substantially reduced DRV trough levels (ratio 0.45), AUC (0.86) and half life (0.56). Nevertheless, DRV levels were well above the EC_{50} for wild-type virus. The investigators suggested a daily regimen of DRV/r 900100 mg + EFV 600 mg for an NRTI-sparing regimen in treatment-naïve patients (*AAC* 2010;54:2775). This study was performed before 400 mg formulation of DRV was available; standard once-daily dose of 800/100 mg may be adequate.

PREGNANCY: Category C. Data are inadequate to recommend for pregnant women (2010 DHHS Perinatal HIV Guidelines). Case reports

■ TABLE 5-27: **Dose Adjustments for Concurrent Use of DRV with Other Antiretrovirals**

Drug	Effect on co-admin drug	Effect on DRV AUC	Dose
RAL	—*	C_{min} ↓36%	Clinical significance unknown. Use standard dose – good virologic suppression
ddI	—	—	ddI requires empty stomach so separate dosing; take ddI 1 hr before or 2 hrs after DRV/r
TDF	AUC ↑22%	—	No dose adjustment
EFV	AUC ↑21%	C_{min} ↓31%	DRV/r 600/100 po bid or consider DRV/r 800-900/100 mg qd (PI-naive patients)
NVP	AUC ↑27%	—	Standard doses both drugs
ATV/r	—	—	Standard DRV/r + ATV 300 mg qd yields comparable AUC to ATV/r when administered alone
IDV/r	↑23%	↑24%	Dose not established
LPV/r	AUC↑37%	AUC ↓50%	Dose not established; avoid
SQV/r	—	AUC ↓25%	Dose not established; avoid
FPV, NFV, TPV	?	?	Not studied; Avoid co-administration
RTV	—	↑14-fold	Standard regimen: DRV/r 600/100 mg bid or DRV/r 800/100 mg qd
ETR	AUC ↓37%	—	Combination is well established
MVC	↑ 4x	—	MVC 150 mg bid

* indicates no clinically-significant effect

indicate low levels of DRV in pregnancy (*Antiviral Ther* 2010; *AIDS* 2009;23:1923; *Antiviral Ther* 2008;13:839; *Antiviral Ther* 2010;15:677), but all 7 of these cases successfully prevented vertical transmission. A more recent report using once-daily dosing with DRV/r 800/100 mg showed trough levels >1400 ng/mL in the second and third trimesters (*AIDS* 2010;24:1083).

DAUNORUBICIN CITRATE LIPOSOME INJECTION

TRADE NAME: *DaunoXome* (Gilead Sciences)

NOTE: Liposomal doxorubicin (*Doxil*), 20-30 mg/M² every 2 wks, is equally as effective.

FORM AND COST: Vials containing equivalent of 50 mg daunorubicin at $340.00/50 mg vial

CLASS: Daunorubicin encapsulated within lipid vesicles or liposomes

Drug Information

INDICATIONS AND DOSES: (FDA labeling): First-line cytotoxic therapy for advanced HIV-associated Kaposi's sarcoma (KS). Pegylated liposomal doxorubicin plus ART is often considered the preferred treatment for moderate to advanced KS (*AIDS* 2004;20:1737). Indications and treatment options: see pg. 532. Administer IV over 60 minutes in dose of 40 mg/M^2; repeat every 2 wks. CBC should be obtained before each infusion and therapy withheld if absolute leukocyte count is <750/mL. Treatment is continued until there is evidence of tumor progression with new visceral lesions, progressive visceral disease, >10 new cutaneous lesions, or 25% increase in the number of lesions compared with baseline. Dose adjustment for hepatic impairment: bilirubin 1.2-3 mg/dL: 3/4 of a normal dose; bilirubin >3 mg/dL: 1/2 of normal dose.

CLINICAL TRIALS: See pg. 532-535. Controlled trials comparing liposomal doxorubicin (*Doxil*) or liposomal daunorubicin vs. chemotherapy show better response and less toxicity with *Doxil* and *DaunoXome*, which are considered equivalent (*J Clin Oncol* 1996; 14:2353; *J Clin Oncol* 1998;16:2445; *J Clin Oncol* 1998;16:683). A randomized trial of pegylated liposomal doxorubicin vs. paclitaxel in 73 patients with advanced Kaposi's sarcoma showed similar response rates (56% vs. 46%) and similar 2 year survival rates (79% vs. 78%) (*Cancer* 2010; 116:3969). Liposomal daunorubicin is substantially less expensive compared to liposomol doxorubicin.

PHARMACOLOGY: Mechanism of selectively targeting tumor cells is unknown. Once at the tumor, daunorubicin is released over time.

SIDE EFFECTS

- **Granulocytopenia** and **mucositis** are the most common toxicities requiring monitoring of the CBC (*Clin Cancer Res* 2001;7:3040).

- **Cardiotoxicity** with decreased ejection fraction and congestive failure is the most serious side effect. It is most common in patients who have previously received anthracyclines or who have pre-existing heart disease. Cardiac function (history and physical examination) should be evaluated before each infusion, and LVEF should be monitored when the total dose is 320 mg/M^2, 480 mg/M^2, and every 160 mg/m^2 thereafter.

- **The triad of back pain, flushing, and chest tightness** is reported in 14%; this usually occurs in the first 5 minutes of treatment, resolves with discontinuation of the infusion, and does not recur with resumption of infusion at a slower rate.

- **Other:** Alopecia, foot-hand syndrome (painful desquamating dermatitis of hands and feet), erythrodyesthesia and hyperpigmented lesions on mucous membranes of the mouth and lines on nails (*Dermatol Online* 2008;14:18).

- Care should be exercised to avoid drug extravasation, which can cause tissue necrosis.

Drug Information

5

DRUG INTERACTIONS: Additive bone marrow suppression with AZT, ganciclovir, and pyrimethamine; monitor closely with co-administration.

PREGNANCY: Category D. Studies in rats showed severe maternal toxicity, embryolethality, fetal malformations, and embryotoxicity.

ddl – see Didanosine (pg. 236)

DELAVIRDINE (DLV)

TRADE NAME: *Rescriptor* (Pfizer)

CLASS: NNRTI

FORMULATIONS AND REGIMENS

- **Forms:** Tabs, 100 mg and 200 mg tabs – $350.57/mo
- **Regimens:** 100 mg tabs – 400 mg tid, dispersed in ≥3 oz water (slurry). 200 mg tabs – 400 mg tid, take intact

FOOD EFFECT: None

ANTACIDS AND BUFFERED ddl: Separate dosing by ≥1 hr

RENAL FAILURE: Standard dose

HEPATIC FAILURE: No recommendation; uses with caution

ADVANTAGES: Virtually none. Some uncommon NNRTI mutations increase DLV susceptibility; clinical significance is unknown. DLV increases levels of some PIs.

DISADVANTAGES: Limited efficacy data; requires tid dosing; limited experience

CLINICAL TRIALS

- **Study 0071** showed equivalence between DLV + ddl vs. ddl monotherapy with regard to CD4 response and viral load. **ACTG 261** found DLV+AZT, DLV+ddl, and AZT+ddl to be equivalent with respect to VL suppression. In an as-treated analysis of **protocol 0021-2** at 52 weeks, 70% of patients receiving DLV+AZT/3TC had VL <400/mL accompanied by CD4 count increases of 49-135/mm³. The viral load results were superior to those achieved with AZT/3TC or DLV+AZT. In **protocol 0073** DLV (600 mg bid) + NFV (1250 mg bid) + ddl ± d4T produced a good virologic response at 40 weeks. **Protocol 0081** was a pilot study of DLV+AZT/3TC+SQV using varying doses of DLV (600 mg bid or 400 mg tid) and SQV (1400 mg bid or 1000-1200 mg tid). Pharmacokinetic and virologic studies favored DLV 600 mg + SQV 1400 mg bid; at 24 weeks VL was <400 c/mL in 83% of 24 patients receiving this combination (*HIV Clin Trials* 2001;2:97-107).

PHARMACOLOGY

- **Bioavailability:** Absorption is 85%; there are no food restrictions.

Food reduces absorption by 20%. Antacids, buffered ddI, and gastric achlorhydria decrease absorption. Separate buffered medications and antacids by ≥1 hr.

- **Distribution:** CSF: Plasma ratio=0.02. DLV ranks class 3 in the 4 class scoring system for CNS penetration (*Neurology* 2011;76:693).
- **T½:** 5.8 h
- **Elimination:** Primarily metabolized by hepatic cytochrome P450 (CYP3A4) enzymes. DLV inhibits cytochrome P450 CYP3A4 and inhibits metabolism of IDV, NFV, RTV, and SQV. Excretion is in urine (50%) and stool (44%). The standard dose is recommended in renal failure.
- **Dose reduction in renal or hepatic failure:** None; consider empiric dose reduction with severe liver disease.

SIDE EFFECTS: <u>Rash</u> noted in about 18%; 4% require drug discontinuation. Rash is diffuse, maculopapular, red, and predominantly on upper body and proximal arms. Erythema multiforme and Stevens-Johnson syndrome have been reported. Duration of rash averages 2 wks and usually does not require dose reduction or discontinuation (after interrupted treatment). Rash accompanied by fever, mucous membrane involvement, swelling, or arthralgias should prompt discontinuation of treatment. Increased transaminase levels are less frequent and severe than with NVP. Other side effects include headache.

BLACK BOX WARNING: None

DRUG INTERACTIONS: Inhibits cytochrome P450 enzymes. The following drugs should not be used concurrently: **Terfenadine, rifampin, rifabutin, simvastatin, pitavastatin, lovastatin, ergot derivatives, astemizole, cisapride, midazolam, alprazolam, triazolam, H2 blockers, and proton pump inhibitors.** Other drugs that either probably or definitely have increased half-life when given with DLV: **Clarithromycin, quinidine, amiodarone, bepridil, lidocaine, propafenone, sirolimus, tacrolimus, cyclosporine, flecainide, atorvastatin, warfarin, sildenafil, and other ED medications;** sildenafil should not exceed 25 mg/48 hrs; vardenafil should not exceed 2.5 mg/24 hrs. **Ethinyl estradiol** levels decrease 20%; use alternative or additional method of birth control. **Ketoconazole** levels increase 50%. There is no change in DLV with methadone. Drugs that decrease levels of DLV: **Carbamazepine, phenobarbital, phenytoin, rifabutin** and **rifampin.** Absorption of DLV is decreased with antacids, buffered ddI (administer ≥1 hr apart), **H₂ blockers, and proton pump inhibitors. Colchicine:** may increase colchicine level. Consider decreasing colchicine dose.

PREGNANCY: Category C. Ventricular septal defects in rodent teratogenicity assay; placental passage studies show a newborn:maternal drug ratio of 0.15. DLV is not recommended for use in pregnancy due

5 Drug Information

to concerns about teratogenicity in animals and lack of experience in patients (2010 DHHS Perinatal HIV Guidelines). The Pregnancy Registry shows birth defects with 19/404 (4.7%) first trimester exposures (accessed 2/1/2011). The expected rate without ART is 2.7%)

d4T – see Stavudine (pg. 378)

DESYREL – see Trazodone (pg. 406)

DIDANOSINE (ddl)

TRADE NAMES: *Videx* and *Videx EC* (Bristol-Myers Squibb) and generic
CLASS: Nucleoside analog reverse transcriptase inhibitor (NRTI)
FORMULATIONS, REGIMENS AND COST:

- **Forms**
  - □ Enteric coated caps (*Videx EC*): 125, 200, 250, and 400 mg
  - □ Generic ddl EC: 125, 200, 250 and 400 mg
  - □ Pediatric powder 2 gm (4 oz) and 4 gm (8 oz)

- **Regimens**
  - □ Weight <60 kg, 250 mg qd. With TDF, ddl 200 mg qd.
  - □ Weight >60 kg, 400 mg qd. With TDF, ddl 250 mg qd. ddl+TDF combination is generally not recommended; see warnings.
  - □ Powder: <60 kg: 167 mg bid; >60 kg: 250 mg bid.
  - □ Take 30 min before a meal or >2 hrs after a meal.

- **AWP:** (for 400 mg/d) $442.44 (brand)/mo – $368.72 (generic)/ mo. Note: Pharmacy purchase price of generic is much lower than AWP.

- **Combinations**
  - □ ddl+d4T: Increased risk of mitochondrial toxicity with increased rates of lactic acidosis, pancreatitis and peripheral neuropathy (*AIDS* 2007;21:2455; *JAIDS* 2006;43:556; *AIDS* 2003;17:2045). Avoid co-administration
  - □ ddl+ABC: Excessive rates of virologic failure, possibly due to selection of K65R mutation by both drugs
  - □ ddl+TDF+NNRTI: High rates of virologic failure and blunted CD4 response. Avoid combination (*CID* 2005;41:901; *AIDS* 2004; 18:459; *Antivir Ther* 2005;10:171).

TDF increases intracellular levels of ddl, risking ddl toxicity and poor immune recovery with a blunted CD4 response (*AIDS* 2005;19:1987).

Drug Information

This is reduced with proper dose adjustment of ddI, but even the modified dose has been associated with excessive rates of virologic failure, best documented when combined with NNRTIs (see drug interactions) (*AIDS* 2005;19:213; *CID* 2005;41:901). As a consequence the 2011 DHHS Guidelines and the 2010 IAS-USA guidelines (*JAMA* 2010;304:321) have recommended avoidance of ddI+TDF+NNRTI. The European Agency for Evaluation of Medicinal Products recommend avoiding TDF+ddI completely (www.mmhiv.com/link/EAEMA-ddi-TDF).

FOOD EFFECT: Food decreases ddI EC levels 55%; must take >30 min before or ≥ 2 h after meal.

RENAL FAILURE: See table 5-28

HEPATIC FAILURE: Standard dose

FINANCIAL ASSISTANCE: 800-272-4878 (8 AM-5 PM CST Mon.-Fri.)

ADVANTAGES: Once daily therapy; extensive experience and, active against some AZT- and d4T-resistant strains depending on the number of TAMs.

DISADVANTAGES: Need for empty stomach; toxicity profile including pancreatitis, neuropathy, and other mitochondrial toxicities; restricted use with TDF and d4T, and contraindicated with ribavirin. Limited data in regimens not including AZT or d4T. Potential for cross-resistance with TDF and ABC. Possible association with non-cirrhotic portal hypertension

RESISTANCE: L74V and K65R are the most important resistance mutations. The L74V mutation results in cross-resistance to ABC, and the K65R mutation causes cross-resistance with ABC and TDF. Susceptibility to ddI is decreased with the accumulation of multiple TAMs: NRTI resistance is associated with the presence of ≥ 3 of the following: 41L, 67N, 210W, 215Y/F, and 219Q/E. M184V reduced phenotypic susceptibility, but does not cause clinically significant resistance unless combined with other mutations.

CLINICAL TRIALS: ddI has been included in numerous trials in combination with 3TC, d4T, FTC, and AZT.

- **ACTG 384** compared AZT/3TC vs. ddI+d4T, each in combination with NFV or EFV, in 908 participants (*NEJM* 2003;349:2293). At a median follow-up of 2.3 years, virologic outcomes were superior with EFV+AZT/3TC compared with EFV+ddI+d4T or to either NRTI combination with NFV. Treatment-limiting toxicity, especially peripheral neuropathy, was significantly greater with ddI+d4T. ddI should not be paired with d4T based on this and other studies demonstrating excessive rates of peripheral neuropathy, lactic acidosis and pancreatitis (BMS warning letter to providers, 1/5/01).

- **Jaguar:** ddI intensification after virologic failure resulted in a median decrease in VL of 0.5 $\log_{10}$ c/mL at week 4 (*JID* 2005;191:840). The extent of decrease in VL correlated with TAMs: 0-1 TAMs, 0.8-1.0 $\log_{10}$ c/mL; 2 TAMs, 0.7 $\log_{10}$ c/mL; ≥ 3 TAMs, no significant

5 Drug Information

response. The L74V mutation also predicted failure to respond. Clinical cut-offs were defined in this study using the *PhenoSense* assay. Those with a fold-change (FC) ≤1.3 had the best response to addition of ddI; those with FC between 1.3 and 2.2 had an intermediate response; and those with FC ≥2.2 had minimal response (*JID* 2005; 191:840).

- **FTC-301A:** Participants taking ddI + FTC with EFV experienced potent virologic suppression (78% had VL <50 c/mL at 48 weeks) (*JAMA* 2004;292:180).

- **GESIDA 3903:** This trial compared ddI+3TC with AZT/3TC (in combination with EFV). At 48 weeks, ddI+3TC was noninferior to AZT/3TC (70% and 63% had VL <50 c/mL, respectively) (*CID* 2008;47:1083).

- **ACTG 5175 (PEARLS trial):** This multinational randomized trial compared 3 treatment regimens in 1,571 treatment-naïve patients randomized to: AZT/3TC+EFV or ddI+FTC+ATV or TDF/FTC+EFV. The ddI+FTC+ATV arm was stopped by the DSMB due to an excessive rate of virologic failure at week 72. Among the remaining 1,045 participants on AZT/3TC vs. TDF/FTC, CD4 increase and virologic response were comparable at 184 weeks, but there were fewer serious ADRs with TDF/FTC (Campbell. 2011 CROI:Abstr. 149LB).

- **NUCREST:** This study examined the relative efficacy of recycling NRTIs in 719 patients with virologic failure and at least one NRTI resistance mutation. The overall response rate with recycling was 65% and was highest with ddI+3TC (*HIV Clin Trials* 2010;11:294).

PHARMACOLOGY

- **Bioavailability:** Tablet – 40%; powder – 30%; food decreases bioavailability by 47% with buffered ddI, 27% with ddI EC. Take all formulations on an empty stomach. They scored "0" for CNS penetration in the comparative merits of ART agents (*JAIDS* 2009;52:56) – Class 2 in the 4 class CNS penetration scoring system (*Neurology* 2011;76:693).

- **T½:** 1.5 h

- **Intracellular T½:** 25-40 h

- **CNS penetration:** CSF levels are 20% of serum levels (CSF: plasma ratio=0.16-0.19) (see pg. 550t).

- **Elimination:** Renal excretion: 50% unchanged in urine. Renal failure, see chart pg. 239.

SIDE EFFECTS

- **Black box warnings:** 1) **Pancreatitis**, 2) **Lactic acidosis** and 3) **Fatal lactic acidosis** with ddI/d4T. Note that the relative risk of mitochondrial toxicity is correlated with affinity for mitochondrial DNA polymerase gamma. The rank order is ddI > d4T > AZT (ABC,

■ TABLE 5-28: Dose Adjustment for ddI with Renal Failure

Wt	CrCl (mL/min)			
	> 60	30-59	10-29	< 10
>60 kg	400 mg/d	200 mg/d	150 mg/d	100 mg/d
<60 kg	250 mg/d	150 mg/d	100 mg/d	75 mg/d

TDF, 3TC and FTC have minimal risk) (*HIV Clin Trials* 2009;10:306; *Top HIV Med* 2008;16:127; *J Biol Chem* 2001;276:40847).

- **Pancreatitis (Black box FDA warning):** Reported in 1-9% (7-9% in the pre-HAART era; <1% in the HAART era). ddI-associated pancreatitis is fatal in 6% (*JID* 1997;175:255). The frequency of pancreatitis is dose-related. Risk factors for ddI-associated pancreatitis include renal failure, alcohol abuse, morbid obesity, history of pancreatitis, hypertriglyceridemia, cholelithiasis, endoscopic retrograde cholangio-pancreatography (ERCP), and concurrent use of ribavirin, d4T, 3TC, TMP-SMX, anti-TB agents, allopurinol, or pentamidine (*Int J STD AIDS* 2008;19:19). A review of pancreatitis in the EuroSIDA cohort with 9678 patients failed to show a pancreatitis risk associated with ddI unless it was combined with d4T (*AIDS* 2008;22:47). Pancreatitis has been reported with ddI in the absence of d4T, but this side effect with ddI alone or d4T alone has nearly disappeared.

- **Peripheral neuropathy** with pain, numbness, and/or paresthesias in extremities. Frequency is 5-12%; it is increased significantly when ddI is given with d4T, hydroxyurea, or both (*AIDS* 2000;14:273). Onset usually occurs at 2-6 mos of ddI therapy and may be persistent and debilitating if ddI is continued despite symptoms.

- **GI intolerance** with buffered powder are common. The EC formulation is preferred because it causes fewer GI side effects. An alternative to buffered ddI is ddI pediatric powder reconstituted with 200 mL water and mixed with 200 mL *Mylanta DS* or *Maalox* extra strength with anti-gas suspension in patient's choice of flavor. The final concentration is 10 mg/mL, and the usual dose is 25 mL.

- **Cardiovascular risk:** A review of NRTIs for risk of mycardial infarction by D:A:D showed recent ddI use was associated with a relative risk of 1.41 (*JID* 2010;201:318). ddI is also associated with significant elevations in LDL-cholesterol levels (*AIDS* 2011;25:185). The D:A:D analysis found a strong association between ddI treatment and cardiovascular events (*JID* 2010;201:318). The mechanism is unclear.

- **Hepatitis** with increased transaminase levels. A study of liver stiffness evaluated by elastography showed the highest rates (16%) were associated with ddI therapy (*Antiviral Ther* 2010;15:753).

5 Drug Information

- **Non-cirrhotic portal HTN** resulting in esophageal variceal bleeding, liver failure and death. Causal association not clearly established.

- **Miscellaneous:** Rash, bone marrow suppression, hyperuricemia, hypokalemia, hypocalcemia, hypomagnesemia, optic neuritis, and retinal changes

- **Class adverse effect: Lactic acidosis** and severe hepatomegaly with hepatic steatosis caused by mitochondrial toxicity (see pg. 132). The most frequent cause is ddl+d4T which should be avoided, especially in pregnancy (Black box FDA warning), based on reports of at least two fatal cases. Didanosine can cause **lipoatrophy**, which is also believed to be mediated by mitochondrial toxicity (see pg. 128).

DRUG INTERACTIONS

- **Tenofovir:** ddl+TDF co-administration is not recommended by the authors. DHHS and IAS-USA guidelines recommends avoiding ddl-TDF + NNRTI combination. Concurrent use of TDF and ddl results in a 48-64% increase in the ddl AUC (*Curr Med Chem* 2006;13:2789), and this results in an increased risk of ddl-associated side effects, including lactic acidosis and pancreatitis. The recommendation is to reduce the ddl dose, but this has been complicated by suspiciously high failure rates, especially when used in NNRTI-based ART (*Antivir Ther* 2005;10:171). A second concern is high risk for selection of K65R and high rates of virologic failure with selection of K65R (*AIDS* 2005;19:1695; *AIDS* 2005;19:1183; *Antiviral Ther* 2005;10:171). A third concern has been raised by several reports of blunted CD4 response with this combination when the ddl dose is not adjusted (*AIDS* 2005; 19:569; *AIDS* 2005;19:1107; *AIDS* 2005;19:695).

- **Drugs that cause peripheral neuropathy** should be used with caution or avoided: d4T, EMB, INH, vincristine, gold, disulfiram, or cisplatin.

- **Atazanavir:** Food with ATV+ddl EC results in reduced ddl exposure and requires separate administration. Poor virologic efficacy in ACTG 5175. This was a trial comparing EFV+AZT/3TV, ATV+ddl+FTC and EFV/TDF/FTC that was stopped prematurely by the DSMB due to excessive failure rates with ATV+ddl+FTC (*NIAID Bulletin* 5/27/08).

- **Tipranivir:** Separate administration by 2 hrs.

- **Methadone** reduces AUC of buffered ddl by 41%; use ddl EC which is not effected (*JAIDS* 2000;24:241).

- **Allopurinol** increases ddl concentrations. This combination is contraindicated (FDA warning 6/19/09).

- **Oral ganciclovir** increases ddl AUC by 100% when administered 2 hrs after ddl or concurrently. Monitor for ddl toxicity and consider dose reduction.

- **Ribavirin** increases intracellular levels of ddl and may cause serious toxicity; avoid combination (*Antiviral Ther* 2004;9:133). This combination is contraindicated (FDA warning 6/19/09).

- **Buffered formulation (powder)**: IDV, TPV, DLV, ATV, NFV, ketoconazole, tetracyclines, fluoroquinolones give >2 hrs. before ddl (buffered formulation).

CAUTION: FDA warning for **ddl + ribavirin** based on 23 cases of pancreatitis and/or lactic acidosis (with some fatalities); this combination is contraindicated. **TDF** increases levels of ddl; dose reduction to 250 mg qd (for >60 kg) or 200 mg qd (for <60 kg). **d4T + ddl** is contraindicated in pregnant women and should be avoided when possible in all patients.

PREGNANCY: Category B. The 2010 DHHS Guidelines for Antiretroviral Drugs in Pregnant Women recommend ddl with another NRTI as an "alternative" to AZT/3TC. Relevant studies have shown no harm in rodent teratogen and carcinogenicity studies; placental passage in humans shows newborn:maternal drug ratio of 0.5; and pharmacokinetics are not altered in pregnancy (*JID* 1999;180:1536). The combination of ddl and d4T should be avoided in pregnancy due to excessive rates of lactic acidosis and hepatic steatosis (*Sex Transm Infect* 2002;78:58). The Pregnancy Registry showed birth defects in 19/404 (4.7%) first trimester exposures for reporting through 7/20/2010. This exceeds the expected rate of 2.7%, but it is not statistically significant and no consistent pattern was observed. The 2010 DHHS Guidelines on Use of Antiretriviral Agents in Pregnant Women recommend ddl as an "alternative".

DIFLUCAN – see Fluconazole (pg. 276)

DOXYCYCLINE

TRADE NAMES: *Vibramycin* (Pfizer), *Doryx* (Warner Chilcott), and generic

FORMS AND COST: 50 mg cap, 100 mg tab at $1.41. IV form 100 mg at $18.55

CLASS: Tetracycline antibiotic

INDICATIONS AND DOSE: 100 mg po bid

- *C. trachomatis:* 100 mg po bid x 7 days.
- **Bacillary angiomatosis:** 100 mg po bid x ≥3 mos; lifelong with relapse
- **Syphilis (primary, secondary, and early latent) in patients with contraindication to penicillin:** 100 mg bid x 14 days + close monitoring
- **Respiratory tract infections (sinusitis, pneumonia, otitis):** 100 mg bid x 7-14 days

PHARMACOLOGY

- **Bioavailability:** 93%. Complexes with polyvalent cations (Ca^{++}, Mg^{++},

Drug Information

5

Fe^{++}, Al^{+++}, etc.), so milk, mineral preparations, cathartics, and antacids with metal salts should not be given concurrently. Administer doxycycline 2 hrs before cations.

- **T½:** 18 hrs

- **Elimination:** Excreted in stool as chelated inactive agent independent of renal and hepatic function.

- **Dose modification with renal or hepatic failure:** None

SIDE EFFECTS: GI intolerance (10% and dose-related, reduced with food), diarrhea; deposited in developing teeth – contraindicated from mid-pregnancy to term and in children <8 years of age (Committee on Drugs, American Academy of Pediatrics); photosensitivity (exaggerated sunburn); *Candida* vaginitis; "black tongue;" rash; esophageal irritation.

DRUG INTERACTIONS: Chelation with cations to reduce oral absorption (administer doxycycline 2 hrs before cations); half-life of doxycycline decreased by carbamazepine, cimetidine, phenytoin, barbiturates; may interfere with oral contraceptives; potentiates oral hypoglycemics, digoxin, and lithium.

PREGNANCY: Category D. Use in pregnant women and infants risk hepatotoxicity and may cause retardation of skeletal development and bone growth; tetracyclines localizes in dentin and enamel of developing teeth to cause enamel hypoplasia and yellow-brown discoloration. Tetracyclines should be avoided in pregnant woman.

DRONABINOL

TRADE NAME: *Marinol* (Unimed Pharmaceuticals)

FORMS AND COST: Gel-caps: 2.5 mg at $5.89, 5 mg at $12.26, 10 mg at $22.51

CLASS: Psychoactive component of marijuana

INDICATION AND DOSE: For anorexia associated with weight loss (also used in higher doses as antiemetic in cancer patients). Long-term therapy with dronabinol has led to significant improvement in appetite but no significant weight gain in three controlled trials (*J Pain Sympt Manage* 1995;10:89; *AIDS Res Hum Retroviruses* 1997;13:305; *Psychopharmacology* 2010;212:675). The latter study with a crossover design also showed improvement in sleeping and mood. Another randomized trial showed smoked cannabis reduced chronic pain (p=0.3) (*Neurology* 2007;68L515). It should be noted that the beneficial effects often required higher than the recommended doses of dronabinol and when weight gain is achieved, it is primarily due to an increase in body fat (*J Pain Symptom Manage* 1997;14:7; *AIDS* 1992; :127). The need for high maintenance doses is more likely in patients who are chronic marijuana users (*Psychopharmacology* 2010;212:675).

RECOMMENDATIONS FOR MANAGEMENT:

- Standard dose: 2.5 mg bid (before lunch and before dinner)

Drug Information

242

- <u>CNS symptoms</u> (dose-related mood high, confusion, dizziness, somnolence) usually resolve in 1-3 days with continued use. If these symptoms are severe or persist, reduce dose to 2.5 mg before dinner and/or administer at bedtime.
- <u>Dose escalation:</u> If tolerated and additional therapeutic effect desired, increase dose to 5 mg bid.
- <u>High dose:</u> 10 mg bid is occasionally required, especially for control of nausea.

PHARMACOLOGY

- **Bioavailability:** 90-95%
- **T½:** 25-36 h
- **Elimination:** First-pass hepatic metabolism and biliary excretion; 10-15% in urine.
- **Biologic effects post-dose**
  - □ Onset of action: 0.5-1.0 h, peak 24 h
  - □ Duration of psychoactive effect: 4-6 h; appetite effect: ≥24 hrs

SIDE EFFECTS (dose-related)

- 3-10%: CNS with "high" (euphoria), somnolence, dizziness, paranoia, GI intolerance, anxiety, emotional lability, confusion
- Low doses (10-20 mg/d) are well tolerated; 30 mg/d is poorly tolerated. There is minimal effect on cognitive function (*Psychopharmacology* 2005;181:170).
- Others: Depersonalization, confusion, visual difficulties, central sympathomimetic effects, hypotension, palpitations, vasodilation, tachycardia, and asthenia

BLACK BOX WARNINGS: None

DRUG INTERACTIONS: Sympathomimetic agents (amphetamines, cocaine) – increased hypertension and tachycardia; anticholinergic drugs **(atropine, scopolamine), amitriptyline, amoxapine, and other tricyclic antidepressants** – tachycardia, drowsiness. There is no effect on PI levels (*Ann Intern Med* 2003;139:258).

WARNINGS: Dronabinol is a psychoactive component of *Cannabis sativa* (marijuana).

- **Schedule II (CII):** Potential for abuse (see Table 5-3, pg. 179). Use with caution in patients with psychiatric illness (mania, depression, schizo-phrenia), with cardiac disorder (hypotension), and in elderly patients. Caution should also be exercised in patients concurrently receiving sedatives and/or hypnotics and in patients with history of or current substance abuse.
- **Warn patient of the following:**
  - □ CNS depression with concurrent use of alcohol, benzodiazepines, barbiturates.

Drug Information

5

- Avoid driving, operating machinery, etc. until safety and tolerance is established.
- Mood and behavior changes.
- Food increases AUC 28%. Avoid meals with >40-60 gm fat, especially during the first 2-4 wks, which is the time of the greatest CNS effect.

PREGNANCY: Category C

EFAVIRENZ (EFV)

TRADE NAME: *Sustiva* (Bristol-Myers Squibb), *Stocrin* (Merck)

CLASS: NNRTI

FORMULATIONS, REGIMENS AND COST:

- **Forms:** Caps 50 and 200 mg; tabs 600 mg. Combination tab: *Atripla* (EFV/TDF/FTC 600/300/200 mg)
- **Regimens:** 600 mg qd or *Atripla*, preferably in the evening on an empty stomach. Administration on empty stomach may reduce CNS side effects.
- **AWP:** *Sustiva* $663/mo, *Atripla* $1858.15/mo
- Some studies have found that lower doses (200 or 400 mg qd) can improve tolerance without loss of potency by screening for genetic changes that prolong the half life (*JID* 2011;203:246) or by therapeutic monitoring (*Antivir Ther* 2011;16:189)

FOOD EFFECT: Take on empty stomach or with a low-fat meal; a concurrent meal with 40-60 gm of fat increases AUC >30% and peak level 40-50%, which may increase side effects. The recommendation to take on an empty stomach applies primarily to the initial weeks of treatment, when CNS side effects are greatest.

RENAL FAILURE: Standard dose (EFV)

HEPATIC FAILURE: No recommendations; use with caution

PATIENT ASSISTANCE PROGRAM: 800-861-0048 (7 AM-7 PM) CST Mon.-Fri.)

INDICATIONS AND DOSE: EFV-based ART is a favored regimen for treatment-naïve patients without pregnancy potential (pg. 90). The standard dose is 600 mg qd, usually in combination with TDF/FTC, taken in the evening to reduce the CNS side effects that are common in the first 2-3 wks. **Discontinuation:** To reduce risk of NNRTI resistance, the recommendations for planned discontinuation of EFV-based ART are to stop EFV and continue two NRTIs 1-2 wks ("staggered discontinuation") or to substitute PI-based ART for one month "substituted discontinuation" (see pg. 117). Timing: EFV is usually taken in the evening so that major CNS effects go unnoticed during sleep. However, morning dosing is safe, effective and preferred by some patients due to sleep disturbances (*Scand J Infect Dis* 2006;38:1089).

<u>CNS penetration</u>: Levels in CSF are 0.26-1.2% plasma levels. On the 4 class ranking system for CNS penetration EFV ranks category 3 (Letendre. 17th CROI 2010:Abstr. 172) (see pg. 550).

ADVANTAGES: EFV-based ART is superior or noninferior to all comparators for viral suppression in multiple clinical trials (Table 5-29); sustained activity with 5-year follow-up; once daily therapy; long half-life produces pharmacologic barrier to resistance, low pill burden; "triple therapy" available as a one-pill daily dose.

DISADVANTAGES: High rate of CNS effects in first 2-3 wks; single mutation confers high-level NNRTI resistance and does not impair fitness; potential for teratogenicity if used in pregnancy; long and variable half-life complicates discontinuation with risk of resistance.

- **Durability:** Retrospective analysis of 3,565 patients given various ART regimens found that EFV was the most likely to show sustained viral suppression (*JID* 2005;192:1387).

CLINICAL TRIALS: See Table 5-29.

- **ACTG 5142:** A seminal study that compared EFV-based vs. LPV/r-based ART in treatment-naïve patients. Entry criteria were VL >2000 c/mL and any CD4 count. Results are summarized in Table 5-30 (*NEJM* 2008;358: 2095). Conclusions from this study were that: 1) EFV-based ART was virologically superior to LPV/r-based ART, 2) LPV/r was superior with respect to drug options lost due to resistance after failure and in the magnitude of the CD4 count increase, 3) EFV/thymidine analogues were associated with more lipoatrophy and 4) triglyceride elevation was greater with EFV+LPV/r than when combined with a thymidine analog NRTI (Table 5-30).

- **Comparison with NVP: 2NN.** This trial randomized 1147 treatment-naïve patients to receive EFV, NVP qd, NVP bid, or EFV+NVP, each in combination with 3TC+d4T (*Lancet* 2004;363:1253). By ITT analysis at 48 weeks, the frequency of virologic suppression to <50 c/mL was: EFV – 70%, NVP bid – 65.4%, NVP once daily – 70% and NVP/EFV – 62.7%. EFV and NVP were comparable, but NVP did not meet FDA criteria for non-inferiority to EFV (*Lancet* 2004;363:1253). The only significant difference in virologic outcome was between EFV and EFV+NVP. The median increase in CD4 count was 150-170/mm^3 in all four groups. NVP therapy was implicated in 2 drug-related deaths. A Cochrane Database Review compared EFV and NVP when combined with 2 NRTIs and concluded they were equivalent in antiviral activity but had different side effects (*Cochrane Database Syst Rev* 2010;12:CD004246)

- **ACTG 364** enrolled 195 patients who failed treatment with NRTIs but were naïve to PIs and NNRTIs. Participants received one to two NRTIs + NFV, EFV, or NFV/EFV. VL was <50 c/mL in 22%, 44%, and 67%, respectively at 40-48 wks. The superior results with EFV vs. NFV were statistically significant (*NEJM* 2001;345:398).

5 Drug Information

Study	Comparison	N	Dur (wk)	VL < 50	VL < 200-400
DuPont 006 (*NEJM* 1999;341:1865)	EFV+AZT/3TC	154	48	64%*	70%
	IDV+AZT/3TC	148		43%	48%
	IDV+EFV	148		47%	53%
ACTG 384 (*NEJM* 2003; 349:2293)	EFV+AZT/3TC	155	48	—	88%*
	EFV+ddI+d4T	155		—	63%
	NFV+AZT/3TC	155		—	67%
	NFV+ddI+d4T	155		—	68%
	NFV+EFV+AZT/3TC	182		—	84%
	NFV+EFV+ddI+d4T	178		—	81%
GS-903 (*JAMA* 2004;292:191)	EFV+TDF+3TC	299	48	78%	82% (68%)
	EFV+d4T+3TC	301	144	74%	79% (62%)
CLASS (*JAIDS* 2006;43:284)	APV/r+ABC/3TC	96	48	59%	75%
	d4T+ABC/3TC	98		60%	81%
	EFV+ABC/3TC	97		72%	80%
2NN (*Lancet* 2004;363:1253)	EFV+3TC+d4T	400	48	70%	—
	NVP+3TC+d4T	387		65%	—
GS-FTC 301A (*JAMA* 2004;292:180)	EFV+FTC+ddI	286	60	78%*	81%
	EFV+d4T+ddI	285		59%	68%
INITIO (*Lancet* 2006;368;287)	EFV+ddI+d4T	288	192	74%*	—
	NFV+ddI+d4T	805		62%	—
	EFV+NFV+ddI+d4T	280		62%	—
ACTG 5095 (*NEJM* 2004;350:1850)	EFV+AZT/3TC ± ABC	765	32	83%*	89%
	AZT/ABC/3TC	382		61%	74%
BMS 034 (*JAIDS* 2004;36:1011)	ATV+AZT/3TC	286	98	32%**	70%
	EFV+AZT/3TC	280		37%**	64%
GS-934 (*NEJM* 2006;354:251)	TDF/FTC+EFV	255	48	80%*	84% (71%)*
	AZT/3TC+EFV	254	144	70%	73% (58%)
ESS 30009 (*JID* 2005;192:1921)	ABC/3TC+TDF	102	12†	—	†
	ABC/3TC+EFV	169	48	71%	75%
CNA 30024 (*CID* 2004;39:1038)	EFV+AZT/3TC	325	48	69%	71%
	EFV+ABC/3TC	324		70%	74%
EFV 30021 (*CID* 2004;39:411)	EFV+AZT/3TC bid	378	48	63%	65%
	EFV+AZT bid+3TC qd	276		61%	67%

Drug Information

■ TABLE 5-29: **Comparative Trials of EFV-based ART in Treatment-naïve Patients** *(Continued)*

Study	Comparison	N	Dur (wk)	VL <50	VL <200-400
CNA 30021(*JAIDS* 2005;38:417)	EFV+ABC/3TC bid	386	48	68%	—
	EFV+ABC/3TC qd	384		66%	—
ACTG 5142(*NEJM* 2008;358:2095)	LPV/r+3TC+(d4T or AZT)	250	96	77%	86%
	EFV+3TC+(d4T or AZT)	253		89%*	93%
	LPV/r (533/133 mg bid)+EFV	253		83%	92%
MERIT (*JID* 2010;201:797)	EFV + 2 NRTIs	361	48	65%	73%
	MVC + 2 NRTIs	360		69%‡	71%
STARTMRK (*JAIDS* 2009;52:350)	EFV+TDF/FTC	282	96	78%	—
	RAL+TDF/FTC	160		84%	—
ECHO/THRIVE (IAC 2010: LBPE17)	EFV + 2 NRTI	682	48	82%	—
	TPV + 2 NRTIs	686		83%	—
ACTG 5202 (*Ann Intern Med* 2011;154:445)	ATV/r+ (TDF/FTC or ABC/3TC)	702	96	—	83%
	EFV+ (TDF/FTC or ABC/3TC)	698		—	85%

* Superior to comparator arm (*P*<0.05).

** Low value compared to other studies attributed to failure to use optimal transport medium.

† Arm terminated early due to high failure rate when analysis at >8 weeks of treatment showed virologic non-response in 49% of the TDF group vs. 5% of the EFV group.

‡ Post-hoc analysis showed equivalence of regimens when adjusted for MVC recipients who acquired X4 virus between screening and treatment initiation.

- **FOTO:** 60 patients with durable viral suppression on TDF/FTC/EFV were randomized to continue this regimen or to take it for 5 consecutive days (Monday-Friday) followed by a 2-day interruption (Saturday & Sunday) (Five On, Two Off, or "FOTO"). At 24 weeks, there were no virologic failures (VL >50 c/mL) among 25 patients in the FOTO arm. At that time the control arm receiving daily therapy was switched to the FOTO regimen. At 48 weeks, virologic response was good with: 1) no blips associated with FOTO; 2) strong patient preference for the FOTO regimen and 3) EFV levels <1000 ng/mL at a mean of 60 hrs after dosing in 52% in the FOTO arm vs. 10% in the standard treatment arm (not associated with virologic failure) (*HIV Clin Trials* 2007;8:19; Chen C. 5th IAS 2009;Abstr. MOPEB063).

- **ECHO and THRIVE:** See rilpivirine, pg. 366.

- **MERIT:** This study compared bid MVC vs. EFV, each combined with AZT/3TC, in 721 treatment-naïve patients. At 48 weeks, the MVC regimen was "not inferior," but this was due to more adverse reactions requiring discontinuation in the EFV arm (13.6% vs. 4.2%)

5 Drug Information

and more virologic failures in the MVC arm (11.9% vs. 4.2%) (*JID* 2010;201:803) (see pg. 320). A subsequent reanalysis of the MERIT results (MERIT ES) excluded patients who had R5-tropic virus at baseline using the original *Trofile* assay but who were subsequently found to have dual/mixed-tropic virus by the enhanced sensitivity assay (Trofile ES) (*HIV Clin Trials* 2010;11:125-32. In this analysis, virologic results were similar with superior tolerability and CD4 increases in the MVC arm, leading to the approval of MVC for treatment-naïve patients.

- **Switch studies**

  □ **SWITCH-EE trial:** Participants were receiving EFV+2 NRTIs, with tolerance of the regimen and VL <50 c/mL. At entry the patients were randomized to receive continued EFV or switch to ETR, and then at 6 weeks were switched to the alternative, NNRTI with continuation of the NRTI backbone. The analysis of patient preference showed those who continued EFV preferred that agent (15/21, 71%) and those who started with ETR preferred ETR (16/17, 94% (p <0.0001). The ETR recipients had lower total cholesterol and LDL cholesterol levels (p=<0.000) (*AIDS* 201;25:57). Switch to **RPV** (see pg. 366).

  □ **DMP 049** was a study of patients who were responding well to PI-based ART regimens with VL <50 c/mL and were randomized to continue the PI-based regimen or switch to EFV (*JAIDS* 2002;29[suppl 1]: S19). At 48 weeks, VL was <50 c/mL in 97% of the EFV arm and 85% of the PI continuation arm.

  □ **ALIZE-ANRS-099** was a randomized trial of switch to EFV+FTC+ddl qd vs. continued PI-based ART in patients with viral suppression. At 12 mos outcomes were comparable among the 355 patients for viral suppression (*JID* 2005;191:830). At 4 years 68% remain on the regimen and 57% had VL <50 c/mL.

  □ **AI266073** queried patients' preference when randomized to switch to TDF/FTC/EFV or continue the original regimen after achieving viral suppression on a PI-based regimen. 80% preferred the TDF/FTC/EFV regimen (*AIDS Patient Care STDS* 2010;24:87).

  □ **Toxicity:** There are **multiple studies** that address the issue of lipodystrophy complicating PI-based ART to determine the effect of changing to EFV-based ART vs. continuation of the original regimen. A review of 14 such studies with 910 patients (*Topics HIV Med* 2002;10:47) showed virologic failure in only 6 patients. Effects on triglycerides and cholesterol were variable, and lipodystrophy was rarely reversed. One report found that adding pravastatin was a more effective strategy than switching ART (*AIDS* 2005;19: 1051).

  □ **ACTG 5142R:** The NRTI-sparing combination most extensively studied is LPV/r 533/133 mg bid + EFV 600 mg/d, in ACTG 5142 (see Table 5-30). Intent-to-treat analysis found that 83% of

Drug Information

■ TABLE 5-30: **ACTG 5142: EFV+2 NRTIs vs LPV/r+2 NRTIs vs EFV+LPV/r in Treatment-naïve Patients** (*NEJM* 2008;358:2095)

96-Week Results	EFV n=253	LPV/r ‡ n=250	EFV+LPV/r n=253
VL <50 c/mL	89%*	77%	83%
Not failed wk 96	76	67	73
CD4 count (median)	241	285*	268
Resistance †			
NNRTI	18/33 (48%)	2/52 (4%)*	27/39 (69%)
PI (major)	0	0*	2/39 (6%)
NRTI – 184V	8/33 (24%)	7/54 (14%)	1/39 (3%)
Metabolic study			
Triglyceride (>750 mg/dL)	6%	16%	34%
Total cholesterol (mg/dL)	+ 33	+ 33	+ 33
LDL Cholesterol (mg/dL)	+ 21	+ 26	+ 26
Lipoatrophy	32%	18%*	18%*

* P= <0.5: EFV superior to LPV/r for virologic failure; LPV/r superior to EFV for CD4 increase, resistance mutations and lipoatrophy.

† Resistance reported for no. resistance mutation/no. strains tested in patients with virologic failure.

‡ LPV/r dose = 533/133 mg

LPV/r/EFV recipients had VL <50 c/mL at 96 weeks. Recommendations for the dose adjustment with the tablet formulation is uncertain because the studies were done using the capsule formulation of LPV/r 533/133 bid (*AAC* 2003;47:350). With the tablet formulation, most recommend 6 tabs/d (600/150 mg bid) in patients with PI resistance, but standard dose (400/100 bid – 4 tabs/d) in patients with no PI resistance. See pg. 122-123.

◻ **A5116** was a randomized, open-label switch study of LPV/r (533 mg/133 mg bid) + EFV (600 mg qd) vs. EFV+2 NRTI in subjects who received at least 18 mos of a 3- or 4-drug PI- or NNRTI-based regimen as a first regimen, had plasma VL <200 c/mL and no documented phenotypic resistance. Among 236 participants, EFV + 2 NRTIs was superior in terms of viral suppression (14 vs. 7) and tolerability (20 vs. 6 discontinuations) (p <0.0015) (*AIDS* 2007;21:325).

◻ **Other NRTI-sparing regimens** containing EFV include EFV 600 mg qd + FPV/r 1400/300 mg qd (PI-naïve only) or EFV 600 mg qd + FPV/r 700/100 mg bid. EFV combined with ATV is more complicated, because the unboosted ATV AUC is reduced 74% with EFV. The recommended regimen is EFV 600 mg qd on an empty stomach and ATV/r 400/100 mg qd on a full stomach.

Drug Information

5

RESISTANCE: The K103N mutation is most common and causes high-level resistance to EFV as well as NVP and DLV. This may be present as a "minority quasispecies" at baseline that is detected only with allele-specific PCR and can lead to rapid virologic failure (*CID* 2009;48:239). In one study of clinical samples, K103N was detected with conventional genotypic testing in 10.5% and by allele-specific PCR only) in 14%. A systematic review of the literature (1974-Dec. 2010) found the most common low frequency resistance mutations were 103N and 181C, and these were associated with significantly higher rates of virologic failure with EFV-based regimens (*JAMA* 2011;305: 1327; *J Med Virol* 2009;81:1983). The K103N mutation does not reduce HIV fitness, so there is no benefit with continuation of EFV, and there is possible harm, since continuation is likely to select for more NNRTI mutations that could reduce effectiveness of ETR. Other major RT mutations associated with reduced susceptibility are RT codon mutations 181C/I, 188L, 190S/A, and 225H. The 181C/I mutation is not selected by EFV, but it contributes to low-level EFV resistance. Detection of this mutation as a minority variant using allele-specific PCR found that a minority 181C mutation was associated with a 3-fold risk of EFV failure in ACTG 5095 (*AIDS* 2008;22:2107; *AIDS* 2007; 21:813).

PHARMACOLOGY

- **Oral bioavailability:** Not known. High-fat meals increase absorption of both capsule and tablet forms by 39% and 79%, respectively, and should be avoided in patients who are experiencing CNS side effects. Serum levels are highly variable likely due to CYP2B6 polymorphisms and this variation explains some of the variations in virologic response (*AAC* 2004;48:979).

- **T½:** 36-100 h depending on the CYP2B6 genotype of the host (*CID* 2007;45:1230).

- **Distribution:** Highly protein-bound (>99%); CSF levels are 0.25-1.2% plasma levels, which is above the IC_{95} for wild-type HIV (*JID* 1999;180:862). Virologic failure correlates with levels <1.1 mg/L (12 th CROI, Boston, Feb. 2005;Abstr. 80). EFV is category 2 in the 4 category CNS penetration score (*Neurology* 2011;76:693) (see pg. 550).

- **Elimination:** Metabolized by the cytochrome P450 metabolic pathway, primarily CYP2B6 and, to a lesser extent, CYP3A4. Studies of poly-morphisms at codon 516 of the CYP2B6 gene have shown significant differences that correlate with half-life, drug levels, and CNS toxicity (*CID* 2006;42:401; *CID* 2007;45:1230). Depending on these genetic differences in the plasma half-life of EFV, the duration of therapeutic levels vs. wild-type HIV (>46 ng/mL) varies from 5.8 days to 14 days, the frequency of therapeutic levels lasting >21 days ranged from 5-29%, and median plasma levels of EFV at 24 hrs ranged from a median of about 3000 ng/mL with the GG genotype at codon 516 to >9000 ng/mL with the TT genotype (*CID* 2006;42:401; *CID* 2007;45:1230). Prolonged half-life and high levels are more common in African-Americans due to higher revalence of the TT genotype (*AAC* 2003;47:130). The substantial variations in EFV levels shown by these data complicate drug discontinuation and correlate with CNS side effects. One group has used these (CY2B6 polymorphism) data to reduce standard EFV dosing to 200-400 mg qd with substantial reduction CNS toxicity in 10 of 14 patients (*CID* 2007;45:1230). The drug induces its own metabolism so that duration of treatment is an important variable.

- **Dose modification with renal or hepatic disease:** No dose modification (*AIDS* 2000;14:618; *AIDS* 2000;14:1062). More frequent monitoring is advocated when given with hepatic disease.

SIDE EFFECTS

- **Switch in patients with NVP-induced rash or hepatotoxicity:** A meta-analysis of 13 reports with 239 patients found that 30 (13%) developed a recurrence of the rash when switched to EFV (*Lancet Infect Dis* 2007;7:722). Review of 11 patients with NVP-induced hepatoxocity found no recurrences (*Lancet Infect Dis* 2007;7:733).

- **Rash:** Approximately 15-27% of EFV recipients develop a rash, which is usually morbilliform and does not require discontinuation of the drug. More serious rash reactions that require discontinuation are blistering and desquamating rashes, noted in about 1-2% of patients, and Stevens-Johnson syndrome, which has been reported in 1 of 2,200 EFV recipients. The median time to onset of the rash is 11 days, and the duration with continued treatment is 14 days. The frequency with which discontinuation is required is 1.7% compared with 7% given NVP, 4.3% given DLV and 2% given ETR.

- **CNS** side effects have been noted in up to 52% of patients but are sufficiently severe to require discontinuation in only 2-5%. Symptoms are noted on day 1 and usually resolve after 2-4 wks. They include confusion, abnormal thinking, abnormal dreams, impaired concentration, depersonalization, , and dizziness. Other side effects include somnolence, insomnia, amnesia, hallucinations, and euphoria. Patients need to be warned of these side effects before starting therapy and should also be told that symptoms improve with continued dosing and infrequently persist longer than 2-4 wks. A substudy of **ACTG A5097** provided periodic neuropsychiatric testing of 170 EFV recipients for 184 wks (*HIV Clin Trials* 2009;10:343). CNS side effects declined to baseline levels at 4 wks, and long term follow-up found that the majority had no residual neuropsychologic deficits, although a small number had high scores for stress, anxiety and unusual dreams. There is evidence that the CNS toxicity is dose related (*JAIDS* 2009;52:240; *CID* 2007;45:1230) based on correlation with serum levels and response to dose reduction, although some studies do not support this correlation (*Antiviral Ther* 2005;10:489;

5 Drug Information

Antiviral Ther 2009;14:75). It is recommended that the drug be given in the evening on an empty stomach during the initial weeks of treatment, because a high-fat meal increases absorption by up to 80%. There is a potential additive effect with alcohol or other psychoactive drugs. Patients need to be cautioned to avoid driving or other potentially dangerous activities if they experience these symptoms. Two studies with extensive neurocognitive analyses showed no evidence that EFV was associated with an increase in serious mental health problems (*Ann Intern Med* 2005;143:714; *CID* 2006;42:1790), although serious disorders have been reported including severe depression in 2.4% (Bristol-Myers Squibb letter to providers, March 2005), and another cohort study showed the odds ratio for cognitive impairment with EFV was 4.0 (p=0.008) (*Neurology* 2011;76:1403). A review of 843 patients given EFV in EuroSIDA found that 138 (16%) stopped the drug due to CNS toxicity (*Antiviral Ther* 2009;14:75). In a retrospective review of ACTG 5095, 9% of patients intolerant of EFV were switched to NVP with resolution of EFV-associated reactions (*CID* 2010;51:365). One report indicated safety and effectiveness if switching from EFV to NVP in patients with CNS toxicity; 41 of 47 experienced resolution of CNS symptoms (46th ICAAC 2008;Abstr. 1236). Switching from EFV to ETR is another within-class change that has been successful in a randomized trial (*AIDS* 2011;25:65). Another option is dose reduction of EFV (600-400 mg) based on plasma concentrations (*JAIDS* 2009;52:240; *CID* 2007;45:1230) or based on genetic analysis for variants that determine EFV metabolism, half life and risk of CNS toxicity (CYP3A4, CYP2A6 and CYP2B6) (*JID* 2011;203:246).

- **Hyperlipidemia:** The D:A:D study found that EFV is associated with increased triglyceride and total cholesterol levels; these effects were greater for EFV compared to NVP (*JID* 2004;189:1056). D:A:D did not find a risk of cardiovascular disease associated with NNRTI use (*NEJM* 2007;356:1723). ACTG 5142, a large trial comparing EFV and LPV/r-based ART in treatment-naïve patients, found similar changes in lipids (LDL cholesterol and triglyceride changes), but lipid levels were greatest in those given both agents (*NEJM* 2008;358:2095). Lipid levels were more favorable with ATV/r than EFV in ACTG 5202 (*Ann Intern Med* 2011;154:445-56.)

- **False-positive urine cannabinoid (marijuana) test:** This occurs with the screening test only, and only with the Microgenic's *CEDIA DAU* Multilevel THC assay. Confirmatory tests are negative (*World* 1999;96:7).

- **False-positive benzodiazepine test:** (*Triage 8, Drug Screen Multi 5*).

- **Increased transaminase levels:** Levels >5 x ULN in 2-8% (*Hepatology* 2002;35:182; *HIV Clin Trials* 2003;4:115). Frequency is increased with hepatitis C or with use of concurrent hepatotoxic drugs. Hepatotoxicity is less frequent and less severe than seen

Drug Information

with NVP; grade 3-4 in 12% given NVP vs. 4% given EFV in one study of 298 patients (*HIV Clin Trials* 2003;4:115). The mechanism is unknown. Discontinuation of EFV is recommended if hepatotoxicity is symptomatic (infrequent) or ascribed to hypersensitivity, or if the transaminase levels are >10x ULN in the absence of other causes (grade IV) (*Clin Liver Dis* 2003;7:475).

- **Vitamin D deficiency:** This is a possible association from the SUN study with an OR of 2.0 (*CID* 2011;52:396). Consequences are unclear. See pg. 64.

BLACK BOX WARNINGS: None.

DRUG INTERACTIONS: EFV both induces and, to a lesser extent, inhibits the cytochrome P450 CYP3A4 enzymes *in vitro*. Enzyme induction has been observed in the majority of PK studies.

CONTRAINDICATED DRUGS FOR CONCURRENT USE: Astemizole, terfenadine, rifapentine, midazolam, triazolam, cisapride, pimozide, ergot alkaloids, St. John's wort and bepridil.

PIs: See Table 5-31.

OTHER DRUGS WITH SIGNIFICANT INTERACTIONS: EFV may reduce concentrations of **phenobarbital, phenytoin,** and **carbamazepine;**

■ TABLE 5-31: **EFV - PI Interactions and Dose Recommendations**

PI	AUC co-admin. drug	EFV AUC	Recommendation
IDV	↓31%	No change	IDV 1000 mg q8h + EFV 600 mg qhs or IDV 800 mg bid + RTV 200 mg bid + EFV 600 mg qd
NFV	↑20%	No change	NFV 1250 mg bid + EFV 600 mg qd
SQV	↓62%	↓12%	Consider SQV/r 1000/100 mg bid
SQV/RTV	↓60%	No change	SQV/r 1000/100 bid + EFV 600 mg qd;
LPV/r	↑36%*	No change	LPV/r 500/125 bid or 400/100 bid (treatment naïve); LPV/r 600/150 bid (treatment experienced)
ATV	↓74%	No change	ATV/r 400/100 mg qd + EFV 600 mg qd; unboosted ATV not recommended; ATV/r + EFV not recommended in ARV-experienced patients.
FPV	C_{min} ↓ 36%	No change	FPV/r 700/100 mg bid + EFV 600 mg qd or FPV/r 1400/300 mg qd + EFV 600 mg qd
TPV	↓ 31%	No change	TPV/r 750/200 mg bid + EFV 600 mg qd
DRV	↓13%	↑21%	Limited data; consider DRV/r 600/100 mg bid + EFV 600 mg qd; consider TDM
RTV	↑ 20%	↑ 20%	Standard doses
MVC	↓ 45%	No change	MVC 600 mg bid; EFV 600 mg qd
RAL	↓ 36%	No change	Standard dose

* Compared to standard dose LPV/r

Drug Information

5

monitor levels of anticonvulsant. **Rifampin** decreases EFV levels by 25%; rifampin levels are unchanged: some advocate higher doses of EFV (800 mg/d for persons >60 kg); a pharmacologic study found that concurrent use in patients with HIV and TB resulted in highly variable EFV levels but good clinical outcomes (*JAC* 2006;58:1299). However, most studies have suggested that the standard 600 mg dose is adequate, including the N2R trial designed to examine this issue (*CID* 2009;48:1752). Another option is to take EFV with a 40-60 gm fat meal, which will substantially increase EFV AUC. **Rifabutin** has no effect on EFV levels, but EFV reduces levels of rifabutin by 35%; with concurrent use, the recommended dose of rifabutin is 450 mg qd or 600 mg 3x/wk plus the standard EFV dose (*MMWR* 2002;51[RR-7]:48). **Rifampin** preferred with EFV co-administration. Concurrent use with **ethinyl estradiol** not affect or slightly increased. **Levonorgestrel** AUC increases 56% with EFV. A second form of contraception is recommended This is particularly important due to the teratogenic effects of EFV. EFV reduces **methadone** levels by 52%; titrate methadone levels to avoid opiate withdrawal. EFV also decreases levels of **buprenorphine** by 50% but may be preferred to methadone in opiate-dependent patients since no withdrawal symptoms were observed (*J Phar Biomed Anal* 2007;44: 188). EFV decreases **simvastatin** AUC by 58%, **atorvastatin** AUC by 43%, and **pravastatin** AUC by 44%. An increase in statin dose may be needed, but do not exceed the maximum dose (*JAIDS* 2005;39:307). **Atorvastatin, pravastatin or rosuvastatin** may be preferred. Monitor carefully when using **warfarin** with EFV. There is a 46% incidence of rash reactions when combining EFV and **clarithromycin**, and levels of clarithromycin are decreased 39%; consider **azithromycin**. **Voriconazole** (see pg. 413). **Diltiazem** AUC decreased 69%. Titrate to effect; **Sertraline** AUC decreased 39%. Titrate to effect; **Bupropion** AUC decreased 55%. Titrate to effect. **Atovaquone/proguanil:** Atovaquone AUC decreased 75% and proguanil AUC decreased 43%. Consider alternative for malaria and PCP prophylaxis.

Interactions and dose recommendations for EFV in combination with selected **other antiretrovial agents** are listed in Table 5-31.

PREGNANCY: Category D. This drug caused birth defects (anencephaly, anophthalmia, and microphthalmia) in 3 of 20 gravid cynomolgus monkeys. There have been seven reports of neural tube defects in infants born to women with first-trimester exposures to EFV (*Arch Intern Med* 2002;162:355; *AIDS* 2002; 16:299; Ely. 15th CROI 2008;Abstr. 624; Bristol-Myers Squibb letter to providers, March 2005). The Antiretroviral Pregnancy Registry (through July 2010) showed birth defects in 21/717 (2.8%) live births with first trimester exposures. These include one case each of sacral aplasia, meningomyelocele, hydrocephalus, facial clefts and anophthalmia. A review of 344 women who conceived on EFV-based ART in West Africa found no congenital malformations (*JAIDS* 2011;56:183). The 2010 DHHS Guidelines for

Use of Antiretroviral Drugs in Pregnancy recommend avoidance of EFV in the first trimester, and women with childbearing potential should be warned of this risk to assure there is adequate birth control. Safety in the second or third trimester is not established but should be safe since the neural tube has closed. The 2010 DHHS Guideline pregnancy statement is that "use after the first trimester can be considered if, after consideration of alternatives, this is the best choice." Pregnant women exposed to EFV should be registered at www.APRegistry.com (Antiretroviral Pregnancy Registry), or call 800-258-4263 (8:30 AM-5:30 PM EST, Mon-Fri).

EMTRICITABINE (FTC)

TRADE NAME: *Emtriva* (Gilead Sciences)

CLASS: NRTI

FORMULATIONS, REGIMENS AND COST:

- **Forms:** FTC – caps 200 mg; TDF/FTC (*Truvada*) – tab 300/200 mg; EFV/TDF/FTC (*Atripla*) – tab 600/300/200 mg; RPV/TDF/FTC (*Complera*) tab 25/300/200 mg; oral solution 170 mL bottle with 10 mg/mL

- **Regimens:** FTC, 200 mg qd or 240 mg oral solution qd; *Truvada*, 1 tab qd; *Atripla*, 1 tab hs on empty stomach; *Complera*, 1 tab qd with a meal

- **AWP:** FTC, $467.45/mo; *Truvada*, $1,195.15/mo; *Atripla*, $1,858.15/mo; 170 mL bottle (1700 mg) at $110.58; *Complera*, $TBA

FOOD EFFECTS: None

RENAL IMPAIRMENT: Dose adjustment for CrCl: 30-49 mL/min, 200 mg q48h; 15-29 mL/min, 200 mg q72h; <15 mL/min or dialysis, 200 mg q96 . Adjust *Truvada* CrCl 30-49 mL/min; 1 tab q48h; but avoid co-formulation at <30 mL/min. Do not use *Atripla* with CrCl <50 mL/min.

HEPATIC FAILURE: No dose adjustment

PATIENT ASSISTANCE: 1-800-226-2056 (9 am-8 pm EST, Mon.-Fri.)

ADVANTAGES: Potent antiretroviral activity, well tolerated, no food effect, longer intracellular half-life than 3TC, once-daily dosing, coformulated with RPV/TDF (*Complera*), TDF (*Truvada*) and TDF/EFV (*Atripla*). No risk of accumulating additional mutations after 184V with continued use. Delays TAMs. Possible decreased risk of K65R with TDF/FTC vs. TDF/3TC and decreased risk of M184V with TDF/FTC vs. AZT/3TC. Active against HBV. May be less prone to the 184V resistance mutation compared to 3TC (*HIV Clin Trials* 2011;12:61)

DISADVANTAGES: Rapid selection of 184V RT mutation in non-suppressive regimen with substantial loss of activity. Activity against HBV sometimes complicates HIV treatment decisions. Associated with skin hyperpigmentation (uncommon).

Drug Information

5

3TC COMPARISON: Similar to 3TC in activity against HIV, loss of most activity and rapid selection of M184V mutation, prolonged intracellular half-life and activity against HBV (*AAC* 2004; 48:3702; *CID* 2006; 42:126). May be less likely to select for M184V mutation than 3TC, and emergence of K65R with TDF/FTC may be less likely than with TDF+3TC.

CLINICAL TRIALS

- **GS-301A** was the FDA registration trial using FTC (200 mg qd) vs. d4T, each in combination with ddI+EFV in 571 treatment-naïve patients. At 60 weeks, VL <50 c/mL was achieved in 76% of FTC recipients compared to 54% in the d4T group (*P* <0.001), and the CD4 count at 48 wks was greater with FTC, a mean of 153/mm^3 vs. 120/mm^3 (P=0.02) (*JAMA* 2004;292:180).

- **GS-303** was a 3TC equivalence open label trial in which 440 patients receiving 3TC as a part of ART were randomized to continue bid 3TC or to switch to FTC. At 48 weeks, virologic failure occurred in 7% of FTC recipients and 8% of 3TC recipients (*AIDS* 2004;18:2269).

- **Protocol 350**, a continuation study, found equivalent rates of viral suppression for GS-303 participants for an additional median follow-up of 152 wks (*AIDS* 2004;18:2269).

- **ALIZE-ANRS-099:** Switch study in 355 patients randomized to continue PI-based ART or switch to FTC+ddI+EFV once daily. At 48 wks, 87% and 79% had a VL <50 c/mL with EFV vs. PI/r-based ART, respectively (*p* <0.05) (*JID* 2005;191:830).

- **GS-903:** A randomized, double-blind study in which 602 treatment-naïve patients received either TDF or d4T in combination with 3TC+EFV. Virologic suppression (<50 c/mL) was equivalent through 144 wks. K65R emerged in 8 and 2 patients in the TDF and d4T arms, respectively. Lipids more favorable in TDF arm, and lipoatrophy more common with d4T. Renal safety profile similar between arms (*JAMA* 2004;292:191-201).

- **GS-934:** See also pg. 390. 517 treatment-naïve patients were randomized to receive EFV+AZT/3TC or EFV+TDF/FTC. At 144 wks, more patients experienced virologic suppression in the TDF/FTC arm by ITT analysis, 71% vs. 58% <400 c/mL. The difference was explained primarily by the higher proportion of discontinuations due to adverse events in the AZT/3TC arm (9% vs. 4%), most of which were due to anemia (*NEJM* 2006; 354: 251). No K65R mutations were observed, and M184V was less common with TDF/FTC than with AZT/3TC (*JAIDS* 2006;43:535).

- **Hepatitis B**: FTC is considered equivalent to 3TC for activity against HBV (*AIDS* 2011;25:73; *CID* 2010;51:1201) and is approved for that indication. One study found that resistance by YMDD mutants was delayed with FTC compared to 3TC (*AIDS* 2005;19:221). Another study found no dedectable HBV DNA levels with FTC monotherapy in 65% of patients at 24 weeks (*AAC* 2006;50: 1642). Current recommendations are that TDF/FTC or TDF/3TC-based ART be used in co-infected patients who require treatment of HBV regardless of the need for HIV treatment. If the decision is to treat HBV without treating HIV, the agents used to treat HBV should be one that is inactive against HIV: interferon, adefovir, or telbivudine (2011 DHHS HIV Treatment Guidelines; *CID* 2006;43:904).

RESISTANCE: Non-suppressive therapy with FTC results in the rapid selection of the M184V mutation, which confers high-level resistance to 3TC and FTC, modest decreases in susceptibility to ABC and ddl, and increased susceptibility to TDF, AZT, and d4T. K65R or multiple TAMs reduce activity of FTC 3- to 7-fold. With maximum selective pressure, the TDF/FTC combination produces mutants with the K65R and M184V genotype *in vitro* (*AAC* 2006;50: 4087); although K65R has not been observed in clinical trials (GS-934 and Abbott 418) using this combination. All of these changes apply to 3TC as well. A comparison of results for resistance in three trials showed the frequency of the 184V mutation with viral failure was greater with 3TC compared to FTC (36% vs. 19%) (*HIV Clin Trials* 2011;12:61).

PHARMACOLOGY

- **Bioavailability:** 93% for the capsule and 75% for the solution; not altered by meals
- **Levels:** C_{max} 1.8 ± 0.7 µg/mL; C_{min} 0.09 µg/mL
- **Distribution:** Protein-binding <4%, concentrated in semen
- **T½:** plasma, 10 h; intracellular, 39 h (*AAC* 2004;48:1300).
- **Elimination:** 13% metabolized to sulfadioxide and glucoronide metabolites. Unchanged drug and metabolites are renally eliminated.

SIDE EFFECTS:

Black Box Warnings:

- Lactic acidosis: Rare and only when used with other NRTI, usually a thymidine analogue
- Flare of HBV when FTC is discontinued in co-infected patients

Generally well tolerated with minimal toxicity. Occasionally, patients note nausea, diarrhea, headache, asthenia, or rash; about 1% discontinue the drug due to adverse effects. **Lactic acidosis and hepatic steatosis**, including fatal cases, have been reported with nucleosides. Rare patients who do not tolerate FTC will tolerate 3TC (*JAC* 2006;58:227). **Skin hyperpigmentation** has been noted primarily on palms and soles in 3% and almost exclusively in Africans and African-Americans. FTC is active against HBV, so discontinuation may result in **HBV exacerbation**.

DRUG INTERACTIONS: None of clinical consequence are known.

PREGNANCY: Category B. The 2010 DHHS Guidlines on Use of Antiretroviral Drugs in Pregnancy list FTC as an alternative to 3TC to be used in combination with another NRTI as the NRTI backbone.

5 Drug Information

Pharmacokinetic studies in pregnancy show FTC levels are modestly lower (Best, 15th CROI;Abstr. 629). The data for birth defects with FTC exposure in the Pregnancy Registry is 16/542 (3.5%) which compares to 2.7% without ART exposure (Last updated 7/20/2010).

ENFUVIRTIDE (ENF, T20)

TRADE NAME: *Fuzeon* (Roche-Trimeris)

FORMULATION: Single-dose vials with 108 mg ENF as lyophilized powder (sufficient for 90 mg dose) to be reconstituted with 1.1 mL sterile water. ENF is packaged in a 30-day kit containing 60 single-use vials of ENF, 60 vials of sterile water for injection, 60 reconstitution syringes (3 cc), 60 administration syringes (1 cc), and alcohol wipes.

ADULT DOSE: 90 mg (1mL) SC q12h into upper arm, anterior thigh, or abdomen with each injection given at a site different from the preceding injection site.

STORAGE: The kit can be stored at room temperature. However, once ENF powder has been reconstituted, it must be refrigerated at 36-46°F (2-8°C) and used within 24 hrs.

COST: $3,154.10/mo or $37,969/year (AWP). Cost-effective analysis is estimated at $69,500/life-year saved (*JAIDS* 2005;39:69).

PATIENT ASSISTANCE: 800-282-7780

ADVANTAGE: Novel mechanism of action, potent antiviral activity, virtually no resistance in patients not previously treated with this drug, well studied with well documented in vivo activity in heavily treatment-experienced patients.

DISADVANTAGES: Requirement for twice daily subcutaneous injections, local reactions at injection sites and rapid development of resistance with virologic failure. ENF is the most expensive ART agent. The main concern is the effect on quality of life.

MECHANISM OF ACTION: ENF binds to HR1 site in the gp41 subunit of the viral envelope glycoprotein and prevents conformational change required for viral fusion and entry into cells. Discontinuation of ENF in 25 patients with ENF resistance resulted in an increase in VL with decrease in resistance; retreatment with ENF led to undetectable virus by week 16 (*JID* 2007;195:387)

CLINICAL TRIALS

- **TORO-1 (North America and Brazil) and TORO-2 (Australia and Europe):** Pooled data presented to the FDA were from 2 randomized, controlled, open-label studies involving 995 treatment-experienced patients with virologic failure (*NEJM* 2003;348:2175; *NEJM* 2003; 348:2186) (Table 5-32). ENF plus an optimized background regimen (OBR) was superior to an OBR alone. Patients had a baseline VL of 5.2 $\log_{10}$ c/mL, a mean of 12 prior antiretroviral agents, and 80-90% had ≥5 resistance mutations to NRTIs, NNRTIs, or PIs. The VL change from baseline to week 24 was -1.52 $\log_{10}$ c/mL for patients in the ENF arm compared to -0.73 $\log_{10}$ for patient receiving only the OBR (P<0.0001). As expected, patients with 2 or more active antiretrovirals, based on history and genotype or phenotype resistance testing, were more likely to achieve a VL <400 c/mL.

■ TABLE 5-32: **TORO-1 and -2, 48- and 96-week Results**

Results		ENF/OBR	OBR
48 weeks		n=661	n=334
NEJM 2003;348:2175 and *JAIDS* 2005;40:404	VL <400 c/mL	34%*	12%
	VL <50 c/mL	18%	8%
	CD4 count (mean)	+91 cells/mm³	+45 cells/mm³
96 weeks		n=368	—
(AIDS Pat Care STDs 2007;21:533)	<400 c/mL	27%	—
	<50 c/mL	18%	—
	CD4 count	+166	

* P <0.001 compared to results in control arm

- **Other salvage studies:** ENF has shown to increase efficacy of other salvage regimens as summarized in Table 5-33.
- **ENF switch: EASIER-ANRS-138** was a randomized trial comparing continuation of ENF-based ART with substitution of RAL for ENF (N=170). At 24 weeks, switch to RAL was associated with significant improvements in pain, social functioning and physical activity scores (*HIV Clin Trials* 2010;11:283).

■ TABLE 5-33: **Summary of Salvage Trials with and without ENF***

Trial	Agent	*N*	Control	Study Agent	Study Agent + ENF
RESIST (*Lancet* 2006;368:466)	TPV/r	1,483	10%	23%	36%
POWER (*Lancet* 2007;369:1169)	DRV/r	255	15%	44%	58%
MOTIVATE (*NEJM* 2008;359:1442)	MVC	1,048	19%	42%	63%
BENCHMRK (*NEJM* 2008;359:339)	RAL	521	34%	57%	80%

* Results are % with VL <50 400 c/mL at 48 weeks

Drug Information

5

DRUG RESISTANCE AND CROSS-RESISTANCE: Resistance to ENF occurs rapidly with nonsuppressive therapy and is associated with mutations in the HR1 region of gp41 at codons 36, 37, 38, 39, 40, 42, and 43 (*J Virol* 2005;79:4991). These mutations reduce fusion efficiency, resulting in reduced fitness; mutations at codons 36 and 38 emerge rapidly (*AIDS* 2006;20:2075; *JAIDS* 2006;43:60), usually within 2 wks with incomplete viral suppression. Mutations in gp41 codons 36-43 were noted in 98% of patients with virologic failure in TORO-1 and -2 (*AIDS Res Human Retroviruses* 2006;22:375). These mutations do not cause cross-resistance with other entry inhibitors such as CCR5 and CXCR4 inhibitors. Discontinuation of ENF in patients with ENF-resistant strains results in a moderate increase in VL and disappearance of ENF mutations within 16 wks (*JAIDS* 2006;43:60; *JID* 2007; 195:387). A case report showed selection of ENF-resistant HIV-1 in CSF led to loss of viral suppression in plasma (*CID* 2010;50:387)

CURRENT STATUS: The introduction of new antiretroviral agents in 2005-08 (DRV, TPV, ETR, RAL, MVC) largely supplanted the need for ENF, and many receiving ENF were switched to alternative agents for improved quality-of-life. Thus, the demand for ENF has decreased substantially (*HIV Clin Trials* 2010;11:283; *HIV Clin Trials* 2009;10:432; *JAC* 2009;64:1341; *JAIDS* 2009;52:382). A potential contemporary use in patients with drug susceptible HIV infection is the need for parenteral therapy.

PHARMACOKINETICS

- **Absorption:** Well absorbed from subcutaneous (SC) site with an absolute bioavailability of 84.3%. Following 90 mg SC, the mean C_{max} was 5.0 mcg/mL, C_{min} was 3.3 mcg/mL, and AUC was 48.7 mcg/mL•hr. Virologic failure is associated with C_{trough} levels <2.2 mcg/mL (*JAC* 2008;62:384).

- **Distribution:** Vd=5.5L. Levels in CSF are nil (*Antiviral Ther* 2008;13:369; *Neurology* 2011;76:693) (see pg. 550t).

- **Protein binding:** 92%

- **Metabolism:** After SC injection, the drug is completely absorbed and largely catabolized, but about 17% is converted to an active deaminated form. Metabolism is not influenced by cytochrome P450 (*Clin Pharmacokinet* 2005;44:175).

- **T½:** 3.8 h

DOSING WITH RENAL FAILURE: No dose adjustment (*CID* 2004;39:119).

DOSING WITH HEPATIC INSUFFICIENCY: No data; usual dose.

DRUG INTERACTIONS: None. *In vitro*, enfuvirtide did not inhibit or induce the metabolism of CYP3A4, CYP2D6, CYP1A2, CYP2C19 or CYP2E1 substrates. Does not interact with TPV/r, DRV/r, RAL, ETR, MVC, SQV/r, RTV, or rifampin (*JID* 2006; 194:1319).

Drug Information

ADVERSE DRUG REACTIONS

- **Injections site reactions:** A review by the FDA of 663 ENF recipients found the injection site reactions occurred in 98%, including pain (96%; severe pain in 11%) induration (90%; severe in 57%), erythema (91%), nodules or cysts (80%) and/or pruritis (65%). Duration of the reaction was >3 days in 41% and >7 days in 24%. Treatment was discontinued in 7% due to these reactions (Gibbs N. 12th CROI, Boston, Feb. 2005:Abstr. 837). Successful desensitization has been reported (*CID* 2004;39:110). Injection site reactions can be managed by rotating sites and massaging the area after injection. Excisional biopsies of these lesions show inflammation resembling granuloma annulare with most of the inflammatory and collagen changes in areas where ENF was injected. These changes were noted even when there was no clinical reaction, which suggests a hypersensitivity reaction (*Am Acad Dermatol* 2003;49:826). A randomized study to evaluate 3 delivery systems (27 gauge needle, 31 gauge needle or needle-free injection device). At week 12, 85% of participants selected to use the needle-free device (*Antiviral Ther* 2008;13:449)

- **Occasional ADRs:** Bacterial pneumonia (event rate per 100 patient-years in trials was 4.68 in the treatment arm vs. 0.61 in controls). Relationship to ENF is unclear (*JAC* 2010;65:138).

- **Rare ADRs:** Hypersensitivity with rash, nausea, vomiting, chills, fever, hypotension, and elevated transaminase, glomerulonephritis, thrombocytopenia, neutropenia, eosinophilia, fever, hyperglycemia, Guillain Barré syndrome, sixth nerve palsy, elevation in amylase and lipase (for rare ADRs, a causal relationship is not established).

BLACK BOX WARNING: None

PREGNANCY/BREASTFEEDING RISKS: Category B. Not teratogenic in animal studies. There are no data concerning safety or pharmocokinetics in pregnancy. Does not cross the placenta (limited data) (*AIDS* 2006;20:297). Breastfeeding not recommended. The 2010 DHHS Guidelines for Anti-Retroviral Treatment in Pregnancy does not recommend ENF due to inadequate data.

ENTECAVIR

TRADE NAME: *Baraclude*

FORMS AND COST: 0.5 mg and 1.0 mg tabs at $30.58, 0.05 mg/mL solution (210 mL) at $642.20

INDICATION: Chronic HBV infection with evidence of active disease. One study found that switching from 3TC to entecavir in monoinfected patients resulted in an increase in HBV suppression and no evidence of HBV resistance (*Hepatol Int* 2010;4:594). See Table 5-34.

■ TABLE 5-34: **Response of Chronic HBV to Entecavir Treatment**

	A1463022 HBeAg Pos		A1463027 HBeAg Neg	
	Entecavir	3TC	Entecavir	3TC
Dose/d	0.5 mg	100 mg	0.5	100 mg
Sample size	314	314	296	287
Histologic Improvment	72%*	62%	70%*	61%
Undedectable HBV DNA	67%*	36%	90%*	72%

* Superior to treatment with 3TC (*P* <0.05) (package insert; *NEJM* 2006;354:1011; *NEJM* 2006;354:1001)

DOSE REGIMEN: NRT-naïve patients – 0.5 mg po qd on empty stomach (2 hrs before or after food). For 3TC-refractory patients – 1 mg po qd on empty stomach.

Use in HIV/HBV co-infection: Entecavir is generally considered one of the best drugs for HBV infection (*CID* 2010;51:1201). A 2010 meta-analysis of 20 studies of outcome at one year from clinical trials of HBV infection found that TDF and entecavir are the most effective agents for initial treatment (*Gastroenterology* 2010;139:1218), but the use of entecavir in HBV/HIV co-infected patients is complicated because it has *in vitro* and *in vivo* activity against HIV as well as HBV. Use in co-infected patients has been associated with a significant decrease in HIV viral load and emergence of the 184V RT resistance mutation (*NEJM* 2007; 356:2614; *AIDS* 2007; 21:2365). It should not be used in HIV/HBV co-infected patients unless it is part of a fully-suppressive ART regimen.

RESISTANCE: *In vitro* tests show that 3TC-resistant strains are 8- to 30-fold less sensitive to entecavir (see Table 5-35). Resistance to entecavir can emerge during treatment but is infrequent and requires additional RT mutations (*AAC* 2004; 48:3498). HBV strains from patients who failed entecavir are resistant to 3TC, but sensitive to adefovir. One trial of entecavir in HIV/HBV co-infected patients with HBV rebound showed a good response to entecavir with a mean decrease of 3.5 $\log_{10}$ c/mL in HBV DNA levels (*AIDS* 2008;22:1779). See pg. 507.

PHARMACOLOGY

- **Bioavailability:** 100% for both oral solution and tablet forms when taken on an empty stomach. If taken with a fatty meal, the C_{max} is decreased 45% and AUC is decreased 18-20%.

- **T½:** 24 h (*J Clin Pharmacol* 2006;46:1250); intracellular: 15 hrs.

- **Elimination:** Entecavir does not induce or inhibit the P450 metabolic pathway. It is eliminated predominantly by renal clearance.

DRUG INTERACTIONS: None established

ADVERSE REACTIONS

- Similar to 3TC in comparative trials for 48 wks

Drug Information

	3TC-refractory cases	
	Entecavir n = 124	3TC n = 116
Histologic improvement	55%*	28%
Ishak fibrosis score improved	34%*	16%
HBV DNA Undectectable (<300 c/mL)	19%*	1%
Mean Viral load change (log_{10} c/mL)	-5.1%*	-0.5
ALT normal (<1 x ULN)	61%*	15%
HBeAg seroconversion	8%	3%

* Superior to treatment with 3TC (P <0.05) (package insert; *NEJM* 2006;354:1011; *NEJM* 2006;354:1001)

- Rare, major severe reaction is lactic acidosis with steatosis, including fatalities (class effect, causal relationship with entecavir unknown)
- Exacerbation of HBV when entecavir is discontinued

PREGNANCY: Category C – not recommended for co-infected patients since drugs active vs. both HIV and HBV are needed. Report exposures during pregnancy to www.apregistry.com/

EPIVIR – see Lamivudine (pg. 304)

EPO – see Erythropoietin

EPZICOM – see Abacavir (pg. 179) and Lamivudine (pg. 304)

ERYTHROPOIETIN (EPO)

TRADE NAME: *Procrit* (Ortho Biotech)

FORMS AND COST: Vials with 2000, 3000, 4000, 10,000, 20,000, and 40,000 units. Standard dose of 40,000 U/wk costs $777.60.

PATIENT ASSISTANCE PROGRAM: 800-553-3851

PRODUCT INFORMATION: Recombinant human erythropoietin (rHU EPO) is a hormone produced by recombinant DNA technology. It has the same amino acid sequence and biologic effects as endogenous erythropoietin, which is produced primarily by the kidneys in response to hypoxia and anemia. It acts by stimulating the proliferation of marrow RBC progenitor cells.

Drug Information

5

INDICATIONS: Serum erythropoietin level <500 milliunits/mL plus anemia ascribed to HIV infection, or to medications, including AZT (*Ann Intern Med* 1992;117:739; *JAIDS* 1992;5:847).

DOSE RECOMMENDATIONS: See pg. 521. Although the FDA-approved dose for initial therapy is 10,000 units 3x/wk, the standard starting dose used in clinical practice is 40,000 units/wk, and trials investigating every-other-week dosing demonstrated good clinical efficacy (*CID* 2004;38:1447). Dosing for patient with ESRD on HD: 50-100 u/kg 3x/wk. Onset of action is within 1-2 wks, reticulocytosis is noted at 7-10 days, increases in hematocrit are noted in 2-6 wks, and desired hematocrit is usually attained in 8-12 wks. Response is dependent on the degree of initial anemia, baseline EPO level, dose, and available iron stores. Transferrin saturation should be ≥20%; serum ferritin should be ≥100 ng/mL. If levels are suboptimal, supplement with iron. (Some experts advocate routine iron supplementation in all patients taking EPO.) If after 4 wks of therapy the Hb rise is <1 g/dL, dose may be increased to 60,000 units SQ weekly. After an additional 4 wks, if Hgb does not increase by at least 1 g/dL from baseline value, discontinue EPO therapy. After achieving the desired response (i.e., increased Hgb or Hct level or reduction in transfusion requirements), titrate the dose for maintenance. Target Hb is 10-11.3 gm/dL. When dosed to target a Hgb level of 13.5 gm/dL there is a significant risk of cardiovascular compli-cations compared to a target of 11.3 g/dL (*NEJM* 2006;355:2085 and 2144; FDA warning, Nov. 22, 2006) – death 7.3% vs. 5% (p=0.07) and congestive heart failure 9% vs. 6.6% (p=0.07). Keep dose steady or reduce by 25% when Hb >12 gm/dL. Reduce dose by 25% if Hgb increases >1 gm/dL in any 2-wk period and hold if Hgb is >13 g/dL or Hct >40%, and re-initiate with a 25% reduction when Hgb is less than 11 g/dL. With failure to respond or suboptimal response, consider iron deficiency, occult blood loss, folic acid or B12 deficiency, or hemolysis.

EFFICACY: A trial using EPO in 1,943 HIV-infected patients with HCT <30% used an initial dose of 4,000 units SQ 6 d/wk, and mean weekly doses ranged from 22,700-32,500 units/wk (340-490 units/kg/wk). Response to treatment, defined as an increase in baseline HCT by 6 percentage points (i.e., 30-36%) with no transfusions within 28 days, was achieved in 44%. Transfusion requirements were significantly reduced from 40-18% at 24 weeks and the average hematocrit increased from 28-35% at 1 year. Subset analysis demonstrated that this response was independent of AZT administration (*Int J Antimicrob Ag* 1997;8:189). In one study anemia was a risk factor for death, and this risk was decreased with EPO (*CID* 1999;29:44).

PHARMACOLOGY

- **Bioavailability:** EPO is a 165-amino acid glycoprotein that is not ab-sorbed with oral administration. IV or SC administration is required; SC is preferred.

- **T½:** 4-16 h
- **Elimination:** Poorly understood but minimally affected by renal failure.
- **Dose adjustment in renal or hepatic failure:** None

SIDE EFFECTS: Increased risk of cardiovascular complications when targeting a Hgb level of 13.5 gm/dL compared to 11.3 g/dL (*NEJM* 2006; 355:2085). The 2007 FDA black box warning recommends EPO dose adjustment to the lowest level that avoids the requirement for transfusions and not to exceed a hemoglobin of 12 gm/dL (FDA Advisory, March 9, 2007). Other side effects are infrequent and not severe. Headache and arthralgias are most common; less common are flu-like symptoms, GI intolerance, diarrhea, edema, and fatigue. Hypertension is an uncommon complication that has been noted more frequently in patients with renal failure. EPO is contraindicated in patients with hypertension that is uncontrolled. The most common reactions noted in the therapeutic trial with 1,943 AIDS patients were rash, injection site reaction, nausea, hypertension, and seizures.

PREGNANCY: Category C. Teratogenic in animals; no studies in humans.

ETHAMBUTOL (EMB)

TRADE NAME: *Myambutol* (Lederle) and generic

FORM AND COST: 100 and 400 mg tab; 400 mg tabs at $0.72/tab

PATIENT ASSISTANT PROGRAM: 800-859-8586

INDICATIONS AND DOSE: Active tuberculosis or infections with *M. avium* complex (MAC) or *M. kansasii* (see Table 5-36; pg. 465-475). **Ethambutol dosing for MAC:** 15 mg/kg/d + macrolide. One report based on pharmacokinetics suggests a dose of 50 mg/kg 2x/wk can be considered for MAC bacteremia (*AAC* 2010;54:1728).

PHARMACOLOGY
- **Bioavailability:** 77%
- **T½:** 3.1 h
- **Elimination:** Renal

■ TABLE 5-36: **Ethambutol Dosing for Tuberculosis (2008 IDSA/NIH/CDC Guideline for Prevention and Treatment of HIV Associated Opportunistic Infections)**

Dosing interval	Weight		
	40-55 kg	56-75 kg	76-90 kg
Daily	800 mg	1200 mg	1600 mg
2x/wk	2000 mg	2800 mg	4000 mg
3x/wk	1200 mg	2000 mg	2400 mg

Drug Information

5

- **Dose modification in renal failure:** CrCl >50 mL/min – 15-25 mg/kg q24h; CrCl 10-50 mL/min – 15-25 mg/kg q24h-q36h; CrCl <10 mL/min – 15-25 mg/kg q48h

SIDE EFFECTS: Dose and duration-related ocular toxicity (decreased acuity, restricted fields, scotomata, and loss of color discrimination) with 25 mg/kg dose (0.8%), hypersensitivity (0.1%); peripheral neuropathy (rare); GI intolerance (*Drug Saf* 2008;31:127; *Expert Opin Drug Saf* 2006;5:615). Ocular toxicity usually improves when the drug is dis-continued, but recovery is often partial (*Brit J Ophthal* 2007;91:895).

WARNINGS: Patients to receive EMB in doses of 25 mg/kg or higher should undergo a baseline screening for visual acuity and red-green color perception; this examination should be repeated at monthly intervals during treatment (*MMWR* 1998;47[RR-20]:31).

DRUG INTERACTIONS: Aluminum-containing antacids may decrease absorption.

PREGNANCY: Category C. Teratogenic at high doses in animals; no reported adverse effects in women with >320 case observations. Avoid in first trimester if possible.

ETRAVIRINE (ETR)

TRADE NAME: *Intelence* (Tibotec Pharmaceuticals)

CLASS: Second generation non-nucleoside reverse transcriptase inhibitor

PATIENT ASSISTANCE: 1-800-652-6227

FORMULATIONS, REGIMENS AND COST:

- Formulations: 100 mg and 200 mg tabs
- Dose: 200 mg po bid with food
- Price (AWP): $919.78/mo
- Storage: Room temperature
- **Once daily ETR:** A pharmacokinetic trial found that once daily administration produced a lower C_{min}, but was >50-fold higher than the IC_{50} of wild-type HIV with or without concurrent DRV (*AIDS* 2009;23:2289; *Antivir Ther* 2010;15:711).

DRUG INTERACTION WARNING: ETR should not be given in combination with any other NNRTI, unboosted PI, TPV/r, FPV/r or ATV/r

FOOD EFFECT: Take with food – type of food is not relevant

RENAL FAILURE: No data; standard dose likely appropriate since renal excretion is minimal. Minimal removal with dialysis (*AIDS* 2009;23:740).

HEPATIC FAILURE: Child-Pugh Class A and B: Standard dose; class C: One report of a very high ETR level (3,257 ng/mL) and prolonged half

Drug Information

life (237 hrs) in a patient with decompensated liver disease (*AIDS* 209;23:1293).

ADVANTAGES: Activity against most HIV strains that are resistant to first generation NNRTIs (EFV and NVP), pharmacologic barrier to resistances. Some advantages compared to EFV: reduced CNS toxicity and safety in the first trimester of pregnancy (but no human data).

DISADVANTAGES: Recommended regimen is bid dosing with food (although PK allows once daily dosing); high incidence of rash (9%). Concurrent use of TPV, ATV and FPV are not recommended; reduced activity with poor ETR mutation score.

RESISTANCE: ETR is active against most but not all EFV or NVP-resistant virus. Resistance to ETR can be determined by phenotype or by genotype analysis using one of two weighted scoring systems.

- The **Tibotec system** predicted virologic response in the DUET trials (*AIDS* 2010; 24:503):
  - *3 points:* 181I/V
  - *2.5 points:* 101P, 100I, 181C, 230L
  - *1.5 points:* 138A, 106I, 190S, 179F
  - *1 point:* 90I, 179D, 101E, 101H, 98G, 179T, 190A
    - 0-2 points predicts a 74% response,
      2.5-3-5 points predicts a 52% response, and
      >4 points predicts a 38% response.

- The **Monogram scoring system** predicts phenotypic susceptibility:
  - *4 points:* 100I, 101P, 181C/I
  - *3 points:* 138A/G, 179E, 190Q, 230L, 238N
  - *2 points:* 101E, 106A, 138K, 179L, 188L
  - *1 point:* 90I, 101H, 106M, 138Q, 179D/F/M, 181F, 190E/T, 221Y, 225H, 238T
    - A score of >4 is associated with reduced susceptibility

Note: The FDA also included other IAS-USA mutations, but unclear clinical significance compared to other NNRTIs.

CLINICAL TRIALS:

- **DUET-1 & -2:** ETR + DRV/r + OBR vs. placebo + DRV/r + OBR (N=1203): See pg. 226. Enrollment requirements were virologic failure on current ART regimen with VL >5,000 c/mL + genotypic resistance to first generation NNRTIs and at least 3 primary PI mutations. At 48 weeks, outcome was superior with ETR vs. placebo for viral suppression to <50 c/mL by ITT analysis (61% vs. 39%) (Table 5-22) (*Lancet* 2007; 370:29). At 96 weeks, VL was <50 c/mL in 57% of 599 patients in the ETR arm and 36% of the 604 patients in the placebo arm (p <0.0001) (*Antiviral Ther* 2010;15:1045). The mean increase in CD4 count was 128 cells/mm^3 in ETR recipients vs. 86 cells/mm^3 in placebo recipients. A subset analysis of patients with

5 Drug Information

virologic failure suggested that ETR protected against DRV resistance (*AIDS* 2010;24:921). See pg. 226.

- **ANRS-139 (TRIO):** Criteria for entry were VL >1000 c/mL, treatment-naïve to DRV, RAL and ETR, and the following: >3 PI resistance mutations, virologic failure with NNRTIs, treatment susceptibility to DRV and <3 of the following DRV mutations: 11I, 32I, 33F, 47V, 50V, 54L/M, 73S, 76V, 84V and 89V. Treatment was with RAL 400 mg bid, ETR 200 mg bid and DRV/r 600/100 bid with or without ENF and NRTIs. At 48 weeks 86% of 100 participants had a VL <50 c/mL; the median CD4 count increase was 108 cells/mm^3. Grade 3-4 adverse reactions were reported in 15 (15%) (*CID* 2009;49:1441). Among 14 virologic failures, 3 had ETR resistance mutations (*AIDS* 2010;24:2651). A pharmacokinetic study of TRIO participants found that the addition of ETR increased trough levels of DRV by 71% and RAL by 34% (*JAIDS* 2010; 24:2581). See pg. 258.

- **EFV to ETR SWITCH for CNS TOXICITY:** This phase IV, double blind, placebo-controlled trial randomized patients with grade 2-4 CNS toxicity plus VL <50 c/mL to ETR-based ART or continued EFV-based ART (Waters L. 2010 IAS, Vienna;Abstr. LBPE19). At 12 weeks, all 38 participants maintained viral control and ETR-recipients experienced a significant reduction of grade 2-4 CNS toxicity, especially abnormal dreams and insomnia. Lipids also improved.

- **SENSE:** Randomized trial of 157 treatment-naïve patients given ETR or EFV, each with 2 NRTIs. The 12-week results showed virologic suppression to <400 c/mL was achieved in 87.9% of ETR recipients compared to 93% with EFV (p=NS) and CD4 count increases were similar (146 vs. 121/mm^3). Drug rela ted adverse events were much more common with EFV (17% vs. 46%, p <0.001) (*AIDS* 2011;25:335).

- **SWITCH EFV → ETR (SWITCH-EE):** Pharmacokinetic studies indicate that this switch does not require dose adjustment of ETR (*JAIDS* 2009;52:222). See SWITCH-EE trial (EFV → ETR and ETR → EFV) pg. 248.

PHARMACOKINETICS: (Package insert)

- **Absorption:** Bioavailability is unknown. Fasting decreases exposure by 50%; ETR should be taken with food but the content of the meal does not appear to be important. Median trough 275 ng/mL (range is 81-2980).

- **Distribution:** Protein binding – 99%. ETR CNS penetration effectiveness score is 2 (*Neurology* 2011;76:693). See pg. 550.

- **Metabolism:** Metabolized by CYP3A4, CYP2C9 and CYP2C19. ETR does not induce or inhibit its own metabolism.

- **Elimination:** Primarily stool with <1.2% recovered in urine. Clearance is reduced with HCV or HBV co-infection but no dose adjustment is recommended. Standard dose is recommended for

Child Pugh Score A & B and there are inadequate data for category C.

- **T1/2** = 41±20 hrs. No difference is noted in pharmacokinetics based on gender, race or age (18-77 years).

SIDE EFFECTS: Severe side effects: Contact Tibotec (1-877-732-2488) and/or FDA 1-800-FDA-1088 or www.fda.gov/medwatch.

- Most serious – Severe cutaneous reactions including Stevens-Johnson syndrome and erythemia multiforme (These are rare).

- Most common: Rash and nausea

- Number of discontinued treatments due to ADR in clinical trials: 2%

- Rash: Rate in registration trials was 9% vs. 3% in controls. Rash was noted in 19% of participants in DUET-1 and -2 (21% vs. 12% in ETR vs. placebo recipients) and was the most common adverse event prompting discontinuation (*JAIDS* 2010;53:614). This included two cases of Stevens-Johnson Syndrome. The early access experience and most controlled trials report discontinuation due to rash in 1.3-2%. Rashes are most common in women, most common at week 2 and infrequent after week 4. Patients with rash due to EFV or NVP generally tolerated ETR, and most rashes resolved in 1-2 wks with continuation of ETR.

- GI Intolerance: Rates of nausea, vomiting, diarrhea and abdominal pain in registration trials was 2-5% for each GI side effect and not different from controls

- Hepatoxicity: Grade > 3 hepatotoxicity (ALT or AST >5 x ULN) in 2-3% in registration trials, but rates were 4 x higher with HBV or HCV co-infection. Data from DUET-1 and -2 showed no increase in hepatotoxicity rates in patients with HBV or HCV coinfection (*JAC* 2010; 65:2450).

- Lipids: Grade ≥ 3 LDL-C (>190 mg/dL) and triglyceride >750 mg/dL were noted in 5-7% in registration trials.

- Psychiatric: Grade ≥3-0.2%; signficantly less than EFV.

DRUG INTERACTIONS: See Tables 5-37 and 5-38.

- ETR is a substrate for CYP3A4, 2C19 and 2C9 and undergoes glucuronidation *in vitro*; it is an inducer of CYP3A4, 2B6. and Phase II enzyme and an inhibitor of 2C9 and 2C19.

- Switches from EFV to ETR are anticipated due to resistance or intolerance. This switch has potential pharmacologic complications due to the long half-life of EFV and its prominent impact on hepatic cytochrome CYP450 enzymes, especially CYP3A4. A trial of co-administration found significantly lower ETR levels, with ETR ratios of AUC-0.71, C_{max} 0.78, C_{trough} 0.67. The authors concluded that the CYP3A4 induction effect of EFV lasted at least 2 wks after discontinuation, but the decrease in ETR levels was probably not clinically significant (*JAIDS* 2009;52:222) (see pg. 248).

- An extensive drug interaction report from the sponsor reports the following drug interactions (*Clin Phamacokinet* 2011;50:25):
  - Drugs with no clinically significant effect on ETR: **atorvastatin, clarithromycin, methadone, omeprazole oral contraceptives, paroxetine, ranitidine** and **sildenafil**.
  - Drugs that have no clinically significant interactions: **azithromycin** and **ribavirin**.
  - Caution advised with: **Digoxin** (follow levels); **rifabutin** in presence of some **PI/r; clarithromycin** (use azithromycin for MAC); **atorvastatin** (dose adjustment); **clopidogrel** (dose adjustment); **diazepan** (lower diazepam dose or alternative); **dexamethasone**: caution or alternative; **cyclosporine**.
  - Not recommended: **Carbamazepine, phenyloin, rifampin, rifapentine, St. John's wort**.

PREGNANCY: Category B. Studies of ETR in pregnant women are inadequate to recommend use or dose although preliminary data suggest pharmacokinetics similar to those of non-pregnant women (*AIDS* 2009;23:434; *Antiriviral Ther* 2010;15:677). The 2010 DHHS Guidelines on Antiretroviral Agents for Pregnant Women classify ETR as "insufficient data to recommend use."

■ TABLE 5-37: **ETR Drug Interactions with ART (AUC)**

Co-agent	AUC ETR	Co-admin drug (AUC)	Recommendation
TDF	↓ 19%	↑ 15% (NS)	Standard dose
EFV	↓ 41%	May ↓	Avoid
NVP	↓ 55%	May ↓	Avoid
MVC	↓ 36%	↓ 53%	MVC 600 mg bid (if not co-administered w/ a PI)
MVC + DRV/r	↓↓	↑ 110%	Decrease MVC 150 mg bid
NFV	↓	May ↑	No data – avoid
ATV	↑ 50%	↓ 17%	Avoid
ATV/r	↑ 30%	↓ 14%	Avoid, but clinical significance unclear
FPV/r	NC	↑ 69%	Avoid, but clinical significance unclear
DRV/r	↓ 37%	↑ 15%	Standard doses; extensive data
LPV/r	↓ 30-45%	↓ 18%	Standard doses
TPV/r	↓ 76%	↑ 18%	Avoid
SQV + LPV/r		NC	Standard doses
RTV (high dose)	↓ 46%		Avoid
IDV	↑ 50%	↓ 46%	Avoid
RAL	↑ 10%	↓ 10%	Standard doses

NC = No significant change

Drug Information

■ TABLE 5-38: **ETR Drug Interactions with Other Drugs**

Class	Agent	Effect on co-administered drug or ETR
Statin	Atorvastatin	↓ AUC statin 37%; use standard dose and monitor response
	Lovastatin	Statin may be ↓
	Simvastatin	Statin may be ↓
	Rosuvastatin	Considered preferred; standard dose; no interaction
	Pravastatin	Considered preferred; standard dose; no interaction
Anti-mycobacterial agents	Rifampin	Significant ↓ ETR-avoid
	Rifabutin	Rifabutin AUC ↓ 17%; ETR↓ 37% Rifabutin 300 mg/d and ETR standard dose if no PI/r used. Do not co-administer DRV/r or SQV/r. With LPV/r use RBT 150 mg every other day or 3x/week. For the treatment of TB, most experts recommend 150 mg qd with PI/r. Consider rifabutin TDM.
Gastric agents	Omeprazole	ETR AUC ↑ 41%; standard dose
	Ranitidine	ETR AUC ↓ 14%; standard dose
Antibiotics	Clarithromycin	ETR AUC ↑ 42%; Clarithromycin AUC ↓ 39% MAC – use azithromycin S. pneumoniae – use azithromycin
Methadone	Methadone	No change; standard doses
Anti-arrhythmia drugs	See comment	Amniodarone, bepridil, disopyramide, flecainide, lidocaine, mexiletine, propafenone, quinidine – may ↓ with ETR co-administration; use with caution.
Anticonvulsants	Phenobarbital, Phenytoin, Carbamazepam	ETR levels ↓↓– avoid Anticonvulsant levels may ↓ also
Erectile dysfunction	Sildenafil	Sildenafil AUC ↓ 57%; titrate to effect
Ethinyl Estradiol		Ethinyl estradiol AUC ↑ 22%, significance unclear; consider barrier method
Steroids	Dexamethasone	↓ ETR levels may ↓ – consider alternative steroid
Antifungal	Azoles (See pg. 208)	ETR AUC ↑ 86% with fluconazole. ETR AUC ↑ 36% with voriconazole. ETR levels may ↑ with other azoles. Standard dose with caution – voriconazole, fluconazole and posaconazole. Itraconazole levels may ↓ and voriconazole levels ↑14%; monitor levels and consider dose adjustment
Antidepressants	St. John's wort	May significantly ↓ ETR - Avoid
	Paroxetine	No change. Standard dose.
Immuno suppressants	Cyclosporin, Tacrolimus, Sirolimus	May ↓ immunosuppressants; Monitor levels closely
Anti-platelet	Clopidogrel	May ↓ the efficacy of clopidogrel. Avoid
Anti-coagulation	Warfarin	May ↑ INR; Monitor closely

5 Drug Information

FAMCICLOVIR – see Acyclovir (pg. 186)

FENOFIBRATE – see also Gemfibrozil (pg. 293)

TRADE NAME: *Tricor* (Abbott Laboratories), *Antara* (Reliant), *Lofibra* (Gate), *Triglide* (Sciele Pharmaceutical, Inc.)

FORMS: *Tricor* tabs, 48 and 145 mg; *Lofibra* caps 67 mg, 134 mg, 200 mg, *Antara* caps, 43 and 130 mg

COST: 48 mg tab at $1.72, 145 mg tab at $5.16

CLASS: Fibrate

INDICATIONS AND DOSES: Fibrates have documented evidence of reducing risk of cariovascular disease in patients who have dyslipidemia without HIV infection, and they have documented benefit for reducing triglycerides and increasing HDL in HIV-infected patients (*Expert Opin Drug Metab Toxicol* 2010;6:995). The usual indication is hypertriglyceridemia, especially levels of >500-700 mg/dL. Starting dose 48 mg qd then increase if necessary at 4-8 wk intervals; maximum dose – 145 mg qd; some authorities consider this the usual dose (*CID* 2006;43:645). Take as a single daily dose with meal. Fenofibrate is by far the most prescribed fibrate in the US with 73% of the market (*JAMA* 2011;305:1221) Gemfibrozil is second with 11%.

MONITORING: Triglyceride levels – discontinue use if ineffective after 2 mos at 145 mg qd (maximum dose). Warn patients to report symptoms of myositis and obtain CPK if there is muscle tenderness, pain, or weakness. Monitor AST + ALT – discontinue if there is an otherwise unexplained CPK increase to $\geq$3x ULN.

CLINICAL TRIALS: ACTG 5087 compared fenofibrate 200 mg/d and pravastatin 40 mg/d in 194 HIV-infected patients with dyslipidemia. At 48 weeks most patients required the addition of the alternative agent. Both drugs were well tolerated, and the combination produced substantial benefit, but <10% of patients achieved the goals set by the National Cholesterol Education Program (NCEP) at 1 year (*AIDS Res Human Retroviruses* 2005;21:757). See pg. 144.

Another trial compared fenofibrate to pioglitazone in patients with metabolic syndrome attributed to PI-based ART (*CID* 2005;40:745). Pioglitazone improved insulin resistance, reduced triglyceride levels, and increased levels of HDL cholesterol, and fenofibrate did not significantly alter lipids or insulin resistance (*CID* 2005;40:745). Other studies have found that fenofibrate has a significant benefit in reducing triglyceride levels in patients with ART-associated hyperlipidemia (*Am J Med Sci* 2004;327:315; *CID* 2006;43:645).

PRECAUTIONS: Avoid or use with caution with gallbladder disease, hepatic disease or renal failure with CrCl <50 mL/min.

Drug Information

PHARMACOLOGY

- **Bioavailability:** Good, improved 35% with food.
- **T½:** 20 h
- **Elimination:** Renal – 60%; fecal – 25%
- **Renal failure:** 54 mg qd; increase with caution due to risk of myopathy, and monitor CPK.

SIDE EFFECTS

Hepatic: Dose-related hepatotoxicity with increased transaminase levels to >3x ULN in 6% receiving doses of 134-201 mg qd; most had return to normal levels with drug discontinuation or with continued treatment.

- **Influenza-like syndrome**
- **Rash, pruritus, and/or urticaria** in 1-3%
- **Myositis:** Warn patient about symptoms of muscle pain, tenderness, and/or weakness, especially with fever or malaise. Measure CPK and discontinue if significantly typical symptoms occur.
- **Rare:** Pancreatitis, agranulocytosis, cholecystitis, eczema, thrombocytopenia.

DRUG INTERACTIONS

Oral anticoagulant: Potentiates warfarin activity; **Cholestyramine** and **colestipol** – bind fenofibrate – take fenofibrate >1 hr before or 4-6 hrs after bile acid binding agent; **Statins** – increase risk of rhabdomyolysis with renal failure.

PREGNANCY: Category C

FENTANYL

TRADE NAME: *Duragesic* (Janssen), *Fentanyl Oralet* (Abbott Laboratories), and generic

FORMS AND COST:

- Injection-fentanyl citrate, 50 µg/mL/2/ mL vial at $0.48
- Buccal (transmucosal) lozenge – 200, 300, and 400 µg
- Transdermal
  - 25 µg/h (10 cm²) *Duragesic* 25: $14.43
  - 50 µg/h (20 cm²) *Duragesic* 50: $26.38
  - 75 µg/h (30 cm²) *Duragesic* 75: $40.23
  - 100 µg/h (40 cm²) *Duragesic* 100: $52.81

CLASS: Opiate; Schedule II controlled substance

INDICATIONS: Chronic pain requiring opiate analgesia

Drug Information

5

DOSING RECOMMENDATIONS (TABLE 5-39 AND 5-40):

- Dose depends on desired therapeutic effect, patient weight, PI interactions and most importantly, existing opiate tolerance. The initial dose in opiate-naïve patients is a system delivering 25 µg/hr. Cachectic patients should not receive a higher initial dose unless they have been receiving the equivalent of 135 mg of oral morphine.

- **Maintenance**: Most patients are maintained with patch applications at 72-hr intervals. Adequacy of analgesia should be evaluated at 72 hrs. The dose should be increased to maintain the 72-hr interval if possible, but application every 48 hrs is another option. Supplemental opiates may be required with initial use to control pain and to determine optimal fentanyl dose. The suggested conversion ratio is 90 mg of oral morphine/24 hrs to each 25 µg/hr labeled delivery. To convert patients who currently receive opiate therapy, see Table 5-39 and Table 5-40.

APPLICATION INSTRUCTIONS: The protective liner-cover should be peeled just prior to use. Apply is to a dry, non-irritated, flat surface of the upper torso by firm pressure for 30 seconds. Hair should be clipped, not shaven, and the skin cleansed with water (not soaps or

■ TABLE 5-39: **Fentanyl Dose Conversion Chart**

Generic Name	Equianalgesic Dose (mg)	
	Parenteral	Oral
Codeine	120	200
Fentanyl	0.1	NA
Hydrocodone	NA	20
Hydromorphone	1.5	6-7.5
Meperidine	75-100	300
Morphine	10	30-40
Oxycodone	NA	15-30
Propoxyphene (napsylate salt form)	NA	200

■ TABLE 5-40: **Equivalence of Fentanyl Patches and Oral Morphine Sulfate**

Oral MS/day	Fentanyl (µg/hour)	Oral MS/day	Fentanyl (µg/hour)
45-134 mg	25	495-584 mg	150
135-224 mg	50	675-764 mg	200
225-314 mg	75	855-994 mg	250
315-404 mg	100	1035-1124 mg	300

Drug Information

alcohol that could irritate skin) prior to application. Avoid external heat to the site because absorption is temperature-dependent. Rotate sites with sequential use. After removal, the used system should be folded so the adhesive side adheres to itself and flushed in the toilet.

NOTE: Buccal (transmucosal) form should be used only with monitoring in the hospital (OR, ICU, EW) due to life-threatening respiratory depression. Use in AIDS is primarily restricted to management of chronic pain in late-stage disease using the transdermal form. This drug should not be used for the management of acute pain.

PHARMACOLOGY: Transdermal fentanyl systems deliver an average of 25 µg/hr/10 cm^2 at a constant rate. Serum levels increase slowly, plateau at 12-24 hrs, and then remain constant for up to 72 hrs. The labeling indicates the amount of fentanyl delivered per hour. Peak serum levels for the different systems are the following: Fentanyl – 25: 0.3-1.2 ng/mL, 50: 0.6-1.8 ng/mL, 75: 1.1-2.6 ng/mL, and 100: 1.9-3.8 ng/mL. After discontinuation, serum levels decline with a mean half-life of 17 hrs. Absorption depends on skin temperature and theoretically increases by one-third when the body temperature is 40° C. In acute pain models, the 100 µg/hr form provided analgesia equivalent to 60 mg of morphine IM.

SIDE EFFECTS

- **Respiratory depression** with hypoventilation. This occurs throughout the therapeutic range of fentanyl concentration but increases at concentrations >2 ng/mL in opiate-naïve patients and in patients with pulmonary disease.

- **CNS depression** is seen with concentrations >3 ng/mL in opiate-naïve patients. At levels of 10-20 ng/mL there is anesthesia and profound respiratory depression.

- **Tolerance** occurs with extended courses, but there is considerable individual variation.

- **Local effects** include erythema, papules, pruritus, and edema at the site of application.

- **Drug interactions** include increased fentanyl levels with all CYP3A4 inhibitors (PIs and DLV) given concurrently. The drug is metabolized by cytochrome P450 isoenzyme 3A4 so strong inhibitors of CYP 3A4 will increase fentanyl and risk respiratory arrest. This includes most PIs and especially boosted PIs. Consider morphine with concurrent use with PIs. EFV, NVP, ETR may decrease fentanyl levels. Interaction unlikely with MVC, RAL, ENF and NRTIs.

PREGNANCY: Category C

FILGRASTIM – see G-CSF (pg. 291)

5 Drug Information

FLUCONAZOLE

TRADE NAME: *Diflucan* (Pfizer) and generic

FORMS AND COST: Tabs: 50 mg at $5.31, 100 mg at $8.75, 150 mg at $13.93, 200 mg at $13.64. IV vials: 200 mg at $24.00, and 400 mg at $30.00; oral solution 10 mg/mL (35 mL bottle) at $35.80

PATIENT ASSISTANCE PROGRAM: 800-869-9979

CLASS: Triazole related to other imidazoles – ketoconazole, clotrimazole, miconazole; triazoles (fluconazole and itraconazole) have three nitrogens in the azole ring.

ACTIVITY: *Candida* – active vs. 95% of all strains in fluconazole-naïve patients except *C. krusei*, many *C. glabrata*, and some *C. tropicalis* and *C. parapsilosis*. Also active against: *Blastomyces, Coccidioidomyces, His-toplasma, Paracoccioidomyces, Sporothrix*, and *Cryptococcus*. Not active against *Aspergillus, Phycomyces, P. boydii*, and *Zygomyces*.

DOSE: See Table 5-41.

FUNGUS-SPECIFIC USES: See Table 5-41, *Candida* pg. 425, cryptococcosis pg. 435 and histoplasmosis pg. 451.

RESISTANCE: Fluconazole is the preferred azole for systemic treatment of candidiasis, but a major concern with long-term use is azole-resistant candidiasis, which correlates with amount of azole exposure and CD4 count <50/mm^3 (*JID* 1996;173:219) (see pg. 427). All oral systemically active azoles predispose to resistance. Some cases involve evolution of resistance by *C. albicans*, and others reflect substitution with non-*albicans* species such as *C. glabrata* or *C. krusei* (*AAC* 2002;46:1723). Resistance is uncommon when fluconazole is used to treat vaginitis (*CID* 2001;33:1069; *Med Mycol* 2005;43:647). Fluconazole-resistant strains of *Candida* can often be treated with caspofungin (*AAC* 2002;46:1723), micafungin (*CID* 2004;39:842), or amphotericin and possibly itraconazole, voriconazole (*CID* 2001;33:1447) or posaconazole. Resistance does not appear to be an issue with Cryptococcal infections (but reports of reduced efficacy with MIC mcg/mL) with the possible exception *C. gatti* (*AAC* 2009;53:309; *J Med Microbiol* 2011;60:961), which is a regional risk in the Pacific Northwest US, British Columbia and South America (*MMWR* 2010;59:865).

CLINICAL TRIALS: Cochrane Library review of 38 trials of treatment of oropharyngeal candidiasis in HIV-infected patients found that 1) fluconazole had a higher cure rate to topical agents (OR = 1:1.7), 2) cure rates for fluconazole and itraconazole were similar (OR = 1.05), 3) mycological cure rates were significantly better with fluconazole and itraconazole than with clotrimazole (OR = 1:1.5 and 1:2.2), and 4) continuous fluconazole was superior to intermittent fluconazole for preventing recurrence of thrush (OR = 0.04) (*Cochrane Database Syst Rev* 2006; CD 003940), but this is generally not recommended due to

■ TABLE 5-41: **Dose Recommendations for Fluconazole**†

Indications	Dose Regimen	Comment
Candidiasis (see pg. 425)		
Thrush		
Acute*	100 mg po qd x 7-14 d	Response rate 80% to 100%, usually within 5 days; may need up to 400-800 mg/day. Maintenance therapy often required in late-stage disease without immune reconstitution. Topical therapy (e.g., clotrimazole) preferred. Chronic treatment: Indication is severe or frequent recurrence. Options are topical agent prn or chronic suppressive oral fluconazole. Risk of fluconazole resistance is increased
Secondary Prevention*	100 mg po 3 x/wk or qd	
Esophagitis		
Acute	100-200 mg po qd or IV up to 400 mg/d x 14-21 d	Relapse rate is 85-90%. Relapse rate is >80% within 1 year in absence of maintenance therapy.
Maintenance	100-200 mg po qd	Maintenance may be required for recurrent esophagitis but increases risk of resistance.
Vaginitis		
Treatment	150 mg po x 1	Response rate 90% to 100% in absence of HIV infection.
Prevention*	Multiple recurrences: 150 mg po qw	Topical azoles generally preferred.
Cryptococcosis (see pg. 435) (CID 2010;50:291)		
Non-meningeal, acute	400 mg/day po x 6-12 mos or amphotericin B + 5FC*	Fluconazole is recommended by the IDSA as the preferred treatment + flucytosine (100 mg/kg/day) for cryptococcal pneumonia
Meningitis		
Acute	1200 mg/d (up to 2000 mg/d) po x10-12 wks or 1200 mg/d ı flucytosino, then maintenance or 1200 mg/d + 5FC x6 wks	Acute treatment with amphotericin B + 5-FC ≥ 2 weeks is preferred
Consolidation (after ampho induction)*	400 mg po qd x 8 wks, followed by maintenance	Continue maintenance until immune reconstitution with CD4 >100-200/mm³ x >6 months.
Maintenance*	200 mg po qd	
Coccidioidomycosis (see pg. 432)		
Meningitis*	400-800 mg IV or po	Preferred for meningeal form.
Non-meningeal		
Acute	400-800 mg po qd	Amphotericin B usually preferred, except with mild disease.*
Maintenance*	400 mg po qd	Itraconazole considered equally effective.
Histoplasmosis (see pg. 451)		
Treatment	800 mg qd	Amphotericin B and itraconazole preferred.

† Sources: *CID* 2000;30:652; *CID* 2010;50:291; 2008 IDSA/NIH/CDC Guidelines for Treatment and Prevention of Opportunistic Infections; and American Thoracic Society (*Am J Respir Crit Care Med* 2011;183:96)

* Preferred agent (2008 CDC/IDSA/NIH OI Guidelines)

Drug Information

5

risk of resistance. The efficacy of fluconazole for the treatment of cryptococcal meningitis appears to be dose related, with doses of 1200 mg/d in one study (*CID* 2008;47:1556).

PHARMACOLOGY: See Table 5-41, pg. 277.

- **Bioavailability:** >90%
- **CSF levels:** 50-94% of serum levels
- **T½:** 30 h
- **Elimination:** Renal; 60-80% of administered dose excreted unchanged in the urine
- **Dose modification in renal failure:** CrCl >50 mL/min – usual dose; 10-50 mL/min – half dose; CrCl <10 mL/min – quarter dose; hemodialysis – standard dose (200-400 mg) after each dialysis.

SIDE EFFECTS: Generally well tolerated. Headache, nausea, and abdominal pain, the most common side effects, are dose-related and most common with >400 mg/d (*JAC* 2006;57:384). GI intolerance (1.5-8%, usually does not require discontinuation); rash (5%); transient increases in hepatic enzymes (5%), increases of ALT or AST to >8x upper limit of normal requires discontinuation (1%); dizziness, hypokalemia, and headache (2%). Reversible alopecia in 10-20% receiving ≥400 mg qd at median time of 3 mos after starting treatment (*Ann Intern Med* 1995;123:354).

DRUG INTERACTIONS: Inhibits cytochrome P450 (2C8/9/19 and 3A4) hepatic enzymes resulting in increased levels of **atovaquone**, some **benzodiazepines, alprazolam, diazepam, midazolam, triazolam, clarithromycin, fentanyl, oral hypoglycemics, phenytoin, warfarin, SQV, rifabutin, cyclosoporine, simvastatin, lovastatin tacrolimus,** and **sirolimus; cisapride, terfenadine** and **astemizole** may cause life-threatening arrhythmias. Fluconazole levels are reduced with **rifampin**; with **rifabutin** there is no effect on fluconazole levels, but rifabutin AUC increases 80%; consider rifabutin TDM. Unlike ketoconazole, voriconazole and itraconazole, fluconazole can be used without dose modification with PIs and NNRTIs except with **NVP,** which increases with NVP levels – monitor for hepatotoxicity and rash or avoid this combination. Effect of RTV boosting of PIs is not well known. **ETR** AUC increased 86% with fluconazole co-administration. Fluconazole increases **AZT** AUC 74% due to decreased AZT glucuronidation; monitor for AZT toxicity. **Fluconazole** may decrease efficacy of **clopidogrel**; avoid (see pg. 208t).

PREGNANCY: Category C. Animal studies show reduced maternal weight gain and embryolethality with dose >20x comparable to doses in humans; sketal and craniofacial abnormalities in infants born to four women given fluconazole in pregnancy. Single dose considered safe for candida vaginitis – topical treatment preferred. Amphotericin B preferred for systemic fungal infection in first trimester if efficacy expected.

Drug Information

FLUCYTOSINE (5-FC)

TRADE NAME: *Ancobon* (ICN Pharmaceuticals) and generic

FORMS AND COST: Caps: 250 mg at $24.68, 500 mg at $47.75

CLASS: Structurally related to fluorouracil

INDICATIONS AND DOSE: See pg. 434. Used with amphotericin B or fluconazole to treat serious cryptococcosis. IDSA guidelines (*CID* 2010; 50:291) and ATS Guidelines (*Am J Respir Crit Care* 2011;183:96) recommend treating cryptococcal meningitis with amphotericin B + flucytosine 100 mg/kg/d in 4 doses for ≥2 wks based on several studies showing benefit of this treatment (reduced rate of relapse and more rapid sterilization of CSF) compared with amphotericin B alone (*CID* 2010;50:345; *NEJM* 1997;337:15; *NEJM* 1992;326:83; *Ann Intern Med* 1990;113: 183; *JID* 1992;165:960; *CID* 1999;28:291). The combination of amphotericin and flucytosine is synergistic against *Cryptococcus in vitro* and *in vivo* (*AAC* 2006;50:113). The combination of fluconazole + 5-FC is also effective, but toxicity at higher 5-FC doses may limit use of 5-FC (*CID* 1994;19:741; *JID* 1992;165:960). Fluconazole (1200 mg/d) + 5-FC (100 mg/kg/d) x 2 wks, followed by fluconazole 800 mg/d resulted in fewer deaths at 2 wks (10% vs. 37%) compared to fluconazole (800 mg) alone (*CID* 2010;50:338). 5-FC (150 mg/kg/d) with fluconazole has been studied for treatment of nonmeningeal cryptococcosis (*CID* 2000;30: 710). Neutropenia and thrombocytopenia are relative contraindications to flucytosine. Multiple trials suggest amphotericin B + 5-FC for 14 days is the most effective induction regimen in patients with a high fungal burden at baseline (*CID* 2008;3:e2870). Flucytosine is concentrated in urine and can be used for *Candida* UTIs (*CID* 2011;52 Suppl 6:S457)

- **Dose:** 25 mg/kg po q6h (100 mg/kg/d)

PHARMACOLOGY

- **Bioavailability:** >80%
- **T½:** 2.4-4.8 h
- **Elimination:** 63-84% unchanged in urine
- **CNS penetration:** 80% of serum levels
- **Dose modification in renal failure:** CrCl >50 mL/min – 25.0 mg/kg q6h; 10-50 mL/min – 25 mg/kg q12-24h; <10 mL/min – 25 mg/kg q24h (use with close monitoring of CBC and 5-FC serum level).
- **Therapeutic monitoring:** Measure serum concentration 2 hrs post-oral dose with goal of peak level of 30-80 µg/mL after 3-5 days.
- **Resistance:** MIC ≥32 mg/mL may be considered resistant

SIDE EFFECTS: Dose-related leukopenia and thrombocytopenia, especially with levels >100 mcg/mL and concurrent use of other marrow-suppressing agents, and in patients with renal insufficiency, which can occur secondary to concurrent amphotericin B therapy; GI intolerance; rash; hepatitis; peripheral neuropathy.

5 Drug Information

PREGNANCY: Category D. – First trimester exposures to doses 400-800 mg/d. New FDA rating 7/3/11 due to rare and distinctive birth defects. This does not apply to low dose used for vaginal yeast infections.

DRUG INTERACTIONS: Drugs that cause bone marrow suppression (e.g. AZT, ganciclovir, pyrimethamine, interferon). Avoid or use with caution.

FLUOROQUINOLONES – see Ciprofloxacin (pg. 214) and Table 5-18 (pg. 216)

FLUOXETINE

TRADE NAME: *Prozac* and *Prozac Weekly* (Eli Lilly) and generic

FORMS AND COST: Caps: 10 mg at $2.60, 20 mg at $2.67, 40 mg at $5.19. Solution 20 mg/5 mL (120 mL bottle) $118.

CLASS: Selective serotonin reuptake inhibitors (SSRI) antidepressant. Other drugs in this class include *Paxil, Zoloft, Celexa*, and *Lexapro*.

INDICATIONS AND DOSE

- **Major depression:** 10-40 mg/d usually given once daily in the morning. Onset of response requires 2-6 wks. Doses of 5-10 mg qd may be adequate in debilitated patients. *Prozac Weekly*: 90 mg/wk.

- **Obsessive-compulsive disorder:** 20-80 mg qd

PHARMACOLOGY

- **Bioavailability:** 60-80%

- **T½:** 7-9 days for norfluoxetine (active metabolite)

- **Elimination:** Metabolized by liver to norfluoxetine; fluoxetine eliminated in urine.

- **Dose modification in renal failure:** None

- **Dose modification in cirrhosis:** Half-life prolonged – reduce dose

SIDE EFFECTS: Toxicity may not be apparent for 2-6 wks. GI intolerance (anorexia, weight loss, nausea) – 20%; anxiety, agitation, insomnia, sexual dysfunction – 20%; less common – headache, tremor, drowsiness, dry mouth, sweating, diarrhea, acute dystonia, akathisia (sensation of motor restlessness).

NOTE: Case reports have suggested an association with suicidal ideation; reanalysis of data showed no significant difference compared with treatment with other antidepressants or placebo (*J Clin Psychopharmacol* 1991;11:166). Nevertheless, the FDA required manufacturers of SSRIs to add a warning label concerning increased risk of suicide with antidepressant initiation.

DRUG INTERACTIONS

- **MAO inhibitors:** Avoid initiation of fluoxetine until ≥14 days after discontinuing MAO inhibitor; avoid starting MAO inhibitor until ≥5 wks after discontinuing fluoxetine (risk is "serotonergic syndrome").

- **Inhibits 2D6 > 2C9; 1A2 > 3A4); Substrate 2C9, 2D6:** May increase levels of tricyclic agents (desipramine, nortriptyline, etc.), phenytoin, digoxin, coumadin, terfenadine (ventricular arrhythmias; avoid), SQV, astemizole (avoid), theophylline, thioridazine (contraindicated), mesoridazine (avoid), haloperidol, carbamazepine and pimozide (avoid).
- **Ritonavir:** Serotonin syndrome has been reported (*AIDS* 2001; 15:1281).
- **Linezolid:** Avoid co-administration. May increase risk of serotonin syndrome. Discontinue fluoxetine or other SSRI 14 days before starting linezolid (*CID* 2006;42:1578), but some advocate a shorter washout period (*CID* 2006;43:180).

PREGNANCY: Category C

FLURAZEPAM – see Benzodiazepines (pg. 207)

FOSAMPRENAVIR (FPV)

TRADE NAME: *Lexiva* (ViiV Healthcare/GlaxoSmithKline); in Europe, *Telzir* (ViiV Healthcare/GlaxoSmithKline)

CLASS: Protease inhibitor (pro-drug of amprenavir)

PATIENT ASSISTANCE PROGRAM: 800-722-9294

FORMULATIONS, REGIMENS AND COST:

- **Form:** 700 mg tab; 50 mg/mL solution (225 mL)
- **Regimen:** Four regimens are FDA-approved
  - □ FPV 1400 mg bid (without ritonavir, PI-naïve only)
  - □ FPV/r 1400/100 mg qd (PI-naïve only) with food
  - □ FPV/r 1400/200 mg qd (PI-naïve only) with food (FPV/r 1400/100 mg qd preferred)
  - □ FPV/r 700/100 mg bid (PI-naïve or experienced) with food
- **AWP:** $1,738.88/mo for 1400 mg bid regimen

FOOD EFFECT: Not significant except with RTV boosting.

EFV: With EFV, use RTV-boosted regimens. If using once daily regimen, increase RTV dose to 300 mg qd (FPV/r 1400/300 mg qd).

RENAL FAILURE: Standard dose

HEPATIC FAILURE: Child-Pugh score: 5-8, FPV 700 mg bid without RTV boosting; >8, avoid FPV

STORAGE: Room temperature, up to 25°C or 77°F

CLINICAL TRIALS: See Table 5-42.

- The **KLEAN** trial (*Lancet* 2006;368:476) was the major comparative clinical trial in treatment-naïve patients. Comparison of FPV/r bid vs. LPV/r bid found nearly identical results at 48 weeks in all important endpoints, including viral suppression to <50 c/mL (66% vs. 65%), CD4 count increase, treatment discontinuation due to adverse events (12% vs. 10%), effect of treatment on lipids, and frequency of treatment-emergent drug resistance. (Note: LPV/r formulation used in this trial was the gel capsule formulation.)

- In the **SOLO** trial, FPV/r 1400/200 qd (with ABC/3TC) was non-inferior at 48 weeks to NFV+ABC/3TC in treatment-naïve patients (*AIDS* 2004;18:1529). Patients who completed SOLO and had viral suppression (<400 c/mL) on FPV/r were followed for up to 142 wks. At 142 weeks, VL was <400 c/mL in 159/211 (75%) and <50 c/mL in 139/211 (66%). The median increase in CD4 cell count was 292/mm³. Resistance tests in 14 virologic failures showed no PI resistance mutations. The most common adverse reactions were

■ TABLE 5-42: **Clinical Trials of FPV in Treatment-naïve and PI-experienced Patients**

Trial	Regimen	N	Wks	VL (c/mL) <400	VL (c/mL) <50
SOLO Treatment-naïve (*AIDS* 2004;18:1529)	FPV/r 1400/200 mg qd + ABC/3TC	322	48	69%	55%
	NFV 1250 mg bid + ABC/3TC	327		68%	53%
NEAT Treatment-naïve (*JAIDS* 2004;35:22)	FPV 1400 mg bid + ABC/3TC	166	48	66%[†]	57%[†]
	NFV 1250 mg bid + ABC/3TC	83		52%	42%
CONTEXT Failure 1-2 PI regimens (6th CROI 2003, Abstr. 178)	FPV/r 700/100 mg bid + 2 NRTIs	107	48	58%	46%[‡]
	FPV/r 1400/200 mg qd + 2 NRTIs*	105			37%
	LPV/r 400/100 mg bid + 2 NRTIs	103		61%	50%[†]
TRIAD Failure > PI regimens (*JAC* 2009;64:398)	FPV/r 700/100 mg bid	24	24		21%
	FPV/r 1400/100 mg bid	24			24%
	FPV 1400 mg bid + LPV/r 533/133 mg bid	20			20%
KLEAN Treatment-naïve (*Lancet* 2006;368:476)	FPV/r 700/100 mg bid + ABC/3TC qd	434	48	73%	66%
	LPV/r 400/100 mg bid + ABC/3TC qd	444		71%	65%
COL100758 Treatment-naive (*AIDS Res Hum Retroviruses* 2009;25:395)	FPV/r 1400/200 mg qd	57	96	53%	53%
	FPV/r 1400/100 mg qd	58		78%[†]	66%
ALERT Treatment-naïve (*AIDS Res Ther* 2008;5:5)	FPV/r 1400/100 mg qd + TDF/FTC qd	45	48	79%	75%
	ATV/r 300/100 mg qd + TDF/FTC qd	49		87%	83%

† Superior to comparator (*P* <0.05)
‡ FPV/r did not meet the FDA criteria for "non-inferiority" criteria compared to LPV/r.
* The once-daily regimen in the CONTEXT trial was dropped due to virologic inferiority

Drug Information

diarrhea (10%), nausea (8%) and increased triglycerides (7%) (*Clin Ther* 2006;28:745).

- **COL100758 Trial:** This was an open- label trial in which 115 treatment-naïve patients were randomized to receive FPV/r 1400/200 mg qd vs. FPV/r 1400/100 mg qd. At 96 weeks, patients receiving RTV 100 mg qd had greater viral suppression to <400 c/mL (78% vs. 53%; p <0.006), lower triglyceride elevations (+27 vs. +48 mg/dL), fewer premature discontinuations for adverse reactions (12 vs. 24) and fewer virologic failures (5 vs. 8). None of the 8 with virologic failures had PI resistance mutations (*AIDS Res Hum Retroviruses* 2009;25:395).

- **LESS Trial:** This was another trial comparing FPV/r 1400/100 vs. FPV/r 1400/200 mg, but in this case the randomization came after achieving virologic suppression (<400 c/mL) on FPV/r 1400/200 mg once daily. At 24 weeks, VL was <50 c/mL in 92% and 94% for the daily RTV dose of 100 mg or 200 mg/d, respectively. Again, the lower dose of RTV was associated with lower triglyceride levels (*HIV Clin Trials* 2010;11:239).

- The **NEAT Trial** found unboosted FPV to be superior to NFV (*JAIDS* 2004;35:22). In a long-term follow-up analysis at 120 weeks in a subset of 211 patients who continued FPV/r qd, 139 (66%) still had VL <50 c/mL (*Clin Ther* 2006;28:745).

- **ALERT Trial:** This was a trial comparing once daily FPV/r (1400/100 mg) vs. ATV/r (300/100 mg), each in combination with TDF/FTC in 106 randomized treatment-naïve patients. At baseline the median VL was 4.9 $\log_{10}$ c/mL in each arm, and baseline CD4 counts were 176 and 205 cells/mm^3. At 48 weeks, VL was <50 c/mL in 40/53 (75%) of FPV/r recipients and 44/53 (83%) of ATV/r recipients by ITT analysis (p=0.34). Changes in lipids were similar (*AIDS Res Ther* 2008;5:5), but median triglyceride levels were higher with FPV/r (150 vs. 131 mg/dL). A subsequent report indicated that 4 FPV and ATV virologic failures had archived resistance strains (*AIDS Res Hum Retroviruses* 2010;26:407)

RESISTANCE: In trials of FPV in PI-naïve patients, the predominant mutations in patients experiencing virologic failure were 32I, 46I/L, 47V, 50V, 54L/M and 84V, all mutations that cause minimal cross-resistance with other PIs except for DRV. The primary PI mutation is I50V, which decreases susceptibility to LPV and DRV, and I84V, a multi-PI resistance mutation. Patients failing FPV/r in the SOLO trial had no PI mutations.

WARNINGS: Hepatic disease; dose modification (see pg. 149, 281).

ADVANTAGES: 1) Potency comparable to LPV/r (*Lancet* 2006;368:476) and ATV/r in treatment-naïve patients; 2) no food requirement if unboosted; 3) may be given once daily with RTV 100 mg (treatment-naïve only); and 4) no significant PI resistance when FPV/r used in treatment-naïve patients.

Drug Information

5

DISADVANTAGE: 1) Once-daily therapy not recommended for PI-experienced patients; 2) no advantage over coformulated LPV/r when given at 700/100 mg bid in terms of efficacy, tolerability or lipid effects; and 3) Once-daily FPV/r (1400/100 mg) is not as extensively studied as once-daily DRV/r or ATV/r.

PHARMACOLOGY

- **Absorption:** Not affected by food; bioavailability not established.
- **Elimination:** APV is an inhibitor, substrate, and likely an inducer of P450 3A4
- **T½:** 7.7 h
- **CNS penetration:** Effectiveness score is 2 in a 4 class system (*Neurology* 2011;76:693) (see pg. 550t).

SIDE EFFECTS : The most common causes for drug discontinuation for adverse reactions (6% in registration trials) are GI intolerance, transaminase elevations and rash.

- **Skin rash:** The common adverse reaction is skin rash, seen in 12-33% of patients (package insert); rash that is sufficiently severe to result in discontinuation in <1%. FPV contains a sulfa moiety, so

■ TABLE 5-43: **Combination of FPV with Other PIs and with NNRTIs**

Drug	Co-admin Drug	FPV	Comment
NVP	↑13%	↑ 29%	Avoid unboosted FPV. Dose FPV/r. 700/100 bid with NVP standard. Limited data (historical comparison *AAC* 2006;50:315)
EFV	↓ 30%	C_{min} ↓ 36%	Increase RTV dose to 300 mg/d (FPV/r 1400/300 QD) with once-daily dosing or use 700/100 mg bid
ATV	↓ 20%	↑ 78%	Avoid; inadequate data
IDV	No data	↑33%	Dose regimens not established
LPV/r	Trough ↓ 53%	Trough ↓ 64%	Avoid since doses are not estialished
DRV	No data	No data	No data; avoid
SQV	No data	↓ 32%	Avoid; inadequate data
ETR	No data	↑ 70%	Avoid; clinical significance unclear
MVC	May ↑	No change likely	MVC 150 mg bid
TPV	No data	↓ 41%	Avoid
NFV	No data	↑ 150%	Avoid; inadequate data
RTV	No data	↑ 100%	1400/200 mg or 1400/100 mg qd or 700/100 mg bid
DLV	↓ 61%	↑ 130%	Avoid co-administration
RAL	No change likely	No change likely	Usual dose

Drug Information

caution is advised with use in patients with a history of severe sulfa allergy, but no increase in rates of rashes was noted in such patients in the registration trials.

- **Cardiovascular disease:** A case control trial (**ANRS-04**) found that FPV treatment was associated with an increased risk of myocardial infarction with an odds ratio of 1.52 (*Arch Intern Med* 2010; 170:1228). This risk was also noted in the D:A:D review. As a result of these reports, the supplier sent a safety advisory in 2009 concerning the potential risk of FPV for acute myocardial infarction and increased cholesterol and triglycerides (12/3/2009).

- **GI intolerance** is most common and includes nausea, vomiting, diarrhea and/or abdominal pain, which are reported in up to 40%, but severe in only 5-10%; diarrhea is less frequent than with NFV (NEAT and SOLO trials). GI side effects with FPV/r were similar to those of LPV/r in the KLEAN trial.

- **Hepatotoxicity:** ALT levels are increased >5x ULN in 6-8%

- **Lipodystrophy:** Observed with FPV.

BLACK BOX WARNING: None

DRUG INTERACTIONS

- The following drugs are contraindicated for concurrent use: **alfuzolin*, amiodarone*, astemizole, bepridil*, cisapride, dihydro-ergotamine, ergotamine, flecainide*, lovastatin, midazolam, pimozide, pitavastatin, propafenone*, quinidine*, rifampin, St. John's wort, simvastatin, terfenadine,** and **triazolam.**

    *Contraindicated with FPV/r.

- The following drugs should be given concurrently with caution:

    Antacids: Decrease FPV 18%: Give 2 hrs before, one hour after or simultaneously with FPV; no data for FPV/r; (PPIs – no effect). **Phenobarbital, phenytoin,** and **carbamazepine** have potential to decrease APV levels and various effects on anticonvulsant levels – monitor anticonvulsant levels and use FPV/r or use alternative anticonvulsant. **Ethinyl estradiol/norethindrone** decrease APV levels; alternative birth control methods should be used. **R-methadone (active)** levels decrease 13% and APV AUC are decreased 25%; no withdrawl symptoms observed. **Paroxetine** AUC ↓55% w/FPV/r titrate. **Alprazolam** should be given with caution. **Rifampin** decreases APV AUC by 82% and should not be used concurrently. **Rifabutin** decreases APV AUC by 15% and FPV increases rifabutin AUC by 193%; use standard FPV dose and rifabutin at 150 mg qd or 300 mg 3x/wk. For the treatment of TB, most experts recommend 150 mg qd with PI/r. Consider rifabutin TDM. FPV/r: 150 mg qod or 150 mg 3x/wk. **Clarithromycin** increases APV AUC by 18%; use standard doses, reduce clarithromycin dose with renal failure. **Voriconazole:** No data but voriconazole level may be decreased with FPV/r (see pg. 413). **Ketoconazole** increased APV

5 Drug Information

AUC by 32% and ketoconazole AUC increases 44%; use standard doses of FPV and do not exceed 200/mg/d ketoconazole. **Atorvastatin** levels increased 150%; maximum daily dose of 10 mg. FPV increases **sildenafil** AUC by 2-11x; do not exceed 25 mg/48 hrs. **Vardenafil** AUC may also be increased – limit dosage to 2.5 mg/24 hrs (2.5 mg/72 hrs with FPV/r) **Fluticasone**: Avoid; consider beclomethasone. **Rosuvastatin:** no interaction. **Colchicine:** FPV increases colchicine levels.

PREGNANCY: Category C. Animal studies showed no embryo-fetal developmental abnormalities. There are inadequate data on safety and pharmacokinetics in pregnancy to recommend use (2010 DHHS Perinatal HIV Guidelines).

FOSCARNET

TRADE NAME: *Foscavir*; generic foscarnet (Hospira Worldwide)

FORMS AND COST: Vials: 6000 mg (250 mL) at $100.33 and 12,000 mg (500 mL) at $98.98

PATIENT ASSISTANCE PROGRAM: 800-488-3247

INDICATIONS AND ACTIVITY: Active against herpes viruses including CMV, HSV-1, HSV-2, EBV (oral hairy leukoplakia), VZV, HHV-6, HHV-8 (KS-related herpes virus), most ganciclovir-resistant CMV, and most acyclovir-resistant HSV and VZV. Also active against HIV-1 and HIV-2 *in vitro* and *in vivo* and has been used for HIV salvage (*Antiviral Ther* 2006;11:561; *J Clin Virol* 2008;43:212; *J Clin Virol* 2010;47:79). The frequency of CMV resistance *in vitro* is 20-30% after 6-12 mos of foscarnet treatment (*JID* 1998;177:770). Clinical effectiveness for CMV retinitis is equivalent to that of ganciclovir (*NEJM* 1992;326:213; *Ophthalmology* 1994;101:1250) but has more treatment-limiting side effects. *In vitro* activity against HHV-8 is good, but results with foscarnet treatment of KS are variable; if KS is a true neoplasm, this treatment is of doubtful utility once malignant transformation has occurred (*Science* 1998;282: 1837).

ADMINISTRATION: Controlled IV infusion using ≤24 mg/mL (undiluted) by central venous catheter or <12 mg/mL (diluted in 5% dextrose or saline) via a peripheral line. No other drug is to be given concurrently via the same catheter. Induction dose of 90 mg/kg q12h is given over ≥2 hr via infusion pump with adequate hydration. Maintenance treatment with 90-120 mg/kg is given over ≥2 hrs by infusion pump with adequate hydration. Many use 90 mg/kg/d for initial maintenance and 120 mg/kg/d for maintenance after re-induction for a relapse. See Tables 5-44, 5-45 and 5-46 for doses and dose adjustments in renal failure.

PHARMACOLOGY

- **Bioavailability:** 5-8% absorption with oral administration, but poorly tolerated

- **T½:** 3 h
- **CSF levels:** 15-70% of plasma levels
- **Elimination:** Renal exclusively

■ TABLE 5-44: **Dose Recommendations for Foscarnet**

Indication	Dose Regimen
CMV retinitis	Induction: 60 mg/kg IV q8h or 90 mg/kg IV q12h x 14-21 days Maintenance: 90-120 mg/kg IV qd*
CMV (other sites)	60 mg/kg IV q8h or 90 mg/kg IV q12h x 14-21 days, indications for maintenance treatment are unclear
Acyclovir-resistant HSV	40 mg/kg IV q8h or 60 mg/kg q12h x 3 weeks
Acyclovir-resistant VZV	40 mg/kg IV q8h or 60 mg/kg q12h x 3 weeks

* Survival and time to relapse may be significantly prolonged with maintenance dose of 120 mg/day vs. 90 mg/day (*JID* 1993;168:444).

■ TABLE 5-45: **Foscarnet Dose Adjustment in Renal Failure for HSV and CMV Infection (in mg/kg)**

CrCl (mL/min/kg)	HSV: Equivalent to 60 mg/kg q12h or 40 mg/kg q8h	CMV: Equivalent to (60 mg/kg q8h)	CMV: Equivalent to (90 mg/kg q12h)
>1.4	40 q8h	60 q8h	90 q12h
>1.0-1.4	30 q8h	45 q8h	70 q12h
>0.8-1.0	35 q12h	50 q12h	50 q12h
>0.6-0.8	25 q12h	40 q12h	80 q24h
>0.5-0.6	40 q24h	60 q24h	60 q24h
-0.4-0.5	35 q24h	50 q24h	50 q24h
<0.4	Not recommended †	Not recommended †	Not recommended †

■ TABLE 5-46: **Foscarnet Maintenance Dose Recommendations**

CrCl (mL/min/kg)	Adjusted dose based on recommendations with normal renal function 90 mg/kg/day (once daily)	Adjusted dose based on recommendations with normal renal function 120 mg/kg/d (once daily)
>1.4*	90 q24h	120 q24h
>1.0-1.4*	70 q24h	90 q24h
>0.8-1.0*	50 q24h	65 q24h
>0.6-0.8*	80 q48h	105 q48h
>0.5-0.6	60 mg q48h	80 q48h
>0.4-0.5	50 mg q48h	65 q48h
<0.4	Not recommended	Not recommended

* Low dose for initial therapy, high dose for relapse

† 38% removal with HD; consider 60 mg/kg post HD (*JID* 1991;64:785)

5 Drug Information

SIDE EFFECTS

- **Dose-related renal impairment:** 37% treated for CMV retinitis have serum creatinine increase to ≥2 mg/dL; most common in second week of induction and usually reversible with recovery of renal function within 1 wk of discontinuation. Monitor creatinine 2-3x/wk with induction and every 1-2 wks during maintenance. Modify dose for creatinine clearance changes. Foscarnet should be stopped for creatinine clearance <0.4 mL/min/kg.

- **Changes in serum electrolytes** including hypocalcemia (15%), hypophosphatemia (8%), hypomagnesemia (15%), and hypokalemia (16%). Patients should be warned to report symptoms of hypocalemia: Perioral paresthesias, extremity paresthesias, and numbness. Monitor serum calcium, magnesium, potassium, phosphate, and creatinine, usually ≥2x/wk during induction and 1x/wk during maintenance. If paresthesias develop with normal electrolytes, measure ionized calcium at start and end of infusion.

- **Seizures:** related to renal failure and hypocalcemia

- **Penile ulcers**

- **Miscellaneous:** Nausea, vomiting, headache, rash, fever, hepatitis, marrow suppression

DRUG INTERACTIONS: Concurrent administration with IV pentamidine may cause severe hypocalcemia. Avoid concurrent use of potentially nephrotoxic drugs such as amphotericin B, aminoglycosides, and pentamidine. Possible increase in seizures with imipenem.

PREGNANCY: Category C. Teratogenic in rodents. Recommend as alternative treatment of life- and site-threatening CMV infections.

FOSCAVIR – see Foscarnet (pg. 286)

FUNGIZONE – see Amphotericin B (pg. 190)

GANCICLOVIR AND VALGANCICLOVIR

TRADE NAME (IV AND ORAL FORMS)

- Ganciclovir: *Cytovene*, IV (Roche) and generic; *Vitrasert*, ocular implant (Bausch & Lomb)

- Valganciclovir: *Valcyte*, PO (Roche) (see Table 4-47)

FORMS AND COST: Ganciclovir: 500 mg vial at $88.36; valganciclovir: 450 mg tab at $49.10; implant: $19,200/implant, $38,400/yr

DOSE RECOMMENDATIONS: See pg. 441-449. Ganciclovir, 5 mg/kg IV q12h x 2 wk (induction), then 5 mg/kg IV qd (maintenance); valganciclovir, 900 mg po q12h x 3 wk (induction), then 900 mg qd (maintenance). Valganciclovir is the preferred oral formulation because it provides blood levels of ganciclovir comparable with those achieved

Drug Information

with recommended doses of IV ganciclovir (*NEJM* 2002;346:1119). Oral ganciclovir should no longer be used, and IV ganciclovir is reserved primarily for seriously ill patients and those who are unable to take oral medications. See Table 5-48 for doses.

■ TABLE 5-47: **Mean AUC with Valganciclovir Compared with IV Ganciclovir in Standard Doses (*NEJM* 2002;346:1119)**

	Valganciclovir	IV Ganciclovir
Induction AUC (µg/hr/mL)	32.8	28.6
Maintenance (µg/hr/mL)	34.9	30.7

■ TABLE 5-48: **Ganciclovir and Valganciclovir Dose Modification in Renal Failure (Induction Dose)**

Ganciclovir (IV Form)		Valganciclovir† (Oral Form)	
CrCl	Dose	CrCl	Dose
>80 mL/min	5 mg/kg q12h	>60 mL/min	900 mg bid
50-79 mL/min	2.5 mg/kg q12h	40-59 mL/min	450 mg bid
25-49 mL/min	2.5 mg/kg q24h	25-39 mL/min	450 mg qd
10-24 mL/min	1.25 mg/kg q24h	10-24 mL/min	450 mg qod (induction); 450 2x/wk (maintenance)
<10 mL/min*	1.25 mg/kg 3x/wk	<10 mL/min	Not recommended

* Hemodialysis: 1.25 mg/kg 3x/wk; give post-dialysis.
† Maintenance dose = 50% of induction dose

PATIENT ASSISTANCE PROGRAM: 800-282-7780

CLASS: Synthetic purine nucleoside analog of guanine

ACTIVITY: Active against herpes viruses including CMV, HSV-1, HSV-2, EBV, VZV, HHV-6, and HHV-8 (KSHV). About 10% of patients given ganciclovir ≥3 mos for CMV will have resistant strains that are sensitive to foscarnet (*JID* 1991;163:716; *JID* 1991;163:1348). The frequency of ganciclovir resistance at 9 mos in patients receiving maintenance IV ganciclovir therapy for CMV show retinitis is 26% (*JID* 1998; 177:770). Ganciclovir is active *in vitro* against HHV-8, but the clinical experience with ganciclovir treatment of KS is variable. A preliminary trial targeting the HHV-8 ORF 36 and ORF 21 lytic genes using high dose AZT (600 mg qid) and valganciclovir (900 mg bid) showed impressive results in 14 patients with Castleman disease (*Blood* 2011;117:6977).

INDICATIONS AND DOSE REGIMEN

■ **CMV retinitis:** A controlled trial of 141 patients randomized to receive IV ganciclovir (5 mg/kg/bid x 3 wks followed by 5 mg/kg qd) vs. oral valganciclovir (900 mg bid x 3 wks followed by 900 mg qd) showed comparable response rates (77% vs. 72% at 4 wks) and median time to progression (125 vs. 160 days) (*NEJM* 2002;346:1119). Oral valganciclovir is now the standard treatment. Multiple trials show that IV ganciclovir, IV foscarnet, IV cidofovir, oral valganciclovir, and the ganciclovir implant are all effective. The most effective systemic treatment in terms of efficacy, convenience and avoidance of toxicity is valganciclovir (*Clin Ophth* 2010;4:111). The preferred contemporary approach is ART used in combination with valganciclovir to prevent systemic CMV disease and contralateral retinitis (*NEJM* 1997;337:83;337:105; *Am J Ophthalmol* 1999;127: 329). Selected patients, especially those with zone 1 retinitis, may receive intra-vitreal injection of ganciclovir or implantation of the ganciclovir sustained release device. Current guidelines for initial management of CMV retinitis are summarized on pg. 441 (*Clin Ophthalol* 2010;4:285.)

Discontinuation of maintenance therapy can be considered in the setting of immune reconstitution with a CD4 count >100/mm^3 for 3-6 mos (*JAMA* 1999;282:1633). The 2008 CDC/NIH/IDSA Opportunistic Infections Guidelines recommendation is to make this decision in consultation with an ophthalmologist based on magnitude and duration of the CD4 response, anatomic location of the lesion, vision in the other eye, and feasibility of ophthalmologic monitoring.

- **Other forms of disseminated CMV:** Ganciclovir or foscarnet are the standard agents to treat CMV esophagitis, colitis, pneumoniitis and neurologic disease (see Table 5-47, pg 289 and pg. 444-447) (*AIDS* 2000;14:517; *CID* 2002;34:101). Recommendations for suspending maintenance therapy with immune reconstitution are unclear for non-ocular CMV, but most will follow the guidelines for CMV retinitis using a CD4 threshold of 100 cells/mm^3 x ≥3 mos (*AIDS* 2001;15:F1). Failures ascribed to lack of CMV-specific CD4 responses with recurrent CMV retinitis have been reported (*JID* 2001;183:1285).

PHARMACOLOGY

- **Bioavailability:** Valganciclovir – 60% absorption with food vs. 6-9% for oral ganciclovir. The valganciclovir formulation is rapidly hydrolyzed to ganciclovir after absorption.

- **Serum level:** Mean peak concentration with IV induction doses is 11.5 µg/mL (MIC$_{50}$ of CMV is 0.1-2.75 µg/mL).

- **CSF concentrations:** 24-70% of plasma levels; **intravitreal concentrations**: 10-15% of plasma levels – 0.96 µg/mL (*JID* 1993;168:1506); with gancyclovir implant, 4.1 mg/mL.

- **T½:** 2.5-3.6 h with IV administration; 3-7 h with oral administration. Intracellular T½: 18 h.

- **Elimination:** IV form: 90-99% excreted unchanged in urine. Oral form: 86% in stool and 5% recovered in urine.

Drug Information

- **Renal failure:** See Table 5-48, pg. 289. Hemodialysis removes 50% of ganciclovir (*Clin Pharmacol Ther* 2002;72:142).

SIDE EFFECTS, IV FORM

- **Neutropenia** with ANC <500/mm³ (25-40%) requires discontinuation of drug or G-CSF in 20%. Discontinuation or reduced dose will result in increased ANC in 3-7 days. Monitor CBC 2-3x/wk and discontinue if ANC <500/mm³ or platelet count <25,000/mm³.

- **Thrombocytopenia** in 2-8%

- **CNS toxicity** in 10-15% with headaches, seizures, confusion,

- **Hepatotoxicity** in 2-3%

- **GI intolerance** 2% (diarrhea)

- **Note:** Neutropenia (ANC <500/mm³) or thrombocytopenia (<25,000/dL) are contraindications to initial use.

SIDE EFFECTS, ORAL FORM: Of 212 patients with CMV retinitis followed for a median of 272 days, 10% developed neutropenia with ANC <500/mm³, hemoglobin <8 g/dL in 12%, diarrhea in 35%, nausea in 23%, and fever in 18% (*JAIDS* 2002;30:392). This is similar to the side effects with oral or IV ganciclovir.

DRUG INTERACTIONS: AZT increases the risk of neutropenia, and concomitant use is not recommended. Other **marrow-toxic drugs** include interferon, sulfadiazine, hydroxyurea, pyrimethamine, TMP-SMX, flucytosine, and cytotoxic agents (vincristine, vinblastine and doxorubicin). Oral and IV ganciclovir increase AUC of **ddI** by 100%; monitor for adverse effect of ddI or consider dose reduction of ddI. (Studies with enteric coated ddI have not been performed.) (*MMWR* 1999;48[RR 10]:48). **Probenecid** increases ganciclovir levels by 50%. Additive or synergistic activity with **foscarnet** *in vitro* against CMV and HSV.

PREGNANCY: Category C. Teratogenic in animals in concentrations comparable to those achieved in humans; should be avoided unless need justifies the risk.

G-CSF (Filgrastim)

TRADE NAME: *Neupogen* (Amgen)

FORMS AND COST: 300 µg in 1 mL vial at $291.24; 480 µg in 1.6 mL vial at $463.74

REIMBURSEMENT ASSISTANCE/APPEAL: 800-272-9376

NOTE: 300 µg vial and 480 µg vial are the only forms available. Pharmacists commonly instruct patients to discard unused portion; the cost-effective alternative is to retain the unused portion in refrigerated syringes for later use. For example, a 75 µg dose = 1 immediate dose and 3 syringes with subsequent doses.

PATIENT INSTRUCTIONS: Subcutaneous injections are usually self administered into the abdomen or upper thighs or in the back of upper arms if injected by someone else. Injection sites should be rotated. The drug should be stored in a refrigerator at 36-46°F.

PRODUCT INFORMATION: A 20-kilodalton glycoprotein produced by recombinant technique that stimulates granulocyte precursors.

INDICATIONS: See pg. 524-525. AIDS patients may tolerate low ANC levels better than cancer patients do in terms of infectious complications (*Arch Intern Med* 1995;155:1965; *Infect Control Hosp Epidemiol* 1991;12:429). G-CSF is "not routinely indicated" for neutropenic patients with HIV infection, according to the guidelines of USPHS/IDSA (*MMWR* 1999;48[RR-10]; *CID* 2000; 30[suppl 1]:S29). Nevertheless, the incidence of bacterial infections appears to be increased 2-3-fold in patients with an ANC <500/mL (*Lancet* 1989;2:91; *Arch Intern Med* 1995;155:1965), and most HIV-infected patients respond to G-CSF. A therapeutic trial in 258 HIV-infected patients with ANC of 750-1000/mm^3 found that G-CSF recipients had 31% fewer bacterial infections, 54% fewer severe bacterial infections and 45% fewer hospital days for these infections, but no mortality benefit (*AIDS* 1998;12:65).

DOSE: Initial dose of G-CSF is 5-10 µg/kg/d subcutaneously (based on lean body weight), usually 5 µg/kg/d. For practical purposes, the dose can be a convenient approximation of the calculated dose using a volume of 1 cc (300 µg), 0.5 cc (150 µg), 0.25 cc (75 µg) or 0.2 cc (60 µg). This may be increased by 1 µg/kg/d after 5-7 days up to 10 mcg/kg/d or decreased 50%/wk and given either daily, every other day, or 2-3x/wk. Monitor CBC 2x/wk and keep ANC >1,000-2,000/mL (*NEJM* 1987;317:593). If unresponsive after 7 days at 10 µg/kg/d, treatment should be discontinued. Usual maintenance dose is 150-300 µg given 3-7x/wk.

PHARMACOLOGY

- **Absorption:** Not absorbed with oral administration. G-CSF must be given IV or SQ; SQ is usually preferred.
- **T½:** 3.5 h (SQ injection)
- **Elimination:** Renal

SIDE EFFECTS: Medullary bone pain is the only important side effect, noted in 10-20%, and is usually manageable with acetaminophen.

RARE SIDE EFFECTS: Mild dysuria, reversible abnormal liver function tests, increased uric acid, and increased LDH.

DRUG INTERACTIONS: Should not be given within 24 hrs of cancer chemotherapy. Lithium may ↑ leukocytosis. Vincristine ↑ peripheral neuropathy (*J Clin Oncol* 1996;14:935).

PREGNANCY: Category C. Caused abortion and embryolethality in animals at 2-10x dose in humans; no studies in humans.

Drug Information

GEMFIBROZIL – see also Fenofibrate (pg. 272)

TRADE NAME: *Lopid* (Pfizer) and generic

FORM AND COST: 600 mg tab at $2.43/tab

CLASS: Antihyperlipidemic; fibric acid derivative (like clofibrate)

INDICATIONS AND DOSE: See pg. 144. Elevated serum triglycerides; may increase LDL cholesterol and cholesterol levels. 600 mg bid po >30 minutes before meal. Meta-analysis found that fibrates decrease total cholesterol by 8% and triglycerides by 30% (*Am J Ther* 2010;17:e182).

MONITORING: Blood lipids, especially fasting triglycerides and LDL cholesterol; if marked increases in LDL cholesterol, discontinue gemfibrozil and expect return of LDL cholesterol to pretreatment levels in 6-8 wks. Gemfibrozil should be discontinued if there is no decrease in triglyceride or cholesterol level at 3 mos. Obtain liver function tests and CBC at baseline, at 3-6 mos, and then yearly. Discontinue gemfibrozil for otherwise unexplained abnormal liver function tests.

PHARMACOLOGY

- **Bioavailability:** 97%
- **T½:** 1.3 h
- **Elimination:** renal – 70%, fecal – 6%
  - □ Hepatic failure: Reduce dosage; use with caution
  - □ Renal failure: Consider reducing dose

PRECAUTIONS: Contraindicated with gallbladder disease, primary biliary cirrhosis, and severe renal failure.

SIDE EFFECTS

- **Blood lipids:** May increase LDL cholesterol and total cholesterol by a mechanism that is poorly understood.
- **Gallbladder:** Gemfibrozil is similar to clofibrate and may cause gallstones and cholecystitis ascribed to increased biliary excretion of cholesterol.
- **Miscellaneous:** GI intolerance, decreased hematocrit and/or WBC (rare)

DRUG INTERACTIONS

- **Gemfibrozil and statins** have resulted in rhabdomyolysis and renal failure; possible increased risk of myositis when used with statins; monitor closely for evidence of myositis with concurrent use (*JAIDS* 2009;52:235; *Ann Intern Med* 2009;150:301). Rosuvastatin AUC increased 90%; use fenofibrate instead.
- **Oral anticoagulants:** May potentiate activity of warfarin.

PREGNANCY: Category C

HALCION – see Benzodiazepines (pg. 207)

HUMATIN – see Paromomycin (pg. 341)

INDINAVIR (IDV)

TRADE NAME: *Crixivan* (Merck)

FORMULATIONS, REGIMENS, COST:

- **Forms:** IDV caps 200, 333 and 400 mg
- **Regimens:** IDV 800 mg q8h; IDV/r, 800/100 mg bid
- **AWP:** $548/mo (IDV 800 q8h)

FOOD: Unboosted, take 1 hr before or 2 hrs after meal, or take with light, low-fat meal. No food restrictions for IDV/r.

FLUIDS: Must take ≥1.5 L/d

RENAL FAILURE: No restrictions but should hydrate well

STORAGE: Room temperature, 15-30°C (59-86°F); protect from moisture

PATIENT ASSISTANCE PROGRAM: 800-850-3430

CLASS: Protease inhibitor

INDICATIONS AND DOSE: This drug played a central role in the early HAART era with extraordinary results in ACTG 320 and Merck Trial 035 (*NEJM* 1997;337:725 & 734). IDV has now been largely replaced by alternative PIs that are more potent, more convenient and less toxic. When used, the standard regimens are IDV/r 800/100 mg bid or 800/200 mg bid (increased risk of renal calculi.

ADVANTAGES: Extensive experience with long-term follow-up; extensive experience in pregnancy.

DISADVANTAGES: Need for q8h dosing on an empty stomach if used without RTV boosting; risk of nephrolithiasis and need for large fluid intake with or without RTV boosting; dermatologic side effects, including dry skin, alopecia, and paronychia; inferior virologic efficacy compared to multiple alternative regimens; IDV and IDV/r are not recommended as first-line therapy by the 2011 DHHS or the 2010 IAS-USA guidelines.

CLINICAL TRIALS: See Table 5-49.

RESISTANCE: Mutations 10I/R/V, 20M/R, 24I, 32I, 36I, 54V, 71V/T, 73S/A, 77I, 82A/F/T, 84V and 90M correlate with reduced *in vitro* activity (*AAC* 1998;42:2775; *Topics HIV Med* 2006;14:125). Substitutions at codons 46, 82, and 84 are major mutations that predict resistance but are not necessarily the first mutations. In general, at least three mutations are necessary to produce phenotypic resistance. The overlap with other PIs is not extensive, but multiple mutations contribute to class resistance (*Nature* 1995;374: 569).

PHARMACOLOGY

- **Bioavailability:** Absorption is 65% in fasting state or with only a light, nonfat meal. Full meal decreases IDV levels 77%; give 1 hr before or

■ TABLE 5-49: **Clinical Trials of IDV in Treatment-naïve Patients**

Trial	Regimen	No.	Dur (wks)	VL <50	VL <200-500
ACTG 320 (*NEJM* 1997;337:725)	IDV 800 mg q8h + AZT/3TC	577	24		60%*
	AZT/3TC	579			9%
Merck 035 (*NEJM* 1997;337:734)	IDV+AZT/3TC	32	52	80%	90%*
	IDV	28		0	43%
	AZT/3TC	31		0	0
Dupont 006 (*NEJM* 1999;341:1865)	EFV+AZT/3TC	154	48	64%*	70%*
	IDV+AZT/3TC	148		43%	48%
	IDV+EFV	148		47%	53%
Merck 060 (*AIDS* 2000;14:367)	IDV+AZT/3TC	52	52		60%*
	AZT/3TC	50			46%
Atlantic (*AIDS* 2003;17:987)	IDV+ddI+d4T	417	48	55%	57%
	NVP+ddI+d4T	394		54%	58%
	3TC+ddI+d4T	396		46%	59%
CNAAB 3005 (*JAMA* 2001;285:1155)	ABC/AZT/3TC	282	48	40%	51%
	IDV+AZT/3TC	280		46%	51%
CNA 3014 (*Curr Med Res J* 2004;20:103)	ABC/AZT/3TC	169	48	60%	66%*
	IDV+AZT/3TC	173		50%	50%
START-1 (*AIDS* 2000;14:1481)	IDV+3TC+d4T	101	48	49%	53%
	IDV+AZT/3TC	103		47%	52%

* Superior to comparator (*P* <0.05)

2 hrs after meal, with light meal or with RTV. Food has minimal effect on IDV when it is coadministered with RTV. CNS penetration is relatively good compared to other PIs (*CNS Drugs* 2002;16:595).

- **T½:** 1.5-2.0 h (serum)

- **C_{max}:** Peak levels correlate with nephrotoxicity and trough levels correlate with efficacy, but levels seem somewhat unpredictable even when IDV is boosted with RTV (*JAIDS* 2002;29:374). Penetration into CSF is moderate (CSF: serum=0.06-0.16) but is superior to that of other PIs and adequate to inhibit IDV-sensitive strains (*AAC* 2000;44:2173), since levels achieved are above the IC_{95} for most HIV isolates (*AIDS* 1999; 13:1227). The ranking in the CNS penetration – effectiveness the highest in a 4 class system (*Neurology* 2011;76:693) (see pg. 550t).

- **Elimination:** Metabolized via CY3A4. Inhibits glucuronidation. Urine shows 5-12% unchanged drug and glucuronide and oxidative metabolites.

- **Dose in renal failure:** Standard dose. This also applies to hemodialysis and peritoneal dialysis (*Nephrol Dial Transplant* 2000;15: 1102).

Drug Information

5

SIDE EFFECTS

- **Asymptomatic increase in indirect bilirubin** to ≥2.5 mg/dL without an increase in transaminases noted in 10-15% of patients. Clinically inconsequential, and rarely associated with jaundice or scleral icterus.

- **Mucocutaneous:** Paronychia and ingrown toenails, alopecia, dry skin, mouth, and eyes (common).

- **Class adverse effects:** Insulin-resistant hyperglycemia, lipodystrophy, hyperlipidemia (increased triglyceride, cholesterol, LDL levels), and possible increased bleeding with hemophilia (*AIDS* 2001; 15:11). IDV use is associated with a substantial increased risk (RR 1.12/year) of cardiovascular disease that is presumably due to its effect on plasma lipids and documented in the D:A:D review (*JID* 2010;201:318). Use of IDV is generally not recommended in patients with hemophilia due to the availability of many alternative PIs.

- **Nephrolithiasis ± hematuria** in 10-28%, depending on duration of treatment, age, RTV boosting, and fluid prophylaxis (*J Urol* 2000;164:1895). The cause is crystallization of the drug with high serum levels and/or dehydration; IDV crystals can be detected in urine of up to 60% of IDV recipients. The frequency of nephrolithiasis with renal colic, flank pain, hematuria and/or renal insufficiency in the ATHENA cohort with 1219 IDV recipients was 8.3/100 patient-years; risk factors included low weight, low mean body mass, regimens with >1000 mg IDV, and warm climate (*Arch Intern Med* 2002; 162:1493). Factors that do not appear to influence risk are CD4 cell count and urine pH. Patients should drink 48 oz of fluid daily to maintain urine output at ≥150 mL/hr during the 3 hrs after ingestion; stones are crystals of IDV ± calcium (*Ann Intern Med* 1997 ;349:1294). Nephrolithiasis usually reflects peak plasma concentrations >10 µg/mL (*AIDS* 1999;13:473). This is most likely with IDV in standard doses or ritonavir-boosted IDV regimens, with the 800/100 mg bid or 800/200 mg bid (*JAIDS* 2002;29:374).

- **Nephrotoxicity:** A retrospective review of renal failure in the ANRS-C03 cohort showed the RR with IDV/r was 2.3 (*HIV Med* 2010;11:308). In a prospective study of 184 IDV recipients, routine urinalysis indicated pyuria in 35%; this was often accompanied by proteinuria, hematuria, and IDV crystals (*JAIDS* 2003;32:135). About 25% with persistent pyuria developed elevated serum creatinine that persisted ≥3 mos after IDV was discontinued. Interstitial nephritis with pyuria and renal insufficiency was previously reported in about 2% of IDV recipients (*CID* 2002;34:1033). Acute renal failure due to IDV is reported, but rare (*AIDS* 1998;12:954). However, a long term study of 1281 patients given ART on average of 7 years showed IDV was the only antiretroviral agent associated with long term renal dysfunction (*CID* 2009;49:1950).

- **Alopecia:** May involve all hair-bearing areas (*NEJM* 1999;341:618)

- **GI intolerance:** Primarily nausea, with occasional vomiting, epigastric distress

- **Less common:** Increased transaminase levels, headache, diarrhea, metallic taste, fatigue, insomnia, blurred vision, dizziness, rash, and thrombocytopenia. Rare cases of fulminant hepatic failure and death. Fulminant hepatitis has been associated with steatosis and an eosinophilic infiltrate, suggesting a drug-related injury (*Lancet* 1997; 349:924). Gynecomastia has been reported (*CID* 1998;27:1539).

BLACK BOX WARNING: None

DRUG INTERACTIONS: IDV is a substrate and inhibitor of CYP4503A4

- **Contraindicated for concurrent use: cisapride, astemizole, midazolam, triazolam, ergotamines, alprazolam, amiodarone, terfenadine pimozide, bepridil, quinidine, alfuzosin, flecainide** and **propafenone. Avoid co-administration: atazanavir, fluticasone, lovastatin, pitavastatin, rifampin, simvastatin,** and **St. John's wort.**

- **Dose modification: Rifabutin** – IDV levels decreased 32% and rifabutin levels increased 2x – reduce rifabutin dose to 150 mg qd or 300 mg 3x/wk and increase IDV dose to 1000 mg tid with IDV/r use standard PI dose and rifabutin 150 mg q24-48h. Consider rifabutin TDM.

- **Azoles:** See pg. 208. **Clarithromycin** levels increase 53%; no dose change; consider decreasing clarithromycin with renal impairment. **Grapefruit juice** reduces IDV levels 26%. **Oral contraceptives**: Norethindrone levels increase 26% and ethinylestradiol levels increase 24%; no change. **Carbamazepine** markedly decreases IDV levels; **Phenytoin** and **phenobarbitol** may decrease IDV levels; avoid or use with close monitoring of IDV levels with IDV/r. IDV increased **Sildenafil** AUC 340% (*AIDS* 1999;13:F10). The maximum recommended dose is 25 mg/48 hrs. **Vardenafil** AUC increased 16x; IDV AUC decreases 30%; dose should be limited to 2.5 mg qd or use alternative; with IDV/r it should be limited to 2.5 mg/3 days. **Tadalafil** AUC increased; use 5 mg initially and do not exceed 10 mg/72 hrs. **Methadone**: no change in methadone levels. **St. John's wort** reduces IDV AUC by 57%; avoid (*Lancet* 2000;355:547). **Vitamin C** (>1 gm/d): decreases IDV C_{min} 32%. **Amlodipine** AUC increased 90%; use with close monitoring. **Colchicine:** IDV increases colchicine levels. **ART agents** (see Table 5-50).

PREGNANCY: Category C. Negative rodent teratogenic assays; Pharmacokinetic studies in PACTG 358 showed that mean levels at 30-32 wks gestation were 74% lower than at 6 wks postpartum. There is concern for this low IDV level and a theoretical concern for the associated hyperbilirubinemia. Boosted IDV (400/100 mg bid) appears to provide adequate trough levels (*AAC* 2008;52:1542). The 2010 DHHS Guidelines on Antiretroviral Drugs in Pregnant Women recommended IDV/r (400/100 bid) as an alternative to LPV/r in the

Drug Information

5

400/100 mg bid dose. The appropriate regimen for pregnancy is not known (2010 DHHS Pregnancy Guidelines; www.mmhiv.com/link/2010-DHHS-Perinatal). Data from the Pregnancy Registry through July 2008 showed birth defects in 6/284 (2.1%) IDV recipients, which is comparable to the 2.7% risk noted in the absence of ART.

■ TABLE 5-50: **Recommendations for IDV in Combination with Other PIs or with NNRTIs**

Agent	AUC	Concurrent Use Regimen
RTV*	IDV ↑ 2-5x	RTV 100 mg bid + IDV 800 mg bid
SQV	SQV ↑4-7x; IDV no effect	Limited data; possible *in vitro* antagonism (*JID* 1997;176:265); avoid
NFV	NFV ↑80%; IDV ↑50%	IDV 1200 mg bid + NFV 1250 mg bid (limited data)
NVP	NVP no effect; IDV ↓28%	IDV 1000 mg q8h or IDV/r + NVP standard
DLV	DLV no effect; IDV ↑40%	DLV 400 mg tid + IDV 600 mg q8h
EFV	EFV no effect; IDV ↓31%	EFV 600 mg qhs + IDV 1000 mg q8h or IDV/r 800/200 mg bid + EFV 600 mg qhs
LPV/r	LPV no change; IDV ↑3x	IDV 600 mg bid + LPV/r 400/100 mg bid
ATV	Combination contraindicated, because both drugs cause indirect hyperbilirubinemia	
FPV	APV↑33%	Regimen not established
TPV	No data	No data; avoid
MVC	**May** ↑ MVC	MVC 150 mg bid + IDV standard
ETR	No data; may ↓ IDV	Inadequate data; avoid

INVIRASE – see Saquinavir (pg. 373)

ISONIAZID (INH)

TRADE NAMES: *Nydrazid, Laniazid, Teebaconin,* and generic; combination with rifampin: *Rifamate,* with rifampin and pyrazinamide: *Rifater* (Aventis)

FORMS AND COST: 50, 100, and 300 mg tabs; $0.15 per 300 mg tab. *Hydrazid* IV – Injections 100 mg/mL 10 mL vial $2.49; INH liquid 50 mg/5 mL (16 oz) $65.10; *Rifamate* – $4.19/tab

COMBINATIONS: Caps with rifampin: 150 mg INH + 300 mg rifampin (*Rifamate*) and tabs with 50 mg INH + 120 mg rifampin and 300 mg PZA (*Rifater*)

INDICATIONS AND DOSES: Prophylaxis and treatment of tuberculosis (see pg. 462-467) is based on 2008 CDC/NIH/IDSA Guidelines for Opportunistic Infections.

■ Treatment of **latent tuberculosis**: INH once daily or twice weekly for 9 mos (if there is no evidence of active TB and no history of treatment for active or latent tuberculosis). The estimated efficacy of INH prophylaxis is a 64% reduction in active TB cases (*Lancet Infect Dis* 2010;10:489). A Cochrane Library review of 12 controlled trials concluded that the treatment of latent TB in patients with HIV reduces the risk of active TB, especially in those with a positive skin test (*Cochrane Database Syst Rev* 2010;20:CD000171).

- Treatment of **active TB**: A multidrug regimen should be started immediately and include INH, RIF or rifabutin, PZA and EMB.

- A review from tuberculosis authorities at the NIH (Bethesda), the Institute of Infectious Diseases and Molecular Medicine (Cape Town) and the MRC (London) (*Lancet* 2011 doi:10. 1016/ j.physletb. 2003.10.071).

  □ The efficacy of INH prophylaxis is well established in persons with a positive skin test and HIV infection.

  □ The protection is about 60%, but the duration is limited.

  □ INH prophylaxis in HIV-infected patients is more effective if given 36 mos vs. 6 mos. The benefit in the trial summarized in the Cochrane Review (above) showed an OR of 0.57 for TB with INH prophylaxis; benefit was limited to patients with a positive skin test, and the risk of drug induced hepatitis or resistance was low. There was increased mortality in the group with INH for 36 mos and negative skin tests that was unexplained and appeared unrelated to drug toxicity.

COMPLIANCE: Adherence concerns have resulted in a preference for DOT in all patients treated for active tuberculosis and for treatment of latent TB with HIV co-infection.

PHARMACOLOGY

- **Bioavailability:** 90%

- **T½:** 1-4 h; 1 h in rapid acetylators

- **Elimination:** Metabolized and eliminated in urine. Rate of acetylation is genetically determined. Slow inactivation reflects deficiency of hepatic enzyme N-acetyltransferase and is found in about 50% of whites and African-Americans. Rate of acetylation does not affect efficacy of standard daily or DOT regimens.

- **Dose modification in renal failure:** Half dose with creatinine clearance <10 mL/min in slow acetylators.

SIDE EFFECTS: A review of 24,221 patients given INH prophylaxis showed adverse events in 132 (0.54%) including rash 61 (0.25%), peripheral neuropathy 50 (0.21%), clinical hepatotoxicity 17 (0.07%) (*AIDS* 2010;24 Suppl 5:S29).

- **Hepatitis:** ALT elevations are noted in 10-20%, clinical hepatitis in 0.6%, and fatal hepatitis in 0.02% (*Am J Respir Crit Care Med* 2003;167:603). The risk of hepatitis increases with increased age, alcoholism, prior liver disease, pregnancy, and concurrent rifampin.

Drug Information

5

One report showed hepatotoxicity rates (defined as an ALT >5 ULN) of 0.15% in 11,141 patients treated for latent TB. It was 1% in those receiving multiple antituberculosis drugs for active TB (*JAMA* 1999;281:1014). 2008 CDC/ATS/IDSA Guidelines for Management of TB in patients with HIV co-infection in the US recommend monitoring for clinical evidence of hepatitis by requiring monthly INH prescriptions contingent on this review. LFTs should be obtained if there are symptoms suggesting hepatitis. If INH is taken for latent TB it should be stopped if the ALT is >3 x ULN with symptoms or >5x ULN without symptoms. Management guidelines with treatment of active TB is provided on pg. 465.

- **Peripheral neuropathy** due to increased excretion of pyridoxine, which is dose-related and rare (0.2%) with usual doses. It is prevented by use of concurrent pyridoxine (10-50 mg qd), which is recommended for patients with HIV co-infection. Overdose of INH may require high doses of pyridoxine (*Pharmacotherapy* 2006; 26:529).

- **Miscellaneous Reactions:** Rash, fever, adenopathy, GI intolerance. Rare reactions: Psychosis, arthralgias, optic neuropathy, marrow suppression.

DRUG INTERACTIONS

- Increased effects of **warfarin, benzodiazepines (midazolam, triazolam), carbamazepine, cycloserine, ethionamide** (may increase INH levels; monitor for INH toxicity), **phenytoin, theophylline**
- INH absorption decreased with **aluminum-containing antacids**
- **Ketoconazole**: Decrease ketoconazole levels (based on case reports)
- **Food:** Decreases absorption
- **Tyramine reaction** (cheese, wine, some fish): Rare patients develop palpitations, sweating, urticaria, headache, and vomiting

PREGNANCY: Category C. Not teratogenic in animals. Possible increased risk of hepatotoxicity; monitor transaminase levels monthly during pregnancy and post-partum. This recommendation also applies to treatment of latent TB. Should give pyridoxine to prevent neuro-toxicity and vitamin K to prevent hemorrhagic disease.

ITRACONAZOLE

TRADE NAME: *Sporanox* (Janssen) and generic

FORMS AND COST: 100 mg caps at $8.90; oral solution with 10 mg/mL (150 mL) at $227.60.

PATIENT ASSISTANCE PROGRAM: 800-652-6227

CLASS: Triazole (like fluconazole) with three nitrogens in the azole ring; other imidazoles have two nitrogens.

ACTIVITY AND PERSPECTIVE: *In vitro* activity against *H. capsulatum, B. dermatitidis, Aspergillus, Cryptococcus, Candida* spp. Strains of *Candida* that are resistant to fluconazole may be sensitive to itraconazole (*AAC* 1994;38:1530). Compared with fluconazole, itraconazole appears to be equivalent for non-meningeal coccidioidomycosis (*Ann Intern Med* 2000;133:676), superior for penicilliosis (*Am J Med* 1997;103:223), inferior for cryptococcosis (*CID* 1999;28: 291), and equivalent for most candidiasis (*HIV Clin Trials* 2000;1:47). Major concerns are somewhat erratic absorption, multiple drug interactions, and cardiotoxicity with congestive heart failure (FDA Health Advisory, 5/09/02).

PHARMACOLOGY

- **Bioavailability:** Caps require gastric acid for absorption; average bioavailability is 55% and improved when taken with food and/or acidic drinks such as colas and orange juice (*AAC* 1995;39:1671). PPIs, H2 blockers and antacids should be avoided. Follow serum levels to ensure absorption. The usual therapeutic level anticipated with a standard dose is 1-10 µg/mL. The liquid formulation is better absorbed and should be taken on an empty stomach. Some consider the liquid formulation to be preferred for all oral itraconazole therapy. The 2011 ATS Guidelines on treatment of fungal infections favor the liquid form due to the widespread use of PPIs, H2 blockers and antacids (*Am J Resp Crit Care Med* 2011;183:96). However, nearly all studies were performed using the capsule formulation, and bioavailability studies have shown substantial variation. Based on these concerns, some authorities prefer the liquid formulation only for thrush – where its topical effect may improve efficacy – for patients with known achlorhydria, and for patients with inadequate serum levels.

- **Reference laboratories for serum levels:**
  - □ Dr. Michael Rinaldi, Dept. of Pathology, Mail Code 7750, University of Texas Health Science Center, 7703 Floyd Curl Drive, San Antonio, TX 78229-3900; telephone 210-567-4131. Cost is $59.
  - □ Specimen should be 2-4 mL serum or plasma obtained 2 hrs post dose after day 5 of treatment sent in frozen state. Results are available in 3 days. Goal is level of ≥1 µg/mL.

DOSE RECOMMENDATIONS: See Table 5-51.

- **T½:** 64 h
- **Elimination:** CYP 3A4 inhibitor and substrate; metabolites include hydroxyitraconazole, which is active *in vitro* against many fungi. Renal excretion is 0.03% of parent drug and 40% of metabolites.
- **Dose modification with renal failure:** None
- **Dose modification with liver disease:** No data. Use with caution. Manufacturer suggests monitoring serum levels.

Drug Information

5

■ TABLE 5-51: **Itraconazole Dose Regimens***

Usual Doses
- **Loading dose:** 200 mg tid x 3 days for serious infections
- **Capsules:** 100-200 mg po qd or bid with food (200-400 mg/day)
- **Oral liquid:** Preferred oral form 100 mg po qd or bid on empty stomach (100-200 mg/day)
- **IV:** 200 mg IV bid x 6 (loading), then 200-400 mg/d po (IV not available in US)

Pathogen	Dose (oral)	Comment
Aspergillosis	(Not recommended)	Voriconazole preferred (see pg. 413)
Blastomycosis	200 mg qd or bid (caps)	
Candidiasis ■ Thrush (see pg. 425) ■ Esophagitis (see pg. 427) ■ Vaginitis (see pg. 428)	■ 200 mg/day (liquid) swish & swallow (S&S) ■ 200 mg/day (liquid) S&S ■ 200 mg/day x 3 days or 200 mg bid x 1 (caps)	As effective as fluconazole, but absorption more erratic and there are more drug interactions (*HIV Clin Trials* 2000;1:47). For fluconazole-resistant *Candida*, options include itraconazole, voriconazole (po or IV), caspofungin (IV), posaconazole po, anidulafungin IV, micafungin IV or amphotericin (IV). Voriconazole is the most predictably active triazole.
Coccidioido-mycosis (see pg. 432)	■ Acute non-meningeal, mild: 200 po tid x 3 days then 200 mg po bid ■ Chronic suppressive treatment: itraconazole 200 mg po bid	■ Non-meningeal form. ■ For meningeal form, fluconazole 400-800 mg/d is preferred.
Cryptococcosis (see pg. 4335)	200 mg qd (caps) tid x 3 days, then bid x 8 weeks, then 200 mg qd maintenance	■ For patients with meningeal form who cannot tolerate fluconazole during maintenance therapy and for non-meningeal cryptococcosis ■ Fluconazole and amphotericin preferred
Dermatophytes (see pg. 493 and FDA warning)	200 mg qd (caps)	■ Tinea corporis and T. cruris: 15 days ■ T. pedis, T. manum: 30 days ■ T. capitis: 4 to 8 weeks
Histoplasmosis (see pg. 451)	■ Acute: 200 mg tid x 3 days, then bid ■ Continuation: 200 mg bid x 12-24 mos. or ■ Maintenance: 200 mg po	■ Preferred azole ■ Amphotericin B preferred for 1-2 wks for initial treatment of severe disseminated histoplasmosis; then itra 200 mg/d x 12 mos. Itraconazole is appropriate for acute phase treatment of those with mild illness
Onychomycosis ■ Fingernails ■ Toenails	200 mg/day (caps) ■ 1 week/month x 2 mos. ■ 1 week/month x 4 mos.	Warn patients of and monitor for cardiotoxicity and hepatotoxicity.
Penicilliosis (see pg. 475)	■ Acute, severe disease: amphotericin B 0.7 mg/kg/d x 2 wks , followed by itraconazole 200 mg bid x 10 wks. ■ Mild disease: 200 mg po bid x 8 wks, followed by 200 mg/d	Preferred azole
Sporotrichosis	200 mg bid	

* Sources: The 2008 IDSA/NIH/CDC Guidelines for Treatment and Prevention of Opportunistic Infections in HIV-infected Adults and Adolescents and 2011 ATS Guidelines for Treatment of Fundal Pulmonary Infections (*Am J Respir Crit Care Med* 2011;183:96)

Drug Information

SIDE EFFECTS

- **Cardiotoxicity:** The negative inotropic effect was noted in animal toxicity studies and in clinical trials an additional 58 cases with CHF reported to the FDA "Drug Watch," (an anecdotal series of cases reported to the FDA and reported by that agency through May, 2001) (*Drug Saf* 2006;29:567).

- **Hepatoxicity:** Elevation of hepatic enzymes in 4%, but clinically significant hepatitis is uncommon (*Lancet* 1992;340:251). Hepatic enzymes should be monitored in patients with prior hepatic disease, and patients should be warned to report symptoms of hepatitis.

- **Other:** Most common side effects are **GI intolerance** (3-10%) and **rash** (1-9% and most common in immunosuppressed patients).

- **Rare:** Infrequent dose-related toxicities include hypokalemia, adrenal insufficiency, impotence, gynecomastia (at doses >600 mg/d), hypertension, and edema. Ventricular fibrillation due to hypokalemia has been reported (*JID* 1993;26:348).

DRUG INTERACTIONS: Impaired absorption of caps with **H2 blockers, proton pump inhibitors, antacids,** or **sucralfate.** Itraconazole is a potent CYP3A4 inhibitor and substrate, resulting in bidirectional inhibition with increased levels of itraconazole and the following interacting drugs: **clarithromycin, erythromycin, DLV, and PIs, especially RTV-boosted PIs. Colchicine** level may be increased. Reduce **IDV** dose to 600 mg q8h and do not exceed 400 mg/d of itraconazole. **NVP** and **ETR** may decrease itraconazole levels; monitor levels. With **DRV/r, TPV/r,** and **LPV/r,** do not exceed itraconazole 200 mg/d. With all PIs, monitor for toxicity. **MVC:** Use 150 mg bid. Should not be given concurrently with **terfenadine, cisapride, pimozide, quinidine, dofetillide, astemizole, alfuzozlin, triazolam, lovastatin, pitavastatin, simvastatin, rifampin, rifabutin, phenytoin, carbamazepine, phenobarbital or ergotamine. Itraconazole** increases levels of **cyclosporine, sirolimus, tacrolimus, oral hypoglycemics, calcium channel blockers,** and **digoxin.** Itraconazole decreases **clopidogrel** efficacy; avoid. See pg. 208t.

Note: Rifabutin: use with caution (increases rifabutin, decreases itraconazole levels by 75%. **Phenytoin, carbamazepine, phenobarbitol** and **rifapentine** decrease intraconazole level; monitor itraconconazole level.

PREGNANCY: Category C. Teratogenic to rats in high doses. Generally not recommended in pregnancy, but some studies have found it to be safe (*Am J Obstet Gynecol* 2000;183:617).

KALETRA – see Lopinavir/Ritonavir (pg. 309)

5 Drug Information

LAMIVUDINE (3TC)

TRADE NAME: *Epivir* (ViiV Healthcare/GlaxoSmithKline)

FORMULATIONS, REGIMENS AND CODT:

- **Forms and regimens**
  - *Epivir* 3TC: 150 mg and 300 mg tabs; 10 mg/mL solution (240 mL bottle). Regimen: 150 mg bid or 300 mg qd – AWP=$457.97/mo
  - *Combivir* AZT/3TC: 300/150 mg. Regimen: 1 bid – AWP=$992/mo
  - *Trizivir* AZT/3TC/ABC: 300/150/300 mg. Regimen: 1 bid – AWP= $1608/mo
  - *Epzicom* 3TC/ABC: 300/600 mg. Regimen: 1 qd – AWP= $1073/mo
  - *Epivir HBV* 100 mg tab at $13.66/tab; *Epivir HBV* 5 mg/mL solution (240 mL) at $163.97.

FOOD: No effect

Combinations to avoid

- 3TC/FTC
- TDF/3TC/ABC
- TDF/3TC/ddI

RENAL FAILURE (Table 5-52)

- TABLE 5-52: **3TC Dosing in Renal Failure**

CrCl	Dose
>50 mL/min	150 mg bid or 300 mg qd
30-49 mL/min	150 mg qd
15-29 mL/min	150 mg, then 100 mg qd
5-14 mL/min	150 mg, then 50 mg qd
<5 mL/min or dialysis	150 mg x 1 then 25 mg qd

HEPATIC FAILURE: No recommendation; usual dose likely

HEPATITIS B: Standard dose is 100 mg qd; coinfected patients should receive the HIV dose of 300 mg qd (or FTC 200 mg qd) + a second agent active against HBV such as TDF in a fully-suppressive HIV regimen regardless of CD4 count if HBV treatment is indicated.

PATIENT ASSISTANCE: 800-722-9294

CLASS: Nucleoside analog reverse transcriptase inhibitor (NRTI)

INDICATIONS AND DOSES

- **HIV:** 3TC or FTC are recommended as components of all initial regimens in the 2011 DHHS Guidelines, the 2010 IAS-USA guidelienes, and virtually all other guidelines. The standard dose is 150 mg bid or 300 mg qd without regard for meals. 3TC is coformulated as *Combivir*, *Trizivir*, and *Epzicom*, which improves convenience and reduces co-pays.

- **Hepatitis B:** 3TC is a potent inhibitor of HBV replication (*NEJM* 2004;350:1118). Several studies have verified activity with HBeAg seroconversion in 22-29%, undetectable HBV DNA in 40-87% of patients coinfected with HBV and HIV (*JID* 1999;180:607; *Hepatology* 1999;30:1302; *CID* 2001;32:963; *CID* 2006;43:904), and improved hepatic histology (*NEJM* 1998;339:61; *Ann Pharamacother* 2010;44:1271; CID 2010;51:1201). Mutations on the YMDD polymerase gene confer 3TC resistance with HIV co-infection at a rate of 15-20% in year 1 and 70-90% by year 4 (*AIDS* 2006;20: 863). These mutations result in HBV virologic failure and, in some cases, a hepatitis flare (*J Clin Virol* 2002;24:173; *Lancet* 1997;349:20; *CID* 1999;28:1032). A second anti-HBV agent should be given to protect against resistance; TDF is a preferred agent if there is no baseline resistance (*CID* 2010;51:201). There are 4 distinct mechanisms of HBV flares with HBV treatment and HIV co-infection: 1) 3TC-resistant HBV, 2) 3TC (or FTC) discontinuation, 3) IRIS or 4) hepatotoxicity of antiretroviral agents. Note that some experts conclude that the preferred drugs for HBV in monoinfected patients are TDF and entecavir (*Clin Gastroenterol Hepatol* 2008;6:1315; *CID* 2010;51:201; *AntivirL Ther* 2010;15:487). See below and pg. 510 for guidance in treating HBV-HIV co-infection (*CID* 2006;43:904).

- **Treatment of HBV only:** With HIV co-infection, TDF can be used only with a fully suppressive HIV regimen; entecavir can also be used only with full suppression of HIV due to the weak activity of entecavir vs. HIV causing the 184V resistance mutation.

- **Treatment of HIV and HBV:** Use TDF+3TC or TDF/FTC as the backbone for a fully HIV suppressive regimen.

ADVANTAGES: Potent activity against HIV, well tolerated, no food effect, may be taken once daily, co-formulated with AZT (*Combivir*), AZT/ABC (*Trizivir*) and ABC (*Epzicom*); active against HBV. 3TC resistance by HIV (M184V) increases susceptibility to AZT, d4T, and TDF, and delays accumulation of TAMs, and may partially reverse their effects. M184V reduces VL by about 0.5 $\log_{10}$ c/mL as a single agent in patients who have drug-resistant virus. Continued administration of 3TC (or FTC) with the M184V resistance mutation results in modest antiretroviral activity and does not select for additional NRTI resistance mutations.

DISADVANTAGES: Single resistance mutation (M184V) occurs early with virologic failure and causes high-level resistance to 3TC and FTC; use in HBV co-infection requires additional agents active against both HIV and HBV. Dose adjustment required with renal failure. May be more likely to select for M184V than FTC; combination of TDF+3TC may select for more K65R than TDF/FTC.

Drug Information

5

RESISTANCE: Monotherapy with 3TC or non-suppressive therapy with 3TC-containing regimens results in the rapid selection of the M184V mutation, which confers resistance to 3TC and FTC. Strains with the M184V mutation have enhanced susceptibility to AZT, d4T, and TDF and a modest decrease in susceptibility to ABC and ddI that is not clinically relevant in the absence of other NRTI mutations. The M184V mutation appears to be associated with persistent anti-HIV activity (mean of 0.5 $\log_{10}$ c/mL) (*JID* 2005;192:1537), presumably due to reduced viral fitness (*New Microbiol* 2004;27 Suppl 2:31; *Expert Rev Anti Infect Ther* 2004; 2:147). K65R and multiple TAMs reduce activity of 3TC 3- to 9-fold. The Q151M complex and the T69 insertion mutation are associated with 3TC resistance as well as with broad multinucleoside resistance. All of these changes are also found with FTC (*JAIDS* 2006;43:567).

CLINICAL TRIALS: There is extensive experience with 3TC combined with AZT, TDF, d4T, and ddI, confirming antiviral potency, excellent long and short-term tolerability, but also early acquisition of the M184V resistance mutation if viral suppression incomplete.

- **ACTG 384** found that AZT/3TC+EFV was superior to ddI+d4T+EFV in virologic suppression and tolerability (*NEJM* 2003;349:2298) (see pg. 237).
- **GS-903** compared TDF vs. d4T, each in combination with 3TC and EFV, for initial therapy. Results at 144 weeks were similar, with 62% and 68% in the d4T and TDF group, respectively, achieving VL <400 c/mL by ITT (M = F) analysis (*JAMA* 2004; 292:194) (see pg. 246t).
- **CNA 30024** compared ABC/3TC vs. AZT/3TC, each with EFV, in 699 treatment-naïve patients. At 48 wks, VL was <50 c/mL in 69% and 70%, respectively by ITT analysis (*CID* 2004;39:1038). This paved the way to coformulation as *Epzicom* (see pg. 180).
- **ESS 30008** compared ABC/3TC twice daily vs. once daily in patients who had viral suppression with ABC/3TC twice daily combined with a PI or NNRTI (*NEJM* 2004;350:1850) (see pg. 181t).
- **Triple nucleoside regimens:** ACTG 5095 compared AZT/3TC/ABC vs. EFV/3TC/AZT ± ABC. See Table 5-4. pg. 181.

PHARMACOLOGY

- **Bioavailability:** 86%
- **T½:** 5-7 h; Intracellular T½: 18-22 h
- **CNS penetration:** 13% (CSF:Plasma ratio=0.11). These levels exceed the IC_{50} and have been shown to clear HIV RNA from CSF (*Lancet* 1998;351:1547). The CNS penetration score is 2 in a 4 class system (*Neurology* 2011;76:693) (see pg. 550t).
- **Elimination:** Renal excretion accounts for 71% of administered dose.

Drug Information

SIDE EFFECTS: Experience with more than 25,000 patients given 3TC through the expanded access program and >8,000 participants in clinical trials has demonstrated minimal toxicity. Infrequent complications include headache, nausea, diarrhea, abdominal pain, and insomnia. Comparison of side effects in 251 patients given 3TC/AZT and 230 patients given AZT alone in four trials (A3001, A3002, B3001, and B3002) indicated no clinical or laboratory complications uniquely associated with 3TC. Pancreatitis has been noted in some pediatric patients given 3TC.

- **Class side effect:** Lactic acidosis and steatosis are listed as toxicities associated with the NRTI class, though it is unlikely that these occur as a result of 3TC therapy (*CID* 2002;34:838).

- **Hepatitis B:** In HIV-infected patients with HBV co-infection, discontinuation of 3TC may cause fulminant hepatic deterioration with increases in HBV DNA levels and ALT (**FDA black box warning**). Monitor hepatic function and clinical course carefully for several months when 3TC is discontinued in patients with HIV/HBV co-infection. Immune reconstitution and development of HBV resistance may also cause a hepatitis B flare (see pg 509).

Black Box Warnings: 1) Lactic acidosis (rare), 2) hepatic failure with chronic HBV infection with immune reconstitution, development of HBV resistance to 3TC or discontinuation of an agent with activity vs. HBV (TDF, 3TC, or FTC). Note that lactic acidosis and mitochondrial toxicity is listed in the black box warning but are very rare, and this drug along with TDF are used as substitutes with NRTI-induced mitochrondrial toxicity as shown in the STACCATO trial (*JAC* 2008;61:1340; *AIDS* 2003;17:2495) (see pg 375).

DRUG INTERACTIONS: TMP-SMX (1 DS daily) increases levels of 3TC; however, no dose adjustment is necessary due to the safety profile of 3TC.

PREGNANCY: Category C. Recommended (with AZT) as the preferred NRTI backbone in the 2010 DHHS Guidelines for Antiretroviral Drugs in Pregnant HIV Infected Women. Special consideration is needed with HBV co-infection. Negative carcinogenicity and teratogenicity studies in rodents; placental passage studies in humans show newborn: maternal drug ratio of 1.0. Studies in pregnant women show that 3TC is well tolerated and has pharmacokinetic properties similar to those of nonpregnant women (*JID* 1998;178:1327; *MMWR* 1998;47[RR-2]:6). Use in pregnancy is extensive; safety is well established, and when combined with AZT, efficacy in preventing perinatal transmission is also well established (*Lancet* 2002;359:1178). The Pregnancy Registry shows birth defects in 113/3754 (3.0%) first trimester exposures, a rate similar to 2.7% for women without ART exposure (www.apregistry.com, accessed 1/20/11).

5 Drug Information

HBV co-infection in pregnancy: the risk of HBV transmission is greatest in the third trimester and correlates with HBV viral load. 3TC and TDF are the best drugs to prevent perinatal HBV transmission (*Curr Hepat Res* 2010;9:147).

LEUCOVORIN (Folinic acid)

TRADE NAME: Generic

FORMS AND COST:

- Oral tabs: 5, 10, 15, and 25 mg tabs; 5 mg tab – $3.25
- Parenteral: 50, 100, and 350 mg; 3 mg/mL; 100 mg – $4.80

CLASS: Calcium salt of folinic acid

INDICATIONS: Antidote for folic acid antagonists

NOTE: Protozoa are unable to utilize leucovorin because they require p-aminobenzoic acid as a cofactor. It does not interfere with antimicrobial activity of trimethoprim or pyrimethamine. Usual use in HIV infected patients is to prevent hematologic toxicity of pyrimethamine. Therapy is usually oral but should be parenteral if there is vomiting, or NPO status.

- **Toxoplasmosis treatment:** Pyrimethamine 50-75 mg qd + leucovorin 10-20 mg qd x 6 wks; maintenance pyrimethamine 50 mg qd + leucovorin 15 mg qd (in combination with sulfadiazine or clindamycin)
- **Toxoplasmosis prophylaxis:** Leucovorin, 25 mg/wk (with dapsone 50 mg/d + pyrimethamine 50 mg/wk)

PHARMACOLOGY: Normal folate levels are 0.005-0.015 µg/mL, levels <0.005 indicate folate deficiency, and levels <0.002 cause megaloblastic anemia. Oral doses of 15 mg qd result in C_{max} of 0.268 µg/mL.

SIDE EFFECTS: Nontoxic in therapeutic doses. Rare hypersensitivity reactions.

PREGNANCY: Category C

LOPINAVIR/RITONAVIR (LPV/r)

TRADE NAME: *Kaletra* (Abbott Laboratories)

CLASS: Protease inhibitor (boosted with coformulated ritonavir)

PATIENT ASSISTANCE: 800-659-9050

FORMULATIONS, REGIMENS AND COST:

- **Forms:** LPV/r 100/25 and LPV/r 200/50 mg tabs at $841.90/mo; LPV/r oral solution, 80/20 mg/mL (160 mL) at $420.95.
- **Regimens:** 400/100 mg bid or 800/200 mg qd (2 tabs bid or 4 tabs qd); oral solution 5 cc bid or 10 cc qd. Oral solution is sometimes

Drug Information

preferred where there is GI intolerance; contains 42% alcohol. Once-daily therapy of 800/200 mg was found therapeutically equivalent to standard bid therapy in treatment-naïve patients and is now FDA-approved, but only for patients with <3 LPV mutations. Once-daily dosing is associated with lower and more variable trough levels (*JID* 2004;189:265), so bid dosing is preferred for treatment-experienced patients. The recommended dose regimen in pregnancy is LPV/r 600/150 mg bid during the second and third trimester. This is 3 200/50 mg tabs bid (*JAIDS* 2010;54:381).

- **AWP:** $877/mo

FOOD: Take tabs with or without food. Take oral solution with food.

RENAL FAILURE: Standard dose

HEPATIC FAILURE: No recommendation; use with caution

STORAGE: Tablets are stable at room temperature. Oral solution is stable until date on label at 2-8°C, and for 2 mos at room temperature (<25°C or 77°F).

ADVANTAGES: Potent antiretroviral activity; durability demonstrated with 7-year follow-up data (*HIV Clin Trials* 2009;9:1); minimal evidence of PI resistance with virologic failure when used as first PI; co-formulated with RTV; efficacy of once daily therapy established; frequently more active against PI-resistant virus than some other approved PIs with the exception of TPV/r and DRV/r; no resistance with failure in patients without prior PI mutations (as with other boosted PIs); preferred PI-based regimen in pregnancy.

DISADVANTAGES: Need for bid dosing in patients with <3 LPV mutations; GI intolerance; hyperlipidemia and other PI-associated metabolic toxicities; need for 200 mg/d RTV (in contrast to ATV/r, DRV/r and FPV/r). Possible association with increased risk of MI.

CLINICAL TRIALS: See Table 5-53.

- **Long-term follow-up:** A EuroSIDA review found that LPV/r had a better record for long-term durability than EFV based on discontinuation rates (*HIV Med* 2011;12:259).

- **Long-term follow-up:** A 6-year follow-up of 63 participants enrolled in a LPV/r trial found that 62 had persistent VL <50 c/mL and a continuing increase in CD4 cell counts with a mean total increase at week 312 of 528/mm³ (*CID* 2007;44:749). The mean CD4 count in those with a baseline count <50/mm³ was 553/mm³. The importance of this long-term follow-up is the admittedly anecdotal demonstration of sustained antiviral activity and continuing immunologic recovery, even for patients who initiated therapy late in the disease course. In a 7-year follow-up of 100 treatment-naïve patients randomized to LPV/r+d4T+3TC, 59% remained on LPV/r-based ART with VL <50 c/mL. Of the 28 with resistance data, none had PI resistance mutations (*HIV Clin Trials* 2008;9:1).

5 Drug Information

■ TABLE 5-53: Clinical Trials of LPV/r in Treatment-naïve Patients

Trial		N	Dur. (wks)	VL <50 c/mL	VL <200-400 c/mL
AB M98-863 (*NEJM* 2002;346: 2039)	d4T+3TC+LPV/r	326	48	67%	75%*
	d4T+3TC+NFV	327		53%	63%
KLEAN (*Lancet* 2006;368:476)	ABC/3TC+FPV/r	434	48	66%	73%
	ABC/3TC+LPV/r	444		65%	71%
AB M02-418 (*JAIDS* 2006;43:153-60)	TDF/FTC+LPV/r bid	75	48	64%	—
	TDF/FTC+LPV/r qd	115		70%	—
ACTG 5142 (*NEJM* 2008;358:2095)	LPV/r+3TC+(d4T or AZT)	250	96	77%	86%
	EFV+3TC+(d4T or AZT)	253		89%*	93%
	LPV/r+EFV	250		83%	92%
GEMINI (*JAIDS* 2009;50:367)	LPV/r+TDF/FTC	135	48	64%	83%
	SQV/r+TDF/FTC	128		65%	80%
CASTLE (*JAIDS* 2010;53:323)	LPV/r+TDF/FTC	440	96	68%	—
	ATV/r+TDF/FTC	443		74%*	—
ARTEMIS (*AIDS* 2009;23:1679)	LPV/r+TDF/FTC	346	96	71%	—
	DRV/r+TDF/FTC	343		79%*	—
M05-730 (*JAIDS* 2009;50:474)	LPV/r 800/200 qd + TDF/FTC	333	48	77%	—
	LPV/r 400/100 bid + TDF/FTC	331		76%	—

* Significantly better than comparator (P <0.05)

- **Once daily LPV/r:** The **M05-730** trial included 633 treatment-naïve patients randomized 3:2 to LPV/r 800/200 mg qd vs. 400/100 mg bid, each in combination with TDF/FTC. At 48 weeks efficacy was comparable for once- vs. twice-daily regimens in terms of viral suppression to 50 c/mL (77 vs. 76%), viral suppression in patients with baseline VL >100,000 and <100,000 c/mL (55% vs. 55%) and CD4 count increase (185 and 194 cells/mm³) (*AIDS Res Hum Retrovir* 2007;23:1505). Lipid changes were similar. Diarrhea was more common with the once-daily regimen (17% vs. 5%) (p=0.01) and was the most common severe adverse event. Adherence was monitored by MEMS and was better with once-daily therapy for prescribed doses taken (99.8% vs. 92.6%). The 96-week results of M05-730 demonstrated that once-daily LPV/r and twice-daily LPV/r had comparable rates of viral suppression to VL <50 c/mL (65% vs. 69%, respectively; P=NS). There were similar increases in CD4 count, similar rates of adverse reactions and no PI resistance mutations (*AIDS Res Hum Retrovir* 2010;26:841).

- **LPV/r monotherapy:** LPV/r monotherapy has been studied in multiple small trials, including one using monotherapy as initial therapy (**MONARK**) and 4 induction-maintenance trials (**OK-04, M03-613, SHCS,** and **KalMO**) that were nearly identical: standard

Drug Information

ART regimens were given for 6 mos, and patients who achieved a VL <50 c/mL at 6 mos were randomized to monotherapy on LPV/r or continued LPV/r-based ART (see Table 5-54 and pg. 122).

□ Patients with LPV/r monotherapy in **M03-613** and **KalMO** had somewhat higher failure rates than controls on triple drug regimens, but they rarely had resistance mutations and resuppressed when NRTIs were added back. Note that the need for reinduction was not classified as failure in these trials. In OK-04 the rate of reinduction was 12/100. The results are summarized in Table 5-54 (see *AIDS* 2008;22:777).

■ TABLE 5-54: **LPV/r Monotherapy**

Study	Criteria	Duration	LPV/r		LPV/r + 2 NRTIs	
			No	VL <50	No	VL <50
MONARK (*AIDS* 2008;22:385)	ART-naïve	48 wks	83	67%	53	75%
OK-04* (*JAIDS* 2009;51:147)	Induction maintenance	96 wks	100	87%	98	78%
M03-613 (*JAC* 2008;61:1359)	Induction maintenance	96 wks	78	50%	77	61%
KalMO (*HIV Clin Trials* 2009;10:368)	Induction maintenance	96 wks	30	80%	30	87%
SHCS (*AIDS* 2010;24:2347)	Induction maintenance	†	42	75%	18	100%
STAR (Bunupuradah. CROI 2011: Abstr. 584)	NNRTI failures (Thailand)	48 wks	100	65%	100	83%

* OK-04 was a trial of LPV/r + AZT/3TC vs. EFV/AZT/3TC
† Study terminated when 6 patient in the monotherapy group had virologic failure

□ The **MONARK** trial randomized treatment-naïve patients with VL <100,000 c/mL and CD4 counts >100/mm³ to treatment initiated with LPV/r or LPV/r+AZT/3TC. At 48 weeks, VL was <50 c/mL in 67% of the monotherapy arm and 75% of the triple therapy arm (Table 5-53) (*AIDS* 2008;22:385). At 96 weeks, 39 of the 83 (47%) assigned to monotherapy had a VL <50 c/mL (*HIV Med* 2010;11:137). Only 3 of 83 actually had VL >400 c/mL, but many changed regimens for other reasons, and the investigators were concerned about low level viremia with monotherapy. They stated that LPV/r monotherapy "cannot be systematically recommended."

□ The **STAR** trial included 200 Thais who failed NNRTI-based regimens and were randomized to receive LPV/r or LPV/r+TDF/FTC. At 48 weeks VL <50 c/mL was achieved in 64% of the monotherapy group compared to 84% in the triple therapy arm (P=<0.01) (Bunupuradah. 2011 CROI;Abstr. 584).

5 Drug Information

- **Swiss HIV Cohort Study:** This study included patients with viral suppression randomized to LPV/r monotherapy (n=62) or continued LPV/r-based ART. Six monotherapy patients failed within 24 weeks. Five had lumbar punctures and all had elevated levels of HIV RNA in the CSF (mean VL >10,000 c/mL). Of the 6 with virologic failure, 5 had symptoms and 4 had neurologic symptoms. The study was stopped and the investigators speculated that monotherapy might be associated with CNS compartment failure (*AIDS* 2010;24:2347).

- A **review of 6 randomized trials** of LPV/r monotherapy concluded that the risk of virologic failure was higher compared to LPV/r + 2 NRTIs (32% vs. 23%) (P=0.04), but the results were comparable when NRTIs were restarted (*AIDS* 2009;23:279). Other concerns have been the use of monotherapy before at least 9 mos of viral suppression, poor adherence (*Antiviral Ther* 2009;14:195) and persistence of high levels in CSF (*AIDS* 2010;24:2347) (see pg. 122t).

- **Treatment-experienced patients**

  - **M98-957** was a salvage trial involving 57 patients who had failed at least two PI-containing regimens. The trial compared two doses of LPV/r (533/133 mg bid and 400/100 mg bid), each combined with EFV. At 72 weeks, ITT analysis showed the VL was <400 and <50 c/mL in 67% and 61%, respectively. Response was correlated with the number of LPV resistance mutations at baseline, with VL <400 c/mL in 91% of those with 0-5 mutations, 71% with 6-7 mutations, and 33% with 8-10 mutations (*Antiviral Ther* 2002;7:165).

  - **M97-765** was a Phase II study in 70 NNRTI-naïve patients with a VL of 1,000-100,000 c/mL (median VL 10,000 c/mL and median CD4 349/mm³) on a PI regimen. Patients received LPV/r + NVP and 2 NRTIs. At 48 weeks, 60% had VL <50 c/mL by ITT analysis (*J Virol* 2001;75:7462).

  - **BMS 043** was an open-label randomized trial comparing unboosted atazanavir (ATV) with LPV/r, both in combination with two NRTIs selected by resistance testing, in 300 patients failing a PI-based regimen with HIV RNA ≥1,000 c/mL (*Curr Med Res Opin* 2005;21:1683). Virologic suppression was superior in the LPV/r arm at 24 weeks (-2.11 vs. -1.57 $\log_{10}$ c/mL, p = 0.032). Virologic suppression to <50 c/mL was found in 54% of those taking LPV/r vs. 38% of those taking ATV by ITT analysis (p = 0.008). Differences between LPV/r and ATV were more pronounced in those with greater antiretroviral experience or resistance.

  - **RESIST:** Subset analysis of TPV/r vs. LPV/r in patients with 3 class failure showed a better virologic response (<400 c/mL) at 24 weeks in patients randomized to TPV/r (116/293, 40%) vs. LPV/r (62/290, 21%) (*Lancet* 2006;368:46) (see pg. 401).

Drug Information

- **ACTG 5143:** Randomized trial of patients with prior PI failure to determine if double boosted PIs (LPV/r + FPV) would achieve viral suppression. The study was stopped prematurely due to lack of trends showing better viral suppression and low PI levels in the dual PI arm (*HIV Clin Trials* 2008;9:9).

- **SWITCHMRK:** Patients with undetectable VL on LPV/r-based ART >3 mos were randomized to RAL vs. remaining on LPV/r. All participants received 2 NRTIs with the assigned "third drug." The analysis for 702 participants at 24 weeks found that the RAL + 2 NRTI recipients had a better lipid profile, but the number with VL <50 c/mL was greater in the LPV/r arm (90% vs. 84%). Non-inferiority was not established, and the study was stopped (*Lancet* 2010;375:396).

- **NRTI-sparing regimens**

  - **ACTG 5142** compared the efficacy of LPV/r 533/133 mg bid + EFV 600 mg qd vs. EFV + 2 NRTIs vs. LPV/r + 2 NRTIs. The NRTI-sparing regimen was effective but associated with higher serum lipids than either of the standard regimens, and also with high rates of NNRTI resistance with failure (*JAIDS* 2007;21:325) (Table 5-29).

  - **A5116** was a randomized trial comparing LPV/r 533/133 mg bid + EFV 600 mg qd vs. EFV + 2 NRTIs in patients with VL <200 c/mL on ART for >18 mos. The latter regimen was superior to the NRTI-sparing regimen in terms of toxicity (17% vs. 5%; P <0.002), and there was a trend toward greater virologic failure in the NRTI-sparing arm (P = 0.09, ITT) (*AIDS* 2007;21:325).

  - **PROGRESS:** LPV/r+RAL vs. LPV/r+TDF/FTC in treatment-naïve patients (Reynes et al.,18th IAS 2010, Vienna;Abstr. MOAB0101). At 48 weeks, patients in the NRTI sparing arm had virolologic response rates (83% vs. 85% <50 c/mL by TLOVR analysis). Two in each group discontinued due to adverse events, and CD4 count increases were similar. Concerns with this study are low baseline VL (mean VL 18,000 c/mL) and small samples size (N=206).

RESISTANCE: The presence of $\geq$6 of the following mutations are associated with decreased activity: 10F/I/R/V, 20M/R, 24U, 32I, 33F, 46I/L, 47V/A, 50V, 53L, 54V/L/A/M/T/S, 63P, 71V/Y, 73S, 82A/F/T/S, 84V, and 90M. Major mutations include 32I, 47V/A and 82A/F/T/S; 84A/C (*AAC* 2002;46:2926; *J Virol* 2001;75:7462). Most patients who receive LPV/r as their first PI have no PI resistance mutations at virologic failure. Mutations 47A and 32I may be associated with high-level resistance (*Topics HIV Med* 2006;14:125). The I50V mutation selected by fosamprenavir causes significant loss of susceptibility to LPV. 63P is common without PI exposure; this mutation combined with other PI resistance mutations has been associated with LPV/r failure (*Topics in HIV Med* 2003;11:92). See pg. 550t.

5 Drug Information

PHARMACOLOGY

- **Bioavailability:** The tablet formulation shows no significant difference in AUC or C_{max} whether given in a fed or fasting state. With the oral solution, there is an AUC increase of 80% when given with a moderate fat meal. The addition of RTV results in a significant increase in LPV concentrations, AUC, and T½ due to inhibition of the cytochrome P450 CYP3A4 isoenzymes. The mean steady-state LPV plasma concentrations are 15- to 20-fold higher than those without RTV. Protein binding is extensive, but there is sufficient CNS penetration to exceed the IC_{50} (*AIDS* 2005;19: 949). The CNS penetration score is 3 in a 4 class system (*Neurology* 2011;76:693).

- **T½:** 5-6 h

- **Metabolism/excretion:** Metabolized primarily by cytochrome P450 CYP3A4 isoenzymes. LPV/r inhibits CYP3A4 isoenzymes, but the effect is less than that of therapeutic doses of RTV, and similar to that of IDV. Based on PK data with APV, LPV/r may be an inducer of CYP3A4 at steady state. Less than 3% excreted unchanged in urine.

- **Renal failure:** No data are available, but usual dose is recommended. LPV/r is not removed with hemodialysis (*AIDS* 2001;15:662).

- **Hepatic failure:** No dose modification recommendations are available. Use with caution in end-stage liver disease.

SIDE EFFECTS: The drug is somewhat less well-tolerated compared to some alternative agents, with 2% discontinuing therapy due to adverse drug reactions in Phase II and III clinical trials through 48 weeks.

- **Diarrhea:** The most common adverse reactions are gastrointestinal, with diarrhea of at least moderate severity in 15-25%. Abdominal pain and nausea is also common and may improve with oral solution.

- **Transaminase levels:** Laboratory abnormalities through 72 weeks included transaminase increases (to >5x normal) in 10-12%.

- **PR and QTc interval prolongation:** Affect on PR interval is similar for most PIs and effect on QT is minimal (*JAIDS* 2011;25:367).

- **Class adverse reactions:** Insulin resistance, fat accumulation, and hyperlipidemia. Clinical trials show triglyceride increases to >750 mg/dL in 12-22%, and cholesterol increases to >300 mg/dL in 14-22% of treatment-naïve patients receiving LPV/r. In HIV-negative men given LPV/r for 10 days, the major effect was an increase in triglyceride levels averaging 83%; there was minimal effect on insulin sensitivity (*AIDS* 2004;18:641). Comparative trials with DRV/r (ARTEMIS) and with ATV/r (CASTLE) demonstrated that LPV/r is associated with significantly greater increases in triglycerides and total cholesterol levels (*JAIDS* 2010;53:323). The D:A:D analysis of 33,308 patients with 580 myocardial infarctions found a relative risk with LPV/r-based ART of 1.3/yr, with 150 events in 37,136 patient-years of LPV/r data (*JID* 2010;20:318). An analysis of 7,053 HIV-

Drug Information

infected patients in Quebec showed LPV/r was associated with a RR of 1.93 for an AMI compared to age matched HIV negative persons (Durand. *JAIDS* 2011;57:175).

- Report of 7 cases of renal or parotid lithiasis (*AIDS* 2004;18:705).

DRUG INTERACTIONS: Antiretroviral agents: See Table 5-55. The major effect is due to the inhibition of CYP3A4 isoenzymes, which results in prolongation of the half-life of drugs metabolized by this route. It is likely an inducer of CYP3A4 and glucuronyl transferase. **Drugs contraindicated for concurrent use: Rifampin, simvastatin, lovastatin, midazolam, triazolam, cisapride, pimozide, derivatives** and **St. Johns's wort, astemizole,** and **terfenadine. Avoid: Bepridil, alfuzosin, amiodarone, flecainide, propafenone, fluticasone, rifapentine,** and **quinidine. Drugs that require a modified dose: Rifabutin** AUC increased 3-fold; with standard LPV dose, rifabutin dose to 150 mg q24-48h. Consider rifabutin TDM. Note that a pharmacokinetic trial of this recommended dose appeared to give inadequate rifabutin exposure with LPV/r (*CID* 2009;49:1305). **Clarithromycin** AUC increased 77%; reduce clarithromycin dose in renal failure; use 50% clarithromycin dose with CrCl 30-60 mL/min and 25% dose with CrCl <30 mL/min. **Methadone** AUC decreased by 53%; monitor for withdrawal (conflicting data on withdrawal symptoms). **Trazodone** AUC increased 240%. Use lowest trazodone dose with close monitoring. **Bosentan:** LPV/r increased bosentan 48-fold on day 4 and 5-fold on day 10 (at steady state). Bosentan 62.5 mg; co-administer only after >10 days of RTV-boosted PI. **Atorvastatin** AUC increased 5- to 6-fold; use lowest dose (10 mg/d) or use alternative, such as pravastatin, or rosuvastatin (5 mg/d). **Pravastatin** levels increased 33%; no dose adjustment. **Azoles:** See pg. 208. **Ketoconazole** levels increased 3-fold; limit to ≤200 mg/d. **Voriconazole:** RTV 200 mg/d reduces voriconazole AUC 40%; avoid or consider TDM. **Itraconazole** levels increased; do not exceed 200 mg/d or monitor levels. **Oral contraceptives:** ethinyl estradiol AUC decreased by 42%; use additional or alternative methods. **Drugs for erectile dysfunction: sildenafil** level increase anticipated; start with 25 mg/48h; **vardenafil:** no data; start with 2.5 mg/72h; **tadalafil:** start with 20 mg and increase to 46 mg qd as tolderated. **Disulfiram:** Oral solution of LPV/r contains alcohol; avoid. **Fluticasone:** May increase levels of fluticasone with decreased serum cortisol levels; avoid coadministration. **Prednisone:** May increase prednisone level; consider dose adjustment with long-term use. **Anticonvulsants:** LPV and phenytoin levels decreased by 33% and 31%, respectively. **Carbamazepine** and **phenobarbital** may decrease serum level of LPV. Consider TDM or use alternative anticonvulsants (i.e., valproic acid, lamotrigine, levetiracetam). **Valproic acid:** May decrease valproic acid; LPV AUC increased 75%. **Lamotrigine:** LPV not affected, but lamotrigine AUC decreased 50%. Titrate to effect. **Atovaquone** levels may be decreased, requiring dose adjustment. **TDF** AUC increase

5 Drug Information

32%; clinical significance unknown; dose adjustment not recommended. **Tacrolimus** half-life increased 10-fold (*Clin Pharmacokinet* 2007;46:941); **sirolimus** and **cyclosporine** T½ may also be increased significantly. **Digoxin** AUC increased 81%; monitor closely. **Bupropion** AUC decreased 46%; titrate to effect.

PREGNANCY: Category C. LPV is the preferred 3rd agent for pregnant women according to the 2010 DHHS Recommendations for Use of Antiretroviral Drugs for Pregnant HIV-1 Infected Women. Most of the pharmacology and clinical trials have used the 133/33 mg LPV/r capsules, which demonstrated suboptimal levels in the 3rd trimester (*AIDS* 2006:20:1931). This led to the recommendation to use 3 tabs (600/150 mg) bid during the third trimester in the 2008 recommendations. The more recent pharmacokinetic studies with the tablet form found a median AUC of 72 ug*h/mL in the 2nd trimester, 97 ug*h/mL with the increased dose in the 3rd trimester and 129

■ TABLE 5-55: **Dose Adjustments for Concurrent Use of LPV/r with Other Antiretroviral Agents**

Drug	Effect on Coadministered Drug	Effect on LPV	Dose Recommendation
EFV	No change	↓36%	EFV 600 mg hs + LPV/r 400/100 mg or 500/125 mg bid bid (treatment-naïve) or 600/150 mg bid (treatment-experienced). LPV/r qd not recommended
IDV	C_{min} ↓45%	No change	IDV 600 mg bid + LPV/r 400/100 mg bid
ETR	↓17%	↓18%	Standard doses
NVP	No change	C_{min} ↓55%	NVP standard + LPV/r 400/100 mg bid (treatment-naïve) or 600/150 mg bid (treatment-experienced). LPV/r 500/125 mg bid can be considered. LPV/r qd not recommended
SQV	↑	↑	SQV 1000 mg bid + LPV/r 400/100 mg bid*
NFV	↑25%	↓27%	Data insufficient; avoid coadministration
ATV	C_{min} ↑45%	No change	Dose: ATV 300 mg qd + LPV/r 400/100 bid
FPV	C_{min} ↓4%	C_{min} ↓53%	No clear dose recommendation. Avoid or consider FPV 1400 mg bid + LPV/r 600/150 mg bid.
DRV	AUC ↓50%	AUC ↑53%	Avoid.
TPV	—	AUC ↓55%	Avoid.
MVC	↑4x	—	MVC dose 150 mg bid
RAL	Interaction unlikely	—	Standard dose
TDF	TDF AUC ↑32%	No change	Clinical significance unknown. Use standard dose.

* Shows synergy *in vitro* (*AAC* 2002;46:2249).

Drug Information

ug*h/mL 2 wks postpartum (*JAIDS* 2010;54:381). Based on these observations, the 2010 DHHS Pregnancy Guideline recommendation is 2 tabs bid (standard dose) until 30 wks gestation and then 3 tabs bid with return to the standard dose at discharge. The Pregnancy Registry reported birth defects in 6/267 (1.9%) first trimester exposures, which is less than the background rate without LPV exposure (1/1/2011).

LOTRIMIN – see Clotrimazole (pg. 220)

MARAVIROC (MVC)

TRADE NAME: *Selzentry* (ViiV/GlaxoSmithKline; *Celsentri*)

FORMS AND COST: 150 and 300 mg tabs, AWP is $18.36 (for 150 mg and 300 mg); $1101.42/mo

CLASS: CCR5 antagonist entry inhibitor: MVC binds the transmembrane co-receptor of R5-tropic virus to prevent its interaction with the V3 loop of gp120. This blocks viral entry (*AIDS* 2009;23:1931).

PHARMACOLOGY:

- Absorption – 32%; food effect – minimal; T1/2 10 hrs;
- Excretion – stool (75%), urine (20%), pharmacokinetics – substrate for CYP3A and Pgp (*CID* 2009;47:236).
- CNS penetration score is 3 in a 4 class system (*Neurology* 2011;76:693).

STANDARD DOSE: 300 mg po bid with or without food

NOTE: Dose varies based on concurrent meds

- Strong CYP 3A4 inhibitors +/- CYP3A4 inducer (which includes all PIs other than TPV/r): 150 mg bid
- No dose adjustment based on concurrent use of drugs that are not strong inducers or inhibitors of CYP3A including ENF, NVP, RAL, TPV/r: 300 mg bid
- Strong CYP 3A4 inducers including EFV, ETR and rifampin without use of PI; MVC 600 mg bid

Renal failure: Renal excretion accounts for <25% of clearance. 1) CrCl < 30 mL/min or HD: Reduce dose to 150 mg bid if signs of postural hypotension and 2) CrCl < 30 mL/min + co-administration of CYP3A inhibitor. Avoid.

Hepatic failure: Limited data show minimal effect. No dose adjustment.

STORAGE: Room temperature

INDICATIONS: HIV-infected patients with: 1) R5 virus only as shown by a co-receptor tropism assay (see pg. 48); and 2) virologic failure and resistance to multiple antiretroviral agents.

ADVANTAGES: 1) Active against R5-tropic HIV strains, including strains resistant to other antiretroviral agents, 2) established efficacy in patients with multiple drug exposure and treatment failure (MOTIVATE trials), 3) no food effect and 4) overall outcome similar to EFV for treatment naïve patients without EFV side effects (MERIT trial). Recommended as an acceptable alternative when combined with AZT/3TC in treatment-naïve patients (2011 DHHS Guidelines and 2010 IAS-USA Guidelines).

DISADVANTAGES: 1) Requirement for pre-treatment screening with expensive co-receptor tropism assay; 2) twice-daily dosing; 3) limited experience with this agent and class; 4) need for caution with pre-existing liver disease , including chronic hepatitis B or C; 5) studied only with AZT/3TC for initial therapy; and 6) drug interactions requiring dose adjustment.

RESISTANCE: Failure occurs by two distinctive mechanisms:

- Selection of pre-existing X4 or dual/mixed (D/M) tropic HIV that escaped detection on baseline tropism screening (*J Virol* 2006;80: 4909). These accounted for 60% of MVC failures using the original *Trophile* assay. The enhanced susceptibility topism assay (*Trofile* ES) is more sensitive (99.7%) at detecting X4- or D/M-tropic virus present at low levels. R5 strains remain susceptible to MVC in this case. Prevalence of R5 virus is 80-90% in treatment naïve patients (*JID* 2005;192:466; *JID* 2005;191:866) and 50-60% in treatment-experienced patients (*JID* 2006;194:926; *CID* 2007;44: 591).

- MVC resistance is attributed to mutations in the V3 loop of the HIV envelope (gp120), usually with mutations at multiple sites that result in a reduction in maximal percent inhibition rather than a fold increase in IC_{50} seen with other antiretroviral agents (*Top HIV Med* 2007;15:119). Polymorphisms 4L, 11R and 19S are associated with reduced response.

- HIV strains resistant to MVC by these mechanisms do not show cross resistance to ENF, which blocks HIV entry by a completely different mechanism (and should be additive or synergistic with MVC). There is no cross resistance between MVC and other classes of antiretroviral agents (*AAC* 2005;49:4751). Analysis of R5-V3 sequences in 498 treatment-naïve HIV-infected patients demonstrated a baseline prevalence of resistance of < 5% (*JAC* 2010;65:2502).

CLINICAL TRIALS

- **MOTIVATE-1 and -2:** Phase III trials of MVC (300 mg qd or bid) plus optimized background therapy (OBT) vs. OBT in highly treatment experienced patients. Enrollment criteria: R5 virus, 3 class exposure, and treatment failure with VL >5,000 c/mL. Randomization was 2:2:1 for MVC 300 mg bid, 300 mg qd, or OBR. Results at 48 weeks for

■ TABLE 5-56: **48-Week Results of MOTIVATE-1 & -2 Comparing OBR vs. MVC + OBR (2-dose Regimens)**

	MVC qd n = 414	MVC bid n = 426	OBR alone n = 209
Baseline			
CD4 count (mean)	187/mm³	196/mm³	189/mm³
HIV VL (mean log$_{10}$ c/mL	4.9	4.9	4.9
<2 active drugs OBR	66%	65%	70%
Results			
VL <50 c/mL	46%	43%	17%
VL <400 c/mL	52%	56%	23%
ADR with discontinuation	5%	5%	5%
AST >5x ULN	4%	4%	3%

■ TABLE 5-57: **MERIT Trial of MVC vs. EFV, Each with AZT/3TC in Treatment-naïve Patients (Post-hoc Analysis) at 48 Weeks** (*JID* 2010; 201:803)

	MVC n = 311	EFV n = 303
Baseline		
CD4 median (cells/mL)	254	236
Viral load (log$_{10}$ c/mL)	4.88	4.85
Results (48 wks)		
Discontinuation due to lack of efficacy	29 (9.3%)	12 (4.0%)*
Adverse events	13 (4.2%)	43 (14.2%)*
CD4 count change (cells/mm³)	+212	+171

* P <0.05

1,049 randomized patients are summarized in Table 5-56 (*NEJM* 2008;359:1429). The 96-week data showed VL < 50 c/mL in 39% and 41% of patients treated with MVC once or twice daily, respectively (*JAIDS* 2010;55:558). Among those with VL<50 c/mL at 48 weeks, virologic suppression (<50 c/mL) was maintained in 81% of those randomized to receive once-daily MVC and 87% of those receiving twice-daily MVC.

■ **MERIT:** MVC vs. EFV in treatment-naïve patients. Participants had R5-tropic virus at baseline and were randomized to receive MVC or EFV, each in combination with 2 NRTIs. Of 1,277 participants 895 began therapy with either MVC+AZT/3TC or EFV+AZT/3TC. Results are summarized in Table 5-57 based on the post hoc analysis (MERIT ES) that corrected for erroneous *Trophile* assays at baseline (*JID* 2010;201:803). In the 96-week follow-up of MERIT, virologic suppression (<50 c/mL) was maintained in 63% of the EFV arm and

5 Drug Information

59% of the MVC arm; time to loss of virologic response (TLOVR) in responders was 61% with EFV and 61% with MVC; median CD4 count increase (cells/mm³) was 171 with EFV and 212 with MVC; and discontinuations for adverse events were 16% with EFV and 6% with MVC (*HIV Clin Trials* 2010;11:125). These results showed EFV-based ART had somewhat better virologic outcomes (that was not statistically significant) and MVC showed better tolerance (*HIV Clin Trials* 2011;12:24).

- **DUAL/MIXED-TROPIC VIRUS STUDY (A4001029):** This was an exploratory, randomized, blinded, placebo-controlled trial to determine the safety and efficacy of MVC treatment in patients with D/M-tropic HIV. Entry criteria were the same as for MOTIVATE-1 and -2, and participants were randomized 1:1:1 to receive MVC twice daily + OBR or MVC once daily + OBR or OBR alone (*JID* 2009; 199:1638). Athough MVC was not virologically effective in this population, there was no decline in CD4 count. These results suggest that the switch to X4 virus is a consequence of disease progression rather than a cause (*JID* 2011;203:237).

NRTI-SPARING: See pg. 122-123.

- **A4001078 - MVC 150 mg qd+ATV/r 300/100 mg qd vs. ATV+TDF/FTC:** A pilot trial of a NRTI-sparing regimen in 120 treatment-naïve patients with a mean baseline CD4 count of 351 cells/mm³ and median VL 4.6 $\log_{10}$ c/mL (Mills A. 2010 IAS, Vienna;Abstr. THLBB203). At 24 weeks, the MCV+ATV/r arm had a numerically lower response rate (80 vs. 89%; p=NS) and more treatment-limiting side effects (16% vs. 8%).

- **MVC/RAL/ETR:** A prospective study of 28 triple-class failure patients given RAL 400 mg bid, MVC 600 mg bid, and ETR 200 mg bid, 26 (92%) had VL <50 c/mL at 48 weeks (*AIDS* 2010;24:924).

- **INTENSIFICATION:** The goal was to determine the potential value of the immunomodulary properties of MVC. Patients (n=45) with CD4 counts <350 cells/mm³ and VL <48 c/mL (*PloS One* 2010;5:e13188) were randomized to add MVC or placebo. MVC increased activation of T cells in the gut and blood but had no effect on the CD4 count (Hunt P. CROI 2011:Abstr.153LB). Treatment intensification also failed to reduce CSF viral load (*JAIDS* 2010;55:590).

PHARMACOLOGY (*JAIDS* 2006;42:183; *Nat Med* 2005;11:1170; *JAIDS* 2006;42:183).

- **CNS penetration** shows a CSF:plasma ratio of 0.09, and CSF showed no detectable HIV in all 9 patients with VL <40 c/mL (*JAIDS* 2010;55:606).

- **Bioavailability:** 25-35%, no dose adjustment with or without food

- **T1/2:** 14-18 hrs

- **Excretion:** 25% metabolized by CYP3A4 and 11% hydroxylated. Unchanged drug and metabolities are excreted via the GI tract

Drug Information

accounting for 76%. About 25% is renally excreted. MVC with a CYP3A4 inhibitor is not recommended in patients with CrCl <30 mL/min. Renal clearance accounts for <25% of total clearance.

DRUG INTERACTIONS (TABLES 5-58A AND B)

- MVC does not inhibit or induce CYP3A4 so it does not alter levels or require dose changes of concurrent agents that use the P450 metabolic pathway.

- Concurrent use of drugs that induce CYP3A4 include **EFV** which decreases MVC AUC by 45%, **rifampin** which decreases the AUC by 63% and **ETR** which decreases MVC 53%. The dose of MVC to compensate for this difference is 600 mg bid. Other CYP3A4 inducers include **barbiturates, carbamazepine, phenytoin, primidone** and **St. John's wort**; avoid or increase MVC dose (600 mg bid).

- Concurrent use of drugs that inhibit CYP3A4, including all **boosted PIs** other than TPV/r, increase MVC AUC 2-8-fold; the dose of MVC should be 150 mg bid. Other drugs that inhibit CYP3A4 include **azoles** (ketoconazole, itraconazole), **erythromycin, clarithromycin**, and **nefazodone** – reduce dose (MVC 150 mg bid). Some SSRIs, **diltiazem, verapamil, amiodarone, cimetidine**, and **fluvoxamine** –

■ TABLE 5-58A: **Maraviroc ART Drug Interactions**

Drug	Effect of Interaction	Recommendations/Comments
NVP	MVC serum concentration is not significantly affected	MVC 300 mg bid + SD NVP if no PI is used
EFV	MVC AUC decreased by 45%	MVC 600 mg bid if no PI is used
ATV	MVC AUC increased 3.6x with ATV/r; MVC increased 5x	MVC 150 mg bid with ATV or ATV/r
TDF	No significant change in MVC concentrations	MVC 300 mg bid
SQV/r	MVC AUC increased 732%	MVC 150 mg bid
LPV/r	MVC AUC increased 283%	MVC 150 mg bid
ATV/r	MVC AUC increased 388%	MVC 150 mg bid
TPV/r	No significant interation	MVC 300 mg bid
LPV/r + EFV	MVC AUC 2.5 5x	MVC 150 mg bid
ETR	MVC AUC decreased 53%	MVC 600 mg bid
ETR + DRV/r	MVC AUC increased 210%	MVC 150 mg bid
FPV, FPV/r, IDV, DLV	Unknown. Anticipate MVC AUC increase	MVC 150 mg bid
RTV	MVC AUC increases 2.6x with RTV 200 mg/d	MVC 150 mg bid
DRV/r	MVC AUC increased 344% with co-administration	MVC 150 mg bid

5 Drug Information

■ TABLE 5-58B: **Maraviroc Non-ART Drug Interactions**

Drug	Effect of Interaction	Recommendations/Comments
Carbamazepine	MVC AUC may significantly decrease with carbamazepine	MVC 600 mg bid, or consider alternative anticonvulsant (i.e. valproic acid or levetiracetam)
Clarithromycin	May increase MVC serum concentrations	MVC 150 mg bid
Erythromycin	May increase MVC serum concentrations	MVC 150 mg bid
Ethinylestradiol	No significant interaction	MVC 300 mg bid. Consider additional barrier contraception.
Itraconazole	May increase MVC serum concentrations	MVC 150 mg bid
Ketoconazole	MVC AUC increased 5-fold with co-administration.	MVC 150 mg bid
Levonorgestrel	No significant interaction	MVC 300 mg bid. Consider an additional barrier contraception
Nefazodone	May increase MVC serum concentrations	MVC 150 mg bid
Phenobarbital	MVC AUC may significantly decrease with phenobarbital co-administration	MVC 600 mg bid, or consider alternative anticonvulsant (i.e. valproic acid or levetiracetam)
Phenytoin	MVC AUC may significantly decrease with phenytoin co-administration	MVC 600 mg bid, or consider alternative anticonvulsant (i.e. valproic acid or levetiracetam).
Rifabutin	Modest impact on MVC serum concentrations	MVC 300 mg bid (No data)
Rifampin	MVC AUC decreased 66% with co-administration	MVC 600 mg bid- (Limited clinical data)
Sulfamethoxazole-trimethoprim	MVC AUC increased 10%	MVC 300 mg bid

may also increase MVC levels, but there are no dose recommendations. If potent inducers are used with potent inhibitors, use MVC at 150 mg bid (*e.g.*, EFV+ATV/r+MVC dosed 150 mg bid).

ADVERSE DRUG REACTIONS: The drug is usually well tolerated. The most common ADRs are **GI intolerance** with **diarrhea** (22%), **nausea** (18%), **headache** (14%) and **fatigue** (12%), but many of these reactions were noted in a comparable number of placebo recipients. The most important ADR in trials has been **postural hypotension**, which may occur more frequently in those without dose adjustment with concurrent use of a CYP3A4 inhibitor and those with renal failure or with initial dosing using higher doses (e.g., 600 mg daily), before enzyme induction has occurred. Consider dose escalation. Grade 3-4

Drug Information

hepatotoxicity has been reported in 3-5% and sometimes follows a pruritic rash with eosinophilia. This was an early concern with MVC, but an analysis of 2,350 recipients found only 2 cases of severe hepatotoxicity, and both were confounded by other factors (*AIDS* 2010;24:2743). In clinical trials there was a significant increase in **URIs** in MVC recipients (5% vs. 2%), but other infections do not appear to be increased. There was concern that decreased immune surveillance due to CCR5 blockade would promote **lymphomas**, but that has not been the experience to date. The 96-week data from the MOTIVATE-1 & -2 and MERIT trials with 1499 MVC recipients showed no increase in **cancer** rates (Walmsley, 2010 IAS;Abstr. TUPE0157). The CCR5 receptor plays a role in the pathophysiology of **West Nile Virus infection**, so there a theoretical possibility that MVC could increase this risk (*JID* 2010;201:178), but this has not been seen clinically. It is emphasized that this is a relatively new class of antiretroviral agents, so the long-term experience is limited. The first CCR5 antagonist (aplaviroc) was withdrawn due to severe hepatotoxicity, which has not been a subsequent concern with MVC as noted above (*AIDS* 2010;24:2473). The same applies to malignancy (*Eur J Med Res* 2007;12:409). MVC appears to be **"lipid neutral"** and may reduce levels of **immune activation** better than EFV according to a substudy of MERIT (*PLoS One* 2010;5:e13188).

BLACK BOX WARNINGS: Severe hepatotoxicity that may be preceded by a pruritic rash and eosinophilia suggesting a systemic allergic reaction.

PREGNANCY: Category B. Experience in humans is very limited. Not recmmended by the 2010 DHHS Guidelines for Pregnant Women with HIV Infection because safety and pharmacokinetics have not been established.

MARINOL – see Dronabinol (pg. 242)

MEGACE – see Megestrol acetate (below)

MEGESTROL ACETATE

TRADE NAME: *Megace* (Bristol-Myers Squibb) and generic

FORMS AND COST: Tabs: 20 mg at $0.65, 40 mg at $1.23. Oral suspension: 40 mg/mL at $144/240 mL

PATIENT ASSISTANCE: 800-272-4878

CLASS: Synthetic progestin related to progesterone

INDICATIONS: Appetite stimulant to promote weight gain in patients with HIV infection or neoplastic disease.

USUAL REGIMEN

Drug Information

5

- **Oral suspension:** 400 mg/d (20 mL in one daily dose), up to 800 mg/d.
- **Tablets:** 400-800 mg/d (suspension usually preferred).

EFFICACY: A controlled trial of 271 patients with HIV-associated wasting found that those given megestrol 800 mg qd gained a mean of 4 kg more than placebo recipients. (*Ann Intern Med* 1994;121:393). However, most of the weight gain was fat. Another study showed that the increase in caloric intake was not sustained after 8 wks (*Ann Intern Med* 1994;121: 400). Published data for use in HIV infection are available only for men. A review of appetite stimulants for patients with cystic fibrosis came to no clear conclusions, but provided the best supportive data for megesterol compared to dronabinol, mirtazapine and cyproheptadine (*J Hum Nutr Diet* 2007;20:526). Megestrol can cause hypogonadism, so it may require discontinuation or a replacement dose of testosterone in men (200 mg q2wk) or anabolic steroids and resistance exercises (*NEJM* 1999;340:1740).

PHARMACOLOGY

- **Bioavailability:** >90%
- **T½:** 30 h
- **Elimination:** 60-80% excreted in urine; 7-30% excreted in feces.

SIDE EFFECTS

- **Most serious** are **hypogonadism** (which may exacerbate wasting), **diabetes**, and **adrenal insufficiency**.
- **Most common** are **diarrhea, impotence, rash, flatulence, asthenia** and **hyperglycemia** (5%).
- **Less common or rare** include carpal tunnel syndrome, thrombosis, nausea, vomiting, edema, vaginal bleeding, and alopecia; high dose (400 mg to 1600 mg/d) – hyperpnea, chest pressure, mild increase in blood pressure, dyspnea, congestive heart failure.
- A review of **FDA reports of adverse drug reactions** with megestrol included 5 cases of Cushing syndrome, 12 cases of new-onset diabetes, and 17 cases of possible adrenal insufficiency (*Arch Intern Med* 1997;157:1651). One report suggested a 6-fold increase in the risk of deep venous thrombosis (*J Am Med Dir Assoc* 2003;4:255). Another review reported an association with osteonecrosis (*JAIDS* 2000;25:19).

DRUG INTERACTIONS: Not a substrate of CYP3A4. No signficant drug-drug interactions.

PREGNANCY: Category D. Progestational drugs are associated with genital abnormalities in male and female fetuses exposed during first 4 mos of pregnancy.

MEPRON – see Atovaquone (pg. 204)

METHADONE

TRADE NAME: *Dolophine* (Roxane) and generic

FORMS AND COST: Tabs: 5 mg at $0.10, 10 mg at $0.14. Usual yearly cost of medication for methadone maintenance averages $180.

CLASS: Opiate schedule II. The FDA restricts physician prescribing for methadone maintenance to those licensed to provide this service and those attached to methadone maintenance programs. However, licensed physicians can prescribe methadone for pain control.

INDICATIONS AND DOSES

- **Detoxification** for substantial opiate abstinence symptoms: Initial dose is based on opiate tolerance, usually 15-20 mg; additional doses may be necessary. Daily dose at 40 mg usually stabilizes patient; when stable 2-3 days, decrease dose 20% per day. Must complete detoxification in <180 days or consider maintenance.

- **Maintenance** as oral substitute for heroin or other morphine-like drugs: Initial dose 15-30 mg depending on extent of prior use, up to 40 mg/d. Subsequent doses depend on response. Usual maintenance dose is 40-100 mg/d, but higher doses are sometimes required. Most states limit the maximum daily dose to 80 mg to 120 mg/d, but doses may be increased due to drug-drug interactions (especially with EFV and NVP).

- **Note:** During first 3 mos, and for all patients receiving >100 mg/d, observation is required 6 days/wk. With good adherence and rehabilitation, clinic attendance may be reduced for observed ingestion 3 days/wk with maximum 2-day supply for home administration. After 2 years, clinic visits may be reduced to 2x/wk with 3-day drug supplies. After 3 years, visits may be reduced to weekly with a 6-day supply. In a trial of Directly Administered Antiretroviral Therapy (DAART) with observed ART at the time methadone was given, adherence with supervised doses was strongly associated with virologic success (*AIDS Patient Care STDs* 2007;21:564).

- **Pain control:** 2.5-10.0 mg po q3-4h or 5-20 mg po q6-8h for severe chronic pain in terminally ill patients.

PHARMACOLOGY

- **Bioavailability:** >90% absorbed

- **T½:** 25 h. Duration of action with repeated administration is 24-48 h, but anlagesic T1/2 is shorter.

- **Elimination:** Metabolized by liver via CYP450 2B6>2C19>3A4. Parent compound excreted in urine with increased rate in acidic urine; metabolites excreted in urine and gut.

DRUG INTERACTIONS: See Table 5-59.

■ TABLE 5-59: **Drug Interactions with Methadone** (See Review: *Curr HIV/AIDS* 2010;7:152)

Drug	Effect on Methadone	Effect on Coadministered Drug	Comment
NRTIs			
ABC	AUC ↓22%	↓ Peak	Dose adjustment unlikely
AZT	None	AUC ↑43%	Monitor for AZT toxicity
3TC	No effect	—	Standard doses
ddI	None	ddI EC – no change	ddI EC preferred
d4T	None	AUC ↓23%	No dose adjustment
TDF	No effect	No effect	Standard doses
DLV	No data; may ↑	No effect	Use standard DLV dose; monitor for methadone toxcity.
NNRTIs			
EFV	AUC ↓52%	No data	Likely to need ↑ methadone dose
NVP	AUC ↓41%	No effect	Withdrawal common
ETR	None	No effect	No dose adjustment; monitor for withdrawal
PIs			
DRV/r	AUC ↓16%	↓	Monitor for withdrawal
FPV/r	AUC ↓16%	↓25%	Monitor for withdrawal
SQV/r	↓10-20% with SQV/r	No effect	Dose SQV/r 1000/100 bid
ATV	No effect	No effect	ATV: No empiric dose adjustment ATV/r: No data; monitor
TPV/r	↓48%	No effect	Empiric dose adjustment; monitor, may need methadone increase.
IDV	No effect	No effect	Standard doses
LPV/r	AUC ↓25-50%	↓	Monitor dose increase (conflicting data)
NFV	AUC ↓40%	No effect	Monitor. Withdrawal rare.
Other			
MVC	No data	No data	Interaction unlikely
RAL	No effect	No effect	Usual dose
Fluconazole	↑30%	No effect	Monitor for methadone toxicity,
Rifampin	↓↓	No effect	Need ↑ methadone dose
Rifabutin	No effect	No effect	No dose adjustment
Phenytoin, carbamazepine, phenobarbitol	↓↓	No effect	May need ↑ methadone dose

Drug Information

- **Acute toxicity:** CNS depression (stupor or coma), respiratory depression, flaccid muscles, cold skin, bradycardia, hypotension. **Treatment:** Respiratory support ± gastric lavage (even hours after ingestion due to pylorospasm) ± naloxone (respiratory depression may last longer than naloxone duration of action – repeated dosing may be needed; may precipitate acute withdrawal syndrome).

- **Chronic toxicity:** Tolerance/physical dependence with abstinence syndrome following withdrawal – onset at 3-4 days after last dose of weakness, anxiety, anorexia, insomnia, abdominal pain, headache, sweating, and hot-cold flashes. **Treatment:** Detoxification.

- QTc prolongation

PREGNANCY: Category C. Avoid during first 3 mos and use spar-ingly, in small doses, during last 6 mos.

MYCELEX – see Clotrimazole (pg. 220)

MYCOBUTIN – see Rifabutin (pg. 362)

MYCOSTATIN – see Nystatin (pg. 340)

NEBUPENT – see Pentamidine (pg. 346)

NELFINAVIR (NFV)

TRADE NAME: *Viracept* (ViiV Healthcare)

CLASS: Protease inhibitor

FORMULATIONS, REGIMENS AND COST.

- **Forms:** Tabs, 250 and 625 mg; oral powder, 50 mg/mL (144 gm) at $74.15

- **Regimens:** 1250 mg bid (tabs); 25 cc bid (oral solution)

- **AWP:** $844.20/mo

FOOD: Increases levels 2-3x; take with food, preferably a fatty meal

RENAL FAILURE: Standard dose

HEPATIC FAILURE: No recommendation; use with caution

STORAGE: Room temperature, 15-30°C

PATIENT ASSISTANCE: 800-777-6637

ADVANTAGES: Extensive experience; well tolerated in pregnancy

DISADVANTAGES: Reduced potency compared to most other regimens; need for concurrent fatty meal; diarrhea; inability to effectively boost levels with RTV

5 Drug Information

CLINICAL TRIALS: See Table 5-60.

■ TABLE 5-60: **Clinical Trials of NFV in Treatment-naïve Patients**

Trial	Regimen	N	Duration (wks)	VL <50	VL <200-400
COMBINE (*Antiviral Ther* 2002;7:81)	NFV+AZT/3TC	70	48	50%	60%
	NVP+AZT/3TC	72		65%*	75%*
SOLO (*AIDS* 2004;18:1529)	FPV/r (1400/200 qd) +AZT/3TC	322	48	56%	68%
	NFV (1250 bid)+AZT/3TC	327		42%	65%
NEAT (*JAIDS* 2004;35: 22)	FPV 1400 bid+AZT/3TC	166	48	58%	66%*
	NFV 1250 bid+AZT/3TC	83		42%	51%
ACTG 384 (*NEJM* 2003; 349:2293)	EFV+AZT/3TC	155	48	–	88%*
	NFV+AZT/3TC	155		–	67%
	NFV+EFV+AZT/3TC	178		–	84%
INITIO (*Lancet* 2006;368:287)	EFV+ddI+d4T	188	192	74%	–
	NFV+ddI+d4T	162		62%	–
	EFV+NFV+ddI+d4T	155		62%	–
Abbott M98-863 (*NEJM* 2002;346:2039)	LPV/r+d4T+3TC	326	48	67%*	75%*
	NFV+d4T+3TC	327		52%	63%
BMS 008 (*JAIDS* 2004;36:684 and *Reyataz* pkg insert)	ATV+d4T+3TC	181	48	33%	67%
	NFV+d4T+3TC	91		38%	59%

* Superior to comparator (P <0.05)

RESISTANCE: The primary resistance mutation is D30N, which is associated with phenotypic resistance to NFV but not to other protease inhibitors (*AAC* 1998;42:2775). However, the L90M mutation can also occur and, unlike 30N, it confers cross-resistance to all PIs except TPV/r and DRV/r. Other less important or secondary mutations are 10F/I, 36I, 46I/L, 71V/T, 77I, 82A/F/T/S, 84V, and 88D/S.

PHARMACOLOGY

■ **Bioavailability:** Absorption with meals is 20-80%. Fatty meal increases absorption 2- to 3-fold.

■ **T½:** 3.5-5.0 h (serum)

■ **CNS penetration:** No detectable levels in CSF (*JAIDS* 1999;20:39) (see pg. 550t)

■ **Excretion:** Primarily by cytochrome P450 CYP2C19 (major) and CYP3A4 (minor). Inhibits CYP3A4. Only 1-2% is found in urine; up to 90% is found in stool, primarily as a hydroxylated metabolite designated M8, which is as active as NFV against HIV (*AAC* 2001;45:1086).

Drug Information

- **Dose modification in renal or hepatic failure:** None. NFV is removed with hemodialysis so that post dialysis dosing is important (*AIDS* 2000;14:89). The drug is not removed by peritoneal dialysis (*JAC* 2000;45:709).
- **Dose modification with hepatic failure:** With severe liver disease, consider therapeutic drug monitoring. It appears that autoinduction of NFV metabolism is blunted in severe liver disease, and there is also a reduction in the M8 active metabolite. Standard doses may yield high or low levels.

SIDE EFFECTS

- **Diarrhea:** About 10-30% of recipients have a secretory diarrhea, characterized by low osmolarity and high sodium, possibly due to chloride secretion (7th CROI, San Francisco, 2000:Abstr. 62). Management strategies include use of several over-the-counter, inexpensive ($4-10/mo) remedies, including oat bran (1500 mg bid), psyllium (1 tsp qd or bid), loperamide (4 mg, then 2 mg every loose stool up to 16/d), or calcium (500 mg bid). Some respond to pancreatic enzymes (1-2 tabs with meals) at a cost of $30-111/mo (*CID* 2000;30:908).
- **Class adverse effects:** Lipodystrophy, increased levels of triglycerides and/or cholesterol, hyperglycemia with insulin resistance and type 2 diabetes, osteoporosis, and possible increased bleeding with hemophilia (*HIV Med* 2006;7:85).

DRUG INTERACTIONS

Drugs that should not be given concurrently: simvastatin, lovastatin, rifampin, astemizole, terfenadine, cisapride, pimozide, midazolam, triazolam, ergot derivatives, St. John's wort, amiodarone, quinidine, and **proton pump inhibitors.**

Drugs that require dose modifications: anticonvulsants (phenobarbital, carbamazepine, phenytoin); oral contraceptives; sildenafil (not to exceed 25 mg/48 hrs); **rifabutin** (decrease rifabutin dose to 150 mg/d and increase NFV dose to 1000 mg tid); **methadone** (no dose change); **statins** (use pravastatin or rosuvastatin); **clarithromycin** (reduce clarithromycin dose in renal failure; CrCl <30 mL/min); **azoles** (see pg. 208); **PIs and NNRTIs** (see Table 5-61); **colchicine:** NFV increases colchicine level; **buprenophine:** no significant effect. Use standard dose.

■ TABLE 5-61: **Nelfinavir Combinations with PIs and NNRTIs**

Drug	Recommendation
RTV, SQV, FPV, IDV	Inadequate data
NVP, EFV, RAL	Standard doses
LPV/r, DRV/r, ETR, TPV/r	Avoid combination
MVC	MVC 150 mg bid

Drug Information

PREGNANCY: Category B. Animal teratogenic studies negative; long-term animal carcinogenicity studies show increased tumors in rats given ≥300 mg/kg; placental passage not known. Experience to establish safety in pregnancy is extensive. The pregnancy registry shows birth defects in 45/1182 (3.8%) exposures (www.apregistry.com, accessed 1/1/2011). The 750 mg tid dose produced variable levels in pregnant women that were generally lower than in non-pregnant women. The 1250 mg bid regimen produced adequate levels except for variations in the third trimester (*CID* 2004;39:736). The 2010 DHHS Guidelines on ART in Pregnant Women recommend NFV as an alternate PI in a dose of 1250 mg bid.

NEUPOGEN – see G-CSF (pg. 291)

NEVIRAPINE (NVP)

TRADE NAME: *Viramune* and *Viramune XR* (Boehringer Ingelheim)

CLASS: Non-nucleoside reverse transcriptase inhibitor (NNRTI)

FORMULATIONS, REGIMENS AND COST:

- **Forms:** Tabs, 200 mg; oral solution, 50 mg/mL (240 mL bottle at $133.02); *Viramune XR* tabs. 400 mg.

- **Regimens:** 200 mg qd x 2 wks, then 400 mg/d using immediate release tab 200 mg bid or XR tab 400 mg qd. After treatment interruption >7 days should restart with the 200 mg/d regimen. If rash appears during the lead-in period, delay dose escalation until after the rash has resolved, and rule out hepatitis. The lead-in dosing regimen of 200 mg qd should not be continued beyond 28 days. No dose escalation when switching from EFV to NVP; start with NVP 400 mg qd (*AIDS* 2004;18:572). A 400 mg extended release forumulation (NVP-XR) for once daily dosing is in development.

- **AWP:** $614.24/mo (200 mg tab); $20.47/tab or $614.24/30 tabs (1 mo supply); price neutral with the prior formulation.

WARNINGS: 1) Avoid initiation of NVP in women with CD4 count >250/mm³ and men with a CD4 count >400/mm³ due to high rates of symptomatic hepatitis; 2) see guidelines for discontinuing NVP at pg. 117.

FOOD: No significant effect

RENAL FAILURE: Patients on dialysis should receive an additional dose of 200 mg following each dialysis treatment.

HEPATIC FAILURE: Contraindicated in patients with moderate or severe liver disease (Child-Pugh B or C).

DISCONTINUATION OF NVP-BASED ART:

The concern is NVP monotherapy if all antiretroviral drugs are stopped

Drug Information

simultaneously due to the long half-life of NVP. A pharmacokinetic study found that NVP could be detected in 83% if NVP recipients one week after the drug was stopped and 25% at 2 wks (*AIDS* 2007; 21:733). The recommendation is to continue the NRTI "backbone" for an additional 7-10 days (2011 DHHS Guidelines). Another option is to substitute a boosted PI for NVP for 2-4 wks before stopping therapy.

PATIENT ASSISTANCE: 800-556-8317 (7:30 am-5:30 pm CST, Mon.-Fri.)

ADVANTAGES: Extensive experience; 2NN trial suggests antiviral potency nearly comparable to EFV; no food effect; fewer lipid effects than EFV; relatively inexpensive third agent. A safe and effective agent for perinatal transmission prevention in resource-limited setting. A Cochrane Library review (2010) concluded that EFV and NVP are equally effective (with two NRTIs) for initial treatment (*Cochrane Database Syst Rev* 2010;8:12:CD004246). A retrospective review of the EuroSIDA database also showed long-term durability of NVP was comparable to that of EFV and LPV/r (*HIV Med* 2010;12:259).

DISADVANTAGES: High rates of serious hepatotoxicity in treatment naïve women with baseline CD4 counts >250/mm^3, high rates of rash, including TEN and Stevens-Johnson syndrome; single resistance mutations often eliminate all therapeutic value; cross-resistance to ETR more likely after failure of NPV than of EFV; single dose for prevention of perinatal transmission may cause resistance. Efficacy data for EFV are more extensive.

CLINICAL TRIALS: Table 5-62

- **2NN:** This is the pivotal study comparing EFV and NVP (see Table 5-62). ITT analysis at 48 weeks showed similar results for NVP bid and EFV, with VL <50 c/mL in 65% and 70%, respectively. The difference was not statistically significant, but the trial failed to show non-inferiority according to the FDA definition. The incidence of clinical hepatitis in NVP qd, NVP bid, EFV and NVP+EFV was 1.4%, 2.1%, 0.3% and 1.0%, respectively. There was more hepatotoxicity in NVP recipients (9.6% vs. 3.5%), and two deaths were attributed to NVP toxicity (*Lancet* 2004;363:1253). NVP given once daily caused more hepatotoxicity (13.6%) and EFV+NVP was inferior virologically compared to EFV alone.

- **NEWART TRIAL:** 152 treatment-naïve patients with baseline CD4 counts <250 cells/mm^3 (females) or <400 cells/mm^3 (males) were randomized to NVP (standard dose) or ATV/r, each with TDF/FTC (*JAIDS* 2010;13:Suppl 4:P4). At 48 weeks, VL was <50 c/mL in 61% (NVP) and 65% (ATV/r).

- **ARTEN:** Treatment-naïve patients with appropriate baseline CD4 counts (<250/mm^3 for women or <400/mm^3 for men) were randomized to NVP+TDF/FTC vs. ATV/r+TDF/FTC (Johnson M. 2009 ICAAC;Abstr. H924C). NVP recipients were in two dose regimens, 400 mg qd or 200 mg bid. The randomization was 1:1:1, but data for

5 Drug Information

the two NVP arms were combined and showed comparable results at 48 weeks, with VL <50 c/mL in 67% vs. 65% of NVP vs. ATV/r recipients, respectively (Table 5-62). The rate of failure with twice-daily dosing was 13% and for once-daily dosing it was 11%. VL decay and time to treatment response were significantly better for NVP recipients. The mean increase in CD4 counts at one year was 193 cells/mm^3 in both groups. The rate of treatment related discontinuations, including discontinuation due to adverse events and investigator-defined lack of efficacy, was greater with NVP (13.6% vs. 3.6%). The most common NVP-associated side effect was rash, but there were no grade 4 rashes.

- **VERxVE**: This trial compared the new 400 mg extended release NVP formulation given once daily (*Viramune* XR) to the previously available 200 mg immediate-release formulation given twice daily to 1013 treatment-naïve patients. Both groups received once-daily TDF/FTC. Criteria for inclusion were absence of baseline resistance and CD4 count <250/mm^3 (women) and <400/mm^3 (men). The median baseline VL was 4.7 log$_{10}$ c/mL, and the mean CD4 count was 228 (Gath J. 18th IAC, 2010, Vienna, THBB 202; Gath J. 50th ICAAC 2010:Abstr. H1808). The 48-week results showed viral

■ TABLE 5-62: **NVP Trials in Treatment-naïve Patients**

Trial	Regimen	N	Duration (wks)	VL <50	VL <200-500
Atlantic (*AIDS* 2000;15:2407)	NVP+ddI+d4T	89	48	54%*	58%
	IDV+ddI+d4T	100		55%*	57%
	3TC+ddI+d4T	109		46%	59%
COMBINE (*Antiviral Ther* 2002;7:81)	NVP+AZT/3TC	72	48	65%	75%
	NFV+AZT/3TC	70		50%	60%
2NN (*Lancet* 2004;363:1253)	NVP 400 mg qd+3TC+d4T	220	48	70%	
	NVP 200 mg bid+3TC+d4T	387		65%†	
	EFV+3TC+d4T	400		70%	–
	EFV+NVP+3TC+d4T	209		63%†	
ARTEN (49th ICAAC, 2009;Abstr. H924C)	NVP+TDF/FTC	376	48	67%	–
	ATV/r+TDF/FTC	193		65%	
NEWART (*JAIDS* 2010; 13[S4]:P4)	NVP+TDF/FTC	75	48	61%	–
	ATV/r+TDF/FTC	77		64%	
VERxVE (Gathe. ICAAC 2010:Abstr. H204)	NVP IR+TDF/FTC	506	48	65%	–
	NVP XR+TDF/FTC	505		80%†	–

* Superior to comparators (*P*<0.05). The *P*-value in COMBINE was 0.06.
† NVP did not meet the non-inferiority criteria

suppression (<50 c/mL) nonsignificant superior results with the XR formulation: 81% vs. 76%, for all participants and 73% vs. 71% for the subset with a baseline VL >100,000 c/mL. Pharmacology studies showed the trough levels for the XR formulation were lower for once-daily XR vs. twice-daily IR but were >13-fold higher than the IC_{90} for wild type HIV.

- **Switch therapy**

  □ **Switch from EFV- to NVP-based ART due to intolerance to EFV:** In ACTG 5095, switching from EFV to NVP was allowed in patients who could not tolerate EFV. The switch was due to EFV-associated CNS toxicity in 47 patients, rash in 18 and "other" in 5. The median CD4 count at the time of switch was 323 cells/mm³. Resolution of CNS symptoms was noted in 46 of 47 with CNS toxicity and 6 of 15 with rash. Of 70 who switched, 15 (21%) subsequently discontinued NVP due to adverse reactions, including 10 due to grade 3-4 hepatotoxicity and 41 of 67 (67%) achieved viral suppression at 24 weeks (*CID* 2010;50:787).

  □ **Switch from PI- to NVP-based ART:** A review of data concluded that "a switch from a PI-based regimen to one containing NVP can be accomplished safely while main-taining virologic suppression ... with no immunologic cost ... and an overall benefit in the metabolic milieu" (*HIV Med* 2006;7:537). The switch is associated with good virologic control and rapid improvement in blood lipid changes and insulin resistance with half the patients experiencing positive changes in lipodystrophy (*AIDS* 1999;13:805; *JAIDS* 2001;27:229; *AIDS* 2000;14:807).

  □ **The ATHENA study** was a review of 125 patients who switched to NVP-based ART compared with 321 who continued PI-based ART. All participants had achieved VL <500 c/mL on PI-based ART. Treatment failure due to toxicity requiring a regimen change (36%) or virologic failure (6%) was greater in the PI continuation group (*JID* 2002;185:1261).

  □ **NVP vs. EFV switch:** Retrospective analysis of 162 patients on PI-based ART who had virologic failure or a request for regimen simplification and were given either EFV- or NVP-based ART. Results showed those switched for simplification maintained virologic control at 48 weeks, and the two drugs were comparable. For salvage, virologic control was achieved in 13/58 (22%) of NVP recipients and 19/49 (38%) of EFV recipients (*HIV Clin Trials* 2003; 4:244).

  □ **NEFA:** A trial in which 460 patients receiving PI-based ART were randomized to switch to ABC, NVP, or EFV plus 2 NRTIs. At 48 weeks, virologic failure occurred in 13%, 10%, and 6% for these 3 groups, respectively (*P* = 0.1). Lipodystrophy did not change in any of the groups (*NEJM* 2003;349:1036).

□ **High baseline viral load:** In an analysis of six reports of 416 NVP recipients, viral suppression to <500 c/mL was observed in 83% and 89% of those with baseline viral loads above and below 100,000 c/mL, respectively *(HIV Clin Trials* 2001;2:317).

□ **TENOR:** Single arm study of 70 patients receiving initial therapy or switching for intolerance of another regimen. Regimen was once daily NVP (400 mg)+TDF/FTC. At 72 weeks the regimen was continued in 52 (74%) and of these patients VL was <400 c/mL in 84% *(Eur J Med Res* 2009;14:516).

RESISTANCE: Monotherapy is associated with rapid and high-level resistance with primary RT mutations 103N, 100I, 181C/I, 188C/L/H, and 190A resulting in an increase in the IC_{90} of >100-fold *(JAIDS* 1995; 8:141; *JID* 2000;181:904). Cross-resistance with EFV is almost universal. NVP is more likely than EFV to select for ETR-resistant virus, because of the possibility of the Y181I/C mutations. NVP resistance is challenging in two distinct clinical settings, both related to the relatively long half-life and the low genetic barrier to resistance mutations:

The more extensive studies involve resistance associated with **single-dose NVP for preventing perinatal transmission**, which is a common strategy in developing countries. HIVNET 012 found that this was highly effective in perinatal transmission prevention, but resistance mutations were noted using standard assays in 19% of women. In PACTG 316 14/95 women (15%) who received intrapartum NVP developed NVP resistance mutations 6 wks postpartum *(JID* 202;186:181). Subsequent studies using real-time PCR to detect minority species, with a detection limit of 0.2%, found that K103N was present in an additional 40% *(JID* 2005;192:16). The frequency is clade-specific: clade C, 69%; clade D, 36%; clade A, 19% *(JAIDS* 2006;42: 610). **Resistance mutations are also observed in the infants born to exposed mothers and in strains recovered from breast milk** *(JID* 2005; 192:1260). The clinical implications of these observations are unclear, but in one study, women with perinatal NVP exposure who were subsequently treated with NVP-based regimens had a poorer virologic response compared to women who had not been previously exposed to NVP *(NEJM* 2004;351:217). A more recent report suggests that the NNRTI mutations were no longer detected even in the minority pool after 6-12 mos *(NEJM* 2007;356:135). See pg. 160-161.

PHARMACOLOGY

- **Bioavailability:** 93%; not altered by food, fasting, ddl, or antacids.

- **T½:** 25-30 hrs

- **CNS penetration:** CSF levels are about 45% of peak serum levels (CSF: plasma ratio=0.45). The CNS penetration effectiveness is the highest – class 4 *(Neurology* 2011;76:693).

- **Breast milk:** Significant concentrations are transferred into breast milk (3TC is also transmitted but AZT is not) *(AAC* 2009;53:1170).

Drug Information

- **Metabolism:** Metabolized by cytochrome P450 (CYP3A4) to hydroxylated metabolites that are excreted primarily in the urine, which accounts for 80% of the oral dose. NVP autoinduces hepatic CYP3A4, reducing its own plasma half-life over 2-4 wks from 45 hrs to 25 hrs (*JID* 1995;171:537).

- **Dose modification with renal or hepatic failure:** NVP is extensively metabolized by the liver. NVP is contraindicated in moderate and severe liver disease due to hepatotoxicity. NVP metabolites are largely eliminated by the kidney with <5% unchanged in the urine. No dose adjustment is required for patients with renal impairment. Patients on dialysis should receive an additional dose of 200 mg following each dialysis treatment (NVP package insert, Section 8.6, 6/2008).

SIDE EFFECTS

- **Black Box Warning:**
  - Severe, life threatening and in some cases fatal hepatoxicity (see below)
  - Severe, life threatening and in some cases fatal skin reaction (see below)

- **Hepatotoxicity:** Early hepatotoxicity usually occurs in the first 6 wks and appears to be a hypersensitivity reaction. It may be accompanied by drug rash, eosinophilia, and systemic symptoms (DRESS syndrome). This reaction differs from "transaminitis" noted with PIs and EFV in that it is more likely to progress to liver necrosis and death even with early detection and occurs primarily with high baseline CD4 counts, especially in women. The rate of symptomatic hepatitis in women with a baseline CD4 count $\geq$250 cells/mm^3 is 11% compared to 0.9% in women with lower CD4 counts at baseline. Men also have an increased risk with a CD4 count $\geq$400 cells/mm^3, but the rates are lower, 6.4% vs. 1.2%. Chronic hepatitis B or C do not appear to be risk factors (*JID* 2005;191:825). The mechanism of this reaction is not known, but the association with high CD4 counts suggests an immune mechanism and a genetic predisposition (*CID* 2006;43:783). There have been at least 6 deaths in pregnant women given continuous NVP-based ART (*JAIDS* 2004;36:772). 2011 DHHS Guidelines recommend that NVP not be given to treatment-naïve women with a baseline CD4 count >250 cells/mm^3 or men with a baseline CD4 count of >400 cells/mm^3. Also, the CDC issued a warning against using NVP for PEP based on reports of two HCW with severe hepatitis, including one who required a liver transplant (*Lancet* 2001; 357:687; *MMWR* 2001;49:1153). This concern does not apply to the single dose of NVP given at delivery to prevent perinatal transmission or to persons who have a high CD4 count on other ART regimens who are switching to NVP-based ART. NVP recipients may also develop hepatotoxicity later in the course of treatment, a form of hepatitis that is more benign and similar to hepatitis seen with other anti-HIV drugs. This hepatitis is characterized by an elevation in transaminase levels, it is usually asymptomatic, the frequency is about 10%, and it is more common in those with chronic HBV or HCV co-infection (*CID* 2004;39:1083). Management guidelines for the severe early form include frequent monitoring of hepatic function in the first 12-18 wks, warning the patient, and prompt discontinuation of NVP if this diagnosis is considered. Guidelines for the later asymptomatic transaminitis are unclear, but many recommend discontinuation of NVP if the ALT is >5 or 10x the ULN (*Hepatology* 2002;35:182). It should be noted that frequency of hepatotoxicity is highly variable in different geographic areas, but most large series report rates of grade 3 hepatoxicity or hepatic enzyme elevations >3-5-fold above ULN at 4-13% and some find no gender difference or CD4 associated risk (*JAIDS* 2004;35:495; *HIV Med* 2010;11:650; *JID* 2005;191:825; *Drug Saf* 2007;30:1161; *HIV Med* 2008;9:221; *HIV Med* 2010;11:334).

- **Rash:** Rash is seen in about 17%. It is usually maculopapular and erythematous with or without pruritus and is located on the trunk, face, and extremities. Some patients with rashes require hospitalization, and 7% of all patients require discontinuation of the drug, compared with 4.3% given DLV, 1.7% given EFV and 26% given ETR (package insert, PDR). Frequency of severe (Grade 3-4) rash in the 2NN trial was 6% in patients with a CD4 count >200/mm^3 and 1-2% in those with a CD4 count <200/mm^3 (*AIDS* 2005;19:463). Indications for discontinuation of an NNRTI due to rash are rash accompanied by fever, blisters, mucous membrane involvement, conjunctivitis, edema, arthralgias, or malaise. Steroids are not effective (*JAIDS* 2003;33:41). Stevens-Johnson syndrome and TEN have been reported, and at least three deaths ascribed to rash have been reported with NVP (*Lancet* 1998;351:567). There is evidence that this NVP-induced rash results from NVP-stimulated CD4 cells that produce IFN-gamma (*J Pharmacol Exp Ther* 2009;331:836). Patients with rash should always be assessed for hepatotoxicity, as the two may occur together. A review of 122 patients with NVP rashes who were switched to EFV showed EFV-associated rashes in 10 (8%), but the rate of EFV rash was 20% among those whose NVP rashes were "severe" (*HIV Med* 2006;7:378).

- **Lipid effects:** The D:A:D study indicates that NVP increases HDL cholesterol, reduces the total:HDL cholesterol index and does not increase the risk for cardiovascular events (*Drugs* 2006;66:1971).

DRUG INTERACTIONS: NVP, like rifampin, induces CYP3A4. Maximum induction takes place 2-4 wks after initiating therapy.

- **Drugs that are contraindicated or not recommended for concurrent use: Rifampin, ketoconazole, St. John's wort, rifapentine, and atazanavir.**

- **Use with antiretroviral agents:** Table 5-63
- NVP may significantly decrease the serum concentrations of **amiodarone, carbamazepine, clonazepam, cycophosphamide, cyclosporin, diltiazem, disopyramide, ergotamine, ethosuximide, fentanyl, itraconazole, lidocaine, nifedipine, posaconazole, sirolimus, tacrolimus, verapamil,** and **voriconazole.** Use with close monitoring – **warfarin.**

■ TABLE 5-63: **Dose Recommendations for NVP + PI Combinations**

PI	PI Level	NVP Level	Regimen Recommended
IDV	↓28%	No change	IDV 1000 mg q8h +NVP standard
RTV	↓11%	No change	Standard doses
SQV	↓25%	No change	Recommend SQV/r 1000/100 mg bid
NFV	↑10%	No change	Standard doses
FPV	↓25%	may ↓ or ↑	FPV/r 700/100 mg bid + NVP standard dose (*Antimicrob Ag Chemother* 2006;50:3157).
LPV/r	LPV ↓55%	No change	LPV/r 400/100 mg bid (treatment-naïve) or 600/150 mg bid (treatment-experienced). Consider LPV/r 500/125 mg bid
ATV	↓	↑	Do not co-administer ATV with NVP as NVP ↓ ATV exposure and potential toxicity with ↑ NVP exposure.
TPV	may ↓ or↑	may ↓ or ↑	Standard; TPV/r 500/200 mg bid + NVP 200 mg bid. Limited data.
DRV	No change	↓27%	DRV/r 600/100 mg bid, standard NVP. Limited observational data.

- **Drugs that require dose modification with concurrent use: Oral contraceptives:** NVP decreases AUC for ethinyl estradiol by about 30% (*JAIDS* 2002;29:471); alternative or additional methods of birth control should be used. **Clarithromycin:** NVP reduces clarithromycin AUC by 30% but increases levels of the 14-OH metabolite, which is active against *H. influenzae* and *S. pneumonia*, but consider azithromycin for MAC. NVP levels increased 26%. Use standard doses and monitor or use azithromycin. **Fluconazole** increases NVP 2-fold. Monitor for toxicity. **Ketoconazole:** AUC and C_{max} levels of ketoconazole are decreased 72% and 44% respectively. NVP increases 15-30%: not recommended. **Voriconazole:** no data, but significant potential for decrease of voriconazole and/or increase of NVP serum level. **Rifabutin:** AUC increased 17%; no dose alteration. **Rifampin:** NVP AUC and C_{max} decreased more than 50%; there is also concern about additive hepatotoxicity (NVP + rifampin in standard doses has been found to be virologically inferior vs. HIV (*JAMA* 2008;300:530). If co-administration is needed, initiate w/ NVP

Drug Information

5

400 mg/d (CROI 2010;abstract 602). **Phenobarbital, phenytoin, carbamazepine:** no data; monitor anticonvulsant levels; NVP concentrations may be decreased. **Methadone:** NVP reduces AUC of methadone by about 50%; opiate withdrawal is a concern and has been reported; methadone dose increases are variable but average 15-25% (*CID* 2001;33:1595). **Statins:** no data; may decrease lovastain and simvastatin levels; consider pravastatin or rosuvastatin. **Buprenorphine:** no significant change; use standard dose.

PREGNANCY: NVP is used extensively in resource-limited countries for prevention of perinatal HIV transmission and the data addressing multiple issues are also extensive. The two forms of NVP-based treatment are:

- Short term peripartum prophylaxis that usually consists of a single 200 mg dose of NVP to the mother at the onset of labor and a single 2 mg/kg dose to the infant at 48-72 hrs (*JID* 1998;178:368). This is well tolerated by the mother regardless of the baseline CD4 count and reduces perinatal transmission by about 50% (*Lancet* 1999;354:795). The major concern is the long half life of NVP with a subsequent HIV resistance rate of 19% in HIVNET 012 (*AIDS* 2001;15:1951) and 15% in PACTG 316 (*JID* 2002;186:181). Some studies show that NVP can still be used effectively if ART is delayed 6-12 mos (*NEJM* 2007;356:135; *CID* 2008;46:611). NVP resistance can also be reduced or avoided with a NRTI "tail" (*JID* 2006;193:482; *PloS Med* 2009;6:e1000172).

- Long-term antenatal NVP-based ART: NVP pharmacokinetics are not notably altered during pregnancy (*HIV Med* 2008;94:214). The major concern is the risk of NVP hypersensitivity reactions in women with a baseline CD4 count of >250 cells/mm^3. The reactions include potentially life threatening hepatotoxicity and life threatening hypersensitivity skin reactions including Stevens-Johnson syndrome (*JAIDS* 2004;35:120; *Obstet Gynecol* 2003;101:1094). These reactions including fatal cases have been described with and without pregnancy, and it appears that pregnancy does not increase the risk (*AIDS* 2010;24:109). As a consequence of these observations, the 2010 DHHS Guidelines for Use of Antiretroviral Agents in Pregnancy recommend: 1) NVP-based ART should be initiated in pregnant women only if the baseline CD4 count is <250 cells/mm^3; 2) Pregnant women who have been receiving NVP-based ART can continue this treatment regardless of the CD4 cell count; and 3) the single NVP dose to prevent perinatal transmission is considered safe regardless of the CD4 cell count.

The Pregnancy Registry reporting of the first trimester NVP exposures in the US indicated 25/970 (2.6%) birth defects (data to 7/31/2010).

Drug Information

NORTRIPTYLINE – see also Tricyclic Antidepressants (pg. 407)

TRADE NAMES: *Aventyl* (Eli Lilly), *Pamelor* (Mallinckrodt), and generic

FORMS AND COST: Caps: 10 mg $0.44, 25 mg $0.88, 50 mg $1.45, 75 mg $2.21. Oral suspension: 10 mg/5 mL, 480 mL $182.95.

CLASS: Tricyclic antidepressant

INDICATIONS AND DOSE REGIMENS

- **Depression:** 25 mg hs initially; increase by 25 mg every 3 days until 75 mg, then wait 5 days, and obtain level with expectation of 100-150 ng/dL.

- **Neuropathic pain:** 10-25 mg hs; increase dose over 2-3 wks to maximum of 75 mg hs. Draw serum levels if higher doses used.

PHARMACOLOGY

- **Bioavailability:** >90%

- **T½:** 13-79 hrs, mean 31 hrs

- **Elimination:** Metabolized and excreted renally

SIDE EFFECTS: Anticholinergic effects (dry mouth, dizziness, blurred vision, constipation, urinary hesitancy), orthostatic hypotension (less than with other tricyclics), sedation, sexual dysfunction (de-creased libido), and weight gain.

DRUG INTERACTIONS: The following drugs should not be given concurrently: Adrenergic neuronal blocking agents, clonidine, other alpha-2 agonists, excessive alcohol, fenfluramine, cimetidine, MAO inhibitors, and any drugs that increase nortriptyline levels (cimetidine, quinidine, fluconazole). All PIs and DLV may increase nortriptyline levels. Avoid in patients with QTc prolongation.

PREGNANCY: Category D. Animal studies are inconclusive, and experience in pregnant women is inadequate. Avoid during first trimester, and when possible limit use in the last two trimesters.

NORVIR – see Ritonavir (pg. 370)

NYSTATIN

TRADE NAMES: *Mycostatin* (Bristol-Myers Squibb) and generic

FORMS AND COST: (generic)

- **Lozenges:** 500,000 units at $0.68/lozenge

- **Cream:** 100,000 U/g, 15 g at $2.71; 30 g at $5.96

- **Ointment:** 100,000 U/g, 15 g at $2.12; 30 g at $3.23

- **Suspension:** 100,000 U/mL, (16 oz) at $116.07

- **Oral tabs:** 500,000 units at $0.69/tab

5 Drug Information

- **Vaginal tabs:** 100,000 units at $0.47/tab

PATIENT ASSISTANCE PROGRAM (*Bristol-Myers Squibb*): 800-272-4878

CLASS: Polyene macrolide similar to amphotericin B

ACTIVITY: Active against *C. albicans* at 3 µg/mL and other *Candida* species at higher concentrations.

INDICATIONS AND DOSES

- **Thrush:** 5 mL suspension to be gargled 4-5x/d x 14 days. Disadvantages: *Nystatin* has a bitter taste, causes GI side effects, must be given 4x/d, and does not work as well as clotrimazole troches or oral fluconazole (*HIV Clin Trials* 2000;1:47). Efficacy is dependent on contact time with mucosa.

- **Vaginitis:** 100,000 unit tab intravaginally 1-2x/d x 14 days

PHARMACOLOGY

- **Bioavailability:** Poorly absorbed and undetectable in blood following oral administration

- Therapeutic levels persist in saliva for 2 h after oral dissolution of two lozenges.

SIDE EFFECTS: Infrequent, dose-related GI intolerance (transient nausea, vomiting, diarrhea)

OXANDROLONE

TRADE NAME: *Oxandrin* (BTG)

FORMS: Tabs, 2.5 and 10 mg

COST: Per tab, $5.52 (2.5 mg), $18.75 (10 mg); cost per day (20 mg), $37.76 - $42.40 (Note: IM nandrolone is more cost-effective at $120/mo vs. $900/mo.

PATIENT ASSISTANCE PROGRAM: 866-692-6374

CLASS: Anabolic steroid

INDICATION AND DOSES: Wasting. Prior studies showed a modest weight gain after 16 wks with a dose of 15 mg qd (*AIDS* 1996;10: 1657; *AIDS* 1996;10:745; *Br J Nutr* 1996;75:129). A more recent clinical trial with 262 HIV-infected men with 10-20% weight loss showed increases in body weight. Body cell mass gain was noted with only 40 mg/d, but treatment was associated with significant decreases in total and free testosterone levels, increased LDL cholesterol, and elevated transaminase levels (*JAIDS* 2006;41:304). Natural testosterone esters are preferred for hypogonadal men (*CID* 2003;36[suppl 2]:S73). A comparison of nutrition counseling, nutrition counseling Plus oxandrolone, or nutrition counseling plus resistance training showed oxandrolone was the least cost effective at $55,000/QALY (*AIDS Care* 2007;19:996).

PHARMACOLOGY: Bioavailability is 97%.

SIDE EFFECTS: Virilizing complications primarily in women, including deep voice, hirsutism, acne, clitoral enlargement, and menstrual irregularity. Some virilizing changes may be irreversible, even with prompt discontinuation. Men may experience increased acne and increased frequency of erections. Of particular concern is hepatic toxicity with cholestatic hepatitis; discontinue drug if jaundice occurs or abnormal liver function tests are obtained. Drug-induced jaundice is reversible. Peliosis hepatis (blood-filled cysts) has been reported and may result in life-threatening hepatic failure or intra-abdominal hemorrhage. Miscellaneous side effects: nausea, vomiting, changes in skin color, ankle swelling, depression, insomnia, and changes in libido. Other potential side effects are increased LDL cholesterol and exacerbation of lipoatrophy.

DRUG INTERACTIONS: Increases activity of oral anticoagulants and oral hypoglycemic agents

PREGNANCY: Category X. Teratogenic.

PAROMOMYCIN

TRADE NAME: *Humatin* (Monarch Pharmaceuticals and Caraco) and generic

FORM AND COST: 250 mg cap at $5.67 ($952/21 day course)

CLASS: Aminoglycoside (for oral use)

INDICATIONS AND DOSE: Cryptosporidiosis. 1 g po bid or 500 mg po qid

EFFICACY: See pg. 439. The drug is active *in vitro* and in animal models against *Cryptosporidia* but only at levels far higher than those achieved in humans. There are anecdotal reports of clinical response, but controlled trials show marginal benefit and no cures (*CID* 1992;15: 726; *Am J Med* 1996;100:370). An uncontrolled trial found good results with paromomycin 1 g bid + azithromycin 600 mg qd x 4 wks, then paromomycin 1 g bid (alone) x 8 wks (*JID* 1998;178: 900), and there are anecdotal case reports supporting this regimen (*Parasitol Res* 2006;98:593). At present, there is a consensus that there is no effective chemotherapy for cryptosporidiosis except immune reconstitution with ART. Even modest increases in CD4 counts are effective (*NEJM* 2002;346:1723).

PHARMACOLOGY: Not absorbed; most of the oral dose is excreted unchanged in stool; lesions of the GI tract may facilitate absorption and serum levels may increase in presence of renal failure.

SIDE EFFECTS: GI intolerance (anorexia, nausea, vomiting, epigastric pain), steatorrhea, and malabsorption rare complications include rash, headache; vertigo with absorption and serum levels. There could be ototoxicity and nephrotoxicity with systemic absorption, as with other aminoglycosides.

PREGNANCY: Category C

PEGYLATED INTERFERON – see also pg. 513-519

TRADE NAMES: Peginterferon alfa-2a – *Pegasys* (Roche); peginterferon alfa-2b – *Peg-Intron* (Schering-Plough)

FORMS

- Peginterferon alfa-2a (*Pegasys*) is supplied as a solution ready for injection, which requires refrigeration and is available at a fixed dose of 180 μg per 1 mL solution at $691.19.

- Peginterferon alfa-2b (*Peg-Intron*) is supplied as lyophilized powder to be reconstituted with 0.7 mL saline; several strengths are available based upon body weight (50 mcg at $627.62, 80 mcg at $658.94, 120 mcg at $691.92, 150 mcg at $726.53).

COST: *Pegasys* $33,177/year and *Peg-Intron* $33,212/year. AWP costs for 70-kg patient treated for 48 weeks: Peginterferon + ribavirin approximately $59,900/48 wks.

PATIENT ASSISTANCE PROGRAM: 877-734-2797 (*Pegasys*) and 800-521-7157 (*Peg-Intron*)

PRODUCT: Recombinant alfa-interferon conjugated with polyethylene glycol (PEG), which decreases the clearance rate of interferon and results in sustained concentrations permitting less frequent dosing.

CONTRAINDICATIONS: Autoimmune hepatitis and hepatic failure with Child-Pugh score ≥ 6 before or during treatment. Contraindications to ribavirin: 1) pregnant female; 2) male patient with pregnant partner; and 3) patient with hemoglobinopathies.

INDICATIONS: FDA indications: Treatment of compensated chronic hepatitis C not previously treated with IFN alfa. HIV-HCV co-infected patients are candidates for anti-HCV therapy if they appear to be at high risk for cirrhosis based on evidence of bridging fibrosis and/or necroinflammation plus HCV RNA levels >50 IU/mL (*CID* 2008;47:94). Cure rates with peg-IFN + ribavirin in absence of HIV co-infection are 42-46% for genotype 1 and 76-82% for genotypes 2 and 3 (*Lancet* 2001;358: 958; *NEJM* 2002;347:975) (see Table 5-64). HCV-infected patients with or without HIV are not considered candidates for this treatment if there is active substance abuse, decompensated liver disease, severe, active psychiatric disease, or refusal of therapy (*Ann Intern Med* 2002;136:288). The three major trials of HIV/HCV co-infected patients generally restricted HCV treatment to those with CD4 counts >200/mm³, and all three trials enrolled patients with a median CD4 count >500/mm³. However, a subset analysis of 17 patients with a CD4 count <200/mm³ given peginterferon + ribavirin showed HCV virologic response of 47% compared to 40% in patients with a higher baseline CD4 count (*NEJM* 2004;351:2340). Most authorities recommend HCV treatment with HIV co-infection only with good HIV virologic control and CD4 count >200/mm³ (*Hepatology* 2006;44:S49) but that restriction is no longer rigid (*CID* 2008;47:94). See pg. 383, 513.

New agents for HCV with HCV/HIV: Initial results with new agents for HCV suggest that telaprevir and boceprevir have extensive drug interactions with PIs and NNRIs, but telaprevir can be used in combination with EFV/TDF/FTC, ATV/r+TDF/FTC and RAL (Sulkowski M. 2011, CROI:Abstr. 146LP). Candidates for this therapy should have no contraindications to peg-IFN or ribavirin, stable HIV with VL <200 c/mL and CD4 count >200/mm³, and advanced liver disease; delay for newer drugs anticipated in 2013 is not a good option. See pg. 383, 513.

■ TABLE 5-64: **Results of 4 Clinical Trials of PegIFN + Ribavirin for HCV in Patients with HIV Co-infection**

| | No. Pts | Regimen x 48 weeks | Rate of SVR | |
			Gen 1	Gen 2/3
ACTG A5071 (*NEJM* 2004;351: 451)	66	Peg-IFN 180 mg/wk Ribavirin 600-1000 mg/d Duration: 48 weeks	14%	73%
APRICOT (*NEJM* 2004;351: 451)	289	Peg-IFN 180 mg/wk Ribavirin 800 mg/d Duration: 48 weeks	29%	62%
RIBAVIC (*JAMA* 2004;292:2839)	205	Peg-IFN 180 mg/wk Ribavirin 800 mg/d Duration: 48 weeks	15%	—
PRESCO (*AIDS Res Hum Retro* 2007;23:972)	389	Peg-IFN 180 mg/wk Ribavirin 1000/d (<75 kg) or 1200/d (75 kg) Duration by Genotype: 1 & 4 – 72 wks, 2 & 3 – 48 wks	36%	72%

DOSE: Pegylated IFN (alfa 2a 180 mg (*Pegasys*) or alfa 2b 1.5 mg/kg (*Peg-Intron*) SC/wk plus ribavirin. The ribavirin dose of 800 mg/d is the dose used in most clinical trials of co-infected patients, but higher doses of RBV for genotypes 1 and 4 are now preferred. These doses are: 800 mg/d for patients <45 kg, 1000 mg qd for 45-75 kg and 1200 mg qd for >75 kg. Usual duration is 48 wks in HIV co-infected patients regardless of genotype. With CrCl <60 mL/min, peg-IFN-alfa-2b 1 mg/kg SQ once weekly or peg-IFN alfa 2a 135 mg SQ once weekly + ribavirin 200-800 mg/d in 2 divided doses, starting with low dose and increase gradually (*Hepatology* 2009;49:1335). Some advocate extending the duration of treatment for genotype 1 and 4 to 72 wks (see PRESCO, Table 5-64). The regimen used with concurrent **telaprevir** in the phase 2a trial was peg-IFN-asa 180 µg/week + RBV 800 mg/d for 12 weeks + TVR for 12 weeks followed by peg-IFN-a2a + RBV (see pg. 383).

5 Drug Information

MONITORING

- **Clinical response:** HCV RNA at 12 wks (see pg. 516). Patients without a ≥ 2 $\log_{10}$ c/mL decrease in HCV RNA levels at 12 wks are unlikely to achieve significant viral response, although this does not exclude the possibility of clinical benefit by other criteria (*JAIDS* 2006; 43:504). If HCV RNA is not decreased by at least 2 logs at 12 wks, consider discontinuation (*Gut* 2007;56:1111). Sustained virologic response is defined as undetectable HCV RNA at 24 wks post therapy.

- **Toxicity:** CBC and comprehensive metabolic panel at baseline, 2 wks, then every 6 wks. TSH at baseline and then every 12 wks.

- **Patients with cardiac disease:** EKG at baseline and prn.

- **Women of childbearing potential:** Urine pregnancy testing every 4-6 wks.

PHARMACOLOGY

The differences between the two commercially available peg-IFN products are that *Peg-Intron* (alfa–2b) is a linear chain PEG and *Pegasys* (alfa–2a) is a branched chain PEG. This structural difference results in higher serum level and more prolonged T½ with *Pegasys*. Despite the PK difference, the two products appear to be clinically equivalent. (*NEJM* 2009;361:580).

- **Bioavailability:** Increases with duration of therapy. Mean trough of peg-IFN alfa 2b with 1 μg/kg SQ at week 4=94 pg/mL, at week 48=320 pg/mL. C_{max} mean is 554 pg/mL at 15-44 hrs and sustained up to 48-72 hrs. Compared to non-pegylated IFN, peg-IFN C_{max} is about 10x greater and AUC is 50x greater.

- **T½:** peg-IFN alfa 2a = 77 h; peg-IFN alfa 2b = 40 h (compared with 8 h for non-pegylated interferon).

- **Elimination:** Renal 30% (7x lower clearance than non-pegylated interferon). Eliminated primarily in the bile.

SIDE EFFECTS: Similar to those of IFN; 15-21% in clinical trials discontinue therapy due to adverse reactions (*NEJM* 2004;351:438; *NEJM* 2004;351:451).

BLACK BOX WARNINGS: Depression, serious bacterial infections, autoimmune disorder, ischemic disorders.

- **Neuropsychiatric:** Depression, suicidal or homicidal ideation, and relapse of substance abuse. Should be used with extreme caution in patients with history of psychiatric disorders. Warn patient and monitor. Depression reported in 21-29%. Suicides reported. Active depression with suicidal ideation is a contraindication. EFV given concurrently has been found to increase mood disorders but did not increase the risk of depression in one report of 53 patients (*JAIDS* 2008;49:61).

Drug Information

- **Marrow suppression:** ANC decreases in 70%, <500/mm³ in 1%, platelet counts decrease in 20%, <20,000/mm³ in 1%. Avoid or discontinue AZT.

Laboratory Measurement	Criteria for Dose Reduction to 0.5 µg/mL	Criteria for Discontinuation
ANC*	<750/mm³	<500/mm³
Platelet count	<50,000/mm³	<25,000/mm³

* Leukopenia generally responds to G-CSF, which may be preferred to avoid dose reduction.

- **Flu-like symptoms:** Most common; about 50% will have fever, headache, chills, and myalgias/arthralgias. May decrease with continued treatment. May be treated with NSAIDs or acetaminophen; with liver disease acetaminophen dose should be <2 g/d.
- **Thyroid:** Thyroiditis with hyperthyroidism or hypothyroidism. TSH levels should be measured at baseline and during therapy every 12 wks.
- **Retinopathy:** Obtain baseline retinal evaluation in patients with diabetes, hypertension or other ocular abnormality.
- **Injection site reaction:** Inflammation, pruritus, pain (mild) in 47%.
- **GI complaints:** Nausea, anorexia, diarrhea, and/or abdominal pain in 15-30%.
- **Skin/hair:** Alopecia (20%), pruritus (10%), and/or rash (6%)
- **Miscellaneous:** Hyperglycemia, cardiac arrhythmias, elevated hepatic transaminase levels 2-5x, colitis, pancreatitis, autoimmune disorders, hypersensitivity reactions.

DRUG INTERACTIONS: Avoid co-administration of marrow suppressive agents including AZT and ganciclovir. Ribavirin should not be given with ddI. ABC should also be avoided with ribavirin.

PREGNANCY: Category C. IFN is not recommended in pregnancy (2010 DHHS Guidelines in Pregnancy). Abortifacient potential in primates. Ribavirin is a potent teratogen (Category X) and must be avoided in pregnancy and used with caution in women of childbearing potential and their male sexual partners. Breastfeeding: No data.

PENTAM – see Pentamidine (below)

PENTAMIDINE

TRADE NAME: *Pentam* for IV use; *NebuPent* for inhalation (American Pharmaceutical Partners)

FORMS AND COST: 300 mg IV vial at $94.80; 300 mg *NebuPent* inhalation at $94.80

PATIENT ASSISTANCE PROGRAM: IV and aerosolized pentamidine 888-391-6300

CLASS: Aromatic diamidine-derivative antiprotozoal agent that is structurally related to stilbamidine

INDICATIONS AND DOSES: See pg. 477-481.

- ***P. jiroveci* pneumonia (PCP):** 3-4 mg/kg IV given over ≥1 hr x 21 days. The approved dose is 4 mg/kg, but some clinicians prefer 3 mg/kg. TMP-SMX is preferred (*Ann Intern Med* 1986;105:37; *AIDS* 1992;6:301).

- **PCP prophylaxis:** 300 mg/mo delivered by a *Respirgard II* nebulizer using 300 mg dose diluted in 6 mL sterile water delivered at 6 L/min from a 50 psi compressed air source until the reservoir is dry. TMP-SMX preferred due to superior efficacy in preventing PCP, efficacy in preventing other infections, reduced cost, and greater convenience (*NEJM* 1995;332:693). Aerosolized pentamidine should not be used for PCP treatment (*Ann Intern Med* 1990;113:203). See pg. 67.

PHARMACOLOGY

- **Bioavailability:** Not absorbed orally. With aerosol, 5% reaches alveolar spaces via *Respirgard II* nebulizer. Blood levels with monthly aerosol delivery are below detectable limits.

- **T½:** Parenteral – 6 h

- **Elimination:** Primarily nonrenal but may accumulate in renal failure

- **Dose modification of parenteral form with renal failure:**
    CrCl >50 mL/min – 4 mg/kg q24h;
    10-50 mL/min – 4 mg/kg q24h-q36h;
    <10 mL/min – 4 mg/kg q48h.

SIDE EFFECTS

- **Aerosolized pentamidine:** Cough and wheezing in 30% (prevented with pretreatment with beta-2 agonist), sufficiently severe to require discontinuation of treatment in 5% (*NEJM* 1990;323:769). Other reactions include laryngitis, chest pain, and dyspnea. The role of aerosolized pentamidine in promoting extrapulmonary *P. jiroveci* infection and pneumothorax is unclear. Risk of transmitting TB to patients and health care workers. See pg. 67.

- **Systemic pentamidine:** In a review of 106 courses of IV pentamidine, 76 (72%) had adverse reactions; these were sufficiently severe to require drug discontinuation in 31 (18%) (*CID* 1997;24:854). The most common causes of drug discontinuation were nephrotoxicity and hypoglycemia. A review of PCP treatment efficacy in 3 cohorts with 1188 episodes of PCP showed 3-mo survival rates of 85% with TMP/SMX treatment, 87% with clindamycin+TMP/SMX treatment, 87% with clindamycin+primaquin, and it was 70% for pentamidine (*JAC* 2009;64:1282). The RR of death with pentamidine after

Drug Information

adjusting for confounders was 2.0. A review of 29 clinical studies also concluded that pentamidine was inferior to TMP/SMX and clindamycin/primaquine (*JAIDS* 2008;48:63). **Nephrotoxicity** is noted in 25-50%. It is usually characterized by a gradual increase in creatinine in the second week of treatment but may cause acute renal failure. Risk is increased with dehydration and concurrent use of nephrotoxic drugs. **Hypotension** is unusual (6%) but may cause death, most often with rapid infusions; drug should be infused over ≥60 minutes. **Hypoglycemia**, with blood glucose 25 mg/dL in 5-10%, can occur after 5-7 days of treatment, sometimes persisting several days after discontinuation. Hypoglycemia may last days or weeks and is treated with IV glucose ± oral diazoxide. **Hyperglycemia** (2-9%) and insulin-dependent diabetes mellitus may occur with or without prior hypoglycemia. **Leukopenia and thrombocytopenia** are noted in 2-13%. **GI intolerance** with nausea, vomiting, abdominal pain, anorexia, and/or bad taste is common. Local reactions include sterile abscesses at IM injection sites (no longer advocated) and pain, erythema, tenderness, and induration (chemical phlebitis) at IV infusion sites. **Other reactions** include pancreatitis hepatitis, hypocalcemia (sometimes severe), increased amylase, hypomagnesemia, fever, rash, urticaria, toxic epidermal necrolysis (TEN), confusion, dizziness (without hypotension), anaphylaxis, arrhythmias, including Torsade de pointes.

MONITORING

- **Aerosolized pentamidine:** This is considered safe for the patient but poses risk of TB to healthcare workers and other patients. Patient should be evaluated for TB (PPD, X-ray, and sputum examination if indicated). Suspected or confirmed TB should be treated prior to aerosol treatments. Adequate air exchanges with exhaust to outside and appropriate use of particulate air filters are required. Some suggest pregnant HCWs should avoid environmental exposure to pentamidine until risks to fetus are better defined.

- **Parenteral administration:** Adverse effects are common and may be lethal. Due to the risk of hypotension, the drug should be given in supine position, the patient should be hydrated, pentamidine should be delivered over ≥60 minutes, and BP should be monitored during treatment and afterward until stable. Regular laboratory monitoring (daily or every other day) should include creatinine, potassium, calcium, and glucose; other tests for periodic monitoring include CBC, LFTs, and calcium.

DRUG INTERACTIONS: Avoid concurrent use of parenteral pentamidine with nephrotoxic drugs, including aminoglycosides, amphotericin B, and foscarnet and cidofovir. Amphotericin B – severe hypocalcemia.

PREGNANCY: Category C. Limited experience with pregnant women.

5 Drug Information

PRAVASTATIN

TRADE NAME: *Pravachol* (Bristol-Myers Squibb) and generic

FORMS AND COST: Tabs: 10 mg at $3.21, 20 mg at $2.89, 40 mg at $4.79, and 80 mg at $4.79.

FCLASS: Statin (HMG-CoA reductase inhibitor)

INDICATIONS AND DOSES: Elevated total cholesterol, LDL cholesterol, and/or triglycerides and/or low HDL cholesterol. This is often a favored statin for dyslipidemia associated with PI-based ART due to paucity of drug interactions with PIs with the exception of DRV/r (*CID* 2003;37: 613; *CID* 2006;43:645), although it may be less effective than other statins. For example, a comparative trial vs. rosuvastatin in HIV-infected patients showed better outcome with rosuvastatin (*AIDS* 2010;24:77), and a review in two large HIV clinics suggested atrovastatin and rosuvastatin are preferred due to greater declines in LDL cholesterol (*CID* 2011;52:387; *CID* 2010;51:718). The initial dose is 40 mg qd. If desired cholesterol levels are not achieved with 40 mg qd, 80 mg qd is recommended. A starting dose of 10 mg daily is recommended in patients with a history of significant hepatic or renal dysfunction. Pravastatin can be administered as a single dose at any time of the day (see pg. 142. A report of pravastatin use in HIV-infected patients demonstrated improvements in the atherogenic lipid profile within 12 wks without change in inflammatory markers (*J Clin Lipidol* 2010;4:279). However, another report found pravastatin and rosuvastatin had a highly-significant effect on reduction in CRP levels in HIV-infected patients that was independent of any lipid effect (*AIDS* 2011;25:1123). See pg 43.

MONITORING: Blood lipids at 4-wk intervals until desired results are achieved, then periodically. It is recommended that transaminases be measured prior to the initiation of therapy, prior to the elevation of the dose, and when otherwise clinically indicated. Patients should be warned to report muscle pain, tenderness, or weakness promptly, especially if accompanied by fever or malaise; obtain CPK for suspected myopathy.

PRECAUTIONS: Pravastatin (and other statins) are contraindicated with pregnancy, breastfeeding, concurrent conditions that predispose to renal failure (sepsis, hypotension, etc.) and active hepatic disease. Alcoholism is a relative contraindication.

PHARMACOLOGY

- **Bioavailability:** 14%
- **T½:** 1.3-2.7 h
- **Elimination:** Fecal (biliary and unabsorbed drug) 70%; renal 20%

SIDE EFFECTS

- **Musculoskeletal:** Myopathy with elevated CPK plus muscle tenderness, weakness, or pain + fever or malaise. Rhabdomyolysis

Drug Information

with renal failure has been reported.

- **Hepatic:** Elevated transaminase levels in 1-2%; discontinue if otherwise unexplained elevations of ALT and/or AST are >3x ULN.
- **Miscellaneous:** Diarrhea, constipation, nausea, heartburn, stomach pain, dizziness, headache, skin rash (eczematous plaques), insomnia, and impotence (rare)

PREGNANCY: Category X. Contraindicated.

■ TABLE 5-65: **Pravastatin-ART Drug Interactions**

Antiretroviral agent	Effect on pravastatin	Dose recommendation for pravastatin
NNRTIs		
EFV	↓ AUC 40%	May need higher dose
ETR	No change	Standard dose
PIs		
DRV/r	↑ AUC 81%	Start with lowest dose or use alternative statin
IDV, NFV, TPV/r, NVP, MVC	No data	Standard dose
LPV/r	↑ AUC 33%	Standard dose
SQV/r	↓ AUC 50%	Standard dose; may need higher dose.

Possible interactions with spironolactone, cimetidine, and ketoconazole that reduce cholesterol levels and may effect adrenal and sex hormone production with concurrent use. Itraconazole increases pravastatin AUC and C_{max} 1.7x and 2.5x, respectively. Cholestyramine and colestipol decrease pravastatin AUC 40%; administer pravastatin 1 h before or 4 h after. Niacin and gemfibrozil: concurrent use with pravastatin increases the risk of myopathy. Rare cases of rhabdomyolysis with acute renal failure secondary to myoglobinuria have been reported with pravastatin and other drugs in this class.

PREZISTA – see Darunavir (pg. 223)

PRIMAQUINE

TRADE NAME: Generic

FORM AND COST: 15 mg base tabs (26.3 mg primaquine phosphate) at $1.50

CLASS: Antimalarial

INDICATIONS AND DOSES: *P. jiroveci* pneumonia: Primaquine 15-30 mg (base) qd + clindamycin 600-900 mg q6-8h IV or 300-450 mg po q6-8h. **Note:** The published experience and recommendation is for mild to moderately severe PCP (*Ann Intern Med* 1996;124:792; *CID* 1994; 18:905; *CID* 1998;27:524). A meta-analysis of published reports of PCP patients who failed initial treatment found that the clindamycin-

Drug Information

5

primaquine regimen was superior to all others with responses in 42 of 48 (87%) (*Arch Intern Med* 2001;161:1529). A more recent review 1188 cases of PCP showed the 3-mo survival rate with TMP-SMX treatment was 85%, for clindamycin-primaquine 81% and pentamidine was 76% (p=0.009) (*JAC* 2009;64:1282). The 2009 Guidelines for Prevention and Treatment of Opportunistic Infections in HIV-Infected Adults and Adolescents (www.mmhiv.com/link/2009-OI-NIH-CDC-IDSA) recommends clindamycin-primaquine as an alternative to TMP/SMX for moderate to severe PCP.

PHARMACOLOGY

- **Bioavailability:** Well absorbed

- **T½:** 4-10 h

- **Elimination:** Metabolized by liver

SIDE EFFECTS: Hemolytic anemia in patients with G6PD deficiency; its severity depends on drug dose and genetics of G6PD deficiency. In African Americans, the reaction is usually mild and self-limited or asymptomatic; in patients of Mediterranean or certain Asian extractions, hemolysis may be severe (see pg. 61). Hemolytic anemia may also occur with other forms of hemoglobinopathy. The 2008 IDSA/NIH/CDC Guidelines recommend screening G6PD deficiency prior to use of primaquine "whenever possible" (see pg. 61). Note that the prevalence of G6PD deficiency in >63,000 US troops was 2.5%, and it was particularly high for blacks, Asians and Hispanics (*Mil Med* 2005; 171:905). Warn patient of dark urine as sign and/or measure G6PD level prior to use in susceptible individuals. **Other hematologic side effects:** Methemoglobinemia, leukopenia. **GI:** Nausea, vomiting, epigastric pain (reduced by administration with meals). **Miscellaneous:** Headache, disturbed visual accommodation, pruritus, hypertension, arrhythmias.

PREGNANCY: Category C. Limited experience in pregnant women. There is a theoretical risk of hemolytic anemia if fetus has G6PD deficiency.

PROCRIT – see Erythropoietin (pg. 263)

PYRAZINAMIDE (PZA)

TRADE NAME: Generic

FORM AND COST: 500 mg tab at $1.25 (usually 2 g/d at $5.00/d)

CLASS: Derivative of niacinamide

INDICATION AND REGIMEN: Tuberculosis, initial phase of three to four drug regimen, usually for 8 wks (*MMWR* 1998;47[RR-20]; *MMWR* 2000;49:185). Treatment of latent TB with PZA + rifampin is no longer recommended due to hepatotoxicity (*MMWR* 2003;52:735). For active TB, see pg. 462-470.

Drug Information

TREATMENT WITH *RIFATER* (tabs with 50 mg INH, 120 mg rifampin, and 300 mg PZA)

- <65 kg: 1 tab/10 kg/d
- >65 kg: 6 tabs/d

PHARMACOLOGY

- **Bioavailability:** well absorbed, but absorption is reduced by about 25% in patients with advanced HIV infection (*Ann Intern Med* 1997;127: 289).
- **T½:** 9-10 h
- **CSF levels:** Equal to plasma levels
- **Elimination:** Hydrolyzed in liver; 4-14% of parent compound and 70% of metabolite excreted in urine.
- **Renal failure:** Usual dose unless creatinine clearance <10 mL/min – 12-20 mg/kg/d (increased risk of hyperuricemia).
- **Hepatic failure:** Contraindicated

SIDE EFFECTS: PZA appears to be the major cause of hepatotoxicity in patients with hepatitis as a complication of TB treatment (*Am J Respir Crit Care Med* 2003;167:1472; and 2008;177:1391). Hepatotoxicity occurs in up to 15% who receive >3 gm/d. The risk is increased with HCV co-infection (*Chest* 2007;131:803), transient hepatitis with increase in transaminases, jaundice, and a syndrome of fever, anorexia, and hepatomegaly; rarely, acute yellow atrophy. Monitor LFTs monthly if there are abnormal baseline levels, symptoms suggesting hepatitis, or elevated levels during therapy that are not high enough to stop treatment (ALT <5x ULN). Hyperuricemia is common, but gout is rare. Nongouty polyarthralgia in up to 40%; hyperuricemia usually responds to uricosuric agents. Use with caution in patients with history of gout. Rare – rash, fever, acne, dysuria, skin discoloration, urticaria, pruritus, GI intolerance, thrombocytopenia, sideroblastic anemia.

PREGNANCY: Category C. Not teratogenic in mice, but limited experience in humans. Risk of teratogenicity is unknown. currently recommended for treatment of active TB in US and in WHO guidelines.

PYRIMETHAMINE

TRADE NAME: *Daraprim* (GlaxoSmithKline) and generic

FORM AND COST: 25 mg tab at $1.09

PATIENT ASSISTANCE PROGRAM: 866-728-4368

CLASS: Aminopyrimidine-derivative antimalarial agent that is structurally related to trimethoprim

INDICATIONS AND DOSE REGIMENS: Toxoplasmosis (see pg 486).

- **Primary prophylaxis:** Pyrimethamine 50 mg po/wk + dapsone 50 mg po qd + leucovorin 25 mg/wk or pyrimethamine 75 mg/wk +

5 Drug Information

dapsone 200 mg/wk and leucovorin 25 mg/wk or atovaquone 1500 mg qd ± pyrimethamine 25 mg qd + leucovorin 10 mg qd.

PHARMACOLOGY

- **Bioavailability:** Well absorbed
- **T½:** 54-148 h (average 111 h)
- **Elimination:** Parent compound and metabolites excreted in urine
- **Dose modification in renal failure:** None

■ TABLE 5-66: **Toxoplasmosis Treatment (2008 CDC/NIH/IDSA Guidelines for Opportunistic Infections)**

Acute (≥ 6 weeks)	Maintenance
Preferred	Preferred
Pyrimethamine 200 mg po x 1, then 50 mg (<60 kg) to 75 mg (>60 kg) po/d + leukovorin 10-25 mg/d + sulfadiazine 1 gm (<60 kg) to 1.5 gm (>60 kg) po q6h	Pyrimethamine 25-50 mg/d po + leukovorin 10-25 mg/d po + sulfadiazine 2-4 gm/d po
Alternatives	Alternatives
Pyrimethamine + leukovorin (as above) + 1. Clindamycin 600 mg IV q6h po or IV 2. Atovaquone 1500 mg po bid	Pyrimethamine + leukovorin (as above) + 1. Clindamycin 600 mg po q8h 2. Atovaquone 750 mg po q6-12h
Alternative without pyrimethamine	Alternative without pyrimethamine
1. Atovaquone 1500 mg po bid + sulfadiazine 1.0-1.5 mg po q6h 2. TMP-SMX (5 mg TMP/kg) IV or po bid 3. Atovaquone 1500 mg po bid	1. Atovaquone 750 mg po q6-12h 2. Continue 3. Continue

SIDE EFFECTS: Reversible marrow suppression due to depletion of folic acid stores with dose-related megaloblastic anemia, leukopenia, thrombocytopenia, and agranulocytosis; prevented or treated with folinic acid (leucovorin).

- **GI intolerance:** Improved by reducing dose or giving drug with meals
- **Neurologic:** Dose-related ataxia, tremors, or seizures
- **Hypersensitivity:** Most common with pyrimethamine plus sulfadioxine (*Fansidar*) and due to sulfonamide component of combination
- **Drug interactions:** Lorazepam: hepatotoxicity. AZT, ganciclovir, interferon: additive bone marrow suppression.

PREGNANCY: Category C. Teratogenic in animals, but limited experience has not shown association with birth defects in humans.

Drug Information

RALTEGRAVIR (RAL)

TRADE NAME: *Isentress* (Merck & Co., Inc)

PRODUCT INFORMATION: 800-850-3430

CLASS: Integrase strand transfer inhibitor (InSTI)

FORMULATION AND COST: 400 mg tabs; $18.70/400 mg tabs; $1,121.93/mo

STANDARD REGIMEN: 400 mg po bid with or without food.

- **Renal failure:** GFR 50-80 ml/min – standard; GFR <50 ml/min – standard dose likely but no data.
- **Hepatic failure:** Standard dose for mild to moderate hepatic failure Severe liver disease; standard dose likely, but no data.

STORAGE: Room temperature

INDICATIONS:

- Treatment of HIV infection in combination with other ARV agents in treatment-naïve and ART-experienced patients with evidence of HIV replication despite ongoing ART.
- Treatment of HIV infection in combination with other ARV agents in ART-naïve patients.
- One of the preferred first line ARV regimen (RAL+TDF/FTC) in treatment-naïve patients (2011 DHHS Guidelines and 2010 IAS-USA Guidelines).

ADVANTAGES:

- Potent antiretroviral agent.
- Transmitted resistance is uncommon.
- Relatively low pill burden (2/d) without food requirements.
- Frequency of adverse reactions is low, there are no black box warnings, RTV is not co-administered, there is no significant effect on insulin resistance or blood lipids and no dose-related toxicity has been detected.
- Clinically important drug interactions are infrequent since RAL does not use, inhibit or induce the P450 metabolic pathway.
- More rapid viral load reduction than with other agents (clinical significance unknown).

DISADVANTAGES:

- Long-term experience is limited, so durability of antiviral effect and long-term toxicity are unknown.
- Cross resistance with elvitegravir (investigational integrase inhibitor)
- Must be taken twice daily (once-daily dosing inferior)
- Low genetic barrier to resistance

5 Drug Information

353

RESISTANCE: RAL, elvitegravir (EVG) and dolutegravir (572) have low genetic barriers to resistance and a high level of cross resistance (*JID* 2011:203:1204). There are also variations in resistance mutations that are subtype specific (*J Med Virol* 2011;83:751). Resistance and failure with RAL in subtype B infected patients is associated with primary mutations at Q148 or N155. Mutations here confer significant reduction in activity but the reduction increases when combined with at least one additional mutation, which can emerge rapidly:

- 155H + (74M/R, 92Q, 97A, 138A/K, 140A/S, 151I, 163R, 183P, 226D/F/H, 230R)
- 148K/R/H + (140S/A, 138K)
- 143C/H/R

Note: In a **BENCHMRK analysis** of 94 failures, 64 (68%) had in vitro resistance (*NEJM* 2008;359:355). Of these, 48 (75%) had 2 or more mutations. The **three most common pathways** in 121 RAL failures were 148 K/R/H (48%), 155 H (31%) and H3 C/R (21%) (*JID* 2011; 203:1204). Strains of HIV resistant to RAL are usually sensitive to dolutegravir and resistant to elvitegravir. Allele-specific sequencing prior to treatment with RAL in BENCHMRK participants found that those who subsequently had virologic failure were twice as likely to have a baseline primary or secondary integrase resistance mutation; secondary mutations were most common (*AAC* 2011;55:114).

CLINICAL TRIALS:

- **Treatment-naïve**

  □ **STARTMRK:** 563 treatment-naïve patients were randomized to RAL+TDF/FTC or EFV/TDF/FTC. Baseline data and 48- and 96-week results are summarized in Table 5-67 (*Lancet* 2009;374:796; *JAIDS* 2010;55:39). The study found: 1) rates of viral suppression with VL <50 c/mL were nearly identical (79% vs. 81%); 2) the mean CD4 count increase was significantly greater in the RAL recipients; 3) adverse reactions were significantly more common in EFV recipients; and 4) EFV recipients has significantly higher levels of LDL-cholesterol. Week 96 data from STARTMRK showed viral suppression (<50 c/mL) in 81% and 79% of RAL-recipients and EFV-recipients, respectively. Median CD4 changes were +240 cells/mm^3 (RAL) and 225 cells/mm^3 (EFV). Increases in total cholesterol, LDL-cholesterol and HDL-cholesterol were greater in EFV recipients, and side effects were greater in the EFV recipients (78% vs. 47%), but the rate of serious side effects was similar (12% and 14%) (*JAIDS* 2010;55:39). The 156-week follow-up presented at the 2011 CROI are summarized in Table 5-67. RAL virologic outcome was non-inferior (p <0.001) (Rockstroh J. CROI 2011:Abstr. 542).

  □ **Protocol 004:** This was a Phase II multicenter, double-blind, randomized controlled trial with RAL (doses of 100,200, 400 and

■ TABLE 5-67: **STARTMRK: RAL + TDF/FTC vs. EFV/TDF/FTC in Treatment-naïve Patients: 48-week (*Lancet* 2009; 374:796), 96-week (*JAIDS* 2010;55:39) and 156-week Results (2011 CROI;Abstr. 542)**

	RAL + TDF/FTC n = 281	EFV/TDF/FTC n = 282
Baseline		
Mean VL (c/mL)	103,205	106,215
Mean CD4 count (cells/mm³)	219	217
Results (48 weeks)		
VL <50 c/mL	81%†	79%
CD4 count increase (cells/mm³)	189	163
ADRs		
• Grade 3 or 4	16%	32%*
• LDL-C mean change (mg/dL)	+9	+21
• Triglyceride mean change (mg/dL)	- 4	+40
• CNS Toxicity	29%	61%
• Cancer	3	11
Results (96 weeks)		
VL <50 c/mL	81%	79%
CD4 count increase (median) (cells/mm³)	240	225
ADRs requiring discontinuation	4%	6%
Results (156 weeks)		
VL <50 c/mL	75%	68%
CD4 count increase (median) (cells/mm³)	331	295
ADRs requiring discontinuation	7%	7%

* P= <0.05
† Resistance tests showed RAL resistance mutations in 3 of 6 patients tested

600 mg po bid) vs. EFV 600 mg/d in 198 treatment-naïve patients. Each group received the study drug in combination with TDF/FTC. At 48 weeks, the pooled outcome data for the 4 RAL dose regimens for 160 patients given RAL were similar to the 38 given EFV-based ART (63% vs. 38%) (*JAIDS* 2007;6:125; Gotuzzo. 2010 CROI;Abstr. 514).

□ **SHIELD:** Randomized pilot trial of 35 treatment-naïve patients treated with RAL+ABC/3TC. At 48 weeks, 32/35 (91%) had VL <50 c/mL and 35/35 (100%) had VL <400 c/mL, the median CD4 increase was 247/mm³, and lipid changes were modest (*HIV Clin Trials* 2010;11:260).

□ **PROGRESS:** Treatment-naïve patients randomized to LPV/r+RAL vs. LPV/r+TDF/FTC (see pg. 313).

5 Drug Information

□ **QDMRK:** The goal was to determine if RAL could be given once daily. The study with 770 treatment-naïve patients randomized to RAL 800 mg qd vs. 400 mg bid, each with TDF/FTC (Eron J. 2011 CROI:Abstr. 150LB). At 48 weeks the outcome was worse in the once-daily arm compared to the twice-daily arm, with viral suppression to <50 c/mL in 83% vs. 88%, virologic failure in 14% vs. 9%, integrase resistance mutations in 9 vs. 2, and FTC RAMs in 11 vs. 4. The study was stopped prematurely. The differences between arms was most pronounced in those with baseline VL >100,000 c/mL and those with low RAL levels.

■ **Treatment-experienced**

□ **BENCHMRK:** Trial of safety and efficacy of RAL in 509 treatment experienced subjects with randomized, double-blind, placebo-controlled study design. Entry criteria were age >16 yrs and resistance to ≥1 drug in each class: NRTI, NNRTI and PI. Participants were randomized 2:1 (RAL:Placebo); each group received optimized background therapy (OBT) or RAL + OBT (see Table 5-68A and 5-68B). The 96 week data from BENCHMRK-1 and -2 showed sustained viral suppression (<50 c/mL) in 57% of RAL recipients and 26% of placebo recipients. There were no new RAL-related safety concerns (*CID* 2010;50:605). HIV isolates from 112 RAL failures showed integrase resistance mutations in 73 (65%).

■ TABLE 5-68A: **BENCHMRK-1 & -2: 48- and 96-week Results (*NEJM* 2008;359:339)**

	RAL + OBT n = 462	Placebo + OBT n = 237
Baseline		
CD4 count (median) (cells/mm³)	151	158
VL (log₁₀ c/mL) (median)	4.6	4.6
Years of prior ART (median)	10	10
No. prior ART (median)	12	12
Results: 48 weeks		
VL <50 c/mL*	63%	33%
Baseline VL >100,000 c/mL	48%	16%
CD4 count increase (median) (cells/mm³)	81	11
ADRs requiring discontinuation	2%	3%
Results: 96 weeks		
VL <50 c/mL*	57%	26%
CD4 count increase (median) (cells/mm³)	123	49

* See Table 5-68B for results for VL <50 c/mL by phenotypic and genotypic resistance score of OBT

Drug Information

Genotype score	OBT	RAL + OBT	Phenotype score[†]	OBT	RAL + OBT
0	3%	45%	0	2%	51%
1	37%	67%	1	13%	61%
≥2	62%	77%	2	48%	71%

† Based on the lower/higher cutoff

- **SWITCHMRK:** This was a phase 3 trial designed to determine the safety and efficacy of switching patients with stable viral suppression on LPV/r-based ART to either RAL plus continued NRTIs or to continue the LPV/r-based regimen (*Lancet* 2010;375:396). Analysis at 24 weeks showed persistant viral suppression in 319/352 (91%) on LPV/r vs. 293/347 (84%) on RAL (p <0.05). A post-hoc analysis found that most of the failures in the RAL group had a history of prior virologic failure indicating the importance of combining RAL with two other active drugs (*Lancet* 2010;375:352).

- **ACTG 5262:** The single arm trial with DRV/r+RAL showed a virologic failure rate of 27% at 48 weeks and was stopped prematurely (see pg. 229).

- **SPIRAL:** Open-label trial in which 273 patients with viral suppression (VL <50 c/mL x 6 mos with PI/r-based regimen) were randomized to continue the current regimen or switch to RAL (plus NRTIs). At 48 weeks, 89.2% of patients on RAL and 86.6% of those on a PI/r remained free of treatment failure (p=NS and 96.9%) and 95.1% remained free of virologic failure, respectively (p=NS) (*AIDS* 2010;24:1697). Switching to RAL was associated with improvement in lipid profile.

- **EASIER-ANRS-138:** Multidrug resistant patients receiving ENF-based ART were randomized to continue the current regimen vs. switch to RAL-based ART (*HIV Clin Trials* 2010;11:283). Virologic responses were comparable at 48 weeks, with significant improvement in quality of life.

- **TRIO-ANRS-139:** This is a non-comparative trial with 100 patients with multi-drug resistant HIV (>3 primary PI mutations, >3 NRTI mutations, <3 DRV mutations and <3 NNRTI mutations). Baseline VL was 4.2 $\log_{10}$ c/mL and median CD4 count was 258 cells/mm³. At week 96 there were 5 virologic failures (>50 c/mL), all with low level viremia. See pg. 268.

- **RAL intensification:** 30 patients with VL <50 c/mL for >1 year on ART were randomized to RAL intensification (400 mg bid) vs. placebo. At 4 and 24 weeks, RAL intensification had no significant impact on: 1) VL using a single copy assay; 2) measures of T cell

Drug Information

5

activation; 3) CD4 count or 4) gut-associated lymphoid tissue (GALT) (Hiroyu-Hatano, et al. 2010 CROI;Abstr. 101LB.

- **NRTI-Sparing:** See Table 4-22A (pg. 124) and Table 4-22B (pg. 125)
  - □ **SPARTAN ATV + RAL:** Pilot study of a NRTI-sparing regimen in treatment-naïve patients using ATV 300 mg + RAL 400 mg bid vs. ATV/r+TDF/FTC once daily. By 24 wks, there were 6 virologic failures in the ATV+RAL arm, including 5 with RAL resistance and 13 (21%) with grade 4 hyperbilirubinemia. Jaundice was also common in this group. The pilot trial was stopped at 24 weeks based on these findings (Kozal M. 2010 IAS, Vienna:Abstr. THLBB204).
  - □ **PROGRESS RAL + LPV/r:** See pg. 313.
  - □ **A5262 RAL + DRV:** See pg. 229.

PHARMACOLOGY:

- **Absorption:** Absolute bioavailability not established; median trough 72 ng/mL (range 29-118).
- **Food Effect:** Delays Tmax, may be taken with or without food.
- **T½:** 9 hrs; intracellular T½: 29 hrs
- **Elimination:** RAL is not a substrate P450 enzyme and it does not inhibit or induce CYP3A4. RAL is eliminated by hepatic glucuronidation; the glucuronidated metabolite is largely eliminated in stool (51%) and urine (32%) (*Drug Metab Dispos* 2007;35:1657). Moderate liver impairment and severe renal disease do not alter pharmacokinetics; severe liver disease has not been studied.
- **CNS Penetration:** 7.3%; CSF levels exceed IC_{50} for wild-type HIV by a median of 4.5-fold. The CNS penetration score is 3 in a 4 class system (*Neurology* 2011;76:693).

ADVERSE DRUG REACTIONS: Few dose related side effects. Doses up to 1600 mg/d were generally well tolerated (*Clin Pharmacol The*r 2008;83: 293). There were no adverse events that were significantly more frequent in the RAL recipients than placebo recipients in BENCHMRK-1 and -2 (*NEJM* 2008;359:339). The frequency of **hepatotoxicity** in STARTMRK and BENCHMRK with 743 RAL recipients showed grade 3/4 liver enzyme elevations were infrequent except with HBV and/or HCV coinfection with rates of 2.6-4.0% (Rockstroh. 2010 CROI;Abstr. Q125). The frequency of **malignancies** in BENCHMRK -1 and -2 was 16/461 (3.5%) in RAL recipients at 48 weeks compared to 4/178 (2.6%) in placebo-recipients for an OR=1.5. The difference did not persist, but post FDA-approval surveillance for malignancies is being carried out. Data from >6000 patients with >3900 patient-years of RAL exposure showed no association (*Ann Pharm* 2010;44:42). Phase 2 trials found that 6% of RAL recipients had grade 3-4 elevations of **CPK** and there have been case reports of **rhabdomyolysis** (*JAIDS* 2007;46:125; *Ann Pharm* 2010;44:42; *AIDS* 2008;22:1382). The **lipid changes** at 48 weeks in STARTMRK showed significantly greater mean increases in

EFV recipients for total cholesterol (+33 vs. +10 mg/dL) and triglyceride levels (+37 vs. -3 mg/dL). Body composition changes were similar (*JAIDS* 2010;55:39). A case of reversible **cerebellar ataxia** has been reported (*AIDS* 2010;24:2757).

DRUG INTERACTIONS: See Table 5-69. RAL is not a substrate, inducer or inhibitor of the CYP3A4 metabolic pathway. It is consequently not expected to alter pharmacokinetics of PIs, NNRTIs, methadone, statins, azoles, tacrolimus, oral contraceptive or erectile dysfunction agents. Nevertheless, some possibly important interactions are noted regarding RAL pharmacology. **Rifampin** decreases RAL levels; avoid or use RAL 800 mg bid (*AAC* 2009;53:2852). Doubling the RAL dose may not compensate for the low trough levels (*JAC* 2010;65:2485), although a limited clinical experience suggests the double dose RAL performs well (*JAC* 2011;66:951). **Rifabutin** has no clinically significant effect on RAL levels (*J Clin Pharmacol* 2011;51:943). **Omeprazole** significantly increases RAL levels presumably due to increased solubility at high pH levels (*Drug Metab Dispos* 2007;35:1657). With regard to antiretroviral agents, the drugs that decrease RAL levels the most are **TPV/r, MVC** and **EFV** (*Ann Pharm* 2010;44:42; *AAC* 2008;52:4338), but the changes are not sufficient to alter dosing. Anecdotal cases of substantial reductions in RAL AUC with concurrent

■ Table 5-69: **RAL Drug Interactions**

Agent	Effect on RAL	Recommendation
Rifampin	RAL AUC ↓40%	Avoid combination. Consider RAL 800 mg bid w/co-administration
Rifabutin	RAL AUC ↓19%	Standard dose rifabutin; RAL 400 mg bid
Phenobarbitol	May decrease RAL	Avoid; use valproic acid or levetiracetam
Phenytoin	May decrease RAL	Avoid; as above
Omeprazole	RAL AUC ↑3x	Standard doses
TDF	RAL AUC ↑49%	Standard doses
TPV/r	RAL AUC ↓24% RAL Cmin ↓55%	Case report of hepatic necrosis reported with co-administration; use with caution
EFV	RAL AUC ↓36%	Standard dose RAL; Cmin RAL not affected
ATV/r	RAL AUC ↑40-70%	Standard doses
RTV	RAL unchanged	Standard doses
ETR	RAL unchanged	Standard doses
LPV/r	RAL Cmin ↓30%	Standard doses
MVC	RAL AUC ↓40%	Standard doses
DRV/r	DRV Cmin ↓36%	Clinical significance unknown. Standard doses
FPV	RAL AUC ↓37% APV AUC ↓36%	Avoid
FPV/r	RAL AUC ↓55%	Clinical significance unknown. Standard doses

5 Drug Information

ETR are reported including virologic failure in four cases (*AIDS* 2009; 27:869). **Oral contraceptive:** No significant interaction. **Methadone:** No significant interaction. Hypersensitivity reactions including DRESS syndrome (drug rash with eosinophilia and systemic symptoms).

PREGNANCY: Category C. No treatment related effects were observed on embryonic or fetal survival in rodents. There are no studies in pregnant woman to document pharmacokinetics or safety. The 2010 DHHS Guidelines on Antiretroviral Drugs in Pregnant HIV-infected women list RAL as "insufficient data to recommend use."

REBETOL – see Ribavirin (below)

RETROVIR – see Zidovudine (AZT, ZDV) (pg. 416)

RIBAVIRIN

TRADE NAME: *Rebetol* and *Rebetron* (combined *Rebetrol/Intron A*) (Schering-Plough); *Copegus* (Roche), *Virazole* (Valeant) inhalation

FORMS AND COST: 200 mg caps at $9.93 per cap; 200 mg tab (*Copegus*) at $10.12 per tab; $5,211/6 gm vial (*Virazole*)

NOTE: Concurrent use with ddI is contraindicated due to increased risk of pancreatitis and/or lactic acidosis. Use with caution when given with AZT (additive anemia) or d4T (potentiation of mitochondrial toxicity). Avoid ABC (potential antagonism).

INDICATION (FDA labeling): Ribavirin in combination with interferon is indicated for treatment of chronic HCV in patients with compensated liver disease who have not previously been treated (see pg. 513).

UNIQUE FEATURES: 1) The mechanism of action against HCV is unknown; 2) Resistance is not an issue; 3) Toxicity as a major concern and 4) It appears necessary for optimal response with HCV treatment.

CONTRAINDICATIONS: Pregnancy in a female patient, pregnancy in the female partner of a male patient, hemoglobinopathies.

REGIMEN: Dose used in therapeutic trials was usually 400 mg bid, but dosage range 1000-1200 mg/d resulted in improved sustained virologic response (SVR) (see pg. 516). Standard dose in absence of HIV co-infection is: <75 kg – 400 mg in a.m., 600 mg in p.m.; >75 kg – 600 mg bid. Dose w/CrCl <60 mL/min: 200-800 mg in 2 individual doses (monitor for toxicity).

CLINICAL TRIALS: Ribavirin has been used to treat HCV for 20 years. It appears to be synergistic with interferon-alfa. The mechanism of action, optimal dose and duration are not well established. Several trials have tested the relative efficacy of HCV treatment using ribavirin + interferon (IFN) vs. IFN alone and show a substantial advantage to including ribavirin. With HIV-HCV co-infection, sustained viral suppression is achieved in 15-25% with genotype 1 and 70-80% with genotypes 2 and 3 (*NEJM* 2004; 351:451; *NEJM* 2004;351:438; *JAMA* 2004;292:2909) (see pg. 518). Compared to HCV mono-infected patients, these rates of SVR are much lower for genotype 1 and comparable for genotypes 2 and 3 (*Lancet* 2001;358:958; *NEJM* 2002;347:975). Initial trials with telaprevir + peg-IFN with or without ribavirin suggest that ribavirin is a necessary component for optimal response (*NEJM* 2009;360:1839). The same applies to boceprevir (NEJM 2011;31:1207). These new PIs (telapravir and bocepravir) will be given with peg-IFN+ribavirin for genotypic 1 and 4. (*NEJM* 2011;364:1272) (see pg. 383-388).

PHARMACOLOGY

- **Oral bioavailability:** 64%; absorption increased with high-fat meal
- **T½:** 30 h
- **Elimination:** Metabolized by phosphorylation and deribosylation; there are few or no cytochrome P450 enzyme-based drug interactions. Metabolites are excreted in the urine. The drug should not be used with severe renal failure.

BLACK BOX WARNINGS: Birth defects, fetal death, hemolytic anemia.

SIDE EFFECTS: About 15-20% of patients receiving ribavirin+IFN discontinue therapy due to side effects. The main side effects are **anemia, cough**, and **dyspepsia**. **Hemolytic anemia** is noted in the first 1-2 wks of treatment and usually stabilizes by week 4. In clinical trials without HIV co-infection, the mean decrease in hemoglobin was 3 g/dL, and 10% of patients had a hemoglobin <10 g/dL. Patients with a hemoglobin <10 g/dL or decrease in hemoglobin ≥2 g/dL *and* a history of cardiovascular disease should receive a modified regimen of ribavirin 600 mg qd. The drugs should be discontinued if the hemoglobulin decreases to ≤8.5 g/dL or if the hemoglobin persists at <12 g/dL in patients with a cardiovascular disease. Erythropoietin (40,000 units SQ every week) is usually effective (*Am J Gastro* 2001;96:2802). Concurrent use of AZT should be avoided whenever possible. Ribavirin is a nucleoside that may cause **mitochondrial toxicity**, especially when combined with other NRTIs that cause mitochondrial toxicity, especially ddI and d4T; 2 of 15 patients given this combination developed lactic acidosis (*Lancet* 2001;357:280). Other side effects ascribed to ribavirin include **leukopenia, hyperbilirubinemia, increased uric acid,** and **dyspnea**.

NOTE: See pegylated interferon, pg. 342, for side effects ascribed to that agent.

DRUG INTERACTION: Increased risk of anemia with **AZT** co-administration; monitor closely (*AAC* 1997;41:1231; *AIDS* 1998;14:1661). In combination with ddI, there is potentiation of **ddI** toxicity due to inhibition of mitochondrial DNA polymerase gamma, resulting in pancreatitis and lactic acidosis (*AAC* 1987;31:1613; *Lancet*

5 Drug Information

2001;72:177). This combination should be avoided. **ABC** may decrease the efficacy of ribavirin (Avoid co-administration).

PREGNANCY: Category X. Potent teratogen. Must be used with caution in women with childbearing potential and in their male sexual partners. Adequate birth control is mandatory.

RIFABUTIN

TRADE NAME: *Mycobutin* (Pharmacia)

FORM AND COST: 150 mg cap at $13.70

PATIENT ASSISTANCE PROGRAM: 800-242-7014

CLASS: Semisynthetic derivative of rifampin B that is derived from *Streptomyces mediterranei*

INDICATIONS AND DOSES

- ***M. avium* complex (MAC) prophylaxis:** 300 mg po qd. Efficacy established (*NEJM* 1993;329:828); azithromycin or clarithromycin is usually preferred (see pg. 71).

- **MAC treatment:** See pg. 459. Sometimes combined with clarithromycin or azithromycin and EMB using 300 mg qd, except in patients treated with PIs or NNRTIs where dose adjustment is recommended (see below).

- **Tuberculosis:** See pg. 462. Preferred over rifampin for use in combination with most PIs or NNRTIs (*MMWR* 2004;53:37). Usual dose for TB treatment and prophylaxis: 300 mg qd, but dose must be adjusted for concurrent use with PIs (see Table 5-70). A meta-analysis of cohort studies and meta-analysis to evaluate rifamycin use in combination with antiretroviral agents suggested excessive rates of relapse with 2 mos of rifamycin compared to 8 mos of treatment (OR 3.6; 95% CI = 1.1-11.7) (*CID* 2010;50:1288).

ACTIVITY: Active against most strains of MAC and rifampin-sensitive *M. tuberculosis*; cross-resistance between rifampin and rifabutin is common with *M. tuberculosis* and MAC.

PHARMACOLOGY

- **Bioavailability:** 12-20%

- **T½:** 30-60 h

- **Metabolism:** Metabolized via CYP3A4 to 25-0-deacetyl-rifabutin (10% of total antimicrobial activity).

- **Elimination:** Primarily renal and biliary excretion of metabolites

- **Dose modification in renal failure:** None

SIDE EFFECTS: Common: **Brown-orange discoloration** of secretions; urine (30%), tears, saliva, sweat, stool, and skin (warn the patient). Infrequent: **rash** (4%), **GI intolerance** (3%), **neutropenia** (2%). Rare: flu-like illness, hepatitis, hemolysis, headache, thrombocytopenia, myositis. **Uveitis**, which presents as red and painful eye, blurred vision, photophobia, or floaters, is dose-related, usually with doses >450 mg qd, or with standard dose (300 mg qd) plus concurrent use of drugs that increase rifabutin levels including most PIs, clarithromycin, and azoles including fluconazole (*NEJM* 1994;330:868). These patients should be evaluated by an opthalmologist are and usually treated with topical corticosteroids and mydriatics.

DRUG INTERACTIONS: Rifabutin induces hepatic microsomal enzymes (cytochrome P450 3A4), although the effect is less pronounced than for rifampin. Dose adjustment for antiretroviral agents when rifabutin is given are summarized in Table 5-70. With EFV, the AUC of rifabutin decreases by a mean of 37%, requiring an increase in rifabutin dose to 450 mg/d (*CID* 2005;41: 1343). Rifabutin reduces the levels of APV (14% decrease), **warfarin, barbiturates, benzodiazepines, beta-blockers, chloramphenicol, clofibrate, oral contraceptives, corticosteroids, cyclosporine, diazepam, dapsone, digitalis, doxycycline, haloperidol, oral hypoglycemics, voriconazole, posaconazole, ketoconazole, phenytoin, quinidine, theophylline, trimethoprim,** and **verapamil**. Drugs that inhibit cytochrome P450 and prolong the half-life of rifabutin: **PIs, erythromycin, clarithromycin** (56% increase), and **azoles** (fluconazole, itraconazole, and ketoconazole). With concurrent rifabutin and fluconazole, the levels of rifabutin are significantly increased, leading to possible rifabutin toxicity (uveitis, nausea, neutropenia) or increased efficacy (*CID* 1996;23;685).

■ TABLE 5-70: **Rifabutin Interactions and Dose Adjustments with ARVs** (2008 NIH/CDC/IDSA Recommendations for Opportunistic Infections and DHHS Guidelines for Use of Antiretroviral Agents in Adults and Adolescents and CDC recommendations [last reviewed 7/1/2010])

ARV	ARV Dose	Rifabutin Dose**
EFV	Standard	450-600 mg/d or 600 mg 2-3x/wk‡
NVP	Standard	300 mg/d or 3 x/wk
ETR	Standard	300 mg/d*
PI/r (all)	Standard	150 mg qod or 3 x/wk‡
FPV†	Standard	150 mg/d or 300 mg 3 x/wk
ATV†	Standard	150 mg qod or 3 x/wk
NFV†	Standard	150 mg qd or 300 mg 3 x/wk
IDV†	1000 mg q8h	150 mg/d or 300 mg 3 x/wk
MCV	600 mg bid	300 mg/d
RAL	Standard	300 mg/d

* Dose assumes no concurrent PI/r. If combined with ETR and rifabutin, SQV/r or DRV/r not recommended due to potential additive decrease in ETR concentrations

** For the treatment of TB, most experts recommend 150 mg qd with PI/r. Consider rifabutin TDM.

‡ Some experts recommend 150 mg qd or 300 mg 3x/week with TDM

† Without RTV boosting

5 Drug Information

COMMENTS

- Rifampin and rifabutin are related drugs, but *in vitro* activity and clinical trials show that rifabutin is preferred for MAC, and rifampin is preferred for *M. tuberculosis*.

- Clarithromycin plus EMB without rifabutin may be the preferred regimen for treatment of disseminated MAC due to the clarithromycin–rifabutin interaction.

- Drug interactions are similar for rifabutin and rifampin, although rifabutin is a less potent inducing agent of hepatic microsomal enzymes.

- Uveitis requires immediate discontinuation of drug and ophthalmology consult.

- All PIs and NNRTIs require a dose adjustment when given with rifabutin except for NVP (see Table 5-70, pg. 362).

PREGNANCY: Category B. Not teratogenic in rats or rabbits. No pharmacologic data or clinical experience in human pregnancy (2010 DHHS Guidelines for ART in pregnant women).

RIFAMATE – see Isoniazid (pg. 299) or Rifampin (below)

RIFAMPIN

TRADE NAME: *Rifadin* (Aventis) and generic; Combination with INH: *Rifamate*. Combination with INH and PZA: *Rifater* (Aventis)

FORMS AND COST: Caps: 150 mg at $2.27, 300 mg at $3.03. *Rifamate*: Caps with 150 mg INH + 300 mg rifampin at $4.19 or $2.39 (generic). *Rifater*: Tabs with 50 mg INH + 120 mg rifampin + 300 mg pyrazinamide at $2.73. IV vials: 600 mg at $139.

INDICATIONS AND DOSE: Tuberculosis (with INH, PZA, and SM or EMB)

- **Dose:** 10 mg/kg/d (600 mg/d max) (see pg. 465-475).

- **DOT:** 600 mg 2x to 3x/wk. (HIV-infected patients with CD4 counts <100/mm)^3 should receive DOT 3x/wk. The rationale is the observation of acquired rifamycin-resistance in trials of HIV-TB co-infected patients with CD4 counts <100/mm^3 treated with rifapentine once weekly or rifabutin twice weekly, each in combination with INH (*Lancet* 1999;343:1843; *MMWR* 2002;51:214).

- **Prophylaxis (alone or in combination with PZA or EMB):** 10 mg/kg/d (600 mg/d max)

- **Antiretrovirals and TB treatment:** See Table 6-8, pg. 467. Rifamycins should be included in any regimen for active TB. Options with ART include:

  □ Rifampin (standard dose) + EFV. Consider increasing EFV dose to 800 mg qd for patient >60 kg.

  □ Rifabutin substitution with IDV, FPV, NFV, LPV/r, SQV, ATV, DRV,

Drug Information

and RTV-boosted regimen in which the RTV dose is ≤200 mg bid (see Table 5-70, pg. 362).

□ Do not delay antiretroviral therapy in patients with CD4 <50 cells/mm^3 (see pg. 464 and 528).

ACTIVE AGAINST: *M. tuberculosis, M. kansasii,* methicillin-sensitive *S. aureus* (use in combination), *H. influenzae, S. pneumoniae, Legionella,* and many anaerobes

PHARMACOLOGY

- **Bioavailability:** 90-95%, less with food. Absorption is reduced by 30% in patients with advanced HIV infection; significance is unknown (*Ann Intern Med* 1997;127:289).

- **T½:** 1.5-5.0 h; average 2 h

- **Elimination:** Excreted in urine (33%) and metabolized

- **Dose modification in renal failure:** None

SIDE EFFECTS

- **Common:** Orange-brown discoloration of urine, stool, tears (contact lens), sweat, skin (warn patient).

- **Infrequent:** GI intolerance; hepatitis (in 2.7% given INH+RIF), usually cholestatic changes in first month of treatment; jaundice (usually reversible with dose reduction or continued use); hypersensitivity, especially pruritus ± rash (6%); flu-like illness in 0.4-0.7% given rifampin 2x/wk with intermittent use – dyspnea, wheezing, purpura, leukopenia.

- **Rare:** Thrombocytopenia, leukopenia, hemolytic anemia, increased uric acid, and BUN. Frequency of side effects that require discontinuation of drug is 3%.

DRUG INTERACTIONS: Extensive, due to induction of hepatic cytochrome P450 (3A4, 2B6, 2C8, 2C9) enzymes (www.mmhiv.com/link/CDC-NCHHSTP). Rifampin should be avoided with all **PIs** and **NNRTIs** except **EFV**. EFV has no significant effect on rifampin levels, but rifampin reduces EFV levels by 20-26%; some recommend EFV 800 mg qd for person >60 kg. Limited experience suggests that **NVP** may not be appropriate due to increased rates of HIV virologic failure. The 2009 CDC/IDSA/NIH OI Guidelines recommend EFV-based ART when rifampin is used (www.mmhiv.com/link/2009-OI-NIH-CDC-IDSA). The CDC previously recommended dosing NVP at 300 mg bid, but this has subsequently been found to be virologically inferior (*JAMA* 2008;300:530), and the dose of 300 mg bid is associated with a higher rate of adverse reactions (*Antiviral Ther* 2008;13:529). With **ETR** there is marked decrease in ETR levels; avoid this combination. The **MVC** AUC decreases 64%; use MVC 600 mg bid (limited clinical data). Rifabutin is preferred. **RAL** level decreased 40-60%; avoid this combination. If co-administration is needed, increase RAL to 800 mg bid (limited clinical data). Consider rifabutin with RAL co-administration (no interaction). The following drugs inhibit cytochrome P450 enzymes and prolong the half-life of rifampin: **clarithromycin, erythromycin,** and **azoles (fluconazole, itraconazole,** and **ketoconazole).** Rifampin decreases levels of **atovaquone, barbiturates, oral contraceptives, corticosteroids, cyclosporine, dapsone, fluconazole, ketoconazole, methadone, phenytoin, theophylline, trimethoprim, sirolimus, tacrolimus,** and many other drugs that are 3A4 substrates. Rifampin should not be used concurrently with **atovaquone, clarithromycin, posaconazole,** or **voriconazole.** With **fluconazole** and **itraconazole** it may be necessary to increase the azole dose. The level of **dapsone** is decreased 7- to 10-fold – consider alternative.

PREGNANCY: Category C. Dose-dependent congenital malformations in animals. Isolated cases of fetal abnormalities noted in patients, but frequency is unknown. Large retrospective studies have shown no risk of congenital abnormalities; case reports of neural tube defects and limb reduction (*CID* 1995:21[suppl 1]:S24). May cause postnatal hemorrhage in mother and infant if given in last few weeks of pregnancy; give prophylactic vitamin K 10 mg single dose to the infant.

RIFATER – see Isoniazid (pg. 299) or Rifampin (above) or Pyrazinamide (pg. 350) (*Ann Intern Med* 1995;122:951)

RILPIVIRINE (RPV)

TRADE NAME: *Edurant* (Janssen Therapeutics)

CLASS: NNRTI

FORMULATION, REGIMENS AND PRICE

FORMS: RPV 25 mg tablet. Price: $1,195 (AWP, 1 mo); RPV/TDF/FTC 25/300/200 mg tab (*Complera*) $2,045.57 (1 mo).

USUAL ADULT DOSE: RPV 25 mg (one tablet) taken once daily with a meal; RPV/TDF/FTC 1 tab qd with a meal

CONCURRENT ART AGENTS

- **Concurrent ART agents:** Standard RPV dose recommended with PI/r, MVC, RAL and NRTI. Co-administration with ddI is complicated by the need to take ddI on an empty stomach, and RPV must be taken with food

- **Hepatic disease:** No dose adjustment needed for mild to moderate (Child-Pugh A and B) hepatic impairment

- **Renal insufficiency:** Use standard dose with close monitoring in patient with ESRD. RPV is unlikely to be removed during hemodialysis and peitoneal dialysis

- **EFV:** RPV should not be given concurrently with EFV; the long EFV T½ and induction properties complicates the EFV→RPV switch. In patients who are virologically suppressed, switching from EFV to RPV is safe (Mills. ICAAC 2011;Abstr. H2-974c).

ADVANTAGES: Potent activity against HIV; well tolerated; once daily administration; relatively few drug interactions; minimal effect on blood lipids; may be used in pregnancy; low pill burden; active against strains with the K103N mutation; once daily, single-tablet coformulation with TDF/FTC (approved August 2011).

DISADVANTAGES: Relatively new so clinical experience is limited; difficult transition from EFV-based ART due to induction of RPV metabolism; low genetic barrier to resistance; a major resistance mutation (E138K) also confers resistance to ETR; increased rates of failure with baseline VL >100,000 c/mL and with suboptimal adherence compared to EFV; reduced pharmacologic barrier to resistance compared to EFV; meal requirement; reduction in bioavailability without gastric acid; contraindicated with PPIs, and dose separation required with H2 blockers and antacids.

CLINICAL TRIALS: The registration trials **ECHO** and **THRIVE** compared RPV to EFV in 1,368 treatment-naïve patients randomized to receive RPV 25 mg or EFV 600 mg qd in combination with TDF/FTC (**ECHO**) or with investigator's choice of TDF/FTC, AZT/3TC or ABC/3TC (**THRIVE**). Criteria for inclusion was a baseline VL ≥5000 c/mL, susceptibility to NRTIs and absence of specific NNRTI mutations. The pooled results at 48 and 96 weeks are summarized in Table 5-71A and 5-71B.

■ TABLE 5-71A: **Pooled Data for ECHO and THRIVE at 48 and 96 Weeks (Package Insert)** (*Drugs Today* 2011;47:5)

Variable	RPV n – 686	EFV n – 682
Baseline data		
Age median (yrs)	36	36
Male	76%	76%
Viral load ($\log_{10}$ c/mL)	5.0	5.0
VL >100,000 c/mL	46%	52%
CD4 count (median, cells/mm³)	249	260
NRTI: TDF/FTC	80%	80%
Results		
VL <50 c/mL	83%	80%
Virologic failure	13%	9%
Failure by baseline VL		
<100,000 c/mL	5%	5%
100,000-500,000 c/mL	20%	11%
>500,000 c/mL	29%	17%
CD4 count (mean, cells/mm³)	+192	+176
Discontinuation due to adverse events	2%	7%
ADR (Grade 2-4)		
Neurological (H/A, dizziness)	4%	10%
Psychiatric (Depression, insomnia, abnormal dreams)	8%	10%
Rash	3%	11%

■ TABLE 5-71B: **Resistance-associated Mutations (RAMs) in Patients with Virologic Failure – Pooled 96-Week Results for ECHO and THRIVE Trials (Cohen CJ. IAS 2011, Rome;Abstr. TULBPE032)**

	RPV	EFV
Number Tested	86	42
Number NNRTI RAMs	46 (53%)	20 (48%)
Predominant RAM	E138K 31 (36%)	K103N 14 (33%)
Number NNRTI RAMs	48 (56%)	11 (26%)
Predominant RAM	M184I 32 (37%)*	M184V 6 (14%)

* The M184I substitution was more frequent than M184V due to a replication advantage when combined with M138K (Hu. 2011 CROI:Abstr. 594). The M184I substitution confers resistance to 3TC and FTC and, combined with E138K, increases resistance to RPV compared to E138K alone.

CONCLUSIONS

- The rate of virologic failure was nearly the same, but there were significantly more failures with a baseline VL>100,000 c/mL.

- Caution or use of an alternative agent is recommended with a baseline VL >100,000 c/mL.

- RPV was better tolerated, with lower frequency of neurologic psychiatric and rash reactions.

- As expected virologic failure was associated with NNRTI and NRTI RAMs. For RPV the dominant RAM was 138K compared to K103N with EFV. This difference will influence NNRTI resistance sequences, especially with ETR, which is active against 103N but has reduced activity with 138K (see below).

RESISTANCE: High level resistance: 101P and 181LV

- Mutations associated with RPV virologic failure V90I, K101E/P, E138K/G. V179I/L, Y181C, V189I, H221Y, F227C/L and M230L. The most common mutation associated with failure is E138K, which increases resistance by 2.8-fold without M184I and 6.7-fold with M184I. With RPV resistance, there is cross-resistance to ETR in 89% and cross-resistance to NVP in 63%.

PHARMACOLOGY

- Food (normal or high fat meal) improves RPV absorption. Fasted condition or high protein drink decreases RPV absorption by 40-50%.

- High protein binding: 99.7%

- RPV undergoes oxidative metabolism via CYP3A4. Parent drug and metabolite are primarily excreted in feces (85%) and urine (6.1%).

- Half-life: 50 hours

SIDE EFFECTS

- **Depressive disorders** including depressed mood, major depression and suicidal ideation. During phase 3 trials the rate of depression, regardless of causality, was 8%; most were mild or moderate in severity. The rate of Grade 3 or 4 depression was 1%.

Drug Information

- **Fat redistribution** including increased visceral fat with central obesity, dorsocervical fat enlargement, breast enlargement and peripheral fat wasting has been observed. The mechanism and causal role of RPV is unclear.
- **Dose dependent QTc prolongation:** (QTc increased 4.8, 10.7, 23.3 milliseconds with 25 mg, 75 mg, 300 mg dose, respectively.
- **Lipids:** There is virtually no impact on serum lipids
- **ECHO and THRIVE trials:** Pooled at 96 weeks (Cohen CJ, *et al.* IAS 2011;Abstr. TULBPE032). RPV was better tolerated than EFV. The relative frequencies of Grade 2-4 toxicities for RPV and EFV, each with TDF/FTC, are summarized in Table 5-71C.

■ TABLE 5-71C: **Side-effects* Noted in ECHO and THRIVE for RPV and EFV**

Results based on week 48 results (*Complera* package insert)	RPV n = 550	EFV n = 546
Symptomatic		
Nausea	1%	2%
Headache	2%	2%
Dizziness	1%	7%
Insomnia	2%	2%
Abnormal dreams	1%	3%
Depressive disorders	1%	2%
Rash	1%	5%
Laboratory changes		
Creatinine elevation >1.3 ULN	<1%	1%
AST elevation >2.5 x ULN	5-6%	10%
LDL-C >160 mg/dL	6%	13%
Total cholesterol >240 mg/dL	4-5%	17%
Triglyceride >500 mg/dL	1-2%	2%

* Grade 2-4 toxicity (DAIDS toxicity range)

DRUG INTERACTIONS

- **RPV should not be co-administered** with several **anticonvulsants** (phenytoin, phenobarbital, oxcarbazepine) **proton pump inhibitors** (omeprazole, pantoprazole, rabeprazole, lansprazole, esomeprazole), more than a single dose of systemic **dexamethasone, St. John's wort, rifampin, rifabutin** or **rifapentine**.
- Avoid co-administration with any other **NNRTI** (e.g., DLV, EFV, ETR, NVP)

Drug Information

5

- **TDF** AUC increased 23%; RPV concentrations not affected.
- **ddl:** no significant interaction if ddl taken 2 hours before RPV; RPV concentrations not affected.
- **DRV/r** and **LPV/r** increase RPV AUC 130% and 52%, respectively; use standard dose.
- **Rifampin** and **rifabutin** decrease RPV AUC by 80% and 46%, respectively. Other CYP 3A4 inducers may also significantly decrease RPV serum concentrations.
- **Omeprazole** decreases RPV AUC 40%. **Proton pump inhibitors** (PPIs) may also significantly decrease RPV absorption and are contraindicated. If acid suppression is needed, **H2 blockers** can be considered; these must be given 12 hrs before or 4 hrs after RPV. Antacid should also be administer >2 hrs before or 4 hours after RPV.
- **Ketoconazole** increases RPV AUC 49%; ketoconazole AUC decreased by 24%.
- **Other azole antifungals** (e.g., fluconazole, itraconazole, posaconazole, voriconazole) may also increase RPV concentrations. Monitor for QTc prolongation and antifungal efficacy.
- **Macrolide antibiotics** (e.g., clarithromycin, troleandomycin, erythromycin) may increase RPV concentrations. Monitor for QTc prolongation. Consider azithromycin with co-administration.
- Avoid RPV co-administration with drugs that can significantly **prolong QTc** (e.g., tricyclic antidepressants, haloperidol, terfenadine, astemizole, sotalol, procainamide, amiodarone, pimozide, disopyramide and high dose methadone)
- **Methadone** No change in Rilpivirine concentrations. (active R-isomer) AUC decreased by 16%; use standard dose and for withdrawal symptoms. Dose adjustment may be needed in some patients. Use standard dose and monitor for withdrawal symptoms.
- **Ethinyl estradiol** AUC increased 14%; and norethindrone decreased 11%. Clinical significance unknown. No change in RPV.
- No significant interaction with **sildenafil**.
- **Atorvastatin** hydroxy metabolites increased by 23-39%. Clinical significance unknown. Use standard dose atorvastatin.

PREGNANCY: Category B. No human data. Not teratogenic and no embryonic toxicity observed in animal studies.

RITONAVIR (RTV)

TRADE NAME: *Norvir* (Abbott Laboratories)

FORMS AND COST: 100 mg soft-gel capsules and tablets at $10.28; Medicaid and ADAP price is $2.14/100 mg cap. Liquid formulation 80 mg/mL at $1,728/240 mL.

PATIENT ASSISTANCE PROGRAM: 800-659-9050 (8 am-5 pm CST, Mon.-Fri.)

STORAGE: Caps can be left at room temperature (up to 25°C or 77°F) for up to 30 days. Oral solution should *not* be refrigerated – store tablet at room temperature.

CLASS: PI

DOSE: Almost always used to boost other PIs. When dose is ≤400 mg/d it is subtherapeutic and should not be considered an antiretroviral agent, hence the designation "/r." The dose is 600 mg bid when used as a single PI, but this is poorly tolerated, not recommended and rarely used. Administration with food improves tolerability but is not required for absorption.

- **Recommended regimens for PI-boosting:** See Table 5-72.

PHARMACOLOGY

- **Bioavailability:** Not well determined. Levels increased from about 4% to ≥15% when taken with meals. CNS penetration: No detectable levels in CSF.

- **T½:** 3-5 h

- **Elimination:** Metabolized by cytochrome P450 CYP3A4 >2D6. RTV is a potent inhibitor of cytochrome P450 CYP3A4>2D6, and an inducer of CYP3A4 and CYP1A2 at steady state.

- **Dose modification in renal or hepatic failure:** Use standard doses for renal failure. With hemodialysis, a small amount is dialyzed: dose post-hemodialysis (*Nephron* 2001;87:186). There are no data for peritoneal dialysis, but it is probably not removed and should be dosed post-dialysis. Consider empiric dose reduction in severe hepatic disease.

- TABLE 5-72: **RTV Boosting of PIs**

PI/r	Dose PI/r Treatment-naïve	Treatment-experienced	AUC PI (-fold increase)*
ATV/r	300/100 mg qd	300/100 mg qd	2.4
DRV/r	800/100 mg qd	600/100 mg bid or 800/100 mg qd if no DRV mutations	14
FPV/r	1400/100-200 mg qd 700/100 mg bid	700/100 mg bid	4
IDV/r	800/100 mg bid		2-5
LPV/r	400/100 mg bid 800/200 mg qd	400/100 mg bid 800/100 mg qd	15-20
SQV/r	1000/100 mg bid	1000/100 mg qd	20
TPV/r		500/200 mg bid	11

* Based on data from Ogden RC and Flexner CW, eds, *Protease Inhibitors in AIDS Therapy* at 166-71, 173 (NY: M Dekker, 2001) and 2011 DHHS Guidelines.

Drug Information

5

SIDE EFFECTS: The most frequently reported adverse events with full dose therapy are GI intolerance (nausea, diarrhea, vomiting, anorexia, abdominal pain, taste perversion), circumoral and peripheral paresthesias, and asthenia. GI intolerance is dose-related and may be severe (*JAIDS* 2000;23:236) and can improve with continued administration for ≥1 mo. Hepatotoxicity with elevated transaminase levels is dose-related and there appears to be a modestly increased risk with hepatitis B or C co-infection (*JAMA* 2000;238:74; *JAIDS* 2000;23:236; *CID* 2000;31:1234). Laboratory changes include elevated triglycerides, cholestrol, transaminases, CPK, and uric acid as well as a prolonged QTc and PR interval w/ RTV 400 mg bid.

- **Class adverse reactions:** Insulin-resistant hyperglycemia, fat accumulation, elevated triglycerides and cholesterol, and possible increased bleeding with hemophilia. Hypercholesterolemia and triglyceridemia may be more frequent and severe with full dose RTV compared with other PIs (*JAIDS* 2000;23:236; *JAIDS* 2000;23:261). Much of the effect on lipids is attributed to the higher levels of the concurrent PI caused by RTV, rather than by RTV per se; the effect may be due to both.

DRUG INTERACTIONS: RTV is a potent inhibitor of cytochrome P450 enzymes, including CYP3A4 and 2D6, and can produce large increases in the plasma concentrations of drugs that are metabolized by those mechanisms. Most data on the extensive drug interactions summarized below is largely based on data generated for FDA approval when the standard dose is 600 mg bid (*CID* 1996;23:685). Relevance with current doses of 100-400 mg/d is sometimes unclear.

- **Use with the following agents is contraindicated: alfuzosin, amiodarone, astemizole, bepridil, cisapride, flecainide, lovastatin, midazolam, ergot alkaloids, pimozide, propafenone, quinidine, simvastatin, terfenadine, triazolam, St. John's wort, rifapentine,** and **voriconazole** (with ≥400 mg/d RTV), or high-dose **sildenafil.**

- **Should not be used** in patients with prolonged QTc at baseline and with drugs that can prolong QTc (**salmeterol, type I and II antiarrhythmics, erythromycin, pitavastatin**).

- **Fluticasone:** RTV increased fluticasone AUC 350-fold, resulting in an 86% decrease in plasma cortisol AUC. Cushing syndrom and adrenal suppression reported. FDA warning: avoid use concurrently only if benefit outweighs risk (consider alternative such as beclomethasone).

- **Drugs that require dose modification: Clarithromycin** AUC increased 77% (*CID* 1996;23: 685); reduce clarithromycin dose for renal failure. **Methadone** levels are decreased by 36% with high dose RTV; monitor for withdrawal. **Desipramine** levels are increased by 145%; decrease desipramine dose. **ddl, buffered form**, reduces absorption of RTV and should be taken ≥2 hrs apart or use ddl EC. **Ketoconazole** levels are increased 3-fold; do not exceed 200 mg ketoconazole/d. **Itraconazole:** no data, but concern with itraconazole doses >400 mg/d; monitor itraconazole levels. **Rifampin** reduces RTV levels 35%; limited data on combination use and concern for hepatotoxicity. **Rifabutin** levels increased 4-fold; rifabutin dose of 150 mg q24-48h. Consider rifabutin TDM with standard RTV dose for all PI/r regimens. **Ethinyl estradiol** levels decreased by 40%; use alternative or additional method of birth control. **Theophylline** levels decreased by 47%; monitor theophylline levels. **Phenobarbital, phenytoin, and carbamazepine** interaction anticipated; carbamazepine toxicity reported. Monitor anticonvulsant levels. **Sildenafil** AUC increased 11-fold; do not use >25 mg/48 hrs; **Vardenafil** levels increased 49x; do not exceed 2.5 mg q72h. **Tadalafil** increased 129%; do not exceed 10 mg/72 h. **Trazodone:** RTV increase trazodone AUC 2.4-fold causing nausea, dizziness, hypotension and syncope. Use with caution and consider lower dose of trazodone. A potentially fatal reaction has been reported with **MDMA (Ecstasy)** (*Arch Intern Med* 1999;159:2221). **Voriconazole** AUC decreased 82% with RTV 400 mg bid; RTV AUC unchanged. Avoid combination with RTV ≥400 mg bid. Low-dose RTV (100 mg bid) decreases voriconazole AUC by 39%. Use with close monitoring and consider voriconazole TDM; alternative antifungal preferred. **Atorvastatin** levels increased 450% with RTV; use lowest atorvastatin dose, or use pravastatin or rosuvastatin. **Pravastatin** levels decreased 50% with concomitant RTV; may need increased pravastatin dose based on lipid response. **Lovastatin** and **simvastatin** are contraindicated. Calcium channel and beta-blockers concentration may increase. Use with close monitoring (see pg. 144). **Colchicine:** RTV increases colchicine level.

PREGNANCY: Category B. Negative rodent teratogenic assays; placental passage studies in rodents show newborn:maternal drug ratio of 1.15 at midterm and 0.15-0.64 at late term. LPV/r is the preferred PI-based regimen. Data from the Pregnancy Registry indicates birth defects in 10/476 (2.1%) first trimester exposures. This is below the expected rate (Accessed 3/1/08).

SAQUINAVIR (SQV)

TRADE NAME: *Invirase* (hard-gel capsule) (Roche). The *Fortovase* formulation was discontinued in February 2006.

FORMULATIONS AND REGIMENS

FORMS: *Invirase:* 200 mg hard gel caps and 500 mg film-coated tabs.

REGIMENS: Give only with RTV, SQV/r 1000/100 mg bid (2000/100 mg once-daily investigational not FDA-approved).

COST: AWP $1,057.13/mo (price does not include RTV boosting)

FOOD: Take within 2 hr of a meal

Drug Information

RENAL FAILURE: Standard regimen

HEPATIC FAILURE: With mild hepatic disease, use standard regimen. No data for moderately severe or severe liver disease; use with caution.

STORAGE: Room temperature, 15-30°C

PATIENT ASSISTANCE PROGRAM: 800-282-7780 (8 am-6 pm Mon.-Fri.)

CLASS: PI. Note that most studies were performed with the *Fortovase* formulation, which is no longer available.

- *Invirase* **vs.** *Fortovase* **formulations of SQV:** The first PI approved by the FDA was *Invirase*, the hard-gel formulation of SQV. Later, *Fortovase* soft-gel formulation was introduced (but no longer available), which showed equivalence to IDV/r in treatment-naïve patients in **MaxCMin-1** (*JID* 2003;188:635). **MaxCMin-2** compared SQV/r (*Fortovase*) 1000/100 mg bid to LPV/r in a mixed population of treatment-experienced and -naïve patients (*Antiviral Ther* 2005;10:735; *HIV Med* 2007;8:529). At 48 weeks, there was no significant difference in virologic outcome and a better lipid profile in SQV recipients. However, a significantly greater number in the SQV/r group discontinued treatment due to GI intolerance.

  A comparison of the *Invirase* and *Fortovase* for-mulations indicated that *Invirase* was better tolerated and, with RTV boosting, had a better pharmacokinetic profile (*HIV Med* 2003;4:94). *Fortovase* was discontinued and a new 500-mg hard-gel cap of *Invirase* became available to reduce the pill burden.

- **GEMINI:** This was a 48-week Phase 3 trial in 337 treatment-naïve patients with CD4 counts <350/mm^3 and VL >10,000 c/mL randomized to either SQV/r (*Invirase*) 1000/100 mg bid or LPV/r 400/100 mg bid, each in combination with TDF/FTC. The ITT analysis at 48 weeks for 337 participants is summarized in Table 5-73 (*JAIDS* 2009;50:367).

■ TABLE 5-73: **SQV/r (***Invirase***) vs. LPV/r in Treatment-naïve Patients (GEMINI Trial)**

	LPV/r n = 170	SQV/r n = 167
VL <400 c/mL	75%	73%
VL <50 c/mL	64%	65%
CD4 increase (mean) (cells/mm^3)	178	204
Discontinuation for ADR	12	5
Virologic failure	3%	7%
New PI mutations	0	1
Elevated LDL-C	24%	34%
Lipid elevation: Statin Rx	7	6

Drug Information

This interim analysis supports the conclusion that this SQV/r regimen appears virologically equivalent to LPV/r, possibly with less GI intolerance and hyperlipidemia.

- **STACCATO** (*Lancet* 2006;368:459): In this trial of SQV/r (1500-1600/100 qd) plus 2 NRTIs, participants were randomized to treatment interruption (TI) or continuous therapy (CT) at a ratio of 2:1 (TI:CT). Criteria for entry were a CD4 count >350/mm³ and a VL <50 c/mL. Those in the TI group discontinued ART when the CD4 count was >350/mm³. Mean duration of treatment was 21.9 mos; the TI group received 12 wks of continuous ART at the end of treatment. Median CD4 increase was 459/mm³ for the TI group (n = 284) vs. 655/mm³ for the CT group (n = 148; P <0.05) and rates of 7% and 8%, respectively, for achieving VL <50 c/mL. A major difference between this study and the SMART study is the CD4 count threshold for treatment interruption, 350 cells/mm³ in STACCATO and 250 cells/mm³ in SMART.

RESISTANCE: Major resistance mutations selected with *in vitro* passage are L90M (most common; 3-fold in IC_{50}) and G48V (less common and 8-fold increase IC_{50}). Mutations noted in isolates with reduced susceptibility that emerged during treatment with *Invirase* include 48V and 90M and the following secondary mutations: 10I/R/V, 54V/L, 71V/T, 73S, 77I, 82A, and 84V. Treatment-naïve patients with virologic failure with SQV/r usually have no PI resistance mutations (*Antiviral Ther* 2006; 11:631).

PHARMACOLOGY

- **EC_{50}:** 50 ng/mL. C_{min} with SQV/r 1000/100 mg bid is usually >500 ng/mL (*JAC* 2005;56:908).

- **Bioavailability:** Absorption of SQV is not influenced by food when taken with RTV. There is essentially no CNS penetration (CSF:serum ratio is 0.02). SQV is category 1 (poor) in the 4 class CNS penetration scoring (*Neurology* 2011;76:693). AUC and trough levels are significantly higher in women compared to men (*JID* 2004;189:1176).

- **Pharmacokinetics:** Current dosing recommendations are based on pharmacokinetic studies in volunteers using the *Invirase* formulation. SQV/r regimens of 1000/100 mg bid and 2000/100 mg qd give desirable C_{min} and AUC values (*JAC* 2004;54:785). The 2000/100 mg qd regimen resulted in a higher AUC (82 vs. 55 mg•h/L) but lower C_{min} (0.28 vs. 1.02 mg/L) than the bid regimen (*JAC* 2004;54:785).

- **T½:** 1-2 h

- **Elimination:** Metabolism is by cytochrome P450 isoenzymes CYP3A4 and CYP3A5 in the liver and gut (*Clin Pharmacol Ther* 2005; 78:65). 96% biliary excretion; 1% urinary excretion

- **Storage:** Room temperature.

5 Drug Information

- **Dose modification in renal or hepatic failure:** Use standard dose for renal failure. The drug is not removed by hemodialysis (*Nephron* 2001;87:186) and is unlikely to be removed by peritoneal dialysis. Consider empiric dose reduction for hepatic failure.

SIDE EFFECTS: Gastrointestinal intolerance with nausea, abdominal pain, diarrhea in 5-15%; **headache**, and **hepatic toxicity**; case reports of **hypoglycemia** in patients with type 2 diabetes (*Ann Intern Med* 1999; 131:980). **Class adverse effects** include fat accumulation, insulin resistance, and type 2 diabetes. SQV appears to have a similar effect on blood lipids compared to most other PIs other than ATV (*JID* 2004; 189:1056). In the GEMINI trial the change in total cholesterol was slightly worse with LPV/r and slightly worse with SQV/r for LDL cholesterol (*JAIDS* 2009;50:367). **Dose-dependent prolongation of QT and PR intervals:** The FDA issued a "safety communication" on Feb. 23, 2011 stating concern for data showing that SQV/r (1000 mg/100) given to healthy adults caused a dose-dependent prolongation of the QT and PR intervals. This risk is increased in persons taking other drugs that cause QT prolongation, primarily Class IA (such as quindine or Class III antiarrhythmics (such as amiodarone) or patients who have a history QT prolongation.

The background data are from a placebo-controlled cross-over study in 59 healthy volunteers who were given SQV/r in doses of 1000/100 mg and 1500/100 mg. The corrected QTc for these two dose regimens were 19 and 30 msec, respectively. The PR interval prolongation was >200 msec in 40% and 47% of the subjects, respectively. The specific FDA recommendations:

- An EKG should be obtained before SQV is prescribed.
- Not recommended if: 1) pre-treatment QT >450 msec, 2) refractory decreases with serum hypocalemia or hypomagnesemia, 3) SQV co-administration with other meds that increase QTc and 4) patients at increased risk of AV block.
- Discontinue SQV if an on-therapy EKC at day 3-4 shows a QT interval >450 msec or >20 msec over pretreatment levels.
- A cardiology consultation is recommended if drug discontinuation is considered.
- Patients should be advised to contact a HCW immediately if they develop symptoms of heart block.
- Report adverse events to FDA Med Watch

DRUG INTERACTIONS

- **Drugs that are contraindicated for concurrent use with SQV/r:** **Terfenadine, astemizole, cisapride, triazolam, midazolam, rifampin, pimozide, ergot alkaloids, simvastatin, lovastatin, St. John's wort, alfuzosin, amiodarone, bepridil, flecainide, propafenone, quinidine, rifapentine** and **trazodone.**

■ TABLE 5-74: **SQV/r** (*Invirase*) + **Second PI or NNRTI**

Drug	AUC*	Regimen*
RTV	SQV ↑ 20x, RTV no change	SQV/r 1000/100 bid
IDV	IDV no change, SQV ↑ 4 to 7x	Insufficient data. *In vitro* antagonism
FPV	FPV ↓ 32%, SQV ↓ 19%	Data inadequate; avoid
EFV	EFV ↓ 12%, SQV no change	SQV/r 1000/100 bid
NVP	NVP no change, SQV ↓ 25%	Consider NVP standard dose plus SQV/r 1000/100 bid
ETR	ETR ↓ 33% SQV no change	SQV/r 1000/100 mg bid ETR standard dose
MVC	MVC ↑ 10x	MVC 150 mg bid
NFV	NFV ↑ 20%, SQV ↑ 3 to 5x	SQV 800 mg tid or 1200 mg bid + NFV standard. Dose with *Invirase* not established.
LPV/r	SQV ↑ 3 to 5x, LPV no change	SQV 1000 mg bid + LPV/r 400/100 mg bid
ATV	ATV (RTV effect); SQV ↑ 60%	ATV 300 mg + SQV/r 1600/100 mg qd. Consider ATV 300 mg qd + SQV/r 1500-2000/100 mg qd. Limited data
DRV	DRV ↓ 26%, SQV no change	Avoid co-administration.
TPV	SQV AUC ↓ 76%	Avoid co-administration.

- **Drugs that should be avoided: pitavastatin, salmeterol** and **fluticasone.**

- **Drugs that may require regimen modification: omeprazole** (40 mg/d) given with *Invirase*/r 1000/100 mg bid increased SQV AUC 80% without change in RTV AUC (*AIDS* 2006; 20:1401). **Dexamethasone** may decrease SQV levels. **Phenobarbital, phenytoin**, and **carbamazepine** may decrease SQV levels substantially; monitor anticonvulsant levels or, preferably, use alternative agent. **Ketoconazole** increases SQV levels 3x; standard dose. Monitor for SQV GI toxicity if ketoconazole dose is >200 mg/d. **Itraconazole** has bidirectional interaction with SQV; may need to use reduced dose of itraconazole or to monitor levels and monitor for SQV toxicity. **Clarithromycin** increases SQV levels 177% and SQV increases clarithromycin levels 45%; reduce with renal failure. **Oral contraceptives:** May decrease ethinyl estradiol. Recommend alternative form of contraception. **Sildenafil** AUC increased 2x; use 25 mg starting dose; **tadalafil:** start with 5 mg dose and do not exceed 10 mg/72 h; **vardenafil:** start with 2.5 mg dose and do not exceed 2.5 mg/72 h. **Rifampin** reduces SQV levels by 80%. A volunteer study showed marked elevations in transaminase. Rifampin + SQV/r should not be used (*AIDS* 2006;20:302; Roche letter to care providers, Feb. 2005). **Rifabutin** reduces SQV levels 40%. With any combination of SQV/r use rifabutin 150 mg qod or 150 mg 3x/wk. For the treatment of TB, most experts recommend 150 mg qd with PI/r. Consider rifabutin TDM. **Voriconazole** levels

Drug Information **5**

may decrease with SQV/r 1000/100 mg bid. Monitor for efficacy of and toxicity to both drugs. **Atorvastatin** levels increase 450% with SQV/r; use lowest starting dose of atorvastatin, or use pravastatin. **Pravastatin** levels are reduced 50% by SQV/r; may need to increase pravastatin dose. **Methadone:** with FTV there is a 10-20% reduction in methadone levels; may increase QTc; avoid co-administration. **Colchicine:** SQV/r increases colchicine level. **Garlic supplements** decrease SQV AUC, C_{max} and C_{min} levels by about 50% (*CID* 2002;34:234). Grapefruit juice increases SQV levels. **Other drugs that induce CYP3A4** (phenobarbital, phenytoin, dexamethasone, carbamazepine, and NVP) may decrease SQV levels; these combinations should be avoided if possible. Fluticasone: avoid long-term co-administration. **Tricyclic antidepressant:** may increase QTc; avoid.

- **Interaction with other antiretroviral drugs:** Table 5-74

PREGNANCY: Category B. Studies in rats showed no teratogenicity or embryotoxicity. The PK data suggests SQV/r at 1000/100 mg bid provides good levels in pregnancy (*Antivir Ther* 2009;14:443-50). The 2010 DHHS guidelines recommend SQV/r 1000/100 mg bid as an alternate to LPV/r based on data showing this will give adequate SQV exposure during pregnancy (*Antivir Ther* 2009;14:443). Data are too limited to recommend single daily dose of SQV/r during pregnancy.

SPORANOX – see Itraconazole (pg. 301)

STAVUDINE (d4T)

TRADE NAME: *Zerit* (Bristol-Myers Squibb) and generics

CLASS: NRTI

FORMULATIONS, REGIMENS AND COST:

FORMS: Caps: 15, 20, 30, and 40 mg; oral solution: 1 mg/mL (200 mL bottle)

REGIMENS: For patients weighing >60 kg, 30-40 mg bid; <60 kg, 30 mg bid. *Note:* WHO has endorsed 30 mg as the standard dose for all patients based on concerns for high rates of peripheral neuropathy and lactic acidosis in low resource countries. Review of available data supported use of the lower dose (*Expert Opin Pharacother* 2007;8: 679), although the FDA has not endorsed this change.

COST: $403/mo (d4T 30 mg bid)

FOOD: No effect

RENAL FAILURE: See Table 5-75.

HEPATIC FAILURE: No dose recommendation

PATIENT ASSISTANCE: 800-272-4878

■ TABLE 5-75: **d4T Dosing in Renal Failure**

Wt.	CrCl (mL/min)			
	> 50	26-50	10-25	Dialysis
>60kg	40 mg bid *	20 mg bid	20 mg qd	20 mg qd
<60kg	30 mg bid	15 mg bid	15 mg qd	15 mg qd

* May consider 30 mg bid

CLINICAL TRIALS: There is extensive experience with d4T combined with 3TC or ddI. **ACTG 384** showed that EFV+AZT/3TC had greater activity and less toxicity compared with EFV+ddI+d4T (see Table 5-75) (*NEJM* 2003;349:2293). **GS-903** compared d4T and TDF in 600 treatment-naïve patients who were randomized to receive TDF or d4T, each with 3TC and EFV. Both regimens were highly effective at 3 years, but d4T was associated with more neuropathy, hyperlipidemia, and lipodystrophy than TDF. The **CLASS** trial examined 3 regimens given over 96 wks. All regimens included ABC/3TC with d4T, EFV or FPV/r. At 48 weeks, outcome was superior for EFV+3TC/ABC vs. d4T+ABC/3TC (*JAIDS* 2006;43:284). The **301A** trial showed once daily FTC was superior to d4T when combined with ddI+EFV. **ACTG 384** showed AZT/3TC+EFV was superior to other combinations including d4T+ddI. **AI 454-152** found that d4T+ddI+NFV was equivalent to AZT/3TC+NFV. See Table 5-76.

■ TABLE 5-76: **Trials in Treatment-naïve Patients Comparing d4T with Other Antiretrovirals**

Study	Regimen	N	Dur (wks)	VL <50	VL <200-500
START-1 (*AIDS* 2000;14:1591)	d4T+3TC+IDV	101	48	49%	52%
	AZT/3TC+IDV	103		47%	52%
CLASS (*JAIDS* 2006;43:284)	d4T+ABC/3TC	98	48	81%	81%
	FPV/r+ABC/3TC	96		80%	80%
	EFV+ABC/3TC	97		90%[†]	90%[†]
ACTG 384 (*NEJM* 2003; 349:2293)	d4T+ddI+EFV	155	48		62%
	d4T+ddI+NFV	155			63%
	AZT/3TC+EFV	155			89%[†]
	AZT/3TC+NFV	155			66%
FTC 301A (*JAMA* 2004;292:180)	FTC+ddI+EFV	286	48	78%[†]	81%[†]
	d4T+ddI+EFV	285		59%	68%
GS-903 (*JAMA* 2004;292:191)	TDF+3TC+EFV	299	144	68%[‡]	71%[†]
	d4T+3TC+EFV	301		63%	68%
AI 454-152 (*JAIDS* 2002;31:399)	d4T+ddI+NFV	258	48	33%	55%
	AZT/3TC+NFV	253		33%	56%

† Superior to comparator (*p* <0.05)
‡ TDF+3TC significantly less toxic

Drug Information

5

379

RESISTANCE: *In vivo* d4T resistance is mediated primarily by thymidine analog mutations (TAMs) (e.g., 41L, 67N, 70R, 210W, 215Y/F, 219Q/E), and d4T also selects for these mutations. Mutations at 44D and 118I increase resistance to AZT and d4T in the presence of TAMs (*JID* 2002;185:8998). As with AZT, the M184V mutation increases susceptibility to d4T. The multinucleoside resistance mutations (Q151M complex and the T69-insertion mutation) result in resistance to d4T. This agent sometimes selects for the K65R mutation, especially in patients with non-subtype B virus, although it appears to have minimal effect on d4T susceptibility.

PHARMACOLOGY

- **Bioavailability:** 86% and not influenced by food or fasting
- **T½:** Serum, 1 h. Intracellular T½: 3.5 h
- **CNS penetration:** 30-40% (*JAIDS* 1998;17:235) (CSF: plasma ratio=0.16-0.97). Ranks 2 in the 4 class CNS penetration score (*Neurology* 2011;76:693).
- **Elimination:** Renal – 40%
- **Dose modification in severe liver disease:** No guidelines; use standard dose with caution.

SIDE EFFECTS

- **Mitochondrial toxicity:** d4T is an important cause of side effects attributed to mitochondrial toxicity, including lactic acidosis with hepatic steatosis, peripheral neuropathy, and lipoatrophy. In most studies of lactic acidosis, d4T is the most frequent NRTI accounting for 33 of 34 reported cases for 2000-2001 (*CID* 2002;31:838), and d4T was implicated in the majority of reported cases in resource limited countries in more recent reports (*AIDS* 2007;21:2455; *CID* 2007;45:254; *S Afr Med J* 2006;96;722) (see pg. 132). Frequency is 5-15% but as high as 24% in some early trials. This side effect is dose and duration related, and it appears to be caused by depletion of mitochondrial DNA (*NEJM* 2002;346:811). The relative binding of mammalian mitochondrial DNA is 13-36 times greater for ddI and d4T compared to other NRTIs (TDF, ABC, 3TC, FTC) (*J Biol Chem* 2001;276:40847). As expected the risk of mitochontrial toxicity is substantially increased when d4T is combined with ddI (*AIDS* 2000;14:273). Onset is usually noted at 2-6 mos of treatment and usually resolves if d4T is promptly stopped, although the recovery is generally slow. Peripheral neuropathy due to HIV infection or another drug (INH, metronidazole, B6, vincristine, dapsone, thalidomide) or ddI represents a contraindication to d4T.

  With regard to d4T doses, a systemic review of 9 trials and 6 cohort reports supported 30 mg bid as the standard dose (*Expert Opin Pharmacother* 2007;8:679). This lower dose appears to be comparable in antiviral efficacy based on 5 studies, and there was strong evidence of reduced peripheral neuropathy with the lower dose. There was a trend lower lipid effect and less lipoatrophy, but these findings were less conclusive. WHO has now adopted the 30 mg dose as standard for all patients, and this has been endorsed by PEPFAR (www.pepfar.gov). The FDA has not adopted the 30 mg dose recommendation. See pg 132-134.

◻ **HIV-associated neuromuscular weakness syndrome:** A syndrome of ascending motor weakness characterized by variable changes, including progressive sensorimotor polyneuropathy with areflexia and ascending neuromuscular weakness. EMG and pathology show changes in nerves, muscles or both. Of 69 cases reviewed, 61 were thought to be due to d4T, and many (36%) had onset of symptoms after d4T was stopped. Lactate levels are usually elevated (*AIDS* 2004;18:1403). The weakness was accompanied by lactic acidosis and is presumed to be a result of mitochondrial toxicity. See pg. 538.

◻ **Lipoatrophy and hyperlipidemia:** d4T is associated with lipoatrophy and hyperlipidemia (*CID* 2006;43:645) See pg. 128-131. The lipoatrophy is a cosmetic effect that is most obvious in the malar (cheek) area, extremities and buttocks. These effects persist for prolonged periods after d4T is discontinued, although some studies show slow but significant increase in malar and extremity fat after several months (*AIDS* 2006;20:243; *AIDS* 2004; 18:1029). Serum lipid changes ascribed to d4T are most significant for triglyceride elevations but also for increased LDL cholesterol (*JAMA* 2004;292:191). Reversal of lipid effects is noted with switch to alternative NRTIs such as TDF or ABC (*JAIDS* 2005; 38:263; *AIDS* 2005;19:15; *AIDS* 2006;20: 2043). See pg. 137.

▪ **Other clinical side effects:** Complaints are infrequent and include headache, GI intolerance with diarrhea, or esophageal ulcers.

▪ **Macrocytosis** with MVC >100, which is inconsequential (*JID* 2000; 40:160).

DRUG INTERACTIONS

▪ **NRTIs: AZT** – Pharmacologic antagonism; avoid. **ddI** – increased risk of pancreatitis, lactic acidosis, and peripheral neuropathy.

▪ **Drugs that cause peripheral neuropathy** should be used with caution or avoided: ddI, ethionamide, EMB, INH, phenytoin, vincristine, glutethimide, gold, hydralazine, thalidomide, and long-term metronidazole.

▪ **Methadone** reduces the AUC of d4T by 24%, but this is not thought to be sufficiently severe to require d4T dose adjustment; d4T has no effect on methadone levels (*JAIDS* 2000;24:241).

▪ Use with caution when combined with **ribavirin**.

PREGNANCY: Category C. The pregnancy registry shows birth defects in 19/797 (2.4%) of first trimester d4T exposures compared to overall prevalence of birth defects of 2.7% (www.apregistry.com, accessed

5 Drug Information

Feb. 1, 2010). d4T is listed as an alternative to AZT in the 2010 Guidelines for Antiretroviral Drugs for Pregnant Women. Studies in pregnancy indicate good tolerability and pharmacokinetics (*JID* 2004;190: 2167). d4T + ddI should not be given to pregnant women due to the risk of lactic acidosis and hepatic steatosis (*Sex Trans Infect* 2002;78:58) and should not be given with AZT due to pharmacologic antagonism. **(FDA black box warning.)**

STOCRIN – see Efavirenz (pg. 244)

SULFADIAZINE

TRADE NAME: Generic

FORMS: 500 mg tab at $2.99

CLASS: Synthetic derivatives of sulfanilamide that inhibit folic acid synthesis

INDICATIONS AND DOSES

- **Toxoplasmosis:** Initial treatment 1.0 g po qid (<65 kg) or 1.5 gm po qid (>65 kg); maintenance dose: half of prior dose (in combination w/pyrimethamine and leucovorin) (see pg. 486).

- **Nocardia:** 1 g po qid x ≥6 mos

- **UTIs:** 500 mg-1 g po bid x 3-14 days

PHARMACOLOGY

- **Bioavailability:** >70%

- **T½:** 7-17 h

- **Elimination:** Hepatic acetylation and renal excretion of parent compound and metabolites

- **CNS penetration:** 40-80% of serum levels

- **Serum levels for systemic infections:** goal is 100-150 µg/mL

- **Dose modifications in renal failure:** CrCl >50 mL/min – 0.5-1.5 g q6h; CrCl 10-50 mL/min – 0.5-1.5 g q8-12h (half dose); CrCl <10 mL/min – 0.5-1.5 g q12-24h (one-third dose)

SIDE EFFECTS: Hypersensitivity with rash, drug fever, serum-sickness, urticaria; crystalluria reduced with adequate urine volume (≥1,500 mL/d) and alkaline urine – use with care in renal failure; marrow suppression – anemia, thrombocytopenia, leukopenia, hemolytic anemia due to G6PD deficiency.

DRUG INTERACTIONS: Decreased effect of cyclosporine, digoxin; increased effect of coumadin, oral hypoglycemics, methotrexate, and phenytoin. Use with caution with ribavirin (anemia).

PREGNANCY: Category C. Competes with bilirubin for albumin to cause kernicterus – avoid near term or in nursing mothers.

Drug Information

SULFAMETHOXAZOLE-TRIMETHOPRIM –
see Trimethoprim-Sulfamethoxazole (pg. 409)

SUSTIVA – see Efavirenz (pg. 244)

TELAPREVIR (TVR)

TRADE NAME: *Incivek* (Tibotec)

CLASS: NS3/4 HCV protease inhibitor

FORMULATION: 375 mg tablet; price: AWP price is $19,680 per 168 tabs (this is a 28 day supply).

FDA INDICATION: Indicated for the treatment of HCV (genotype 1) in combination with peg-interferon (IFN) and ribavirin (RBV) in patients with compensated liver disease, including cirrhosis, who are treatment-naïve; or who have been previously treated with IFN-based regimens but had no response, partial response, or relapsed. See pg. 507-513.

ADULT DOSE: 750 mg q8h (must be taken 7-9 hrs apart) with standard fat meal (at least 20 gm of fat) in combination with peg-IFN+RBV for the first 12 wks.

- Peg-IFN+RBV recommended for an additional 12 wks if HCV RNA is undetectable at 4 and 12 wks.
- Peg-IFN+RBV for an additional 36 wks if HCV RNA detectable <1000 IU/mL at 4 and/or 12 wks.
- In patients with prior treatment with peg-IFN+RBV, but only a partial or no response, give an additional 36 wks of peg-IFN+RBV. Treatment discontinuation recommended if HCV RNA >1000 IU/mL at week 4 or week 12.
- **In combination with EFV:** 1125 mg (3 tabs) with standard fat meal
- **In combination with ATV/r:** 750 mg (2 tabs) with standard fat meal
- **In combination with DRV/r, FPV/r, and LPV/r:** TVR is not recommended
- **Dosing with hepatic impairment:** standard dose with Child-Pugh score <7. Not recommended in patients with Child-Pugh score >7.
- **Dosing with renal impairment:** limited data. Standard dose recommended.

PHARMOKINETICS

- **Absorption** increased 237% with standard fat meal (533 kcal with 21 gm fat). C_{max} 3510 ng/mL; C_{min} 2030 ng/mL; AUC 22,300 ng hr/mL. Distribution: widely distributed (Vd=252L). Protein binding: 59-76%
- **Metabolized** via CYP3A4 and non-CYP route. Metabolites are excreted primarily in the feces (82%), exhaled air (9%), and urine (1%). Half-life: 9-11 hrs at steady-state.

5 Drug Information

SIDE EFFECTS: Compared to peg-IFN+RBV-treated patients, rash, pruritus, and anemia occurred more frequently in TVR-treated patients.

- **Rash** (56% vs. 34%); 6% of rash led to TVR discontinuation; **pruritus** (37% vs.23%),

- **Anemia** (36% vs. 17%); occurred during the first 4 weeks with the lowest Hgb level at 12 weeks.

- **Nausea** (56% vs. 23%); **diarrhea** (33% vs. 28%).

- **Anorectal discomfort, hemorrhoids, rectal pruritus** and **burning** (29% vs. 7%)

- **Lymphopenia** of less than 499/mm^3 (15% vs. 5%); **thrombocytopenia** (3% vs. 1% with platelet <50,000/mL)

- **Bilirubin elevation** (4% vs. 2%); **uric acid elevation** common, but less than 1% developed **gout**.

- **Rare cases of severe rash** including Stevens-Johnson syndrome and drug rash with eosinophilia and systemic symptoms (DRESS) have been reported.

RESISTANCE: In patients who did not achieve SVR, emergence of resistance occurs in the majority of cases. V36M/A/L, T54A/S, R155K/T, and A156S/T lead to decreased TVR activity and cross-resistance to boceprevir.

DRUG INTERACTIONS: TVR is a P-gp and CYP3A4 substrate and inhibitor.

- TVR is contraindicated with the following: **alfuzosin, rifampin, ergotamines, cisapride, St John's wort, atorvastatin, lovastatin, simvastatin, pimozide,** high dose **sildenafil** and **tadalafil,** oral **midazolam** and **triazolam.**

- **Ketoconazole:** TVR AUC increased 62%.; ketoconazole AUC increased 46-125% (avoid doses >200 mg/d). **Other azoles** (e.g., itraconazole, posaconazole, voriconazole) concentrations may be increased. Monitor for QTc prolongation and azole concentrations with co-administration.

- **Rifampin:** TVR AUC decreased 92%; contraindicated.

- **Rifabutin:** no data, but TVR may be decreased and rifabutin increased; co-administration not recommended.

- TVR <u>increases</u> concentrations of **alprazolam** (35%), **IV midazolam** (240%; monitor closely), **PO midazolam** (796%; contraindicated), **amlodipine** (179%; all calcium channel blockers may be increased; consider dose reduction with close monitoring), **atorvastatin** (688%; contraindicated by manufacturer), **cyclosporin** (364%), **digoxin** (85%; monitor serum digoxin with dose titration), **tacrolimus** (70-fold; significant dose reduction required with close serum concentration monitoring).

- TVR <u>decreases</u> concentrations of **ethinyl estradiol** (28%), **norethindrone** (11%), **escitalopram** (35%), **active R-methadone**

(29%; monitor with withdrawal symptoms), **zolpidem** (47%; titrate to effect).

- TVR <u>may increase</u> **antiarrhythmic drug** levels (e.g., lidocaine, amiodarone, bepridil, flecainide, propafenone, and quinidine). Use with caution and close monitoring.
- **Macrolides:** clarithromycin, erythromycin and telithromycin concentrations may be increased. May increase risk of QTc prolongation. Consider azithromycin.
- **Warfarin** concentration may be increased or decreased. Monitor INR closely with co-administration.
- **Seizure agents:** carbamazepine, phenobarbital, phenytoin may decrease TVR concentrations. Use with caution. Monitor for TVR therapeutic efficacy and anticonvulsant serum concentrations.
- **Desipramine** and **trazodone** serum concentrations may be increased. Consider low dose TCA and monitor for orthostatic hypotension/syncope.
- **Colchicine** serum concentrations may be increased. For gout flares, 0.6 mg x1, and 0.3 mg 1 hr later (do not redose before 3 days).
- **Steroids:** prednisone, methylprednisolone, inhaled/nasal fluticasone and budesonide serum concentrations may be increased. Avoid co-administration. If systemic corticosteroids needed, consider dose reduction with chronic therapy.
- **Salmeterol** concentrations may be increased; co-administration not recommended due to risk of QTc prolongation; consider formoterol.
- **Dexamethasone** (multiple dose) may decrease TVR concentrations. Use with caution or consider alternative.
- **Bosentan** concentrations may be increased. Use with close monitoring. Consider ambrisentan for pulmonary hypertension.
- Similar to tacrolimus, **sirolimus** and **cyclosporine** serum concentrations can be significantly increased. Dose reduction required with close sirolimus and cyclosporine serum concentrations monitoring.
- **Sildenafil, tadalafil, vardenafil** levels may be increased. Maximum dose recommended with TVR co-administration: sildenafil 25 mg q48h; vardenafil 2.5 mg q72h; tadalafil 10 mg q72h. High dose PDE5 for the treatment of pulmonary hypertension not recommended with TVR.

CLINICAL TRIALS

HCV monoinfection trials – PROVE-1: HV- infected treatment-naïve patients were randomized to receive peg-IFN+RBV x 48 wks or TVR for 12 wks in combination with peg-IFN-alfa-2a and RBV for 12, 24, or 48 wks. Sustained viral response (SVR) was higher (61-67% vs. 41%) when TVR was given for the first 12 wks with peg-IFN-a2a+RBV followed by 24-48 wks peg-IFN-a2a+RBV. In patients with rapid

5 Drug Information

virologic response (RVR), treatment duration can be shortened to 24 wks when TVR is given for the first 12 wks. Pruritus, rash, and anemia were more commonly reported in the TVR-treated patients (*NEJM* 2009;360:1827).

PROVE-2 is a randomized study of TVR and peg-IFN with or without RBV for chronic HCV Infection. RBV is a critical component, with significant improvement in SVR (69% vs 36%) and decreased TVR resistance when RBV was included in the regimen.

Clinical trial with TVR in HIV/HCV co-infected patients (Sulkowski M, 2011 CROI: Abstr. 146LP). The trial compared TVR+peg-IFN-a2a +RBV in patients with HIV infection who were receiving no ART, EFV/TDF/FTC or ATV/r+TDF/FTC. Each group had a control that was given peg-IFN-a2a+RBV alone. All TVR recipients received peg-IFN-a2a 180 µg/wk + RBV 800 mg for 12 wks followed by peg-IFN-a2a+RBV x 36 wks. Dose adjustment for TVR with concurrent use of EFV and ATV/r are those noted under adult dose; all three arms included a control group that did not receive TVR. Results at 12 weeks showed:

Interim results HCV undetected	No ART		EFV/TDF/FTC		ATV/r + TDF/FTC	
	TVR n = 7	Control n = 6	TVR n = 16	Control n = 8	TVR n = 14	Control n = 8
Week 4	5 (71%)	0	12 (75%)	1 (12%)	9 (64%)	0
Week12	5 (71%)	1 (17%)	12 (75%)	1 (12%)	8 (57%)	1 (12%)
Week 4 or 12	3 (43%)	0	10 (62%)		6 (43%)	0

The total responses with TRV combined with ART with undetectable HCV RNA at 4 and 12 wks was 19/37 (40%) compared to 0/22 in the control group given peg-IFN-a2a+RBV alone. Of the TVR recipients, 2 (3%) discontinued the drug due to adverse reactions.

HCV TREATMENT RECOMMENDATIONS FOR HIV/HCV CO-INFECTED PATIENTS

- **Peg-IFN and RBV** remain the standard of care for treatment of HCV infection when there is **genotype 2, 3** or **4 HCV infection** or pharmacokinetic interactions between TVR or boceprevir and other necessary medications including antiretroviral therapy cannot be confidently eliminated or managed (see Pharmacokinetics above). Candidates for TVR need to meet the criteria for peg-IFN+RBV as well as TVR.

- TVR or boceprevir should always be used with peg-IFN for individuals with **chronic genotype 1 HCV infection**. Single agent therapy is contraindicated because TVR or boceprevir resistant viruses are rapidly selected if the medications are used without peg-IFN+RBV. Accordingly, persons with contraindications for peg-IFN and RBV (e.g., pregnancy, ddl use) also have contraindications to TVR- and boceprevir-based therapy. No treatment is needed for persons with a positive HCV antibody but undetectable HCV RNA.

- The benefits of TVR or boceprevir and peg-IFN+RBV treatment are most likely to outweigh the risks for individuals with significant **liver fibrosis** (the equivalent of a metavir fibrosis score 2-4/4). Although HIV/HCV co-infected persons have more rapid progression of liver disease than HIV-uninfected persons and treatment is more efficacious at lower disease stage, experts believe that it is safer to monitor many persons with little or no fibrosis for evidence of progression, while awaiting additional safety and efficacy data in HIV/HCV co-infected persons, as well as a large number of new antiviral agents.

- TVR or boceprevir and/or peg-IFN+RBV treatment should not be used for persons with **liver failure** (decompensated cirrhosis) outside of a research setting. There is evidence that peg-IFN+RBV may exacerbate liver disease once liver failure has occurred as defined as a history of encephalopathy, ascites, bleeding varices or laboratory data showing INR >1.3, albumin <3.4 mg/dl, or direct (conjugated) bilirubin >1 mg/dl (unless unconjugated bilirubin on ATV).

- **HIV infection** should be controlled before treatment with TVR or boceprevir with peg-IFN+RBV, and TVR or boceprevir should not be used with medications with proven or suspected pharmacologic interactions (Table). HIV control is often defined as off ART with CD4 count > 500 cells/mm^3 and HIV RNA <20,000 c/mL or on ART with HIV RNA <200 c/mL.

■ TABLE 5-77: **Interactions between telaprevir (TVR) and ARVs**

ARV	TVR AUC$_{tau}$	TVR C$_{min}$	ARV AUC$_{tau}$	ARV C$_{min}$	Comments
TVR 750 mg q8h with					
ATV/r 300/100 mg qd	↓20%	↓15%	↑17% (NS)	↑85%	
DRV/r 600/100 mg bid	↓35%	↓32%	↓40%	↓42%	Avoid co-administration
FPV/r 700/100 mg bid	↓32%	↓30%	↓47%	↓56%	Avoid co-administration
LPV/r 600/100 mg bid	↓54%	↓52%	↑6% (NS)	↑14% (NS)	Avoid co-administration
TDF 300 mg qd	No change	↑3% (NS)	↑30%	↑41%	
RAL 400 mg bid	↑7% (NS)	↑14%	↑31%	↑78%	
TVR 1125 mg q8h with					
EFV 600 mg qd (w/TDF)	↓18%	↓25%	↓18%	↓10%	
TDF 300 mg qd (w/EFV)	↓18%	↓25%	↑10%	↑17%	

Drug Information

5

- With **TVR**, acceptable regimens include:
  - **ATV/r** 300/100 mg qd + **TDF/FTC** 1 tab qd
  - **EFV** 600 mg qd + **TDF/FTC** 1 tab qd with increased TVR dose to 1125 q8h
    - Although there are no data with **RAL**, drug-drug interaction is unlikely. RAL can be considered in patients unable to take ATV/r- or EFV-based regimen.
  - Boceprevir cannot be recommended for HIV/HCV co-infected persons on ART until pharmacokinetic data are published.
- To minimize the risk of selecting for TVR or boceprevir resistance, patient adherence should be high and the medications should be stopped if HCV RNA is not suppressed.
- To ensure the benefits of treatment are sustained and outweigh the risks, persons should be judged to be at limited risk of reinfection.
- TVR or boceprevir and peg-IFN+RBV treatment is expected to be less efficacious in persons who did not respond to peg-IFN+RBV treatment and/or those with cirrhosis, unfavorable IL28b genotype, or African ancestry. Data regarding use of these agents in HCV treatment-experienced patients is lacking. However, triple therapy response is higher than with peg-IFN+RBV alone, and guidelines for use similar to that in treatment naïve patients should be applied pending availability of additional data.

PREGNANCY: Category B. Not teratogenic in animal studies. No human data, but since TVR is always co-administered with RBV (a known teratogen), use in pregnancy is contraindicated. Excreted in breast milk in rat studies.

TELZIR – see Fosamprenavir (pg. 281)

TENOFOVIR DISOPROXIL FUMARATE (TDF)

TRADE NAME: *Viread* (Gilead Sciences). Combination with FTC: *Truvada* (Gilead Sciences). Combination with FTC+EFV: *Atripla* (Gilead Sciences and Bristol-Myers Squibb). Combination with FTC+RPV: *Complera* (Gilead Sciences).

CLASS: Nucleotide analog reverse transcriptase inhibitor (NtRTI, NRTI)

PATIENT ASSISTANCE PROGRAM: 800-226-2056 (9 am-8 pm EST)

FORMULATIONS AND REGIMENS: TDF: 300 mg tab (1 po qd); *Truvada* (TDF/FTC) 300/200 mg (1 po qd); *Atripla* (EFV/TDF/FTC) 600/300/200 mg (1 po qd); *Complera* (RPV/TDF/FTC) 25/300/200 mg (1 po qd with a meal)

COST: *Viread* $832/mo; *Truvada* $1,195/mo; *Atripla* $1,858/mo; *Complera* $2,045.57/mo

■ TABLE 5-78: **TDF Dose Adjustments for Renal Impairment**

CrCl (mL/min/1.73m²)	TDF	TDF/FTC (*Truvada*)
≥ 50	300 mg qd	1 tab qd
30-49*	300 mg q48h	1 tab q 48 h
10-29*	300 mg q72-96h	not recommended
<10	Inadequate data; Consider 300 mg/wk	not recommended
hemodialysis	300 mg/wk or after 12 hrs of hemodialysis	not recommended

* Note: Most authorities avoid TDF with a creatinine clearance <50 mL/min due to confusion about the contribution of TDF with progression of disease; the exception is with end-stage renal disease.

FOOD: No clinically significant effect on TDF, but fatty meals increase EFV absorption by 40% with coformulated EFV/TDF/FTC.

RENAL FAILURE: See Table 5-78.

HEPATIC FAILURE: No dose change recommended

CLINICAL TRIALS

- **GS-97-901:** Median decrease in VL at 28 days with monotherapy in treatment-naïve patients using 300 mg dose was 1.2 $\log_{10}$ c/mL (*AAC* 2001;45:2733).

- **GS-98-902:** Dose finding/toxicity study using 75, 150, and 300 mg added to antiretroviral regimen in 189 treatment-experienced patients with VL 400-100,000 c/mL. At 48 weeks, the mean VL decrease was 0.62 $\log_{10}$ c/mL among 54 patients receiving 300 mg/d (*JAIDS* 2003;33:15).

- **GS 907:** Placebo-controlled trial in treated patients with VL 400-10,000 c/mL given 300 mg tenofovir. At 24 weeks (n=550), the mean decrease in VL was 0.61 $\log_{10}$ c/mL among tenofovir recipients compared with 0.03 $\log_{10}$ c/mL in placebo recipients.

- **GS-903:** Randomized, placebo-controlled trial comparing TDF vs. d4T, each in combination with 3TC+EFV for treatment of ART-naïve patients (*JAMA* 2004;292:191). By ITT (missing=failure) analysis at 144 weeks, 73% of TDF recipients and 69% of d4T recipients had a VL <50 c/mL (p=NS) (*JAMA* 2004;292:191). The drop-out rate was low, but d4T recipients had higher rates of peripheral neuropathy, higher rates of 184V resistance mutations, lipoatrophy and elevated fasting/levels of total and LDL cholesterol and triglycerides.

- **ESS 30009:** A trial comparing the triple NRTI regimen of TDF+ABC/3TC with EFV+ABC/3TC in 194 treatment-naïve patients. The trial was stopped at 12 weeks due to high rates of virologic failure in the triple NRTI arm (49% vs. 5%); resistance testing showed a high frequency of M184V (100%) and K65R (64%) in 36 with virologic failure (*JID* 2005;192:1821).

5 Drug Information

- **ACTG 5202:** 1,858 treatment-naïve patients were randomized to ABC/3TC vs. TDF/FTC plus either EFV or LPV/r (*NEJM* 2009; 361:2230). The DSMB unblinded the study for the subset of patients with a baseline VL >100,000 c/mL after a medium follow-up at 60 weeks because of a higher rate of virologic failure with ABC/3TC compared to TDF/FTC. The respective failure rates were 14% and 7%; OR 2.33, 95% CI 1.46-3.72; P= <0.001.

- **GS-934:** 517 treatment-naïve patients were randomized to receive co-formulated AZT/3TC+EFV or TDF/FTC+EFV. Results at 48 weeks in 487 participants by modified ITT showed TDF/FTC was superior to AZT/3TC in these categories: virologic suppression to <400 c/mL (77% vs. 68%), mean increase in CD4 count (190 cells/mm^3 vs. 171 cells/mm^3), lower increase in LDL cholesterol (13 mg/dL vs. 20 mg/dL), less limb fat loss, less 184V resistance mutation (2 vs. 9), and fewer drug discontinuations for ADRs (4% vs. 9%) (*NEJM* 2006;354:251; *JAIDS* 2006;43:535). The difference was explained primarily by the higher proportion of discontinuations due to adverse events in the AZT/3TC arm (9% vs. 4%), most of which were due to anemia. At 96 weeks, there was significantly greater limb fat (8.9 vs. 6.9 kg) and a significantly lower number of M184V mutations (2 vs. 7) among patients on TDF/FTC (*JAIDS* 2006;43:535). Results at 144 weeks show TDF/FTC superior to AZT/3TC in viral suppression (71% vs. 58%) and in median total limb fat (7.9 vs. 5.4 kg) (*JAIDS* 2008;47: 74). A subsequent report found TDF and AZT have divergent effects on pro-inflammatory effects including a strong reduction in IL10 by TDF (*JAIDS* 2011;57:265).

- **ASSERT Trial (TDF/FTC vs. ABC/3TC):** Comparisons of these two combinations agents in terms of viral response and toxicity are summarized in Table 5-79. See also pg. 182.

■ TABLE 5-79: **TDF/FTC vs ABC/3TC**

	ACTG 5202 (pg. 100) *NEJM* 2009;361:2230	HEAT (pg. 181) *AIDS* 2009;23:1547	ASSERT (pg. 182) *JAIDS* 2010;55:49 *CID* 2010;51:963
Sponsor	NIH	GSK	GSK
Number	1858	688	385
Trial Design	Double-blind	Double-blind	Randomized
Primary Result	Time to virologic failure (60 wks)	VL<50 c/mL (48 wks)	Toxicity and VL (48 wks)
Result (Duration)	Superior virologic response with TDF with baseline VL >100,000 c/mL (14% vs. 7%)	Viral suppression equal (67% vs. 68%)	• TDF superior in VL <50 c/mL (71% vs. 59%) • No difference in eGFR but TDF showed **more** tubular dysfunction • Greater ↓ in BMD with TDF/FTC than ABC/3TC

Abbreviations: eGFR=estimated glomerular filtration rate; BMD=bone mineral density

Drug Information

- **TDF + ddl:** This NRTI combination should be avoided due to: 1) increased ddl toxicity reflecting increased intracellular ddl concentrations (*J Clin Pharm* 205;45:1360; *CID* 2003;36:1082); 2) blunted CD4 response (*AIDS* 2004;18:459; *AIDS* 2005;19:569; *CID* 2005;41:901); 3) high rates of virologic failure (*AIDS* 2004;13:180; *AIDS* 2005;19:1183; *AIDS* 2005;19:1695 and 4) rapid selection of the K65R resistance mutation (*AIDS* 2005;19:1695; *Antivir Ther* 2005;10:171; *AIDS* 2005;19:213).

- **HBV:** TDF is active against HBV has been FDA approved for that indication and, along with FTC, is considered a preferred agent based on potency and durability (*CID* 2010;51:1201). In patients with HIV and a positive HBeAg, the inclusion of TDF in the HIV regimen results in a decrease of 4-5 $\log_{10}$ in HBV DNA levels, including those with 3TC-resistant strains (*AIDS* 2003;17:F7; *JID* 2003;186:1844; *CID* 2004; 38[suppl2]:S98; *CID* 2003;37:1678; *JID* 2004;189:1185). In a review of literature comparing the 6 FDA-approved drugs for HBV, TDF was the most active and durable in reducing HBV DNA and promoting histologic improvement (*CID* 2010; 51:1201). A report of 426 patients with HBV monoinfection treated with TDF 144 wks showed no HBV resistance and 13 (3%) failures attributed to nonadherence (*Hepatology* 2010;51:73). One report found that prolonged exposure to TDF in patients with HBV-HIV co-infection was associated with increased rates of HBeAg clearance (*HIV Clin Trials* 2009;10:3). The addition of 3TC does not augment TDF activity against HBV, but the addition of TDF to 3TC protects against HBV resistance to 3TC (*JID* 2004;189:1185). FTC is also active against HBV. Practical application of these data is to use coformulated TDF/FTC in patients with HBV-HIV co-infection. See pg. 507.

RESISTANCE: Susceptibility of HIV is decreased in patients with 3 or more thymidine analog mutations (TAMs) that include the 41L and 210W mutations. Susceptibility is maintained with other TAM mutations and increased with 184V. TDF, ddl and ABC select for the 65R mutation, which confers resistance to all three drugs, as well as to 3TC and FTC (*AAC* 2004;48:1413). Resistance testing in 14 patients with virologic failure in GS-903 showed no K65R mutations at 96 wks. There is substantial loss of susceptibility with T69 insertion mutation (*AAC* 2004;48:992); susceptibility is maintained with Q151M complex. Partial phenotypic susceptibility may be maintained despite presence at K65R when M184V is also present. Mutants with K65R and 184V on the same genome were detected in 50% of samples from failures with ddl+TDF+3TC in patients (*Antiviral Ther* 2010;15:437)

PHARMACOLOGY

- **Bioavailability:** 25% (fasting) to 40% (with food); improvement with food, especially high-fat meal , but levels are adequate when taken in a fasting state. CNS penetration is poor; score 1 (lowest) in the CNS penetration score (*Neurology* 2011;76:693)

5 Drug Information

- **T½:** 17 h; intracellular >60 h
- **Elimination:** Renal, glomerular filtration, and active tubular secretion.

DRUG INTERACTION

- **ATV: ATV** AUC is decreased 25%; use standard dose TDF+ATV/r (300/100 mg) qd.
- **ddl EC:** TDF and ddl co-administration is not generally recommended.
- **Miscellaneous: Ganciclovir, valganciclovir, probenicid, and cidofovir** compete for active tubular secretion with increased levels of either tenofovir or the companion drug; monitor for toxicities. **LPV/r** increases levels of TDF 30% with co-administration. This appears to be due to decreased tenofovir clearance, but the mechanism and significance is unclear (*Clin Pharm Ther* 2008;83:265). **DRV:** tenofovir levels and AUC increase by a mean of 20-25% (2011 DHHS Guidelines). Use standard doses but watch for renal toxicity. Several studies suggest that PI-based ART with TDF is associated with a greater decline in renal function than TDF combined with NNRTIs (*JID* 2008;197:7; *AIDS* 2009;23:1971-5).

SIDE EFFECTS

- **GI intolerance** reported, but it is infrequent. Flatulence occurred more often in TDF-treated patients than placebo-treated patients.
- **Nephrotoxicity:** TDF and related drugs (adefovir and cidofovir) may cause renal injury, including the Fanconi syndrome, which is characterized by hypophosphatemia, hypouricemia, proteinuria, normoglycemic glycosuria, and, in some cases, acute renal failure (*JAIDS* 2004;35:269; *AIDS* 2004;18:960; *CID* 2003;37:e174). The mechanism is unclear, but one report suggests mitochondrial toxicity (*Kidney Int* 2010;78:1060). In the early stages this may be asymptomatic or cause myalgias; most resolve when the drug is discontinued (*JAIDS* 2004;35:269). Risk factors are low body weight, pre-existing renal disease (*AAC* 2001;45:2733), and concurrent use of nephrotoxic agents. With TDF there is a dose or TDF exposure relationship, but there were no cases among patients given double dose of TDF (*J Med Virol* 2007;79:105). Combination with ddl may contribute through mitochondrial toxicity and competition for uptake by proximal renal tubular cells (*Mayo Clin Proc* 2007;82:1103). Numerous studies have examined the rate of TDF-associated nephrotoxicity. A large cohort study showed a minimal but statistically significant reduction in creatinine clearance and increase in anion gap with a mean follow-up of 1.7 years; treatment duration was not a significant association (*HIV Med* 2006;7:105). A EuroSIDA review of 6,842 patients showed the risk of chronic renal disease defined as a 25% decrease in CrCl was 2.4/100 person-years compared to 0.7/100 p-y in ART recipients not given TDF. Risks with TDF-associated CRD were increasing age, HBP, HCV and low CD4 count (*AIDS* 2010;24:1667). Others have found lower rates. Analysis

of 600 participants in GS-903 with calculated CrCl >60 mL/min and serum phosphorus ≥2.2 mg/dL at baseline showed no change in mean serum creatinine or phosphorus levels at week 144 (*Nephrol Dial Transplant* 2005;20:743). A longer follow-up of GS-903 found that the difference in median GFR at 7 years in mL/min/1.73 M^2 was 112 in TDF recipients vs. 120 in controls (17th IAC;Abstr. TUPE0057). In another study of 1058 TDF recipients, 9 (0.9%) developed an otherwise unexplained increase in serum creatinine (*JAIDS* 2004;37:1489). Other studies have shown modest declines in creatinine clearance in clinical cohorts (*CID* 2005;40:1194). A review from Johns Hopkins comparing GFR for 201 TDF recipients and 231 given alternative NRTIs (*AIDS* 2009;23:197) showed a slight decline in eGFR in the first 180 days that stabilized from day 180 to720. The change in eGFR was more common with TDF combined with PIs rather than NNRTIs (decrease of 8 mL/min vs. 4 mL/min (*CID* 2005,40: 1194). The conclusion is that TDF may cause nephrotoxicity, but it is infrequent and usually modest in severity and reversible, especially in patients with normal baseline renal function and relatively high baseline CD4 counts (*AIDS* 2010;24:223:2239). Nevertheless, there are anecdotal reports of severe kidney disease, including acute renal failure. See pg. 568-570.

- **Monitoring renal function with TDF treatment** according to the 2011 DHHS Guidelines should include:

  □ Baseline urinalysis and chemistry profile.

  ⊓ Patients with a CrCl <50 mL/min should not receive TDF since progressive deterioration would make it difficult to distinguish the effect of TDF and the primary renal disease; an exception might be the patient with total renal failure.

  □ Renal function monitoring during TDF treatment should include a baseline chemistry profile (for creatinine and creatinine clearance) and a urinanalysis. The chemistry profile should be repeated at 2-8 wks then every 3-6 mos. The urinalysis should be repeated every 6 mos during TDF treatment. More frequent monitoring is recommended with other risks for renal disease such as diabetes or hypertension.

Evaluation for TDF nephrotoxicity should include serum phosphate levels, and urine dipstick for glucose and protein. Glycosuria in a non-diabetic with a normal serum glucose is diagnostic of tubular dysfunction, whereas proteinuria may be due to other causes. Hypophosphatemia is non-specific unless persistent; the fractional excretion of phosphate is a more useful measure of tubular phosphate wasting, and should be calculated in patients with evidence of glomerular or tubular dysfunction.

- **Bone toxicity:** Initiation of many antiretroviral regimens results in a modest non-progressive decline in bone density. Bone density declines observed in TDF-treated patients are generally of greater

5 Drug Information

magnitude than those seen in patients treated with other NRTI. The most comprehensive study with long term follow-up is ACTG A 5224, a substudy of ACTG A5202, in which DXA scans were done sequentially in 269 patients randomized to ABC/3TC or TDF/FTC (*JID* 2011;203:1791). Analysis at 196 wks showed the rate of fractures was 5.4% and was equal by treatment categories. DXA scans showed a decrease in BMD that was 1.4-2.0% greater at 96 wks for TDF/FTC recipients, especially when this was combined with ATV/r. Most of the changes occurred in the first 6 months; the BMD then stabilized and increased at 1-2 yrs (*JID* 2011;203:1705) (see pg. 62, 554).

- **Other:** The incidence of laboratory and clinical adverse events has been similar to placebo in controlled clinical trials.

PREGNANCY: Category B. Studies of high dose TDF exposure in fetal monkeys (doses that produced TDF levels 25-fold higher than in humans) produced a slight reduction in bone porosity and lower levels of insulin-like growth factor (IGF)-1, which regulates linear growth (*JAIDS* 2002;29:207). Continued administration of TDF to the previously exposed infant primates resulted in a significant reduction in growth and reduced bone porosity. Studies in children (and adults) show bone demineralization with chronic use, which is of uncertain significance (*Pediatrics* 2006;118:e711; *AIDS* 2002;16:1257). Pharmacokinetic studies demonstrated a lower AUC in pregnancy but normal trough levels (Mirochnick M. *JAIDS* 2011;Epub Ahead:PMCID PMC 3125419). Due to concerns about bone abnormalities and limited experience, the 2010 DHHS Guidelines on Use of Antiretroviral Agents in Pregnancy recommend TDF use in pregnancy "only after consideration of the alternatives." If used, renal function should be monitored. Concurrent HBV infection is a concern if TDF is discontinued. The Pregnancy Registry through July 2010 showed birth defects in 25/981 (2.5%) first trimester exposures; this is comparable to CDC population-based surveillance data (2.7%).

TELZIR – see Fosamprenavir (pg. 281)

TESTOSTERONE

SOURCE

- Testosterone cypionate (various generic manufacturers)
- Testosterone enanthate (various generic manufacturers)
- Testosterone patch (*Androderm*, Watson)
- Testosterone gel (*AndroGel,* Unimed, *Testim*, Auxilium)
- *Testim* 1% gel
- Testosterone buccal (*Striant*, Columbia Laboratories)

FORMS AND COST: Vials of 100 mg/mL and 200 mg/mL at $16.99/200 mg

- *Androderm* 24-h patch at $5.43/2.5 mg or $5.43/5 mg
- *AndroGel* 5 g packet at $11.15
- *Striant* 30mg at $4.26

INDICATIONS (for men only, except where noted)

- **Hypogonadism:** Normal testosterone levels in adult men are 300-1,000 ng/dL at 8 AM, representing peak levels with circadian rhythm (see pg. 63). Reports from the pre-HAART era showed subnormal testosterone levels in 45% of patients with AIDS and 20-30% of HIV-infected patients without AIDS (*Am J Med* 1988;84:611; *AIDS* 1994;7:46; *J Clin Endocrinol* 1996;81:4108). At that time the frequency of hypogonadism correlated with low CD4 counts and symptomatic HIV (*Am J Med* 1988;84:611). Patients are now living longer, so age-related decline in testosterone levels becomes a complicating factor that generally supersedes the impact of immunosuppression. The CHAMPS study (Cohort of HIV At-risk Aging : Men's Prospective Study) with men age >49 years with and without HIV infection found that hypogonadism (<300 ng/mL) was unrelated to HIV serostatus or CD4 count, but was correlated with a VL >10,000 c/mL (*CID* 2005;41:1794). For indications for testing testosterone levels, methods and interpretation (see pg. 63).

The **usual test indications** in men with HIV infection are symptoms of low libido, low bone mineral density and low BMI despite response to ART. **Recommendations for testosterone therapy** from **the Endocrine society** (*J Clin Endoc Rinol Metab* 2010;95:2536) are "for symptomatic men with classical androgen deficiency syndromes aimed at inducing and maintaining secondary sex characteristics and at improving sexual function, sense of well being and bone mineral density." **Contraindications and precautions** are: 1) breast or prostate cancer; 2) exclude prostate cancer with prostate digital exam or PSA <4 ng/mL (<3 ng/mL in high risk men); 3) hematocrit >50%; 4) severe lower urinary tract symptoms; 5) untreated severe sleep apnea; 6) poorly controlled heart failure; or 7) desire for fertility. The **goal of therapy** is normal free testosterone level, measured in the morning. In men ≥40 years there should be a baseline PSA and a digital exam at 3-6 mos and then according to standard guidelines. In a small placebo-controlled trial of testosterone gel vs. placebo in men >65 years with total serum testosterone levels 100-350 ng/dL; testosterone recipients had increased cardiovascular, respiratory and dermatologic events compared to placebo recipients (*NEJM* 2010;363:109). (Benefits included increased strength). A review of 51 reports (2003-2008) concluded that the only statistically significant adverse effects were an increase in hemoglobin and a small decrease in HDL cholesterol (*J Clin Endocrinol Metab* (2010;95:2560). There was no significant effect on mortality,

5 Drug Information

cardiovascular events or prostate cancer.

Therapeutic trials with testosterone treatment of HIV-infected hypogonadal men show substantial improvements in quality of life with increased libido, reduced fatigue, and reduced depression (*Arch Gen Psych* 2000;57:141; *HIV Clin Trials* 2007;8:412). Benefit has also been shown in eugonadal HIV-infected men receiving twice the physiological dose (200 mg/wk), but long-term toxicity should be considered (*Ann Intern Med* 2000;133:348).

- **Wasting:** Testosterone is an anabolic steroid that may restore nitrogen balance and lean body mass in patients with wasting (*JAIDS* 1996;11:510; *JAIDS* 1997;16:254; *Ann Intern Med* 1998;129:18). A placebo-controlled trial of 51 hypogonadal men with AIDS-associated wasting found that replacement dosing (testosterone enanthate 300 mg IM q3wk) was associated with an average gain of 2.6 kg lean body mass over 6 mos (*Ann Intern Med* 1998;129:18); these results were sustained over 12 mos in an open-label extension (*CID* 1999;31:1240). See pg. 130.

- **Lipodystrophy:** Testosterone may reduce visceral fat and reduce cholesterol; however, studies show minimal effect on body weight or muscle mass (*J Clin Eudocrinol Metals* 2005;90:1531), and risks include reduced HDL cholesterol, hepatotoxicity, and risk of prostatic cancer (*CID* 2002;34:248). See pg. 130.

- **Testosterone for wasting in women:** A placebo-controlled trial of women with HIV infection and androgen deficiency defined as free testosterone ≤3 pg/mL demonstrated substantial benefit from testosterone patches of 300 ug 2 x/wk for ≥18 mos (*AIDS* 2009;23:951). Testosterone was well tolerated. Benefits included increases in BMI, lean mass, bone mineral density and sexual function and decrease in depression.

  - □ Indication: Free testosterone <3 pg/mL; weight <90% of ideal body weight or weight loss >10%.

  - □ Treatment: *Androderm* patch (2.5–5.0 mg patch) 2x/wk

REGIMEN (MEN)

- **Intramuscular:** 200-400 mg IM every 2 wks. The dose and dosing interval may need adjustment; many use 100-200 mg IM every week given by self administration to avoid low levels in the second week; many initiate therapy for wasting with 300-400 mg every 2 wks, with taper to 200 mg when weight is restored, or combine with other anabolic steroids. Replacement doses are 100 mg/wk (*CID* 2003; 36:S73).

- **Transdermal systems:** Advantages are rapid absorption, controlled rate of delivery with less day-to-day variation in testosterone levels, avoidance of first-pass hepatic metabolism, avoidance of IM injections, and possibly less testicular shrinkage. Two delivery systems are available: Skin patches and a topical gel (*Androderm*) are

Drug Information

available in 2.5-5 mg sizes. Serum testosterone levels peak at 3-8 hrs. After 1 month, a morning testosterone level should be obtained. *Androderm* consists of a liquid reservoir containing 12.2 mg testosterone (delivers 2.5 mg/d of testosterone) or 24.3 mg (that delivers 5 mg/d testo-sterone). The usual dose is a system that delivers 5 mg/d. *AndroGel* and *Testim* are rubbed on the skin starting with 5 mg qd. Gel formulations have the advantage of permitting dose titration based on serum testosterone levels.

CONTROLLED SUBSTANCE: Schedule C-III (see pg. 179).

PHARMACOLOGY

- **Bioavailability:** Poor absorption and rapid metabolism with oral administration. The cypionate and enanthate esters are absorbed slowly from IM injection sites.

- **Elimination:** Hepatic metabolism to 17 ketosteroids that are excreted in urine.

SIDE EFFECTS: Androgenic effects include acne, flushing, gynecomastia, increased libido, priapism, and edema. Other side effects include aggravation of sleep apnea, sodium retention, increased hematocrit, possible promotion of KS, and promotion of breast or prostate cancer. In women, there may be virilization with voice change, hirsutism, and clitoral enlargement. Androgens may cause cholestatic hepatitis. Patches are associated with local reactions, especially pruritus and occasionally blistering, erythema, and pain.

DRUG INTERACTIONS: May potentiate action of oral anticoagulants.

PREGNANCY: Category X. Contraindicated.

THALIDOMIDE

TRADE NAME: *Thalomid* (Celgene)

FORM AND COST: 50, 100, and 200 mg capsules; 100 mg cap at $263.23

AVAILABILITY: Thalidomide is FDA-approved for marketing through a restricted distribution program called "System for Thalidomide Education and Prescribing Safety" (STEPS). The STEPS Program is designed to eliminate the risk of birth defects by requiring registration of prescribing physicians, patients, and pharmacists, combined with informed consent, rigorous counseling, accountability, and a patient survey. Only physicians registered with STEPS may prescribe thalidomide. Call 888-423-5436 (option 1) to register and receive necessary forms. **Requirements for prescribing:** 1) agreement to patient counseling as indicated in the consent form; 2) patient consent form with one copy sent to Boston University; and 3) completion of the physician monitoring survey. **Patients are registered if they** 1) agree to use two reliable methods of contraception; 2) have pregnancy tests performed regularly (females); 3) use latex condoms when having sex with women (males); and 4) agree to participate in mandatory and confidential patient survey. **Pharmacies**

Drug Information

5

must register to dispense thalidomide by agreeing to 1) collect and file informed consent forms; 2) register patients by phone or fax; 3) prescribe no more than a 28 day supply within 7 days of the prescription date; and 4) verify patient registry with refills.

PATIENT ASSISTANCE: 888-423-5436 (press 2)

FDA LABELING: Approved for moderate to severe erythema nodosum leprosum and multiple myeloma.

REGIMEN: Usual dose is 50-200 mg/d, most commonly 100 mg hs to reduce sedative side effect. Often start at 100-200 mg qd and titrate down to 50 mg qd or give intermittent dosing (*JID* 2001;183: 343). Doses above 200-300 mg/d are poorly tolerated (*NEJM* 1997; 336:1487; *CID* 1997;24:1223).

MECHANISM: Presumed mechanism for HIV-associated wasting is the reduction in TNF-alpha production (*J Exp Med* 1991;173:699). Thalidomide also has numerous other anti-inflammatory and immunomodulatory properties (*Int J Dermatol* 1974;13:20; *PNAS USA* 1993;90:5974; *Mol Med* 1995;1:384; *J Exp Med* 1993;177:1675; *JAIDS* 1997;13:1047).

CLINICAL TRIALS

- **Aphthous ulcers:** In a placebo-controlled trial using thalidomide (200 mg qd) in patients with oral aphthous ulcers, 16/29 (53%) in the thalidomide arm responded compared with 2/28 (7%) in the placebo group (*NEJM* 1997;336:1489). ACTG 251 was a placebo-controlled trial involving 45 patients given thalidomide (200 mg qd x 4 wks followed by 100 mg qd for responders and 400 mg qd for nonresponders for oral or esophageal ulcers). Among 23 recipients of thalidomide, 14 (61%) had a complete remission in 4 wks, and 21 (91%) had a complete remission or partial response. In another ACTG trial for patients with aphthous ulcers of the esophagus, thalidomide (200 mg qd) was associated with a complete response at 4 weeks in 8 of 11 (73%) (*JID* 1999;180:61). Ulcers usually heal in 7-28 days. The usual dose for aphthous ulcers is 100-200 mg qd, with increases up to 400-600 mg qd if unresponsive; after healing, discontinue or use maintenance dose of 50 mg qd (*J Am Acad Dermatol* 1993;28:271; *Gen Dent* 2007;55:537).

- **Wasting:** Two placebo-controlled trials and three open-label studies demonstrated that thalidomide (daily doses of 50-300 mg qd) for 2-12 wks was associated with significant weight gains. The largest trial showed a dose of 100 mg qd x 8 wks was associated with a mean weight gain of 1.7 kg compared to placebo; half was lean body mass (*AIDS Res Hum Retro* 2000;16:1345). The recommended dose is 100 mg qd because larger doses do not increase weight gain but cause more side effects (*CID* 2003;36[suppl 2]:S74).

- **Miscellaneous Conditions:** HIV-associated complications with a limited but favorable reported experience include refractory colitis (*CID* 2008;47:133), Castleman's disease (*AIDS* 2008;22:1232; *Am J*

Hematol 2006;81:303; *Clin Nephrol* 2004;61:352) and IRIS (*Curr HIV/AIDS Rep* 2009;6:162).

PHARMACOLOGY (*AAC* 1997;41:2797)

- **Bioavailability:** Well absorbed

- **T½:** 6-8 h. Peak levels with 200 mg dose are 1.7 µg/mL; levels >4 µg/mL are required to inhibit TNF-alpha (*PNAS USA* 1993;90:5974; *J Exp Med* 1993;177:1675; *J Am Acad Dermatol* 1996;35:969). It is not known whether thalidomide is present in semen.

- **Elimination:** Nonrenal mechanisms, primarily nonenzymatic hydrolysis in plasma to multiple metabolites. There are no recommendations for dose changes in renal or hepatic failure.

SIDE EFFECTS

- **Teratogenic effects:** Major concern is use in pregnant women due to high potential for birth defects, including absent or abnormal limbs; cleft lip; absent ears; heart, renal or genital abnormalities and other severe defects (*Nat Med* 1997;3:8). Maximum vulnerability is 35-50 days after the last menstrual period, when a single dose is sufficient to cause severe limb abnormalities in most patients (*J Am Acad Dermatol* 1996;35:969). It is *critical* that any woman of childbearing potential not receive thalidomide unless great precautions are taken to prevent pregnancy (pills and barrier protection). Because thalidomide may be present in semen, condom use is recommended for men. Company records indicate that through January 2001, there were 26,968 patients treated, and there were no documented exposures during pregnancy. Several male exposures followed by conception were noted, but none resulted in birth defects.

- **Dose effect:** Teratogenic effects occur even with single dose. Neuropathy, rash, constipation, neutropenia, and sedation are common dose-related side effects found in up to 50% of AIDS patients and are more frequent with low CD4 cell counts (*CID* 1997; 24:1223; *JID* 2002;185:1359).

- **Drowsiness:** Most common side effect is the sedation for which the drug was initially marketed. Administer at bedtime and reduce dose to minimize this side effect. There may be morning somnolence or "hangover."

- **Rash:** Usually pruritic, erythematous, and macular over trunk, back, and proximal extremities. TEN and Stevens-Johnson syndrome have been reported. Re-challenge following erythematous rash has resulted in severe reactions and should only be done with caution.

- **Neuropathy:** Dose-related paresthesias and/or pain of extremities, especially with high doses or prolonged use. This complication may or may not be reversible; it is not known whether the risk is increased by diabetes, alcoholism, or use of neurotoxic drugs including ddI and d4T. Symptoms may start after the drug is discontinued. Neuropathy is a contraindication to the drug, and

5 Drug Information

neurologic monitoring should be performed for all patients.

- **HIV:** Thalidomide may cause modest increase in plasma levels of HIV RNA (0.4 $\log_{10}$/mL) (*NEJM* 1997:336:1487).
- **Neutropenia:** Discontinue thalidomide if ANC is <750/mm³ without an alternative cause.
- **Constipation:** Common; use stool softener, hydration, milk of magnesia, etc.
- **Less common side effects** include dizziness, mood changes, bradycardia, tachycardia, bitter taste, headache, nausea, pruritus, dry mouth, dry skin, or hypotension.

DRUG INTERACTIONS: The greatest concern is in women of child-bearing potential who take concurrent medications, such as rifamycin and possibly PIs and NNRTIs, that interfere with the effectiveness of contraceptive. Barrier of contraception must be used. Concurrent use of drugs that cause sedation or peripheral neuropathy (e.g., ddl, d4T) may increase the frequency and severity of these side effects.

PREGNANCY: Category X (contraindicated).

TIPRANAVIR (TPV)

TRADE NAME: *Aptivus* (Boehringer-Ingelheim)

CLASS: Protease inhibitor

FORMS AND COST: Caps, 250 mg at $10.49/cap, $1,259.57/mo; solution 100 mg/mL as 95 mL bottle (price does not include price of required RTV booster).

PATIENT ASSISTANCE: 800-556-8317

STANDARD DOSE: TPV/r 500/200 mg bid with food

AVOID: With severe liver disease (Child Pugh Score Class B or C) and avoid use in combination with other PIs.

STORAGE: TPV must be used within 60 days if stored at room temperature (up to 25°C or 77°F). Refrigerated TPV caps are stable until date on label.

- **Advantages:** 1) Active against most PI-resistant HIV (*Curr HIV Res* 2010;8:347); 2) established efficacy in salvage therapy (*JAIDS* 2007;45:401).
- **Disadvantages:** 1) Elevated transaminase levels and hyperlipidemia; 2) reduced efficacy with extensive PI resistance (see "Resistance"); 3) multiple drug interactions and inability to combine with other PIs and ETR; 4) RTV 400 mg/d boosting requirement; 5) higher incidence of hepatitis and hyperlipidemia than other PIs; 6) black box warning of potential for intracranial hemorrhage and hepatic failure; 7) bid dosing; and 8) DRV/r is better tolerated and typically active against most PI-resistant virus.

Drug Information

INDICATION: Highly pretreated adults with resistance to multiple PIs and susceptibility to TPV (preferably those with virus more susceptible to TPV than to DRV). It requires RTV boosting and initially was most effective when combined with ENF in ENF-naïve patients.

CLINICAL TRIALS

- **RESIST-1 and -2:** Phase 3 trials of patients who failed at least 2 PI-based regimens, had VL >1000 c/mL and had at least one primary PI mutation and no more than two at codons 33, 82, 84 and 90. RESIST-1 was conducted with 620 subjects in the U.S., Canada and Australia; RESIST-2 was conducted with 539 evaluable patients in Europe and South America. Participants were randomized to receive TPV/r or one of four alternative boosted PI regimens: LPV/r, IDV/r, SQV/r or APV/r (*Lancet* 2006;368:466). The 1159 participants had a median baseline VL of 4.8 $\log_{10}$ c/mL, a median CD4 count of 155 cells/mm^3, and an average of 10 PI resistance mutations. Participants with no virologic response in control arm were allowed to roll over to trial 1182.17, which included TPV/r. The NRTI backbone was individualized. Results are summarized in Table 5-80. Response rates correlated with use of enfuvirtide, higher TPV trough level, baseline phenotype resistance test, and by the "TPV score" (0-2 vs. 5-6), determined by the number of the following PI mutations: 10V, 13V, 20M/R, 33F, 35G, 36I, 43T, 46L, 47V, 54A/M/V, 58E, 69K, 74P, 82L/T, 83D, 84V. Virologic results with these variables are summarized in Table 5-81.

- **BI 1182.52:** This dose-finding study in 216 patients who failed >2 PI-based regimens (CROI 2003:Abstr. 596) showed that patients with ≥3 of 4 PRAMs (PI resistance-associated mutations at codons 33, 82, 84, and 90) had a reduced response. This was the reason for the limitation of ≤2 PRAMs as an entry criterion for RESIST.

- **BI 1182.51:** This study enrolled simultaneously with RESIST but was restricted to the patients with 3 or 4 PRAMs (*JAIDS* 2008;47: 429). Patients were randomized to TPV/r (*n* = 61) or to LPV/r (*n* = 79), APV/r (*n* = 76), or SQV/r (*n* = 75). After 14 days TPV/r was added to the regimens of patients in the other three arms. Patients on TPV/r had a median VL decrease of 1.2 $\log_{10}$ c/mL compared to <0.4 $\log_{10}$ c/mL in each of the other arms; the addition of TPV/r to the other regimens resulted in a substantial boost to viral suppression to a median total decrease of 1.2 $\log_{10}$ c/mL at 4 weeks. The suppression noted above was not sustained, indicating the need for additional active agents. Pharmacokinetic studies of the dual PI-boosted regimens showed that TPV reduced C_{min} of the concurrent PIs by 55-81%, presumably due to P450 and P-gp induction. For this reason, dual-boosted PI therapy with these TPV combinations is not recommended.

5 Drugs

■ TABLE 5-80: **RESIST-1 and -2: Results at 48 Weeks (*Lancet* 2006;368:466)**

	TPV/r *n* = 749	CPI/r* *n* = 737
Baseline[†]		
VL ($\log_{10}$ c/mL) (mean)	4.7	4.7
CD4 count (mean; /mm³)	196	195
PI mutations (median)	10	10
Prior antiretroviral agents (median)	12	12
Results at 48 weeks		
Completed 48 wks	541 (73%)	230 (31%)[‡]
VL <400 c/mL	30.4%	13.8%[‡]
with ENF	43%	19%[‡]
without ENF	27%	13%[‡]
VL <50 c/mL	23%	10%[‡]
Reduction in VL ($\log_{10}$ c/mL) with ENF	-1.14	0.5
CD4 count increase	48/mm³	21/mm³[‡]
Withdrawals for adverse event/100 pt-yr exposure	12.4	10.6
Grade 3/4 events/100 pt-yr exposure[§]	64	64
Results at 96 weeks[#]		
VL <400 c/mL	26.9%	10.9%
VL <50 c/mL	20.4%	9.1%
with ENF	35%	14%

* Comparator PI: LPV/r, IDV/r, SQV/r or APV/r
† All results are mean values unless otherwise indicated.
‡ $P \leq 0.0001$
§ TPV was associated with significantly more grade 3/4 elevations of triglycerides (31% vs. 23%) and ALT (10% vs. 3%).
# 8th Int Congress on Drug Therapy in HIV Infection, Glasgow, 2006, Abstr. P23

■ TABLE 5-81: **Response Correlates in RESIST-1 and -2**

		VL decrease $\log_{10}$ c/mL
TPV score (6 mo)	0-1 mutations	−2.10
	2-3 mutations	−0.89
	4-7 mutations	−0.46
	8-9 mutations	−0.08
Baseline phenotype (48 wks)	IC_{90} fold change 0-3	−1.02
	IC_{90} fold change >3-10	−0.27
ENF (48 wks)	ENF	−1.67
	No ENF	−0.98

Lancet 2006;368:466 and package insert (11/15/06)

Drugs

- **TPV/r vs. LPV/r:** A subset analysis of RESIST-1 compared 24-week results for patients randomized to either TPV/r or LPV/r. Response was significantly better in the TPV/r recipients in terms of VL reduction ≥ 1 $\log_{10}$ c/mL (40% vs. 21%), proportion with VL <400 c/mL (34% vs. 25%) and mean CD4 response (+31/mm^3 vs. +6/mm^3) (*AIDS* 2007;21:2734). Virologic response was greater in both groups when ENF was used concurrently; VL decreased >1 $\log_{10}$ c/mL at 24 weeks in 58% of 293 TPV/r recipients and 26% of 290 LPV/r recipients.

- **Utilize:** Observational study at 40 US sites in which 236 patients failing a PI-based regimen had resistance tests showing 139 (59%) had a PI resistance mutation, and >50% were sensitive to DRV or TPV; other PIs showed that <22% were sensitive (*Curr HIV Res* 2010;8:347). These data suggest that the most predictably active PIs in patients with multiple PI failures are DRV and TPV.

RESISTANCE: Mutations that contribute to resistance are 10V, 13V, 20M/R/V, 33F, 35G, 36I, 43T, 46L, 47V, 54A/M/V, 56E, 69K, 74P, 82L/T, 83D, and 84V (*Topics HIV Med* 2008;16:62; *J Virol* 2006;80:10794). Accumulation of these mutations reduces response. The best response is seen with ≤ 1 TPV mutation. Intermediate response is seen with 2-7 mutations; with ≥ 8 mutations, response is minimal. Nevertheless, some of these are more important. The mutations with the greatest impact on resistance are 74P, 47V, 58E and 82L/T (*AIDS Rev* 2008;10:125). Clinical cutoffs for TPV susceptibility using the *PhenoSense* or *PhenoSense GT* assays are -fold changes of 2 and 8. Corresponding cutoffs using the *VircoTYPE* assay are 1.2 and 5.4. Mutations at 30N, 50V and 88D are associated with TPV hypersusceptibility (*HIV Clin Trials* 2004;5:371; *Expert Rev Anti Infect Ther* 2005;3:9; *Antivir Ther* 2010;15:959).

An alternative TPV-weighted mutation score has been proposed based on at week 8 of treatment (*Antiviral Ther* 2010;15:1011). Mutations are assigned the following score:

- **4+:** 74P, 82 L/T, 83D and 47V
- **3+:** 58E and 84V
- **2+:** 36I, 43T and 54A/M/V
- **1+:** 10V, 33F and 46L
- **-2:** 76V
- **-4:** 50L/V
- **-6:** 54L

Score interpretation:
sensitive=<3; partially sensitive=4-9; resistant=>10

The most common TPV-associated resistance mutations that occur during failed TPV therapy are 10I, 13V, 33V/F, 36V/I/L, 82/T/L and 84V (*AIDS* 2007;21:179). Note that DRV failures are often associated with

5 Drugs

the 54L mutation, which confers with TPV hypersusceptibility (*AAC* 2010;54:3018). Other reports indicate that resistance to both DRV and TPV is rare (*AAC* 2010;54:2479).

PHARMACOLOGY

- **Bioavailability:** Oral absorption is substantially improved with a concurrent high-fat meal. RTV given concurrently increases TPV 29-fold and should always be used in combination with TPV. CNS penetration is poor (*Neurology* 2011;76:693).

- **T½:** 6 h

- **Excretion:** Most of TPV is eliminated in stool; 5% is found in urine.

- **Dose adjustment for renal failure:** None.

- **Dose adjustment for hepatic failure:** Not established. TPV/r is contraindicated with moderate or severe hepatic disease (Child-Pugh class B or C).

- TPV is a substrate of CYP3A4 and Pgp. TPV/r has a net inhibitory effect on CYP3A4 and is a potent inducer of Pgp.

DRUG INTERACTIONS

- **RTV:** RTV 200 mg bid increases TPV levels 29-fold and is required for TPV to achieve therapeutic levels.

- **NRTIs:** Must be dosed ≥2 h before or after ddI EC; ddI AUC decreased by 40%; clinical significance not known. AZT and ABC concentrations decreased by 40-50%; dose adjustment is not established (package insert). No clinically significant interactions with 3TC, d4T, or TDF (2011 DHHS Guidelines).

- **MVC:** No dose adjustment necessary; use standard dose.

- **RAL:** RAL C_{min} ↓55%, but no change in AUC; use standard dose.

- **NNRTIs:** No interaction with EFV or NVP. ETR AUC decreased by 76%; avoid.

- **PIs:** Studies combining PIs with TPV/r showed that the drug induced P450 and Pgp, resulting in a 50-80% reduction in the C_{min} levels of LPV, FPV, ATV, and SQV. Therefore, these PIs should not be co-administered with TPV. There are no data for concurrent administration of NFV, IDV, or DRV, but the assumption is that these drugs will be affected in a similar way.

- **Drugs contraindicated** for concurrent administration: **anti-arrhythmics (amiodarone, bepridil, flecainide, propafenone, quinidine), ergot derivatives, lovastatin, simvastatin, pimozide, rifampin, triazolam, midazolam, St. John's wort, astemizole, terfenadine, cisapride, ranolazine,** and **alfuzosin.**

- **Drugs to avoid: salmeterol, fluticasone** and **pitavastatin.**

- **Other drugs: Alprazolam:** increase alprazolam levels; consider lorazepam, temazepam, oxazepam. **Antacids:** decrease TPV AUC 25-30%; take ≥2 h apart. **Antiplatelet drugs** (ASA, NSAIDs,

Drugs

clopidogrel, tilopidine): May increase risk of bleeding. Avoid co-administration. **Atorvastatin:** atorvastatin AUC increased 9x; use with caution starting with lowest dose (10 mg) and avoiding high doses (e.g., >40 mg/d) or use rosuvastatin (AUC increased 37%; start with 5 mg) or pravastatin. **Buprenorphine:** Norbuprenorphine AUC decreased by 80%. TPV trough decreased by 19-40%. Consider TPV TDM. **Benzodiazepines:** Avoid clorazepate, estazolam, flurazepam; consider lorazepam, oxazepam or temazepam. **Calcium channel blockers:** may increase levels of calcium channel blockers; monitor closely. **Carbamazepine:** Carbamazepine AUC increased 26%; may decrease TPV levels; consider valproic acid, lamotrigine, levetiracetam or topiramate. **Clarithromycin:** increases TPV and clarithromycin levels; no dose adjustment necessary with normal renal function; decrease clarithromycin dose by 75% with CrCl <30 mL/min. and by 50% with CrCl 30-60 mL/min. **Colchicine:** TPV/r increases colchicine level. **Corticosteroids (dexamethasone):** may decrease TPV levels, use with caution. **Cyclosporine:** may increase cyclosporine levels; monitor levels. **ddI EC:** Separate doses of TPV and ddI EC by 2 hrs. **Desipramine:** may increase desiramine, reduce despiramine dose and monitor. **Disulfiram/metronidazole:** TPV caps contain 76% alcohol per 100-mg cap and may cause disulfiram-like reactions; avoid. **Ethinyl estradiol:** EE AUC reduced 50%; use alternative birth control. **Fluticasone:** risk of increased steroid levels; avoid combination; consider beclomethasone. **Flecainide:** flecainide levels increased; avoid or monitor levels. **Fluconazole:** TPV AUC increased 56%; limit fluconazole dose to ≤200 mg/d; monitor LFTs. Consider alternative PI if fluconazole >250 mg is needed (see azoles pg. 208). **Halofantrine** (not available in the US), **lumefantrine:** not recommended; risk of inducing torsades de pointes. **Itraconazole** and **ketonazole:** azole and TPV levels may be increased; consider fluconazole. **Meperidine:** may decrease meperidine levels and increase metabolite normeperidine, which may cause seizures. **Methadone:** decrease R-methadone AUC levels 50%. May need to increase methadone dose. **Metronidazole:** may result in disulfiram reaction. **Nifedipine:** may increase nifedipine levels; avoid. **Paclitaxel:** possible increase in paclitaxel levels; monitor closely. **Phenobarbital:** may decrease TPV levels and increase or decrease phenobarbital levels; consider valproic acid, lamotrigine, levetiracetam, or topiramate. **Phenytoin:** as with phenobarbital. **Rifampin:** decrease TPV levels; avoid. **Rifabutin:** RBT levels increased 2.9x; use RBT 150 mg q24-48h. Consider rifabutin TDM. **Sildenafil:** increased sildenafil levels; limit to ≤25 mg in 48 h. **Tacrolimus:** increased levels of tacrolimus; use reduced doses. **Tadalafil:** ≤10 mg q72h. For the treatment of pulmonary hypertension; start with tadalafil 20 mg/d only after TPV/r has reached steady state (>7 days). **Theophylline:** may increase levels of theophylline; consider therapeutic monitoring. **Vardenafil:** increased

5 Drugs

levels of vardenafil; do not exceed 2.5 mg q72h (with RTV). **Voriconazole:** may decrease voriconazole levels and increase TPV levels; avoid (use amphotericin or caspofungin) or monitor voriconazole levels carefully. See pg. 413.

ADVERSE DRUG REACTIONS: With the exceptions of hepatitis and hyperlipidemia, the side effects profile is similar to that of other PIs. The most common side effects are GI intolerance, headache, hypertriglyceridemia, rash, and fatigue, and increases in transaminase levels (grade 3/4 increases in 8%). **Hepatotoxicity** with clinical hepatitis, sometimes with hepatic failure and death, has been reported. Hepatotoxicity is more common in patients with HBV or HBC co-infection. Indications to discontinue TPV/r based on grade 3/4 transaminase increases are unclear. **GI intolerance** includes nausea (5%) and diarrhea (4-10%). Less frequent side effects are fatigue, headache, and abdominal pain. **Rash:** more common in women (13% vs. 8%). **Hyperlipidemia:** increases in total cholesterol, LDL-C, and triglycerides (Grade 3/4 increases in triglyceride elevations in 31% of RESIST participants who received TPV/r vs. 23% of controls) are common; serum lipid levels should be monitored. **Intracranial bleeding:** includes fatal and nonfatal cases, but did not correlate with abnormal coagulation parameters. Most had recent head surgery, head trauma, or similar risk factors. Review of Boehringer- Ingelheim records found 13 cases, including 8 fatal intracranial hemorrhages in 6,840 HIV infected patients in clinical trials (*J Infect* 2008;57:85). The cause may be related to inhibition of platelet aggregation.

BLACK BOX WARNING: 1) Fatal and non-fatal intracranial hemorrhage and 2) Clinical hepatitis including fatal cases.

PREGNANCY: Category C. The 2010 DHHS Guidelines on Antiretroviral Agents in Preganancy list TPV as "insufficient data to recommend use."

TRAZODONE

TRADE NAME: *Desyrel* (Bristol-Myers Squibb) and generic

FORMS AND COST: Tabs: 50 mg at $0.43, 100 mg at $0.78, 150 mg at $1.46, 300 mg at $5.43.

CLASS: Nontricyclic antidepressant

INDICATIONS AND DOSE REGIMENS

- **Depression**, especially when associated with anxiety or insomnia: 400-600 mg hs. With insomnia, give 50-150 mg hs. Increase dose 50 mg every 3-4 days up to maximum dose of 400 mg qd for outpatients and 600 mg qd for hospitalized patients.
- **Insomnia:** 50-150 mg qhs

PHARMACOLOGY

- **Bioavailability:** >90%, improved if taken with meals
- **T½:** 6 h

Drugs

- **Elimination:** Hepatic metabolism, then renal excretion

SIDE EFFECTS: Adverse effects are dose- and duration-related and are usually seen with doses >300 mg qd; may decrease with continued use, dose reduction, or schedule change.

- **Major side effects:** Sedation in 15-20%; orthostatic hypotension (5%); nervousness; fatigue; dizziness; nausea; vomiting; and anticholinergic effects (dry mouth, blurred vision, constipation, urinary retention). Rare: priapism (1/6000); agitation; cardiovascular; and anticholinergic side effects are less frequent and less severe than with tricyclics.

DRUG INTERACTIONS: LPV/r and RTV increase trazodone levels. Trazodone may increase levels of phenytoin and digoxin; alcohol and other CNS depressants potentiate sedative side effects. Contraindicated with SQV/r.

PREGNANCY: Category C

TRICYCLIC ANTIDEPRESSANTS – see also Nortriptyline (pg. 339 and pg. 558)

Tricyclic antidepressants elevate mood, increase physical activity, improve appetite, improve sleep patterns, and reduce morbid preoccupations in most patients with major depression. The following principles apply:

INDICATIONS

- **Psychiatric Indications:** Major depression – response rates are 60-70%. Low doses are commonly used for adjustment disorders including depression and anxiety. Usual therapeutic dose for depression is 50-150 mg hs for noritriptyline and 100-300 mg hs for amitriptyline.

- **Peripheral neuropathy:** Controlled trials have not shown benefit in AIDS-associated peripheral neuropathy, but clinical experience is extensive and results in diabetic neuropathy are good. If used, choice of agents depends on time of symptoms (*JAMA* 1998;280:1590). Night pain: amitriptyline (most sedating) start with 25 mg hs. Day pain: nortriptyline (less sedating and less of an anticholinergic effect) start with 25 mg hs. Some recommend therapeutic drug monitoring for depression, but generally not for peripheral neuropathy.

DOSE: Initial treatment of depression is 4-8 wks, required for therapeutic response. Initial dose is usually given at bedtime, especially with insomnia or if sedation is a side effect. Common mistakes are use of an initial dose that is too high, resulting in excessive anticholinergic side effects or oversedation. The dose is increased every 3-4 days depending on tolerance and response. Treatment of major depression usually requires continuation for 4-5 mos after response. Multiple recurrences may require long-term treatment.

5 Drugs

SERUM LEVELS: Efficacy correlates with serum levels of nortriptyline when used as an antidepressant. Therapeutic monitoring of drug levels allows dose titration. Target level for nortriptyline is 70-125 ng/dL.

PHARMACOLOGY: Well absorbed, extensively metabolized, long half-life, variable use of serum levels (see below).

SIDE EFFECTS: Anticholinergic effects (dry mouth, dizziness, blurred vision, constipation, tachycardia, urinary hesitancy, sedation), sexual dysfunction, orthostatic hypotension, weight gain, QTc prolongation (with PIs use with caution).

RELATIVE CONTRAINDICATIONS: Cardiac conduction block (avoid with RTV >400 bid). prostatism, and narrow angle glaucoma. Less common side effects: mania, hypo-mania, allergic skin reactions, marrow suppression, seizures, tardive dyskinesia, tremor, speech blockage, anxiety, insomnia, Parkinsonism, hyponatremia; cardiac conduction disturbances and arrhythmias (most common serious side effects are with overdosage).

TRIMETHOPRIM (TMP)

TRADE NAME: Generic

FORMS AND COST: Tabs: 100 mg at $0.68

INDICATIONS AND DOSE REGIMENS

- **PCP** (with sulfamethoxazole as TMP-SMX or with dapsone): 5 mg/kg po tid (usually 300 mg tid or qid) x 21 days
- **UTIs:** 100 mg po bid or 200 mg qd x 3-14 days

PHARMACOLOGY

- **Bioavailability:** >90%
- **T½:** 9-11 hrs
- **Excretion:** Renal
- **Dose modification with renal failure:** CrCl >50 mL/min – full dose; 10-50 mL/min – one-half to two-thirds dose; <30 mL/min – one-third to one-half dose

SIDE EFFECTS: Usually well tolerated; most common – pruritus and skin rash; GI intolerance; marrow suppression – anemia, neutropenia, thrombocytopenia; antifolate effects – prevent with leucovorin; reversible hyperkalemia in 20-50% of AIDS patients given high doses (*Ann Intern Med* 1993;119:291,296; *NEJM* 1993;238:703).

DRUG INTERACTIONS: Increased activity of phenytoin (monitor levels) and procainamide; levels of both dapsone and trimethoprim are increased when given concurrently.

PREGNANCY: Category C. Teratogenic in rats with high doses; limited experience in patients shows no association with congenital abnormalities.

Drugs

TRIMETHOPRIM-SULFAMETHOXAZOLE
(TMP-SMX, cotrimoxazole)

TRADE NAME: *Bactrim* (Roche), *Septra* (Monarch), and generic

FORMS AND COST: TMP/SMX 80/400 mg (SS) tabs at $0.66; 160/800 mg (DS) tabs at $1.09. For IV use: 10 mL vials with 16/80 mg/mL at $10.98/30 mL.

INDICATIONS AND DOSE REGIMENS

- **PCP prophylaxis:** 1 DS qd or 1 SS qd; alternative is 1 DS 3x/wk. Discontinuation of PCP prophylaxis after ART-associated immune reconstitution is safe and avoids significant toxicity (*CID* 2001;33: 1901; *MMWR* 2002;51[RR-8]:4). PCP prophylaxis with TMP-SMX reduces the frequency of bacterial pneumonia and other bacterial infections (*CID* 2006;43:90). See pg. 67.

- **Graduated initiation to reduce adverse effects** (ACTG 268) (*JAIDS* 2000;24:337): Oral preparation (40 mg trimethoprim and 200 mg sulfamethoxazole/5mL) – 1 mL qd x 3 d, then 2 mL qd x 3 d, then 5 mL qd x 3 d, then 10 mL qd x 3 d, then 20 mL qd x 3 d, then 1 TMP-SMX DS tab qd. Alternative schedule: See pg. 411.

- **Desensitization:** See Table 5-82 and 5-83, pg. 411.

- **PCP treatment:** 5 mg/kg (trimethoprim component) po or IV q8h x 21 days, usually 6 DS/d divided q8h (70 kg). A review of 1,188 episodes of HIV-associated PCP in Europe showed TMP-SMX was the most frequent first line agent (81%), had the lowest rate of drug change for failure or toxicity (21%) and the best survival rate (85%) (*JAC* 2009;64:1282). See pg. 477.

- **Toxoplasmosis prophylaxis:** 1 DS qd

- **Toxoplasmosis treatment:** Alternative to sulfadiazine – acute therapy (>6 wks) TMP-SMX 5 mg/kg (TMP) PO or IV bid x ≥6 wks, then maintenance at half dose (*Eur J Clin Microbiol Infect Dis* 1992;11:125; *AAC* 1998;42:1346; *Cochrane Database Syst Rev* 2006;19:CD005420).

- ***Isospora:*** 1 DS po qid x 10 days; may need maintenance with 1-2 DS/d. IDSA recommendation: TMP-SMX 1 DS bid x 7-10 days, then 1 DS 3x/wk or 1 *Fansidar* /wk indefinitely.

- ***Salmonella:*** 1 DS po bid x 5-7 days; treat >14 days if relapsing.

- ***Nocardia:*** 4-6 DS/d x ≥6 mos

- **Urinary tract infections:** 1-2 DS/d x 3-14 days

- **Prophylaxis for cystitis:** ½ SS tab daily

- **Malaria prophylaxis:** TMP-SMX is effective prophylaxis for PCP and has proven highly effective for preventing malaria (*Lancet* 2006;367: 1256). Initial results in malaria-endemic areas shows TMP-SMX prophylaxis for PCP does not select for TMP-SMX resistant malaria (*Ann J Trop Med Hyg* 2006;75:375).

5 Drugs

ACTIVITY: TMP-SMX is effective in the treatment or prophylaxis of infections involving *P. jiroveci*, most **methicillin-sensitive *S. aureus*** (MRSA), >80% of **community-associated MRSA** (USA 300 strains), ***Legionella, Listeria*,** and **common urinary tract pathogens**. TMP/SMX is used preferentially in low resource countries for CNS **toxoplasmosis** with good results (*Am J Trop Med Hyg* 2009;80:583). Some studies show increasing rates of mutations in the dihydropteroate synthase gene of *P. jiroveci* that are associated with increased resistance to sulfonamides and dapsone (*JID* 1999;180:1969); a meta-analysis found that this mutation is associated with prolonged exposure to sulfonamides, but the clinical significance of these mutations in terms of reduced response is unclear (*Emerg Infect Dis* 2004;10:1760). In clinical trials, clinical outcome has not been worse with DHPS mutation when these patients were treated with TMP-SMX (*Lancet* 2001;358: 545; *Emerg Infect Dis* 2004;10:1721; *Proc Am Thorac Soc* 2006;3:655). Current rates of resistance of *S. pneumoniae* to TMP-SMX are about 15-30% (*AAC* 2002;46:2651; *NEJM* 2000; 343:1917), but their significance is questioned (*Proc Am Thoracic Soc* 2006;3:655). A systematic review of the literature suggested that TMP-SMX prophylaxis does not promote resistance to other antibiotics (*CID* 2011;52:1184)

PHARMACOLOGY

- **Bioavailability:** >90% absorbed with oral administration (both drugs)
- **T½:** Trimethoprim, 8-15 h; sulfamethoxazole 7-12 h
- **Elimination:** Renal; T½ in renal failure increases to 24 hrs for trimethoprim and 22-50 hrs for sulfamethoxazole
- **Renal failure:** CrCl >30 mL/min – usual dose; 10-30 mL/min – one-half to two-thirds dose; <10 mL/min – manufacturer recommends avoidance, but one-third to one-half dose may be used for PCP.

SIDE EFFECTS: Noted in 10% of patients without HIV infection and about 50% of patients with HIV. The gradual initiation of TMP-SMX noted above results in a 50% reduction in adverse reactions (*JAIDS* 2000;24:337), suggesting that it is not a true hypersensitivity reaction. The prevailing opinion is that these side effects are usually due to toxic metabolites ascribed to altered metabolism of TMP-SMX with HIV infection. The presumed benefit from gradual initiation is to permit time for enzyme induction. A Cochrane Library review examined three strategies with TMP-SMX reaction: Treat through, rechallenge or desensitize (*Cochrane Database Syst Rev* 2007;CD005646). Best results were achieved with desensitization (see Tables 5-82 and 5-83).

- **Most common:** Nausea, vomiting, pruritus, rash, fever, neutropenia, and increased transaminases. Many HIV-infected patients may be treated despite side effects (GI intolerance and rash) if symptoms are not disabling; alternative with PCP prophylaxis is dose reduction usually after drug holiday (1-2 wks) and/or "desensitization" (see

Drugs

■ TABLE 5-82: **Rapid TMP-SMX Desensitization Schedule**

Time (hour)	Dose (TMP/SMX)	Dilution
0	0.004/0.02 mg	1:10,000 (5 mL)
1	0.04/0.2 mg	1:1,000 (5 mL)
2	0.4/2.0 mg	1:100 (5 mL)
3	4/20 mg	1:10 (5 mL)
4	40/200 mg	(5 mL)
5	160/800 mg	Tablet

■ TABLE 5-83: **8-Day TMP-SMX Desensitization Schedule**

Day	Dilution
1	1:1,000,000
2	1:100,000
3	1:10,000
4	1:1,000
5	1:100
6	1:10
7	1:1
8	Standard suspension – 1 mL 40 mg SMX – 8 mg TMP
9	1 DS tab/day

below). The mechanism of most sulfonamide reactions is unclear, and cause of increased susceptibility with HIV is also unclear.

- **Rash:** Most common is erythematous, maculopapular, morbilliform, and/or pruritic rash, usually 7-14 days after treatment is started. Less common are erythema multiforme, epidermal necrolysis, exfoliative dermatitis, Stevens-Johnson syndrome, urticaria, and Henoch-Schönlein purpura.

- **GI intolerance** is common with nausea, vomiting, anorexia, and abdominal pain; rare side effects include *C. difficile* diarrhea/colitis and pancreatitis.

- **Hematologic side effects** include neutropenia, anemia, and/or thrombocytopenia. The rate of anemia is increased in patients with HIV infection and with folate depletion. Some respond to leucovorin (5-15 mg qd), but this is not routinely recommended.

- **Neurologic** toxicity may include tremor, ataxia, apathy, aseptic meningitis, and ankle clonus (*Am J Med Sci* 1996;312:27).

- **Hepatitis** with cholestatic jaundice and hepatic necrosis has been described.

5 Drugs

- **Hyperkalemia** in 20-50% of patients given trimethoprim in doses >15 mg/kg/d (*NEJM* 1993;328:703). The risk is particularly great with co-administration of beta-blockers.

- **Interstitial nephritis** is more commonly a pseudo-elevation of serum creatinine of ≥17.6% without affecting GFR (*Chemotherapy* 1981; 27: 229).

- **Altered flora:** Chronic administration of TMP-SMX may increase rates of resistance to this and other antibiotics for bacteria in the normal flora including E. coli and S. pneumoniae (*JAIDS* 2008;47:585; *J Infect* 2008;56:171).

PROTOCOL FOR ORAL DESENSITIZATION OR "DETOXIFICATION": See Tables 5-80 and 5-81.

- **Rapid desensitization** (*CID* 1995;20:849): Serial 10-fold dilutions of oral suspension (40 mg TMP, 200 mg SMX/5 mL) given hourly over 4 hrs (see Table 5-80).

- **Note:** A prospective trial showed no difference in outcome with desensitization compared with rechallenge (*Biomed Pharmacother* 2000;54:45)

- **8-day protocol:** Serial dilutions prepared by pharmacists using oral suspension (40 mg TMP, 200 mg SMX/5 mL). Medication is given 4 times daily for 7 days in doses of 1 cc, 2 cc, 4 cc, and 8 cc using the following dilutions:

DRUG INTERACTIONS: Increased levels of oral anticoagulants, phenytoin, and procainamide. Risk of megaloblastic anemia with methotrexate.

PREGNANCY: Category C. The two issues are birth defects with first trimester exposures and hyperbilirubinemia and kernicterus with exposure near delivery. A systematic review of data through July 2005 showed minimal risk of kernicterus with late pregnancy exposures; with first trimester exposures there was "mixed evidence linking first trimester exposures to cleft lips, neural tube defects, cardiovascular defects, and urinary tract defects" (*AIDS Rev* 2006;8:24). The conclusion is that the risk is small and TMP-SMX is considered safe for pregnant women in developing countries as currently recommended by the WHO. In the U.S., recommendation is to use TMP-SMX with caution due to possible kernicterus, although no cases of kernicterus have been reported (*CID* 1995;21[suppl 1]:S24). The 2008 DHHS Opportunistic Infection Guidelines recommend TMP-SMX in pregnancy when indicated, while acknowledging a small increased risk of birth defects associated with first trimester exposure. This should be accompanied by the standard folic acid supplement of 0.4 mg/d; it is unclear if higher doses would provide additional protection. Ultrasound at week 18-20 is recommended due to possible kernicterus, although no cases of kernicterus have been reported (*CID* 1995; 21[suppl 1]:S24).

Drugs

TRIZIVIR – see Zidovudine (pg. 416), Lamivudine (pg. 304), and Abacavir (pg. 179)

TRUVADA – see Tenofovir (pg. 388) and Emtricitabine (pg. 255)

VALACYCLOVIR – see Acyclovir (pg. 186)

VALGANCICLOVIR – see Ganciclovir (pg. 288)

VALCYTE – see Ganciclovir (pg. 288)

VIBRAMYCIN – see Doxycycline (pg. 241)

VIDEX – see Didanosine (pg. 236)

VIRACEPT – see Nelfinavir (pg. 327)

VIRAMUNE – see Nevirapine (pg. 330)

VITRASERT – see Ganciclovir (pg. 288)

VORICONAZOLE

TRADE NAME: *Vfend* (Pfizer)

FORMS AND COST: Tabs: 50 mg at $13.04, 200 mg at $52.17; Vial for IV use: 200 mg at $153.54. Oral suspension (200 mg/5 mL) at $895.84 per 75-mL bottle.

CLASS: Triazole antifungal

REGIMENS

- **Oral:** 300 mg (6 mg/kg) po bid x 1 day (loading dose), then 4 mg/kg (200-300) mg po bid on an empty stomach. Avoid high-fat meal. Usual dose for aspergillosis or severe infections is 300 mg bid; 100-150 mg bid for patients <40 kg. High degree of variability in voriconazole levels attributed to variable metabolism due to age, hepatic disease, genetic polymorphisms and drug interactions, especially omeprazole (*CID* 2008;46:201).

5 Drugs

- **IV:** 6 mg/kg IV q12h x 2 doses (loading dose), then 3-4 mg/kg IV q12h
- **Hepatic failure:** 6 mg/kg q12h x2 doses, then use half-dose 2 mg/kg q12h.
- **Renal failure:** Use standard oral dose.

IN VITRO **ACTIVITY:** Active against most *Candida* species, including many fluconazole-resistant strains. Voriconazole is 16- to 32-fold more active than fluconazole against *Candida* (*JCM* 2007;45:70). Active against >98% of *C. albicans, C. krusei, C. tropicalis,* and *C. parapsilosis* (*AAC* 2002;46:1032; *J Med Microbiol* 2002;51:479; *J Clin Microbiol* 2002;40:852). Very active against most *Aspergillus*; more active *in vitro* than itraconazole (*J Infect Chemother* 2000;6:101; *CID* 2002;34:563; *JCM* 2002;40:2648; *AAC* 2002;46:1032). More recent reviews indicate persistence of good activity (*Med Mycol* 2008;12:1) **Zygomycetes** (mucor) are less susceptible; posaconazole preferred (*AAC* 2002; 46:2708; *AAC* 2002;46:1581; *AAC* 2002;46:1032). Activity against *Scedosporium apiospermum* (*Pseudoallescheria boydii*) is variable (*AAC* 2002;46:62). Most dermatophytes are sensitive (*AAC* 2001; 45:2524). *C. neoformans* is usually highly susceptible with *in vitro* activity superior to both fluconazole and itraconazole but minimal experience clinically (*Eur J Clin Microbiol* 2000;19:317; *AAC* 1999; 43:1463; *AAC* 1999;43:169). Also active *in vitro* against *H. capsulatum, B. dermatitidis,* and *Penicillium marneffei.*

FDA APPROVAL: Voriconazole is approved for treatment of 1) invasive aspergillosis, 2) serious infections caused by *Scedosporium apiospermum* and *Fusarium* spp., 3) esophageal candidiasis, and 4) candidemia in the non-neutropenic host.

CLINICAL TRIAL: Major clinical trial compared voriconazole (6 mg/kg IV q12h x 2 doses, then 4 mg/kg IV q12h x ≥7 days, then oral voriconazole 200 mg bid) with amphotericin B (1.0-1.5 mg/kg/d IV) in 277 patients with invasive *Aspergillus*. Voriconazole had a significantly better response rate (53% vs. 32%), better 12-week survival (71% vs. 58%), and less toxicity (*NEJM* 2002;347:408).

PHARMACOLOGY

- **Oral bioavailability:** 96%; AUC reduced by 24% when taken with high-fat meal
- **Tissue penetration:** Autopsy studies show good penetration into lung, brain, liver, kidneys, spleen and myocardium (*AAC* 2010;2011;55:925). Preliminary data suggest that effective levels are achieved in CSF (*Br J Haematol* 1997:97:663).
- **Loading dose:** Day 1; without loading dose, the maintenance dose requires 6 days to reach steady state.
- **Metabolism:** Metabolized primarily by P450 CYP219>>2C9>3A4 enzymes. >94% of metabolite is excreted in urine; metabolites have little or no antifungal activity; <2% parenteral formulation is excreted in urine. Review of 181 level measurements showed great variation

Drugs

ranging from <1 mg/L in 25% to >5.5 mg/L in 31% (*CID* 2008;46:201). The high levels were associated with omeprazole co-therapy and IV therapy; there was CNS toxicity with high levels that cleared when the drug was stopped.

- **Hepatic failure:** AUC increases 2.3-fold; use 100 mg bid. $T\frac{1}{2}$ = 6-24 hr.
- **Levels:** Target C_{min} >2.05 mcg/mL (*Antimicrob Ag Chem* 2006;50: 1570) and C_{trough} <5.5 mcg/mL (*CID* 2008;46:212).

DRUG INTERACTIONS: Inhibition of P450 enzymes primarily CYP2C19 and to a lesser extent 2C9 and 3A4 (*AAC* 2002; 46:3091). Drug interactions with boosted PIs, NNRTIs and MVC are extensive (*Ann Pharm* 2008/42:698). See pg. 208t.

- **Contraindicated for concurrent use:** (Decreased voriconazole levels: rifampin, rifabutin, carbamazepine, efavirenz, ritonavir (≥400 mg bid), and phenobarbital. Increased concurrent drug levels: sirolimus, terfenadine, astemizole, cisapride, pimozide, quinidine, ergot derivatives
- **Alter dose: Cyclosporine:** increased cyclosporine; use half dose cyclosporine and monitor levels. **Tacrolimus:** increased tacrolimus levels 3-fold; use ⅓ dose tacrolimus; monitor levels. **Warfarin:** may increase prothrombin time; monitor. **Statins:** increased simvastatin lovastatin levels; consider pravastatin, rosuvastatin or atorvastatin. **Benzodiazepines:** midazolam, triazolam, and alprazolam increased levels expected; reduce benzodiazepine dose. **Calcium channel blockers:** nifedipine and felodipine level increases expected; may need dose decrease. **Methadone:** increases methadone's pharmacologically active R-enantiomer by a mean of 47%. There were no cases of withdrawal or detectable overdose among 16 methadone recipients given voriconazole 200 mg qd (*AAC* 2007,51:110). Caution is advised, since reduced dose of methadone may be indicated. **Sulfonylureas:** tolbutamide, glipizide and glyburide level increases expected; monitor blood glucose. **Vinca alkaloids:** increaced vincristine and vinblastine levels expected; dose may be reduced to avoid neurotoxicity. **Phenytoin:** decreased voriconazole 70% and increase phenytoin levels 80%; use voriconazole 400 mg po q12h or 5 mg/kg q12h; monitor phenytoin levels. **Omeprazole:** AUC increased 4-fold; voriconazole C_{max} and AUC increased 15% and 40%, respectively; reduce omeprazole to half dose (*Br J Clin Pharm* 2003;56 Suppl 1:56). **Oral contraceptives:** ethinyl estradiol AUC increased 61%, norethindrone AUC increased 53%; monitor for ADRs related to these oral contraceptives. **Clopidogrel:** may decrease efficacy of clopidogre; avoid. **Colchicine:** voriconazole may increase colchicine leve; consider decreasing colchicine dose.
- **Antiretroviral agents:** See pg. 208t.

5 Drugs

SIDE EFFECTS

- **Visual effects** are most common; 30% in clinical trials; these include altered visual perception, color change, blurred vision, and/or photophobia. Changes are dose related, reversible and infrequently require discontinuing therapy, but patients should be warned.
- **Rash** in 6%, including rare cases of Stevens-Johnson syndrome, erythema multiforme and toxic epidermal necrolysis.
- **Hepatotoxicity:** Elevated transaminases in 13%, usually resolves with continued drug administration. Serious hepatic toxicity is rare, but supplier recommends monitoring liver enzymes.
- **Toxic encephalopathy** attributed to high levels has been reported (*AAC* 2007;51:137; *CID* 2008;46:212). Response has been rapid and complete with stopping the drug.

PREGNANCY: Category D. Teratogenic in rodents and congenital anomalies in rabbits.

XANAX – see Alprazolam (pg. 209)

ZALCITABINE (ddC) This drug has been discontinued.

ZERIT – see Stavudine (pg. 378)

ZIAGEN – see Abacavir (pg. 179)

ZIDOVUDINE (AZT, ZDV)

TRADE NAME: *Retrovir, Combivir* (AZT/3TC), *Trizivir* (AZT/3TC/ABC) (ViiV Healthcare/GlaxoSmithKline), and generic

CLASS: Nucleoside analog reverse transcriptase inhibitor (NRTI)

FORMULATIONS, REGIMENS AND COST:

- **Forms**
  - AZT: 100 and 300 mg tabs; 10 mg/mL IV solution; 10 mg/mL oral solution.
  - AZT/3TC: 300/150 mg tabs (*Combivir*)
  - AZT/3TC/ABC: 300/150/300 mg tabs (*Trizivir*)
- **Regimens:** AZT: 300 mg bid or 200 mg tid; AZT/3TC or AZT/3TC/ABC: 1 tab bid.
- **AWP:** AZT, $297/mo; AZT/3TC, $993/mo; AZT/3TC/ABC, $1,608.36/mo. Generic AZT is now available at $0.50/300 mg tab (*Roxane*) or $30/mo.

Drugs

- **Food:** No effect
- **Renal failure:** CrCl <15 mL/min – 100 mg tid or 300 mg qd. AZT/3TC (*Combivir*) and AZT/3TC/ABC (*Trizivir*) co-formation: not recommended with CrCl <50 mL/min
- **Hepatic failure:** *Trivizir* contraindicated with severe liver disease. AZT, *Combivir:* standard dose.
- **Combination to avoid:** AZT/d4T
- **Combination to use with caution:**
  □ AZT plus ganciclovir or valgancyclovir: marrow suppression
  □ AZT plus ribavirin: Additive anemia; may need EPO
  □ AZT plus EPO: Hold EPO when Hgb >13 g/dl (see EPO)
  □ AZT plus cancer chemotherapy: marrow suppression
- **ACTG 076 protocol:** Intrapartum regimen is 2 mg/kg IV over 1 h, then 1 mg/kg/h until delivery.

PATIENT ASSISTANCE PROGRAM: 800-722-9294

CLINICAL TRIALS: FDA-approved in 1987 based on a controlled clinical trial showing significant short-term benefit in preventing AIDS-defining opportunistic infections and death (*NEJM* 1987;317:185). Early studies (ACTG 019, 076, 175, Concord, etc.) became sentinel reports. Despite 15 years of use, resistance in recently transmitted strains is only about 2-10% (*NEJM* 2002;347:385). AZT is commonly paired with 3TC (*Combivir*), or ABC/3TC (*Trizivir*) as the nucleoside components of ART regimens. Potency of these regimens is well established.

- **ACTG 384** showed that AZT/3TC/EFV was superior to ddI/d4T/EFV (*NEJM* 2003;349:2293), but in **GS-934** TDF/FTC/EFV was superior to AZT/3TC+EFV in terms of viral suppression to <50 c/mL (80% vs. 70%), rates of toxicity, CD4 response at 48 weeks (+90/mm^3 vs. +58/mm^3), and adverse reactions requiring discontinuation (4% vs. 9%; *NEJM* 2006;354:251). Follow-up at 96 weeks demonstrated greater loss of limb fat and more M184V mutations in patients in the AZT/3TC arm (*JAIDS* 2006;43:535). A Cochrane Review comparing AZT and TDF containing ART regimens concluded that TDF was superior in terms of CD4 response, tolerance, adherence and less resistance (*Cochrane Database Syst Rev* 2010;6:CD008740).

RESISTANCE: The thymidine analog mutations (TAMs) are 41L, 67N, 70R, 210W, 215Y/F, and 219Q/E. A total of 3-6 mutations result in a 100-fold decrease in sensitivity. About 5-10% of recipients of AZT + ddI as dual NRTI therapy develop the Q151M complex, and a larger number develop the T69S insertion mutation, both of which confer high-level resistance to AZT, ddI, ddC, d4T, 3TC and ABC. The M184V mutation that confers high-level 3TC resistance delays resistance or improves susceptibility to AZT unless there are multiple TAMs. It may also prevent the emergence of multinucleoside mutations, which are now very uncommon. Analysis of patients with early HIV infection

Drugs

5

indicates that 2-10% have genotypic mutations associated with reduced susceptibility to AZT (*NEJM* 2002;347:385).

PHARMACOLOGY

- **Bioavailability:** 60%; high-fat meals may decrease absorption. CSF levels: 60% serum levels (CSF:plasma ratio=0.3-1.35) (*Lancet* 1998; 351:1547). Another report showed a median CSF concentration of 6% of plasma levels which was 4.3-fold above the IC_{50} for wild-type virus (*Arch Neurol* 2008;65:65: *AIDS* 2009;23:1359). CNS penetration score is highest: rank 4 (*Neurology* 2011;76:693).

- **T½:** 1.1 h; Renal failure: 1.4 h; intracellular: 3 h

- **Elimination:** Metabolized by liver to glucuronide (GAZT) that is renally excreted.

- **Dose modification in renal failure or hepatic failure:** Excreted in urine as active drug (14-18%) and GAZT metabolite (60-74%). In severe renal failure (CrCl <18 mL/min), AZT half-life is increased from 1.1 to 1.4 hrs and GAZT half-life increased from 0.9 to 8.0 hrs. Dosing recommendation: GFR >15 mL/min – 300 mg bid; GFR <15 mL/mm – 300 mg qd; hemodialysis and peritoneal dialysis – 300 mg qd. No dose modification with liver disease.

SIDE EFFECTS

- **Subjective:** GI intolerance, altered taste (dysgeusia), insomnia, myalgias, asthenia, malaise, and/or headaches are common and are dose related (*Ann Intern Med* 1993;118:913). Most patients can be managed with symptomatic treatment.

- **Marrow suppression:** Related to marrow reserve, dose and duration of treatment, and stage of disease (*J Viral Hepatol* 2006;13:683; *HIV Med* 2007;8:483). **Anemia** may occur within 4-6 wks, and neutropenia is usually seen after 12-24 wks. Marrow examination in patients with AZT-induced anemia may be normal or show reduced RBC precursors. Severe anemia should be managed by discontinuing AZT or giving erythropoietin concurrently (see pg. 263, 520). **Neutropenia** and ANC <750/mm³ should be managed by discontinuing AZT or giving G-CSF concurrently (see pg. 291). Most patients with pre-existing HIV-associated anemia have increased Hb with ART that includes AZT, but this response is slower than with other NRTIs (*JAIDS* 2008;48:163).

- **Myopathy:** Rare dose-related complication possibly due to mitochondrial toxicity. Clinical features are leg and gluteal muscle weakness and/or pain, elevated LDH and CPK, muscle biopsy showing ragged red fibers, and abnormal mitochondria (*NEJM* 1990; 322:1098); response to discontinuation of AZT occurs within 2-4 wks. The mechanism is unclear (*Pharmacology* 2008;82:83).

- **Macrocytosis:** Noted within 4 wks of starting AZT in virtually all patients and serves as crude indicator of adherence.

Drugs

- **Class adverse reaction:** Lactic acidosis, often with steatosis, is a complication ascribed to all NRTIs but primarily to d4T and, to a lesser degree, ddI and AZT. This complication should be considered in patients with fatigue, abdominal pain, nausea, vomiting, and dyspnea. Laboratory tests show elevated serum lactate, CPK, ALT and/or LDH, and reduced serum bicarbonate ± increased anion gap. Abdominal CT scan or liver biopsy may show steatosis. This is a life-threatening complication. Pregnant women and obese women appear to be at increased risk. NRTIs should be stopped or there should be a change to NRTIs that are unlikely to cause mitochondrial toxicity such as TDF and ABC. Lipoatrophy, also most commonly associated with d4T or d4T+ddI, also occurs with AZT therapy. In ACTG 384, lipoatrophy was observed in both the ddI+d4T and AZT/3TC arms, but its onset was slower in the AZT/3TC-treated patients. There is also evidence that AZT-induced lipoatrophy may be less reversible than lipoatrophy caused by d4T. See pg. 132-134.
- **Fingernail discoloration** with dark bluish discoloration at base of nail noted at 2-6 wks.
- **Carcinogenicity:** Long-term treatment with high doses in mice caused vaginal neoplasms; relevance to humans is not known.

DRUG INTERACTIONS: Use with caution with **ribavirin** (anemia). Additive or synergistic against HIV with ddI, ABC, IFN-alfa, and foscarnet *in vitro*; antagonism with **ganciclovir** and **d4T**. AZT and d4T should not be given concurrently due to *in vitro* and *in vivo* evidence of antagonism resulting from competition for phosphorylation (*JID* 2000;182:321). Clinical significance of interaction with ganciclovir (in vitro) is unknown. **Methadone** increases levels of AZT 30-40%; AZT has no effect on methadone levels (*JAIDS* 1998;18:435). Marrow suppression usually precludes concurrent use with ganciclovir. Other marrow-suppressing drugs should be used with caution: **TMP-SMX, dapsone, pyrimethamine, flucytosine, interferon, adriamycin, vinblastine, sulfadiazine, vincristine, amphotericin B,** and **hydroxyurea. Probenecid** increases levels of AZT, but concurrent use is complicated by a high incidence of rash reactions to probenecid.

- **Fluconazole, atovaquone, valproic acid may increase AZT levels.**

PREGNANCY: Category C. AZT is advocated as preferred (with 3TC and a third agent) for all pregnant women to prevent perinatal transmission and for maternal health. Exceptions are maternal intolerance or *in vitro* resistance (see pg. 160, 166). The data on efficacy of AZT for preventing prenatal HIV transmission were well established with ACTG 076 (*NEJM* 1994;331:1173). This effect is presumably due to reduction in maternal VL, but also by other mechanisms that are poorly understood (*NEJM* 1996;335:484). More recent studies show that the rates of HIV transmission are far lower with HAART than with AZT monotherapy (0-2% vs. 8.8%) (*JAIDS* 2002;29:484). Extensive pharmacokinetic studies show that AZT levels are not significantly altered by pregnancy so standard doses are advocated (*NEJM* 1994;331:1173).

With regard to infant safety, concerns have been raised regarding hypospadias, vaginal and other tumors and mitochondrial toxicity. One report showed an increased rate of hypospadias (7/752 vs. 2/895 [p=0.007]) (*JAIDS* 2007;44:299), but this risk has not been observed in other studies or in the HIV Pregnancy Registry with over 1,500 cases. Two transplacental carcinogenicity studies in mice showed increases in rates of tumors, especially vaginal cancer (*J Natl Cancer Inst* 1997;89:1602; *Fundam Appl Toxicol* 1997;38:195). The relevance of these studies is not established since doses used produced far higher AZT exposures than are seen clinically, the relevance of such animal models of carcinogenesis is not established, and the HIV Pregnancy Registry has not confirmed the association, with reports on over 1,500 AZT exposures. The rate of birth defects associated with AZT first trimester exposures in the Registry reported through July 31, 2010 was 113/3,534 (3.2%).

An earlier report from France found evidence of mitochondrial toxicity with neurologic consequences in 12 infants exposed to AZT *in utero* (*Lancet* 1999;354:1084). Subsequent reviews with data on 20,000 infants exposed to AZT failed to show any neurologic, immunologic, oncologic, or cardiac complications (*NEJM* 2000; 343:759; *NEJM* 2000;343:805; *AIDS* 1998;12:1805; *JAMA* 1999; 281:151; *JAIDS* 1999;20:464). An expert NIH panel concluded that the benefit of decreasing risk of perinatal transmission exceeded the hypothetical concerns of transplacental carcinogenesis and these complications have not been supported in the Pregnancy Registry as summarized above.

ZITHROMAX – see Azithromycin (pg. 205)

ZOVIRAX – see Acyclovir (pg. 186)

6 | Management of Infections
(Pathogens are listed alphabetically)

Recommendations are based largely on Benson C., et al., 2009 NIH/CDC/IDSA Guidelines for Prevention and Treatment of Opportunistic Infections in HIV-Infected Adults and Adolescents, available online at www.mmhiv.com/link/2009-OI-NIH-CDC-IDSA; American Thoracic Society Guidelines: *Am J Resp Crit Care Med*;2011;183:96-128)

Aspergillus spp.
Invasive Pulmonary or Disseminated Aspergillosis

PRESENTATION: Risks include neutropenia, chronic corticosteroids, broad spectrum antibiotics and prior lung disease. HIV specific risks are CD4 count <100 cells/mm³, prior AIDS-defining diagnosis and lack of ART (*Chest* 1998;114:131; *CID* 2000;31:1253; *Chest* 1998;114:251). There are two recognized clinical forms in AIDS patients:

1) Pneumonia or tracheobronchitis: with pneumonia there is an infiltrate that is diffuse, focal or cavitary; the "halo" or "air crescent" sign on CT scan suggests this diagnosis (*Lancet* 2000;355:423). Clinical symptoms include fever, cough, dyspnea, pleurisy, hemoptysis and /or hypoxemia. With tracheobronchitis, there is an ulcerative or exudative pseudomembrane adherent to the trachea seen by bronchoscopy (*CID* 1993;17:344). Symptoms include cough, fever, dyspnea, stridor and wheezing.

2) Extrapulmonary: Includes meningoencephalitis, osteomyelitis, sinusitis and skin/soft tissue aspergillosis.

DIAGNOSIS: The usual diagnostic criteria are repeated positive culture from a likely clinical source, or typical organisms with dichotomous branching hyphae in respiratory secretions plus typical symptoms, or with histopathology. The most common species is *A. fumigatus*; other reported species in AIDS patients include *A. flavus*, *A. niger* and *A. terreus* (60-65%) (*CID* 2001;33:1824). Assays for galactomannan in serum and BAL fluid are recommended primarily for stem cell transplant recipients; utility in AIDS patients is less well established (*Med Mycol* 2008;14:1; *AIDS* 2007;21:1990). Galactomannan is also detected with *Penicillium marneffei* infections in HIV patients with pulmonary infection (*BMC Infect Dis* 2010;10:44).

Diagnostic criteria from the National Mycosis Study Group are as follows: <u>Definite</u> = positive histology + positive culture, or positive culture from a normally sterile site. <u>Probable</u> = two positive cultures of sputum or one positive bronchoscopy + appropriate host (AIDS, prednisone, ANC <500/mL) (*CID* 2001;33:1824). Halo sign on CT scan is highly suggestive (*Lancet* 2000;355:423).

TREATMENT (*AM J RESP CRIT CARE MED* 2011;183:96)

- **Preferred regimen:** (invasive disease): voriconazole or liposomal amphotericin (see regimens below), until clinical improvement and CD4 >200 cells/mm^3 (*NEJM* 2002; 347:408). Note voriconazole drug interactions with NNRTIs and PIs (see pg. 208t). Options for drug interactions include: 1) therapeutic drug monitoring; 2) use of alternative agents, such as amphotericin, caspofungin or posaconazole; 3) combination therapy with amphtericin B + an azole or echinocandin or an azole + an echinocandin; 4) voriconazole + amphotericin or caspofungin; 5) voriconazole with RAL-based ART; or 6) higher doses of voriconazole.

Regimens*

- □ <u>Primary</u>: Voriconazole 6 mg/kg IV q12h x 1 day then 4 mg/kg q12h IV. After clinical improvement: 200 mg po bid[†] until resolution or stabilization. See pg. 413-416.

- □ <u>Alternative</u>: Liposomal amphotericin B 3-5 mg/kg/d until improved, then voriconazole 200 mg q12h or itraconazole 400-600 mg qd until resolution or stabilization

- □ <u>Salvage</u>: Caspofungin 70 mg IV x 1, then 50 mg IV/d or posaconazole 400 mg po bid

- □ <u>Chronic necrotizing pulmonary aspergillus</u>: Voriconazole 200 mg po bid or itraconazole 400-600 mg qd until resolution or stabiization[†]

  * Duration: Treat until clinical response established and CD4 count >200 cells/mm^3

  † Monitor serum concentrations (azoles).

- **Comments**

  - □ <u>Amphotericin</u> is no longer the preferred drug for invasive aspergillosis in non-AIDS patients based on a large randomized trial showing voriconazole was superior (*NEJM* 2002;347:408). High doses of liposomal amphotericin (10 mg/kg/d vs. 3-5 mg/kg/d) didn't improve outcome (*CID* 2007;44:1289). Preferred agent is voriconazole. A concern with HIV-infected patients is drug interaction between voriconazole and PIs or NNRTIs. See pg. 413-416.

  - □ <u>Voriconazole:</u> A randomized trial in 277 patients with invasive aspergillosis demonstrated that voriconazole was significantly better than amphotericin (1-1.5 mg/kg/d) with higher rates of response (53% vs. 32%) and lower rates of adverse side effects other than visual disturbance in 45% (*NEJM* 2002;347:408). This trial clearly made voriconazole the preferred drug (*Am J Resp Crit Care* 2011;183:96).

- Caspofungin was investigated in 83 patients with invasive aspergillosis, including 71 (86%) who were refractory to alternative treatment. Results were favorable in 37 (45%), including 32/64. An observational study showed a favorable response in 57 of 101 (56%) patients (*BMC Inf Dis* 2010;10:182). Caspofungin is not recommended in the 2011 ATS recommendations for aspergillosis based on "lack of robust data" (*Am J Respir Crit Care Med* 2011;83:96).

- Posaconazole and ravuconazole show excellent *in vitro* activity against *Aspergillus* (*AAC* 2005;49:5136; *JCM* 2006;44:1782). In 107 salvage patients treated with posaconazole (800 mg qd), found a "global response" rate of 42% was reported (*CID* 2007;44:2). A retrospective review of 79 patients given posaconazole (400 mg bid) for chronic pulmonary aspergillosis showed a response rate of 61% at 6 months and 46% at 12 months (*CID* 2010;51:1383). See pg. 208t.

- Chronic necrotizing aspergillosis or "semi-invasive aspergillosis": There are no randomized trials, but case series favor oral voriconazole or itraconazole (*Am J Resp Crit Care Med* 2011;93:96). Initial IV treatment with amphotericin or voriconazole should be considered.

- Duration: The length of treatment has not been well defined. Recommendation is to treat until there is "clinical resolution or stabilization" and the CD4 count is >200 cells/mm^3

RESPONSE: Prognosis with invasive pulmonary disease in AIDS patients is poor without immune reconstitution (*CID* 1992;14:141; *Clin Microbiol Rev* 1999; 12:310). The trials summarized above show response rates of about 20-50% with recommended regimens. Median survival in a review of 110 patients with AIDS was 3 mos (*CID* 2000;3:1253). In a review of 33 reported cases of CNS aspergillosis in AIDS patients, all were fatal; amphotericin was uniformly unsuccessful in these cases (*Medicine* 2000;79:269). Patients unresponsive to amphotericin should be given voriconazole or posaconazole and vice versa. IRIS with a severe bronchial mucus impaction has been reported (*Eur Clin Microbiol Infect Dis* 2005;24:628).

Bartonella henselae and *quintana*
Bacillary Angiomatosis, Trench Fever, Peliosis Hepatitis

RISK: *Bartonella* has 21 species, including 5 that infect people, but disease in HIV-infected patients has been associated only with *B. quintana* and *B. henselae*. The latter is epidemiologically linked to cat exposure possibly through the cat flea as the vector. *B. quintana* is linked to body louse infestation, primarily in homeless people. Control is based on prevention of cat infestation, elimination of fleas, avoidance of cat scratches (*B. henselae*), and avoidance and treatment of body lice (*B. quintana*).

6 Management of Infections

PRESENTATION: *B. henselae* and *B. quintana* cause bartonellosis, which may involve every organ. Most common is bacillary angiomatosis (BA), with red papular skin lesions that resemble Kaposi sarcoma in patients with a CD4 count that is usually <50 cells/mm³ (*CID* 2005;40:1545; *Dermatology* 2000;21:326). Bacillary peliosis causes angiomatous masses in visceral organs, most commonly the liver as peliosis hepatitis (*B. henselae*), and less often endocarditis, eye involvement, transverse myelitis, CNS lesions, and bacteremia presenting as FUO, typically in homeless persons with low CD4 counts (*CID* 2003;37:559). Most HIV-infected patients with bartonellosis have chronic *Bartonella* infection for months or years with BA and intermittent bactermia.

DIAGNOSIS: is established with tissue histology using Warthin-Starry silver stain to detect clusters of organisms. Serology (IFA) is available from the CDC, but cross reactions with other bacteria may be seen, and patients with advanced HIV disease may not generate antibody, so up to 25% are false negatives (*CID* 2003;37:559; *Lancet* 1992;339:1443). PCR is the most sensitive test; these assays are available in some commercial labs (*CID* 2010;51:131; *JCM* 1999; 37:4045). Histology plus PCR is the preferred diagnostic test for pathogen detection in tissue specimens (*JCM* 1999;37:993; *Diagn Microbiol Infect Dis* 2005;53:75). The organism is hard to grow, but this can be sometimes be done using EDTA tubes with lysis centrifugation and incubation for up to 6 wks (*CID* 2003;37:559; *NEJM* 1992;327:1625).

TREATMENT: See *MMWR* 2009;58 RR11;1-166.

Severe cutaneous disease, peliosis hepatis, bacteremia and osteomyelitis: Erythromycin 500 mg po or IV qid or doxycycline 100 mg po or IV bid for >3 mos. The duration of treatment should be 3 mos for BA. Alternative: azithromycin 500 mg po qd or clarithromycin 500 mg po bid (*CID* 1993;17:264; *Pediatr Inf Dis* 1998;17:447). Quinolones , betalactams and TMP-SMX show variable activity and are not recommended.

CNS Infection and severe infections: Doxycycline 100 mg po or IV bid or erythromycin (clarithromycin or azithromycin can be considered) +/- rifampin 300 mg po or IV q12h (if not contraindicated) x ≥4 mos.

- **Comments**
  - □ Prevention: Macrolide for MAC prophylaxis is protective.
  - □ May have severe Jarisch-Herxheimer reaction in the first 48 hrs.
  - □ Duration: Patients should be treated until CD4 is >200 cells/mm³.
  - □ *In vitro* sensitivity tests do not predict response. Lesions can develop in the presence of TMP-SMX, fluoroquinolones and betalactams. These drugs should not be used despite *in vitro* activity.

RESPONSE: The response is usually dramatic for cutaneous bacillary angiotomasis with resolution by one month. Visceral bacillary angiomatosis responds more slowly. Patients who relapse should be retreated for 4-6 mos. With failure to respond or repeated relapses consider alternative agents. IRIS has been associated with lymphadenitis and splenitis, but it is rare (*Medicine* 2002;81:213; *AIDS* 2002;16:1429).

Candida spp.
Thrush (Oral Candidiasis)

PRESENTATION and **DIAGNOSIS:** Pseudomenbraneous candidiasis is most common: white painless plaques on the buccal or pharyngeal mucosa or tongue surface that can easily be scraped off, typically in patients with a risk factor: CD4 <250 cells/mm^3, antibiotics, chronic steroids, etc. The diagnosis is usually based on the appearance of the lesions. The ease of scraping the plaques off distinguishes thrush from oral hairy leukoplakia, which is typically located on the lateral surfaces of the tongue. If lab confirmation is necessary, use KOH prep. Culture is best used for speciation and sensitivity testing in patients with refractory infections (*Medicine* 2003:82:39) but not for diagnosis due to high rates of colonization.

TREATMENT: INITIAL INFECTION

- **Preferred regimen**
  - Fluconazole 100 mg qd po x 7-14 days. Preferred by some since it is better tolerated and more convenient than topical agents (*CID* 2004;35:144)
  - Clotrimazole oral troches 10 mg 5x/d *(HIV Clin Trials* 2000;1:47) until lesions resolve, usually 7-14 days.
  - Nystatin 500,000 units (4-6 mL) gargled 4-5x day or 1-2 flavored pastilles 4-5x/d x 7-14 days.
  - Miconazole mucoadhesive tabs qd (*JAIDS* 2004;35:144; *HIV Clin Trials* 2010;11:186).

- **Regimens for refractory and recurrent infections**
  - Treatment failure with topical agents: fluconazole 100-200 mg po qd
  - Treatment failure with fluconazole: 1) posaconazole oral suspension 100 mg bid x 1, then 100 mg qd (*CID* 2007;44:607); 2) itraconazole soln 200 mg po qd; 3) voriconazole 200 mg po or IV bid; 4) caspofungin 50 mg IV/d; 5) amphotericin B 0.3 mg/kg/d and 6) micafungin 150 mg IV/d. See azoles pg. 208.
  - Recurrent disease: fluconazole 100 mg 3x/wk until CD4 count >200 cells/mm^3 or posaconazole oral solution 100 mg po bid x 1, then 100 mg qd

- **Comments**
  - Oral fluconazole is considered the drug of choice since some

6 Management of Infections

studies show superiority to topical agents, it is better tolerated and is more convienient (*CID* 2004;38:161; *Cochrane Database* 2010;CD003940).

- Posaconazole is as effective as fluconazole, it has a more sustained benefit (*CID* 2006:42:1179), and it is effective in 75% of fluconazole refractory cases (*CID* 2007;44:607). It is expensive – $1500/10 days.

- Itraconazole is as effective as fluconazole but less well tolerated.

- Ketoconazole is not recommended because fluconazole and posaconazole are better tolerated, have more predictable absorption and fewer drug intereactions (*JAC* 2006;57:384)

- Immune reconstitution is highly effective in preventing thrush.

- *In vitro* azole resistance is most common with prolonged prior azole exposure and late-stage HIV infection with CD4 count <50 cells/mm^3 (*CID* 2000;30:749). This is due to a single strain of *C. albicans* that becomes progressively more resistant (*Eur J Clin Microbiol Infect Dis* 1997;16:601) and/or high rates of non-*albicans* species (*Lancet* 2002;359:1135; *HIV Clin Trials* 2000;1:47, *Clin Rev Microbiol* 2000;26:59). The most common non-albicans types are *C. glabrata* and *C. tropicalis* (*Indian J Dermatol* 2009;54:385). Some report good response (48/50) to fluconazole despite *in vitro* resistance (*JID* 1996;174:821).

- Azole drug interactions: Fluconazole can be given with EFV, PIs and boosted PIs except TPV/r and EFV using standard doses; NVP AUC increased 2-fold with fluconazole risking hepatotoxicity (see pg. 208t). Voriconazole AUC decreased 39% with RTV 200 mg qd, and AUC of PIs may be increased; avoid or monitor for toxicity. Voriconazole levels are decreased with EFV by 77% and increased with ETR; use EFV 300 mg qd + voriconazole 400 mg bid (monitor voriconazole levels).

RESPONSE: Most respond within 7-14 days, except with extensive prior azole exposure and CD4 count <50 cells/mm^3 (*CID* 2000;30:749; *CID* 1997;24:28). Failure of fluconazole: 1) Use empiric treatment (see above); or 2) culture to determine *in vitro* sensitivity; empiric therapy with posaconazole or itraconazole solution, which are favored second line agents in 2008 NIH/CDC/IDSA guidelines. Relapses within 3 mos after treatment are common and require intermittent therapy, maintenance therapy, or immune reconstitution.

MAINTENANCE: Optimal prevention is immune reconstitution and avoidance of steroids and antibacterials. Dapsone may be considered for PCP prophylaxis in place of TMP-SMX since the antibacterial activity of TMP-SMX promotes *Candida* growth. Chronic maintenance oral fluconazole or possibly itraconazole are recommended for recurrences that are severe or frequent (*NEJM* 1995;332:700; *Ann Intern Med* 1997;126: 689; *CID* 1998;27:1369). Continuous use is not associated with more resistance than episodic treatment (*CID* 2005;41:1473), but long duration may increase risk of resistance.

- **Preferred regimens**
  - □ Fluconazole 100 mg qd po or 200 mg 3x/wk.
  - □ Itraconazole oral solution 100-200 mg qd on empty stomach.
- **Comments**
  - □ Immune reconstitution is highly effective therapy (*AIDS* 2000;14: 979).
  - □ Resistance: Potential problems with use of continuous or frequent intermittent fluconazole include possible azole resistance, drug interactions, and cost. Risks for azole resistant *Candida* infections are prolonged azole exposure (although this was not shown in ACTG 323), use of TMP/SMX prophylaxis for PCP, and low CD4 count (*JID* 1996;173:219). Some authorities try to avoid continued use of fluconazole except where necessary due to concern for resistance, but supporting data are inconsistent, and the largest controlled trial is not supportive (see ACTG 323 results below).

Esophagitis: See pg. 503-504.

PRESENTATION: Symptoms include diffuse retrosternal pain, dysphagia, and/or odynophagia, usually without fever. Thrush is usually present, and the CD4 count is typically <100 cells/mm³. Cases with typical features are usually treated empirically; rapid response to standard treatment strongly supports this diagnosis. Endoscopy, when performed, shows white plaques on the esophageal mucosa, and histology and culture show *Candida* species. A 2010 report of upper endoscopy in HIV-infected patients noted the expected substantial decrease in *Candida* esophagitis, but a significant increase in the frequency of *H. pylori* infection and GERD (*HIV Med* 2010;11:412).

TREATMENT: INITIAL INFECTION

- **Preferred regimen:** fluconazole 200-400 mg qd po or IV x 14-21 days.
- **Alternative regimens:** See antifungal agents in Chapter 5 for drug interactions with ART agents, including azoles (pg. 208).

Fluconazole-refractory esophagitis

- □ Posaconazole 400 mg po bid
- □ Itraconazole oral solution 200 mg po qd
- □ Voriconazole 200 mg po or IV bid
- □ Caspofugin 50 mg IV qd
- □ Micafungin 150 mg IV qd
- □ Anidulafungin 100 mg IV x1 then 50 mg qd
- □ Amphotericin B 0.6 mg/kg/d IV

6 Management of Infections

MAINTENANCE: Only with relapsing disease

- **Preferred regimen:** Fluconazole 100-200 mg qd.
- **Comments:**
  - □ Consider <u>maintenance therapy</u> in patients with recurrent esophagitis. This may increase the possibility of resistance (*JID* 1996;173:219), but a large comparative ACTG 323 trial showed no difference in rates of refractory candidiasis with continuous versus episodic fluconazole (*CID* 2006;41:1473). Best treatment is immune reconstitution (*JID* 1998;27:1291; *AIDS* 2000;14:23).
  - □ <u>Relapse rate</u> is high in absence of immune reconstitution (*JID* 1998;27:1291; *AIDS* 2000;14:23).
  - □ <u>Fluconazole</u> is preferred over ketoconazole and itraconazole due to more predictable absorption. It is preferred over voriconazole and echinocandins due to greater experience in HIV-infected patients.
  - □ <u>Caspofungin</u> was superior to amphotericin (0.5 mg/kg/d) in one comparative trial (*AAC* 2002;46:451) and comparable to fluconazole in another (*CID* 2001;33:1529).
  - □ <u>Voriconazole</u> 200 mg bid is equivalent to fluconazole for initial treatment *(CID* 2001;33:1447) but hard to give with EFV and PIs.
  - □ <u>Posaconazole</u> (200 mg x 1, then 100 mg qd) was also equivalent to fluconazole in HIV-associated thrush or *Candida* esophagitis (*CID* 2006;42:1179). Neither study demonstrated a clinical or mycologic advantage of the new drug over fluconazole, but treatment of fluconazole-resistant candidiasis is a potential role. EFV decreases posaconazole AUC by 50%; avoid this combination. Posaconazole increases ATV/r AUC by 150% and ATV AUC by 268%; monitor for ATV adverse effects.

RESPONSE: Most (85-90%) patients respond within 7-14 days (*CID* 2004;39:842). For refractory cases: 1) Perform endoscopy to establish diagnosis ± fungal culture for *in vitro* sensitivity tests, or 2) Change therapy: increase fluconazole dose, use alternative azole (voriconazole or itraconazole), or IV treatment (caspofungin, amphotericin or fluconazole). Fluconazole-resistant *Candida* esophagitis will often respond to itraconazole at least temporarily. Many patients relapse after therapy and require maintenance or immune reconstitution.

Vaginitis (*MMWR* 2010;59:RR-12)

DIAGNOSIS: Typical symptoms are mucosal burning and pruritis combined with a creamy yellow-white discharge. Examination shows erythema and yellow-white adherent discharge; 10% KOH prep or gram stain show yeast or pseudohyphae. Most cases are in immunocompetent women. Culture is rarely necessary except to detect a non-*albicans* species (rare) or fluconazole resistance (also rare).

TREATMENT

- **Preferred regimens:** Intravaginal azoles, usually 3-7 days

  □ Over-the-counter for intravaginal application: Butoconazole, clotrimazole, miconazole and tioconazole: These are provided in creams at various concentrations for application for various durations. Use suppliers prescribing instructions.

  □ Prescription agents:

  - Fluconazole 150 mg 1 tab po x 1
  - Butoconazole 2% 5 gm IV* x 1
  - Nystatin 100,000 unit tab IV* qd x 14/d
  - Terconazole 0.4% cream IV* qd x 7/d
  - Terconazole 0.8% cream 5 gm IV* qd x 3/d
  - Terconazole 80 mg supp qd x 3/d
  - *IV=intra-vaginal application

- **Preferred systemic azoles**

  □ Fluconazole 150 mg po x 1.

  □ Itraconazole oral solution 200 mg po qd x 3-7 days

- **Complicated or recurrent** *Candida* **vaginitis**

  □ Topical azole daily x 7 days

  □ Fluconazole 150 mg/wk

- **Comments**

  □ Treatment is identical for women with and without HIV infection.

  □ Clotrimazole, tioconazole, and miconazole are available over the counter. Self-administration advised only if prior diagnosis and typical symptoms.

  □ Azole-resistant strains of *Candida* are rare causes of vaginitis.

  □ Severe disease: Topical azole x 7-14 days or oral fluconazole 150 mg po x 2 separated by 72 hrs.

  □ Pregnancy: Topical azole only.

  □ Probiotic treatment with *Lactobacilli* for prevention shows unconvincing evidence of efficacy (*JAC* 2006;58:266).

RESPONSE: Uncomplicated vaginitis (90% of all cases) responds rapidly. Complicated cases are prolonged or refractory, account for 10% of cases and are treated for >7 days.

MAINTENANCE (with ≥4 episodes/year): Clotrimazole 500 mg vaginal tablet every week, or fluconazole 100-150 mg po every week or ketoconazole 200 mg/wk po or itraconazole 400 mg/mo or 100 mg/wk, all x 6 mos. (Based on recommendations for women without HIV infection.)

Clostridium difficile (*C. difficile* infection or CDI)

FREQUENCY: Analysis of 44,778 HIV-infected persons followed for a mean of 2.6 years found that *C. difficile* was by far the leading bacterial agent of diarrhea, accounting for 607/1150 (54%) of cases with bacterial pathogens detected (*CID* 2005;41:1621). It is unclear whether HIV infection and immunosuppression predispose to CDI or if this simply represents the risk associated with frequent hospitalization and antibiotic exposure (*TOP HIV Med* 2007;15:94; *AIDS* 1994;8:557; *AIDS* 1993;17:109). A review of 3,245 patients with HIV infection discharged from 4 New York City hospitals from 1997-2001 showed 1,120 (35%) had diarrhea and only 23 (0.7%) had CDI (*JAIDS* 2001;31:542).

CLINICAL FEATURES: Watery diarrhea, often with a distinctive odor, fever, hypoalbuminemia, and leukocytosis are common. Nearly all patients have recent (within 2 weeks of onset) exposure to antibacterial agents, especially fluoroquinolones, extended spectrum cephalosporins or clindamycin. Infrequent causes drugs commonly used with HIV infection are TMP-SMX, narrow spectrum betalactams, and rifampin. Antiretrovirals, antivirals, antifungals, dapsone and INH are not implicated. The major risks are advanced age, antibiotic exposure and presence in a hospital or chronic care facility. HIV *per se* is not a clear risk.

■ TABLE 6-1: **Tests for *C. difficile* Infection (CDI) (All Require 1-2 hrs)**

Test	Detection	Comment
EIA	Detects toxin A or A+B	Sensitivity: 70-80%; Specificity >98% Major concern is false negatives
PCR for toxin B gene	Detects toxigenic C. difficile	Sensitivity: >99%; Specificity may be low in hospitalized pts due to high carriage rates of toxigenic *C. difficile*. Requires clinical correlations
Combination (EIA for toxins and EIA for *C. difficile*)	Detects *C. difficile* toxin and *C. difficile*	Two assays *C. difficile* toxin + /*C. difficile* + = CDI *C. difficile* toxin - /*C. difficile* - = No CDI *C. difficile* toxin - /*C. difficile* + may be false negative toxin; need alternate test for toxin

Caveats regarding stool tests for *C. difficile* infection (CDI)

■ Send only diarrheal stools

■ Test only one sample/4-7 days: Repeat tests using same lab method does not improve the yield (unless a different test is used)

■ Clinical correlations are critical

■ Test interpretation depends on test:
  □ toxin assays: problem of false negatives;
  □ PCR: problem of false positives;
  □ combination tests: problems of (+ antigen) and (- toxin); may be false negative toxin test indicating need for alternate toxin assay

NAP-1 STRAIN: In 2003 there was recognition of *C. difficile* cases that were more frequent, more severe, and more refractory to standard treatment (*NEJM* 2005;353:2442; *NEJM* 2005;353:2433; *NEJM* 2005; 353:2503). Clinical features include leukemoid reactions, toxic megacolon, shock, and renal failure. It now appears that many of these cases are caused by a unique strain of *C. difficile* designated NAP-1. This strain produces large amounts of toxin A and toxin B, possibly accounting for the unusual severity of cases (*Lancet* 2005;366:1079) and, unlike the vast majority of prior strains, it is resistant to fluoroquinolones *in vitro*. This may explain the high frequency with which these agents are now implicated (*CID* 2005;41:1254; *Topics HIV Med* 2007;15:94). There is no evidence that this is more or less common with HIV infection. A review of US hospital reports (ICD-9 codes) for 2000-2005 shows the incidence of CDI in hospital admissions increased from 5.5/10,000 in 2000 to 11.2 in 2005 and the mortality rate increased from 1.2% to 2.2% (*Emerg Infect Dis* 2008;14:929).

DIAGNOSIS: Contemporary lab tests are the EIA for *C. difficile* toxins AB (70-80% sensitive), PCR of the toxin B gene (very sensitive, but lacks specificity) and a combination test that simultaneously detect the organism and the toxin (*Ann Intern Med* 2009;151:176; *Infect Control Hosp Epidemiol* 2010;31:S35; *JCM* 2010;48:603) (see Table 6-1).

TREATMENT: Based on the 2010 IDSA/SHEA Guidelines (*Infect Control Hosp Epidemiol* 2010;31:431). All patients: Stop implicated antibiotic, avoid antiperistaltics (loperamide or narcotics) and avoid "the big three" (fluoroquinolones, clindamycin, and broad-spectrum betalactams).

- Mild to moderate disease: (WBC <15,000/mL and creatinine <1.5x baseline): oral metronidazole, 500 mg tid x 10-14 days.

- Serious disease (WBC ≥ 15,000/mL or creatinine > 1.5 x baseline): oral vancomycin 125 mg qid x 10-14 days (*Current Infect Dis Rep* 2009;11: 21; *CID* 2008;47:56).

- Severe and complicated disease (C. *difficile* infection with ileus, hypotension, toxic megacolon, leukemoid reaction, renal failure or ICU requirement): vancomycin 500 mg po qid, but with ileus deliver by N-G tube or per rectum in saline enema combined with IV metronidazole 500-750 mg IV tid. Consider IVIG and colectomy.

- Relapsing disease: First relapse: treat as initial infection. Subsequent relapses: vancomycin 125 mg po qid x 10-14 d, then 125 mg bid x 7 d, then 125 mg qd x 7 d, then 125 mg every 2-3 days for 2-8 wks.

- Infection control: Patients with CDI in acute and chronic care facilities need prompt infection control measures to prevent transmission. These include: 1) single room with bathroom until diarrhea resolves (or cohorting), 2) barrier precautions, 3) hand hygiene with soap and water, 4) terminal room cleaning with 1:10 household bleach and 5) antibiotic stewardship (*Clin Microbial Infect* 2008;14 Suppl 5:2-20; *Infect Control Hosp Epidimiol* 2010;31:431).

6 Management of Infections

RESPONSE: Fever usually resolves within 24 hrs and diarrhea resolves in an average of 5 days. Nearly all patients respond if there is no ileus. About 20-25% have relapses at 3-14 days after treatment stops. Poor prognostic signs are leukemoid reactions, ileus, pseudomembraneous colitis, lactate level >5 mmol/mL, renal failure or sepsis syndrome.

Coccidioides immitis

Coccidioidomycosis (*CID* 2005;41:1174; *Ann NY Acad Sci* 2007; 1111;336; *Am J Respir Crit Care Med* 2011;183:96; *CID* 2010;50:1)

CLINICAL FEATURES: Continues to be a relatively common cause of death in HIV-infected patients in endemic areas (California, Arizona) (*CID* 2006;42:1059). Risk of infection is higher with exposure in endemic areas, and risk of disseminated disease is higher in African-American or Filipino men, women in the second or third trimester of pregnancy and patients with immune deficiency, including those with a CD4 count <250 cells/mm^3 or AIDS. The usual presentation in patients with CD4 counts >250 cells/mm^3 is focal pneumonia, and with CD4 counts <250 cells/mm^3 it is often disseminated disease (90%) or meningitis (10%). Clinical features of disseminated disease include fever, generalized adenopathy, skin nodules or ulcers, hepatitis, bone/joint lesions, or peritonitis. The incidence of symptomatic coccidiodomycosis and its severity has decreased significantly in the HAART era (*CID* 2010;50:1). In a review of 29 cases from 2003-08, mean CD4 count at diagnosis was 369 cells/mm^3 and only two had extrapulmonary disease. The authors concluded that the incidence is substantially lower (about 8-fold in this clinic) in the HAART era and that those with CD4 counts >250 cells/mm^3 and receiving ART can be treated according to standard guidelines for immunocompetent hosts (*MMWR* 2009;58:1).

DIAGNOSIS: The diagnosis is established by 1) positive culture from any clinical specimens; 2) histopathology of tissues showing typical spherules; and 3) positive serology; *C. immitis* complement fixation (CF) serology with a titer >1:16 indicates disseminated disease. With meningitis the usual presentation is fever, lethargy, headache, nausea, and vomiting. CSF shows a mononuclear pleocytosis, glucose <50 mg/dL, and protein that is normal or slightly elevated. The diagnosis is established by positive CF serology in CSF (diagnostic); cultures are usually negative.

INITIAL TREATMENT

- <u>Focal pneumonia:</u> Fluconazole – 400 mg po qd or itraconazole-200 mg po tid x 3 days, then 200 mg po bid.

- <u>Diffuse pneumonia or non-meningeal extra-pulmonary:</u> Liposomal amphotericin B (5 mg/kg/d) or amphotericin B (0.7-1.0 mg/kg/d) IV until clinical improvement, then fluconazole (400 mg qd) or itraconazole (400 mg qd) for at least 1 year and often life long due to high rates of relapse.

- Meningitis: Fluconazole 400-1000 mg qd or itraconazole 400-600 mg qd IV or po; when clinically improved give maintenance fluconazole 400 mg qd or itraconazole 200 mg bid; consider intrathecal amphotericin if triazoles are ineffective. Treat for life due to high relapse rates (see pg. 208t).
- Maintenance therapy: Fluconazole 400 mg qd or itraconazole 200 mg bid.
- **Azole interactions with ART:** See pg. 208.
  - □ Meningitis should be treated with fluconazole (*Ann Intern Med.* 1993;119:28); alternative azoles include itraconazole (but poor CNS penetration) (*JAIDS* 1997;16:100), voriconazole (*CID* 2003; 36:1619; *AAC* 2004;48:2341) or posaconazole (*CID* 2005; 40:1770). Relapses are observed in 80% of cases when azoles are stopped (*Ann Intern Med* 1996;124:305), which is why lifelong treatment is recommended. IV amphotericin is considered ineffective. CF levels suggest response.
  - □ Diffuse pneumonitis or extrapulmonary (25-35%) is common even with CD4 counts >250 cells/mm³ (*Am J Med* 1995;98:249; *Am J Med* 1990;89:282), which is why lifelong treatment is recommended.
  - □ Fluconazole, itraconazole, and posaconazole: A therapeutic trial of fluconazole 400 mg qd vs. intraconazole 200 mg bid in 198 patients with non-meningeal disease found no significant difference; the trend favored itraconazole (*Ann Intern Med* 2000;133:676), although fluconazole is preferred for meningitis (*Ann Intern Med* 1993;119:28). Posaconazole has been effective in cases refractory to other azoles (*Chest* 2007;132:952), but experience is limited.
  - □ Azoles have largely replaced amphotericin, especially for chronic disease (*CID* 2006;42:1289).

RESPONSE: Clinical response is slow (weeks), and relapses are common. Follow CF titer every 12 wks to document response or relapse. Options for non-response include increasing the fluconazole dose, use of an alternative azole or amphotericin, and/or surgical debridement or drainage.

Cryptococcus neoformans
Cryptococcal Meningitis

PRESENTATION: (*NIAID* Mycosis Study Group Recommendations, *CID* 2000;30:710): The usual portal of entry is the lung, and many have pneumonitis, although it may be subclinical. The usual presentation is subacute meningitis with fever, headache, and malaise in a patient with a CD4 count <100 cells/mm³. Some patients are asymptomatic and many have non-meningeal sites of involvement, especially the skin, with vesicular or papular lesions that may resemble molluscum.

6 Management of Infections

CSF analysis should be performed whenever there is evidence of cryptococcal infection.

DIAGNOSIS: The diagnosis of cryptococcal meningitis is usually easy, with positive blood cultures in 50-70%, positive serum cryptococcal antigen in >95%, positive CSF culture in >95%, positive CSF cryptococcal antigen in >95%, and positive India ink in 60-80%. Lumbar puncture usually shows elevated opening pressure (>200 mm H_2O in 75%) and CSF shows increased protein (50-150 mg/dL) and mononuclear pleocytosis (5-100 mg/dL) (*NEJM* 1992;329:83; *NEJM* 1997;337:15).

TREATMENT: See Table 6-2.

- **Elevated intracranial pressure (ICP):** With focal neurologic signs or obtundation, obtain CNS imaging before LP to look for mass lesions that contraindicate LP.

■ TABLE 6-2: **Treatment of Cryptococcal Meningitis** (2008 NIH/CDC/IDSA Guidelines for Prevention and Treatment of Opportunistic Infections in Adults and Adolescents and 2010 IDSA Guidelines [*CID* 2010;50:291])

Preferred regimen [†]	Alternative

Induction (≥2 weeks)[†]
1) Amphotericin B 0.7-1.0 mg/kg/d*
  + flucytosine 25 mg/kg po qid
or
2) lipid amphotericin B 4-6 mg/kg/d
  IV + flucytosine
	Alternatives for induction & maintenance in rank order:
	1) ampho B 0.7-1.0 mg/kg/d, or liposomal ampho B 3-4 mg/kg/d, or ABLC 5 mg/kg/d for 4-6 weeks
	2) ampho B 0.7 mg/kg/d and fluconazole 800 mg/d x 2 wks, then fluconazole 800 mg/d po x >8 wks
	3) fluconazole >800 mg qd po (1200 mg qd favored) and flucytosine 100 mg/kg/d po in 4 divided doses x 6 wks
	4) fluconazole 800-2000 mg qd po x 10-12 wks
	5) itraconazole 200 mg bid po x 10-12 wks

Consolidation [†] (8 weeks) fluconazole 400 mg po qd (6 mg/kg/d)	1) itraconazole 200 mg bid with drug level monitoring 2) ampho B 1/mg/kg/wk IV (less effective than azoles)
Maintenance Fluconazole 200 mg po qd (until pt asymptomatic, initial treatment completed and CD4 count is >100 cells/mm³, VL <50 c/mL x 3 mo antifungal treatment, and antifungal treatment at least 12 mo	Itraconazole 400 mg po qd in 2 divided doses with drug monitoring

* Miscellaneous issues: Start ART in treatment-naïve patients within two weeks of starting antifungal treatment. Consider maintenance treatment if CD4 decreases to <100 cells/mm³

† Document that CSF culture is negative before switching to consolidation phase

□ Management of increased ICP is critical (*CID* 2000;30:47). Increased intracranial pressure (ICP) accounts for >90% of deaths in first 2 wks and 40% of deaths in weeks 3-10 (*CID* 2000;30:47). **Failure to manage elevated ICP is the most common and most dangerous mistake in management** (*CID* 2005;40:477; *CID* 2010;50:291). Specifics (IDSA Guidelines, *CID* 2010;50:291): 1) Determine baseline CSF pressure unless focal neurologic signs or impaired mentation requires delay for CT or MRI; 2) If CSF pressure is >25 cm with symptoms of increased pressure: reduce pressure with LP drainage to 50% if very high or to <20 cm; if persistent elevation >25 cm and symptoms repeat LP daily until pressure and symptoms stabilized >2 days; 3) Consider temporary percutaneous drains or ventriculostomy if daily LP is repeatedly required and 4) Consider permanent VP shunt only if antifungal therapy and conservative methods to control ICP have failed. Note that VP shunts can be placed during active infection.

- ***Cryptococcus gatti*:** This yeast differs from *C. neoformans* in that *C. gattii* occurs in immunocompetent hosts, is less susceptible to standard antifungal agents and is geographically unique. Historically it caused cryptococcosis primarily in the tropical and subtropical areas, but more recently it has caused disease primarily in healthy hosts in British Columbia in Canada and the Northwest US (*JID* 2009;199:1081; *Emerg Infect Dis* 2009;15:1185). In vitro tests with 350 clinical isolates show substantial variability with most strains being susceptible to amphotericin B (MIC 90 <1 µg/mL) and relative resistance to flucytosine (MIC 50 2-4 µg/mL) (*AAC* 2010;54:5139). *C. gatti* can be distinguished from *C. neoformans* by microbiologic and molecular methods (*Med Mycol* 2009;47:561; *Diagn Microbiol Infect Dis* 2010;68:471). A suggested method is the use of canavanine-glycine-bromothymol blue (CGB) medium (*Adv Appl Microbiol* 2009;67:131).

- **Comments**

  ⊓ Repeat LP is indicated only to control elevated ICP and possibly at the end of induction at 2 wks (positive cultures at this time predict worst outcome). Continue induction if positive CSF culture at 2 wks.

  □ Amphotericin B is associated with more rapid clearance of *C. neoformans* than fluconazole (*CID* 2007;45:76). A randomized trial in Malawi comparing fluconazole (1200 mg qd) alone or in combination with flucytosine (100 mg/kg/d) for 14 days followed by fluconazole (800 mg qd) showed more rapid fungal clearance and lower mortality (10% vs. 31% at 2 wks) with the combination (*CID* 2010;50:338).

  □ Flucytosine + amphotericin B produces more rapid clearance than amphotericin alone (*Lancet* 2004;363:1764; *PLoS Med* 2007; 4:e21) and the best clinical outcome (*PLoS One* 2008;3:32870).

Management of Infections

6

Another study found that high dose amphotericin B (1.0 mg/kg) + flucytosine produced even more rapid clearance without increasing the rate of nephrotoxity (*CID* 2008;47:123).

- Flucytosine blood levels should be measured 2 hrs post dose and should not exceed 75 µg/mL (target 30-80 mcg/mL). Reduce dose with renal insufficiency (see pg. 279).

- Fluconazole + flucytosine is less effective than amphotericin (*CID*;2007;45:76) and may be more toxic, possibly due to higher flucytosine doses used (*CID* 1994;19:741; *CID* 1998;26:1362; *CID* 2007;45:76).

- Fluconazole alone: Response appears to be dose related. Doses of 1200 mg qd appear superior to 800 mg qd (*CID* 2008;47:1556).

- Lipid amphotericin: Best data are for *AmBisome* at 4-6 mg/kg/d (*AIDS* 1997;11:1463; *CID* 2005;40[Suppl 6]:S409; *CID* 2007;45: 76) 6 mg/kg recommended for severe disease.

- Fluconazole maintenance (200 mg qd) is superior to amphotericin B maintenance (*NEJM* 1992;326:793) and superior to itraconazole at a dosage of 200 mg qd po (*CID* 1999;28:291).

- Resistance: Amphotericin B resistance is rare or too hard to demonstrate (*AAC* 1993;37:1383; *Clin Microbiol Rev* 2001;14:643; *AAC* 1999;43: 1463). Resistance develops rapidly with flucytosine monotherapy (*Lancet* 2002;359:1135). Fluconazole resistance is rare (*AAC* 1999;43:1856; *AAC* 2001;45: 420). Resistance is more common in Africa; MIC >16 mcg/mL has been associated with reduced efficacy (*AAC* 2000;44:1544).

- Prophylactic fluconazole or itraconazole significantly reduces the frequency of cryptococcal meningitis in patients with CD4 counts <50 cells/mm^3 (*NEJM* 1995;332:700; *CID* 1999;28:1049). This is not recommended due to concern for resistance and drug interactions.

- Clearance of *C. neoformans* from CSF is fastest with amphotericin B + flucytosine, then amphotericin B + fluconazole and then amphotericin B alone (*CID* 2000; 30:710; *NEJM* 1997; 337:15; *Lancet* 2004; 363:1764; *PLoS Med* 2007;4:e21). Amphotericin B + flucytosine sterilizes CSF in 60-90% within 2 wks (*NEJM* 1987;317:334). If flucytosine cannot be given, induction duration w/ amphotericin B is 4-6 wks. Liposomal amphotericin (4 mg/kg/d) eradicated *C. neoformans* from CSF more rapidly than amphotericin B (0.7 mg/kg/d) (*AIDS* 1997;11:1463).

- Consolidation: After induction, use fluconazole 400 mg qd (6 mg/kg/d) x 8 wks.

- Treatment failure: Possible role for posaconazole or voriconazole or higher dose ambisone (6 mg/kg/d).

- Monitoring for drug toxicity: Fluconazole: monitor for hepatotoxicity (rare). Amphotericin B: monitor for nephrotoxicity and electrolyte changes; reduce risk with pre-infusion 500 mL normal saline and reduce symptomatic reactions by pretreatment with acetaminophen and diphenhydramine +/- corticosteroid 30 minutes before amphotericin (steroids are rarely needed). Flucytosine: monitor neutropenia and GI toxicity; 2 hr post-dose blood levels should be <30-80 µg/mL.

□ Serum cryptococcal antigen screening (CRAG) in patients with CD4 counts <100 cells/mm³: a report from Uganda found a positive CRAG test merited therapy in patients with advanced HIV even without clinical evidence of cryptococcosis (*CID* 2010; 51:448).

RESPONSE: Mortality with the recommended 3-phase regimen is 5%, and CSF cultures at 2 wks are sterile in 60-70% (*PLoS One* 2009;4:e5575; *CID* 2000;30: 47; *NEJM* 1997;337:15). Factors that correlate with poor or delayed response are altered mental status at presentation, high fungal load and slow fungal clearance (*CID* 2009;49:702). The major early concern is elevated ICP, which can lead to cranial nerve deficits or herniation and death. Management of elevated ICP with repeated LPs is critical since most deaths are associated with increased ICP (*CID* 2000;30:47). The relapse rate with fluconazole therapy (phase 3) is 2% (*NEJM* 1992; 326:796). Guidelines recommend routine CSF cryptococcal culture at 2 wks. Serum cryptococcal antigen is usually not useful in following response to treatment; CSF antigen may be (*HIV Clin Trials* 2000;1:1). Long-term follow-up of 82 HIV-infected patients with cryptococcal meningitis in the HAART era who survived >3 mos showed a relapse rate of 0.9/100 patient-years. The serum cryptococcal antigen assay is reportedly negative by 48 mos in 71% (*AIDS* 2006;20: 2183). Induction treatment for cryptococcomas recommended using ambisome 6 mg/kg/d + 5 FC; this is followed by 6 wks, then 6-18 mos for consolidation.

TREATMENT FAILURE: Treatment failure is defined by the lack of clinical response, positive CSF culture for *C. neoformans* and/or rising CSF cryptococcal antigen titer at 2 wks. Ensure IRIS is addressed and CSF pressure is controlled. Consider increasing dose of amphotericin. If intolerant of amphotericin preparations, consider fluconazole >800 mg qd + flucytosine 100 mg/kg/d. If flycytosine intolerant, consider amphotericin + fluconazole. Intrathecal amphotericin is rarely needed. Consider testing MIC isolate to fluconazole; if ≥16 mcg/mL consider resistant and use alternative agent.

RELAPSE: Restart induction, test MIC to azoles and consider voriconazole (200-400 mg po bid) or posaconazole (800 mg qd po in 2-4 doses) x 10-12 wks. Therapeutic drug monitoring is recommended with voriconazole and posaconazole.

CRYPTOCOCCAL IRIS AND ART TIMING: ACTG 5164 compared early (ART initiated within 14 days of OI treatment) vs. late ART (ART initiated at completion of OI treatment). This showed an advantage to early ART in terms of AIDS progression or death (14% vs. 24%). The trial included 35 patients with cryptococcosis and this subset showed substantial benefit to early ART (*PLoS One* 2009;4:e5575). However, a review of 101 cases of HIV-associated cryptococcal meningitis in Uganda found a mortality rate of 36% with IRIS vs. 21% in patients without IRIS (*PLoS Med* 2010;7:e1000384).

A review of 12 studies with 598 patients found cryptococcal IRIS in 8-49% (*Lancet Infect Dis* 2010;10:791). The presentation in 171 cases was primarily meningeal (74%), CNS disease (11%), adenopathy (11%), pneumonitis (5%) and multifocal (4%). Median times from ART to presentation ranged 1-10 mos. The reported incidence of ART-associated cryptococcosis (cryptococcosis recognized only after ART) was 0.2-1.6% in 6 studies. A proposed definition of cryptococcal IRIS from this review was: 1) taking ART after cryptococcosis diagnosed, treated and had partial or complete resolution clinically and/or by antigen titer or quantitative culture; 2) occurance within 12 mos of ART with clinical worsening of inflammatory manifestations (meningitis, adenitis, cerebritis, pneumonitis, etc.); and 3) no other likely explanation such as alternative diagnosis or treatment failure (HIV or cryptococcis).

MANAGEMENT RECOMMENDATIONS OF CRYPTOCOCCAL IRIS: (IDSA Guidelines, *CID* 2010;50:291): 1) Do not change antifungal therapy; 2) minor IRIS manifestations: no intervention; and 3) major IRIS symptoms: consider prednisone 0.5-1.0 mg/kg/d or equivalent usually for 2-6 wks. Anti-inflammatory agents have shown impressive results in patients with IRIS presenting as cryptococcal lymphadenitis (*JID* 1998;30:615). Prevention of IRIS might be achieved by delaying initation of ART until the end of induction therapy and CSF culture negative (2-10 wks), but this is ill advised (*PLoS One* 2009;4:e5575).

Pulmonary, Disseminated, or Antigenemia

DIAGNOSIS: Positive culture of blood, urine, and/or respiratory secretions virtually always indicates cryptococcal disease and mandates lumbar puncture to exclude meningitis. Serum antigenemia suggests cryptococcosis, especially with titer >1:8; this test should be confirmed with a fungal blood culture and a LP should be performed to exclude meningitis.

TREATMENT

- **Preferred regimen: For mild-moderate** (absence diffuse pulmonary infiltrates, and absence of severe immunosuppression): fluconazole 400 mg qd po x 6-12 mos. If receiving ART with CD4 >100 cells/mm³ plus antigenemia titer <1:512; consider stopping at one year. For severe disease – treat as for CNS cryptococcosis. For **severe disease** – treat as for CNS *cryptococcus*.

- **Alternative regimen: Cryptococcosis** – non-meningeal and non-pulmonary: For cryptococcemia or disseminated disease (>1:512: treat as CNS cryptococcosis.

Management of Infections

- **Comments**
  - □ Refractory lung and bone lesions may require surgery.
  - □ Non-meningeal sites include lungs, skin, joints, eye, adrenal gland, GI tract, liver, pancreas, prostate, and urinary tract.
  - □ Cryptococcal antigen titer >1:8 confirmed, treat with fluconazole (*CID* 1996;23:827).

Cryptosporidium parvum

Cryptosporidiosis: (See *Clin Microbiol Rev* 1999;12:554; *CID* 2001;32:331; *NEJM* 2002;346:1723)

PRESENTATION: Typical symptoms are acute, subacute, or chronic profuse watery diarrhea often associated with cramps, nausea, and vomiting; about one-third have fever (*Ann Intern Med* 1996;124:429; *CID* 2003;36:903). Stool assays with acid fast stain, IFA, PCR or EIA are sensitive, specific, and nearly equal in diagnostic utility with watery stools (*NEJM* 2002;346:1723; *Acta Trop* 2008;1071:1; *JCM* 2009;47:4060; *BMC Microbiol* 2010;10:11; *JCM* 2011;48:1607). IFA is preferred for formed stool. A single specimen is adequate with severe diarrhea. Repeat sampling is recommended for less severe disease. Patterns of disease with AIDS: 1) asymptomatic carriage (4%); 2) self-limited diarrhea <2 mos (29%); 3) chronic diarrhea >2 mos (60%); 4) fulminant diarrhea with >2 L/d (8%) (*NEJM* 2002;346:1723). The chronic and fulminant form is seen almost exclusively with CD4 counts <100 cells/mm^3. Rates of cryptosporidiosis in HIV infection are greatly reduced in the HAART era (*HIV Med* 2010;11:245).

PREVENTION: See pg. 80.

TREATMENT

- **Preferred regimens**
  - □ ART with immune reconstitution is the only treatment that controls persistent cryptosporidiosis. Resolution usually occurs with CD4 >100 cells/mm^3 and may improve with only modest CD4 increases (*JAIDS* 2000;25:124; *Lancet* 1998;351:256).
  - □ Symptomatic treatment: Fluids including sports rehydration beverages such as *Gatorade*, bouillon, oral rehydration (see comments below) and nutritional supplements; parenteral nutrition is sometimes required. Attempts to restore fluid and nutrients should be accompanied by antimotility agents such as loperamide, paregoric and tincture of opium.
  - □ Antimicrobial: Nitazoxanide (1 gm po bid x 60 days with food) is the only antimicrobial advocated on 2008 NIH/CDC/IDSA OI Guidlines and then only as an "alternative" to symptomatic treatment. (See: *Pediatr Infect Dis* 2008;27:1040; *Parasite* 2008; 15:275). A randomized controlled trial in 52 HIV-infected children with chronic cryptosporidiosis given high dose nitazoxanide or

6 Management of Infections

placebo in Zambia showed no benefit with treatment (*BMC Infect Dis* 2009;9:195).

- **Comments**
  - Antimicrobials: More than 95 drugs have been tried, and none have been consistently successful. (*NEJM* 2002;346:1723; *Lancet* 2002;360:1375). These include rifamycins, paromomycin, azithromycin, and nitazoxanide. One randomized trial of paromomycin (a non-absorbable aminoglycoside) showed a modest but statistically significant improvement in symptoms and oocyte shedding (*CID* 2000;31:1084); two other randomized trials showed no benefit (*JID* 1995;170:419; *BMC Infect Dis* 2009;9:195). A review of 70 AIDS patients given paromycin and antimotility agents was effective in reducing diarrhea in 54 (77%), but the relapse rate was high (*Medicine* 1997;76:118). .
  - Oral rehydration (severe diarrhea): NaCl 3.5 g ($^3/_4$ tsp), $NaHCO_3$ 2.5 g (1 tsp baking soda), KCl 1.5 g (1 cup orange juice or bananas) in 1 liter water. Packets of pre-mixed salts available from Cera Products (888-237-2598) and Jianas Brothers (816-421-2880).
  - Nitazoxanide: 1000 mg po bid with food x 60 days. Efficacy is not clearly established (*JID* 2001;184:103; *Br J Clin Pharmacol* 2007; 63: 387; *Aliment Pharmacol Ther* 2006;24:887). One randomized trials in 60 Zambian children with AIDS showed no significant benefit in terms of clinical response or parasitic clearance (*BCM Infect Dis* 2009;9:195). Another randomized trial in 207 adult patients in Zambia failed to show benefit (*Aliment Pharmacol Ther* 2005;21:757) Nevertheless, nitazoxanide is FDA approved for cryptosporidiosis in immunocompetent children and has modest favorable evidence of efficacy in adults (see Cochrane Library review below). Nitazoxanide shows few adverse reactions and few drug interactions and shows in vitro activity vs. cryptosporidia (*JAC* 2000;45:453), so it may be the best option. However, it should not be used as a substitute for aggressive attempts at immune reconstitution, and evidence supporting efficacy is marginal (*Curr Opin Infect Dis* 2010;23:494).
  - A Cochrane Library review in 2007 concluded "the absence of effective agents" but noted that nitazoxanide reduces parasite load and "should be considered" (*Cochrane Database Syst Rev* 2007; CD004932).

RESPONSE: Cryptosporidiosis in patients with CD4 count >100 cells/mm^3 usually resolves spontaneously after 2-8 wks, as it does with immunocompetent hosts. For AIDS patients with fulminant or chronic, persistent cryptosporidiosis, the goal is immune reconstitution: even modest elevations in CD4 count may result in resolution of symptoms and pathogen elimination (*JAIDS* 1998;12:35; *JAIDS* 2000; 25:124). This is an indication for urgent initiation of ART.

Management of Infections

Cytomegalovirus (CMV)

CMV Retinitis

PRESENTATION: Studies from the pre-HAART era found that about one-third of persons with untreated HIV infection develop CMV retinitis (*Herpes* 2007;14:66), but this complication has decreased dramatically in the HAART era (*AIDS* 2010;24:1549; *Am J Opthal* 2011;151:198). The presenting symptoms are variable and include floaters, field defects, scotomata, or decreased acuity. CD4 count is usually <50 cells/mm^3, and the mean in 1,632 AIDS patients with CMV retinitis was 30 cells/mm^3 (*Amer Acad Ophthal* 2007;114:780). Funduscopic exam shows perivascular yellow-white retinal infiltrates ± intraretinal hemorrhage ("scrambled eggs and ketchup"). Blood cultures, CMV viral load determinations, and antigen assays are often not helpful due to lack of specificity for CMV disease (*JCM* 2000;323:563), but blood cultures may be useful for *in vitro* sensitivity tests in reference labs for patients with relapses. Serum CMV antibody testing is not useful unless negative, since this tends to exclude the diagnosis. The diagnosis is usually made by funduscopic exam by an experienced ophthalmologist (*Ophthal* 2007;14:787). CMV PCR is often positive in vitreous and aqueous humor and is highly specific, but usually unnecessary (*Ophthalmolgia* 2004;218:43).

TREATMENT

- **Preferred regimens**

  - Vision-threatening lesion: Intraocular ganciclovir implant (*Vitrasert*) every 6-8 mos + valganciclovir 900 mg po bid with food x 14-21 days, then 900 mg qd and ART. Some advocate an intravitreous injection of ganciclovir at the time of the diagnosis to provide rapid local treatment during the delay to implant insertion.

  - Peripheral lesions: Oral valganciclovir (above doses) plus ART in treatment-naïve patients.

- **Alternative regimens**

  - Ganciclovir 5 mg/kg IV q12h x 14-21 days, then valganciclovir 900 mg po qd or IV ganciclovir 5 mg/kg/d.

  - Foscarnet 60 mg/kg IV q8h or 90 mg/kg IV q12h x 14-21 days then 90-120 mg/kg once daily.

  - Cidofovir 5 mg/kg/wk IV x 2 wks, then 5 mg/kg every other week with saline hydration and probenecid 2 gm po 3 hrs before cidofovir dose and 1 gm 2 hrs and 8 hrs post dose. Cannot be used in patients with sulfa allergy.

  - Intravitreous injections of ganciclovir and foscarnet When intravitreal therapy is used because of nonavailability of systemic anti-CMV agents, the recommendation is ganciclovir 2 mg in 0.1 mL twice weekly until retinitis is inactive, followed by the same maintenance dose given once weekly. The dose of foscarnet is

6 Management of Infections

2.4 mg in 0.1 mL. These two drugs given by intraocular injection appear equal in efficacy and side effects. The injections are given after subconjunctival lidocaine and epinephrine to reduce pain and bleeding. The intraocular injections are given with an eyelid speculum and topical 5% betadine.

- Interferon (INF-a2b) has been used successfully to treat CMV retinitis (*HIV Clin Trials* 2011;12:118).

- **Comments**

  - Ganciclovir + foscarnet is more effective than either drug alone for preventing relapse, but is usually toxic (*Ach Ophthl* 1996;114: 23)

  - Intraocular ganciclovir implant requires replacement every 6-8 mos in absence of immune reconstitution.

  - Valganciclovir is a prodrug of ganciclovir and provides serum levels comparable with IV ganciclovir at standard doses (*NEJM* 2002;346:1119).

  - *Vitrasert* (intraocular ganciclovir release device) was superior to IV ganciclovir in time to relapse (220 days vs 71 days), but there is increased risk of involvement of the other eye and increased risk of extraocular CMV disease without concomitant systemic anti-CMV therapy (*NEJM* 1997;337:83). Thus, local therapy should be accompanied by systemic anti-CMV therapy such as valganciclovir.

  - ART with effective HIV suppression controls CMV retinitis so that CMV therapy may be unnecessary (*Am J Opthal* 2011; 151:198).

PROGRESSION OR RELAPSE

- **Preferred regimens**

  - Induction dose of the same agent (ganciclovir IV 10 mg/kg/d, foscarnet IV 180-240 mg/kg/d, or valganciclovir 900 mg po bid). Switching to alternative drug for first relapse is generally not advocated unless resistance is suspected (see below) or toxicity is the reason.

  - Late relapse: switch to alternative agent (see below).

  - Discontinue maintenance therapy when CD4 count is >100 cells/mm^3 for 3-6 mos and disease is inactive according to an ophthalmologist. After stopping therapy the patient should be evaluated every 3 mos for relapse or immune recovery uveitis.

  - Follow-up evaluations during treatment include indirect ophthalmoloscopy after induction treatment is discontinued. Retinal photographs provide the optimal method to evaluate response and relapse.

  - Drug resistance in the pre-HAART era was about 25% per person-year and was similar for ganciclovir, foscarnet and cidofovir (*JID* 1998; 177:770; *J Ophthol* 1998; 126:543; *JID* 2003; 187:777; *Antimcrob Ag Chemother* 1998;42:2240). It is about 10% per person-year in the HAART era.

- ☐ Relapse is expected in the absence of immune recovery.
- ☐ Time to relapse varies with definition, use of retinal photographs, and treatments summarized above. Subsequent relapses occur more rapidly.

RESPONSE: The goal of treatment is to stop visual loss. Treatment usually stops progressive blindness, but does not reverse prior damage. Other major complications are involvement in the second eye, retinal detachment and progression of retinitis due to resistance. Ganciclovir resistance is usually due to mutations on the UL97 phosphotransferase gene, causing low-level resistance that can be overcome with the ganciclovir implant, and the UL54 DNA polymerase gene, which confers high-level resistance and cross-resistance to cidofovir and sometimes foscarnet (*JID* 2001;183:333; *JID* 2000;182:1765). The UL97 mutation can be detected by sequence analysis of strains directly from blood (plasma and leukocytes); results are available in <48 hrs instead of the 4 wks required for traditional CMV cultures (*JID* 2006;193:1728). Ganciclovir resistance rates are <10% at 3 mos and 25-30% at 9 mos (*JID* 1998;177:770; *JID* 2001;183: 333; *AAC* 2005;49:873). Thus, relapses in <3 mos are usually not due to resistance; relapses after 9 mos often are. The long-term results are highly correlated with response to ART for both CMV viral response and immune recovery. Sequential analysis of 271 patients with CMV retinitis found that the rate of progression (movement of CMV lesion >750µm or a new lesion) was 0.6 per patient-year with CD4 counts <50 cells/mm^3 compared to 0.02 per patient-year with CD4 counts >200 cells/mm^3. Involvement of the contralateral eye with CMV occurs at a rate of 0.07/person-year and is highly dependent on the CD4 count (0.34/PY with CD4 <50 cells/mm^3) and CMV viral load (*Opthalmology* 2004;111:2232). The risk of retinal detachment in this study was 0.06/person-year with rates that correlated with low CD4 count and area of retinitis involvement. ART conferred benefit even without a CD4 response (*Ophthalmology* 2004;111:2224). Long-term follow-up of 494 eyes with CMV retinitis found that visual acuity at a median of 3.1 years was reduced to ≥20/50 in 29% and ≥20/200 (legal blindness) in 15% (*Ophthalmology* 2006;113:1432). The rate of immune recovery uveitis among those with immune recovery was 17%. A review of 475 eyes in AIDS patients with CMV retinitis showed that the field loss rate decreased 6- to 7- fold from the post-HAART era compared to pre-HAART era.

MAINTENANCE

- **Preferred regimens**
  - ☐ Valganciclovir 900 mg qd; ganciclovir 5 mg/kg IV bid (induction) followed by maintenance with 5 mg/kg IV qd or, preferrably valganciclovir
  - ☐ Intraocular ganciclovir implant every 6 mos + valganciclovir 900 mg qd (AWP $19,200/implant!).

6 Management of Infections

- **Alternative regimens**
  - □ Foscarnet 90-120 mg/kg/d IV.
  - □ Cidofovir 5 mg/kg IV every two weeks.
- **Discontinuation of therapy and relapse:** Discontinue maintenance therapy when the CD4 count is >100 cells/mm³ for 3-6 mos, there is no evidence of active disease according to an ophthalmologist, and regular ophthalmologic follow-up is avialable. Restart prophylaxis when CD4 count is <50-100 cells/mm³. The relative safety of discontinuing therapy when the CD4 count is >100 cells/mm³ has been demonstrated, and most relapses occur when the CD4 count is <50 cells/mm³ (*AIDS* 2000;14:170; *AIDS* 2001;15:23). Relapse rate after discontinuation of anti-CMV therapy is 0.03 per person-year, and is highly correlated with the CD4 count. Relapses with CD4 counts as high as 1250 cells/mm³ appear to reflect a lack of CMV-specific immunity (*JID* 2001;183: 1285; *HIV Clin Trials* 2005;6: 136).

IMMUNE RECOVERY VITRITIS

- **Clinical features:** Inflammation in the anterior chamber and/or vitreous, usually occurring at 4-12 wks after initiating ART (*Arch Ophthalmol* 2003;121:466; *Am J Ophthalmol* 2000;129:634). Incidence is highly variable, from 0.11 per patient-year to 0.86 per patient-year (*Am J Ophthalmol* 2000;129:634; *JID* 1999;179:697). The major risk appears to be the extent of immune dysfunction before starting ART (*CID* 2011;52:409). The lower rate may be due to better CMV suppression before ART was initiated. CMV PCR of aqueous and vitreous humor is usually negative (*Ophthalmalgia* 2004;218:43), and CMV viremia is not found (*HIV Clin Trials* 2005;6:136). This complication was associated with a reduction in visual acuity to 20/50 or worse at a rate of 0.2 per patient-year but a rate of only 0.04 per patient-year for blindness; this figure for blindness is no different from what is seen in patients with immune recovery without uveitis. Further analysis of this database of 494 eyes found that 1) causes of vision loss to <20/200 were zone 1 disease (50%), cataract (30%) and retinal detachment (20%); 2) cataract and cystoid macular edema accounted for 50% of vision loss with long standing CMV retinitis, but only 10% of blindness in all cases (*Opthalmology* 2006;113: 1441).
- **Treatment** usually includes continued ART, an anti-CMV agent plus systemic and local steroids such as intravitreal injection of 0.1 mL triamcinolone 0.4% solution (*Ophthalmol Surg Lasers Imaging* 2003;34:398). About 50% respond.

CMV Extraocular Disease – Gastrointestinal (Usually esophagitis or colitis)

PRESENTATION: <u>CMV esophagitis</u> is characterized by fever, odynophagia ± retrostenal pain that is often well-localized in patients with a CD4 count <50 cells/mm^3 (see pg. 504). <u>CMV colitis</u> presents and fever, weight loss, abdominal pain, diarrhea, and GI bleeding in patients with CD4 counts <50 cells/mm^3. Complications include severe hemorrhage and perforation (*JAIDS* 1991; 4: Suppl:S29)

DIAGNOSIS: The diagnosis of esophagitis or colitis is established with endoscopic visulization of large shallow mucosal ulcers and histopathology showing typical intranuclear and intracytoplasmic inclusion with inflammatory response at the ulcer edge (*JAIDS* 1991;4:S29). Culture or PCR detection of CMV in blood or intestinal biopsies is not diagnostic because many patients have viremia or CMV in tissue without CMV disease. (*Lancet* 2004;363:2116; *AIDS* 1997;11:F21) Serology is not helpful except to make CMV disease unlikely if the IgG antibody level is negative. Similarly, CMV antigenemia is primarily useful for excluding this diagnosis (*World J Gastroenterol* 2011;17:1185).

TREATMENT

- **Preferred regimens**
  - □ Valganciclovir 900 mg po bid with food x 3-4 wks (if symptoms do not interfere with oral meds).
  - □ Ganciclovir 5 mg/kg IV bid x 3-4 wks.
  - □ Foscarnet 60 mg/kg q8h or 90 mg/kg IV q12h x 3-4 wks.
  - □ Consider maintenance therapy: if there is relapse on or after therapy.

- **Comments**
  - □ Ganciclovir and foscarnet are equally effective for <u>CMV colitis</u> (*Am J Gastroenterol* 1993;88:542).
  - □ <u>Duration of treatment</u> is usually 21-28 days or until signs and symptoms have cleared.
  - □ <u>ART</u> should be started without delay
  - □ <u>Valganciclovir</u> provides ganciclovir serum levels comparable with IV ganciclovir and is generally preferred in patients who can swallow.
  - □ Patients with CD4 counts <100 cells/mm^3 should undergo <u>ophthalmologic screening</u> to rule out retinitis.

RESPONSE: CMV esophagitis usually responds within 1-2 wks with decrease in fever and odynophagia. Patients with colitis respond poorly – abdominal pain and diarrhea may not improve or may improve only modestly; viral shedding is markedly reduced. There is a case report of **IRIS CMV colitis** with colonic perforation (*CID* 2008;46:e38).

CMV Neurological Disease

PRESENTATION: CMV neurologic disease includes encephalitis, ventriculoencephalitis and ascending polyradiculomyelopathy.

6 Management of Infections

- Patients with **polyradiculomyelopathy** present with: 1) progressive leg paresis, then bladder and bowel dysfunction and 2) CSF with polymorphonuclear cells and increased protein.

- **Encephalitis** presents with (1) rapidly progressing delirium, cranial nerve defects, ataxia, and nystagmus; (2) CSF with increased protein and a mononuclear pleocytosis; (3) MRI showing periventricular enhancement.

- Patients with **ventriculoencephalitis** have a rapidly progressive neurologic syndrome with focal neurologic defects and MRI showing periventricular enhancement.

DIAGNOSIS: The diagnosis of CMV CNS disease is established by a compatible clinical syndrome + detection of CMV, usually by PCR, in CSF or brain. The sensitivity of CSF PCR is 80% with specificity of 90% (*CID* 2002;34:103). Brain biopsy with histopathology or culture is diagnostic. With radiculomyelopathy CSF shows PMNs.

TREATMENT

- **Preferred regimen**

  - Ganciclovir 5 mg/kg IV bid + foscarnet 90 mg/kg IV bid until symptomatic improvement, then foscarnet 90-120 mg/kg/d IV + valgan-ciclovir 900 mg po bid for life.

  - Immune reconstitution is most important.

- **Alternative regimen:** Ganciclovir 5 mg/kg IV bid x 3-6 wks, then maintenance with foscarnet IV or valganciclovir po.

RESPONSE

- **CMV encephalitis:** In a trial of ganciclovir + foscarnet for CMV encephalitis, median survival was 94 days vs. 42 days in historic controls (*AIDS* 2000;14:517).

- **CMV polyradiculopathy:** Improvement occurs within 2-3 wks (*Neurology* 1993;43:493).

- **Induction therapy** may need to be continued for several months in severe cases with CMV neurologic disease (*CID* 1993;17:32). Maintenance therapy is lifelong.

- **IRIS:** A case of CMV ventriculitis due to immune reconstitution inflammatory syndrome (IRIS) with onset after 3 wks of ART has been reported; the patient responded to foscarnet therapy (*J Neurol Neurosurg Psychiatry* 2005;76:888).

CMV Pneumonitis

PRESENTATION: Symptoms include fever, cough, dyspnea, and interstitial infiltrates.

DIAGNOSIS: Minimum diagnostic criteria include all of the following (*CID* 1996;23:76): 1) pulmonary infiltrates; 2) characteristic intracellular inclusions in lung tissue; and 3) absence of another pulmonary pathogen.

INDICATIONS TO TREAT: CMV pneumonitis in patients with histologic evidence of CMV disease + failure to respond to treatment of other pathogens. Isolation of CMV from respiratory secretions is not diagnostic; true CMV pneumonitis is uncommon.

TREATMENT: Ganciclovir 5 mg/kg IV bid >21 days, foscarnet 60 mg/kg q8h or 90 mg/kg IV q12h >21 days, or valganciclovir 900 mg po bid x 21 days.

- **Comments**
  - Response to ganciclovir is >60% (*CID* 1996;23:76).
  - Indications are unclear for long-term maintenance therapy.

Herpes simplex virus (HSV) (*MMWR* 2006;55[RR-11]:16)

PRESENTATION: The seroprevalence of HSV-2 in patients with HIV infection in the US is 70% and for HSV-1 or -2 it is 95% (*JAIDS* 2004; 35:435). Orolabial and genital HSV are similar in presentation, diagnosis, and management, except for anatomical site of infection. Most patients are asymptomatic but have micro-ulcerations. The usual presentation starts with a sensory prodome at the involved site, followed by rapid evolution of lip/genital papule → vesicle → ulcer → crust. Lesions with advanced AIDS are more severe, more likely to disseminate, more likely to be refractory to therapy and more likely to be acyclovir-resistant.

DIAGNOSIS: The diagnosis is best when there is laboratory confirmation with viral cultures, HSV DNA PCR, or HSV antigen tests. PCR is most sensitive and should be used to screen for HSV-2 infection (*NEJM* 2007;370:2127). Type-specific serology tests are commercially available for asymptomatic patients; those who are seropositive should be counseled about transmission (www.mmhiv.com/link/CDC-STD-Treatment). Condoms reduce HSV transmission (*Ann Intern Med* 2005;143:707), and the use of prophylactic valacyclovir (500 mg bid) by patients coinfected with HIV and HSV may reduce HIV transmission to partners by 50% (*NEJM* 2004;350:11) but does not appear to protect the patient with HSV from acquisition of HIV (*Lancet* 2008;371:2109).

TREATMENT (*MMWR* 2006;55 [R11]:16; 2008 NIH/CDC/IDSA Guidelines for Treatment and Prevention of Opportunistic Infections) (see Table 5-7, pg. 188 and Table 6-3, pg. 448).

- **HSV encephalitis:** Acyclovir 10 mg/kg q8h IV x 21d
- **Severe mucocutaneous disease:** Acyclovir 5 mg/kg q8h IV until improved, then oral acyclovir 400 mg tid or alternative oral agent. Continue until lesions are healed
- **Acyclovir-resistant:** Foscarnet 80-120 mg/kg/d IV in 2-3 divided doses until clinical response
  - Alternatives: Topical cidofovir (1%), topical trifluridine (1%) or topical imiquimod, each for 21-28 days or longer

6 Management of Infections

- **Herpes keratitis:** Trifluridine, 1 drop q2h up to 9x/d for up to 21 days
- **Comments**
  - Acyclovir-resistant HSV is rare in immunocompetent hosts, but should be suspected in immunocompromised patients who do not respond within 7-10 days. In this case lesions should be cultured and HSV strains should be tested for acyclovir susceptibility (*NEJM* 1999; 340:1255; *NEJM* 1999; 325:551). Treatment options include IV foscarnet or topical cidofovir (1% compounded by the pharmacy) or topical trifluridine (1% as *Viroptic*) or topical imiquimod (*JID* 1997; 17:862; *NEJM* 1993; 327:968; *JAIDS* 1996; 12:147; *CID* 2004;39 (Suppl 5);S248).
  - Pregnancy: Treatment with acyclovir should be offered for initial and recurrent HSV during pregnancy, but suppressive therapy is not recommended. Acyclovir is the preferred agent because it has the most extensive experience in pregnancy and appears safe (*Birth Defects Res. A Clin Md Teratol* 2004; 70:201). Women with HSV prodrome or genital lesions at labor should undergo Caesarian delivery. Proplylactic acyclovir beginning at 36 weeks has been recommended for high risk women to prevent HSV outbreaks at labor (*Obstet Gynec* 2003;102:1396; *Am J Obstet Gynecol* 2003; 188:136)
  - HSV and HIV transmission: Genital ulcers including subclinical ulcers are risk factors for HIV transmission (*JAIDS* 2004;35:435; *JID* 2003;187:19; *JID* 2003;187:1513). Studies in Rakai, Uganda and the US have shown that HIV transmission to susceptible partners is increased by 50% when the HIV-negative partner is seropositive for HSV-2 (*NEJM* 2004;350:11; *CID* 2006;43:347). The implication is that HSV suppression in the HIV-negative partner may decrease the rate of HIV transmission (*JID* 2002; 186:1718; *Lancet Infect Dis* 2007;7:249; *NEJM* 2007;356:790; *JID* 2010;201:1164). However, the initial large controlled trial to test this strategy showed no benefit (*Lancet* 2008;371:2109). With regard to the patient with HIV and HSV co-infection, a randomized trial of acyclovir vs. placebo showed acyclovir failed to decrease HIV transmission despite a 73% reduction in genital ulcers and a 0.25 $\log_{10}$ c/mL reduction in HIV VL (*NEJM* 2010;362:427).

- TABLE 6-3: **Recommendations for Treatment of HSV Infections**

Agent	Initial or recurrent	Prophylaxis
Acyclovir	400 mg po tid x 5-14 d[†]	400 mg bid[*]
Famciclovir	500 mg po bid x 5-14 d[†]	500 mg bid[*]
Valacyclovir	1 gm po bid x 5-14 d[†]	500 mg bid[*]

* Recommended with frequent recurrences. Latex condoms also prevent transmission (*Ann Intern Med* 2005;143:707)
† Oral herpes: 5-10 days; genital: 5-14 days

- □ HSV infection and HIV progression: Chronic HSV infection has been implicated as a cause of immune activation and a possible cause of an increase in the rate of HIV progression (*Infect Dis* 2002;186:1718; *JID* 2008;198:241). This is the possible mechanism to explain older studies suggesting a benefit to acyclovir treatment of HIV (*AIDS* 1994;8:641; *JID* 2007;196:1500; *NEJM* 2007;356:790). More recent studies suggest that this anti-HIV effect is modest but real with a reduction in HIV viral load by 0.25 $\log_{10}$ c/mL (*NEJM* 2010;362:427) and a 16% decrease in the rate of HIV disease progression (*Lancet* 2010;375:824).

- □ Acyclovir, famciclovir, and valacyclovir are clinically equivalent for treatment of HSV (*Sex Transm Dis* 1997;24:481; *JID* 1998;178:603; *JAMA* 2001;144:818; *Br J Dermatol* 2001;144:188).

- □ Patient information services recommended by CDC: 800-227-8922, www.ashastd.org.

- □ Allergy to acyclovir is rare but will contraindicate use of famciclovir and valacyclovir. Desensitization has been described (*Ann Allergy* 1993;70:386).

RESPONSE: Early treatment of acute genital HSV shortens duration of mucocutaneous lesions, reduces systemic symptoms, and reduces viral shedding (*Arch Int Med* 1996;156:1729); it does not change probability of recurrence (*Med Letter* 1995;37:117). In HIV-infected patients with refractory disease, suspect acyclovir resistance (*NEJM* 1991; 325:551). Acyclovir-resistant strains are resistant to famciclovir, valacyclovir, and (usually) ganciclovir. Treatment options are topical cidofovir or IV foscarnet (*JID* 1997;17:862, *NEJM* 1993;327:968) or topical trifluridine (*Viroptic* 1%) (*JAIDS* 1996;12:147). **Herpes simplex IRIS** has been described with erosive genital lesions (*HIV Med* 1999; 1:10; *CID* 2006;42:418).

SUPPRESSION

- ■ **Indication:** Severe or frequent recurrent HSV. See above for HSV suppression to prevent HIV transmission.

- ■ **Suppressive regimens:** Table 6-3: acyclovir 400 mg bid, famciclovir 500 mg bid, or valacyclovir 500 mg bid.

Herpes Zoster

PRESENTATION: About 95% of healthy adults are seropositive for VZV, and about 15% of healthy adults develop herpes zoster. Risk factors are advanced age and immunosuppression. The age adjusted risk with HIV infection is 15 times greater than in the general population. The major risks are advanced age and advanced HIV infection, but patients at all CD4 strata are at increased risk, and ART has had minimal effect on incidence (*JID* 1992;166:1153; *JID* 1999;180:1784; *JAIDS* 2005;38:111; *JAIDS* 2005;40:169; *JAIDS* 2004;37:1604). The usual presentation is a painful prodrome in the region of a dermatome that then evolves within days to a characteristic dermatomal vesicular rash that evolves over 3-5 days. In a review of 282 cases in HIV-infected patients with a mean age of 41 years, 67% had disease involving a single dermatome, risk factors were ART (OR = 2.4) and CD4 50-200 cells/mm^3 (OR = 2.7 vs CD4 <50 cells/mm^3), and 18% had post-herpetic neuralgia (*JAIDS* 2005;40:169). The diagnosis is usually made clinically based on the appearance of the lesions. When uncertain, the diagnosis can be confirmed by detecting the organism with swabs or biopsy for culture, DFA stain, histopathology (tissue specimens) or PCR.

- **Major complications:**
  - Progressive outer retinal necrosis (PORN) is associated with rapid vision loss (*Ophthalmology* 1994;101:1488; *AIDS* 2002;16:1045). Most patients have CD4 counts <100 cells/mm^3, the disease is characterized by dermatomal zoster and retinal necrosis (*J Clin Virol* 2007;38:254). Immediate evaluation by an ophthalmologist and high-dose IV acyclovir + foscarnet plus intravitreal antivirals is required (see treatment).
  - Acute retinal necrosis (ARN) with peripheral necrotizing retinitis and vitritis shows a high rate of vision loss that is sometimes due to retinal detachment (*CID* 1998;26:34). This may be seen at any CD4 count.
  - Neurologic VZV syndromes seen rarely in AIDS patients include transverse myelitis, encephalitis, optic neuritis, focal brain lesions, aseptic meningitis, cranial nerve palsies, radiculitis and vasculitic stroke. Caution is necessary in the interpretation of CSF findings, since a mononuclear pleocytosis, with increased protein and positive VZV PCR, may also characterize uncomplicated shingles.
  - Post-herpetic neuralgia:The rate of this often devastating pain syndrome with HIV infection is 10-20% (*JAIDS* 2005;38:111; *JAIDS* 2005;40:169).

TREATMENT

- **Preferred regimens**
  - Dermatomal zoster: Famciclovir 500 mg po tid, acyclovir 800 mg po 5x/d, or valacyclovir 1 g po tid x 7-10 days. Longer if lesions respond slowly (see pg. 186).
  - Severe cutaneous or visceral disease: Acyclovir 10-15 mg/kg IV q8h followed by valacyclovir, famciclovir or acyclovir (above doses) starting when there is clinical improvement and continued until all lesions are cleared.
  - Acute retinal necrosis (ARN): Acyclovir 10 mg/kg IV q8h x 10-14 days followed by valacyclovir 1000 mg po tid x 6 wks
  - Progressive outer retinal necrosis (PORN): Ganciclovir 5 mg/kg IV q12h + forcarnet 90 mg/kg IV q12h + intravitreal ganciclovir 2 mg/0.05 mL and /or foscarnet 1.2 mg / 0.05 mL 2x/wk.

□ Suspected resistance: Foscarnet IV 90 mg/kg bid.

□ Pain control: Gabapentin, tricyclics, carbamazepine, lidocaine patch, narcotics (effective and underutilized).

□ Chicken pox (adult): Valacyclovir 1000 mg po tid or acyclovir 800 mg po 5x/d or famciclovir 500 mg tid x 5-7 days. If severe: acyclovir 10-15 mg/kg IV q8h x 7-10 days with option to switch to oral therapy when afebrile.

- **Comments**

  □ Some authorities recommend corticosteroids to prevent post-herpetic neuralgia (*Ann Intern Med* 1996;125:376), but this is not recommended in HIV infection (2008 NIH/CDC/IDSA OI Treatment Guidelines).

  □ Post-herpetic neuralgia is uncommon in persons <55 years, including AIDS patients.

  □ Foscarnet preferred for acyclovir-resistant cases (*NEJM* 1993; 308:1448).

  □ Comparative trial of oral acyclovir vs valacyclovir showed slight advantage of valacyclovir (*AAC* 1995;39:1546).

RESPONSE: Antiviral therapy of zoster reduces the duration of lesions, reduces the number of new lesions, and reduces systemic complaints, but the benefits are modest and largely limited to those receiving therapy within 24 hrs of onset (*NEJM* 1991;325:1539). For most patients the main concern is pain, including post-herpetic neuralgia, especially in older patients. **IRIS:** Zoster allegedly accounts for 7-12% of IRIS cases, usually about 4 wks after starting ART and usually with a typical course (*Oral Surg Oral Med Oral Path* 2007;104:455; *AIDS* 2008;22:601). Cases have been reported, presenting with transverse myelitis, iritis, keratitis, and typical dermatomal lesions (*AIDS* 2004;18:1218; *CID* 2006;42:418; *Medicine* 2002;81:213).

PREVENTION: See pg. 72-73.

Histoplasma capsulatum: 2011 ATS Guidelines (*Am J Respir Crit Care Med* 2011;183:96)

Histoplasmosis, Disseminated

PRESENTATION: The disease is endemic in the US, especially the Ohio and Mississippi River Valleys, in Puerto Rico and in Latin America. Infection is acquired by inhalation, dissemination without symptoms is common and the infection is controlled by cellular immunity. Patients with HIV infection with CD4 counts >300 cells/mm³ usually have pulmonary disease. With CD4 counts <150 cells/mm³ the usual presentation is disseminated infection that may have been acquired years previously and presents as a multiorgan disease with constitutional symptoms, including fever, weight loss and fatigue, often with lung, marrow, GI tract ± CNS involvement (*Medicine*

6 Management of Infections

1990;69:361; *CID* 2005;40:1122; *Am J Trop Med Hyg* 2005;73:576; *Diagn Microbiol Infect Dis* 2006;55: 195; *Medicine* 2008;87:193).

DIAGNOSIS: Cultures of blood, respiratory tract secretions, marrow, or focal infections are positive in 85% of cases but take 2-4 wks. Cytopathology showing typical budding yeast may provide an early diagnosis (*Cytopathology* 2010;21:240). The most common diagnostic method in cases of disseminated disease is by detection of capsular polysaccharide in urine and blood (*Trends Microbiol* 2003;11:488; *Expert Rev Resp Med* 2010;4:427). Relative sensitivities with disseminated disease for this and other tests reported by MiraVista Diagnostics are: antigen detection in urine – 95%, antigen in serum –85%; culture of multiple sites including blood – 86% (but takes 2-4 wks) and histopathology to show 2-4 um budding yeast-43%. Serology is less useful except in patients with immune competence. The blood and urine antigen assays may be used to follow the course of treatment since antigen levels at 3-4 mo intervals decrease with response and levels increase with relapse. The antigen assay is often positive in BAL fluid with pulmonary involvement (*Chest* 2010;137:623; *CID* 2009;49:1878) and in CSF with meningitis (*Ann Intern Med* 1991;115: 936). This test is available from Mira Vista Labs at 866-647-2847, 317-856-2681, or www.miravistalabs.com. The diagnosis of meningitis can be made by detection of antigen or antibody in CSF.

TREATMENT: See Table 6-4.

- **Comments**
  - ◻ Severe disseminated disease is defined by one or more of the following: temp >39°C, hypotension, pO_2 <70 torr, weight loss >5%, Karnofsky <70, hemoglobin <10 gm/dL, neutrophil count <1000/mL, ALT >2.5 ULN, creatinine >2x ULN, albumin <3.5 gm/mL or other organ dysfunction (*CID* 2000;30:688; *Ann Intern Med* 2002;137:105).
  - ◻ A therapeutic trial of amphotericin B vs. *AmBisome* in AIDS patients showed more rapid defervescence and fewer adverse reactions with *AmBisome* (*AAC* 2001; 45:2354; *Ann Intern Med* 2002;37:154).
  - ◻ 2011 ATS recommendations: Continue itraconazole for > one year and CD4 count of >200/mm³; follow urinary and serum levels of Histoplasma antigen. With chronic pulmonary histoplasmosis: treat with itraconazole 200 mg po bid x 12-24 months and do not monitor antigen levels (*Am J Resp Crit Care Med* 2011;183:96).
  - ◻ Voriconazole and posaconazole (800 mg qd) are usually active *in vitro;* the experience in AIDS patients is limited but favorable (*Trans Infect Dis* 2005;7:109; *JAC* 2006;57: 1235; *JID* 2007;54: 319).
  - ◻ Itraconazole levels are recommended to assure levels of >1 µg/mL and should be measured after >5 days of itraconazole (San

■ TABLE 6-4: Initial Treatment of Histoplasmosis

Preferred	Alternative
Moderately severe or severe	
Liposomal ampho B 3-5 mg/kg/d x 2 wks or until improved. Maintenance: itraconazole 200 mg (soln) po tid x 3d, then 200 mg po bid. Treat until CD4 count is >200/mm³ and treated at least 12 weeks	Amphotericin B 0.7-1.0 mg/kg/d up to 2 gm total followed by itraconazole
Less severe disseminated disease	
Itraconazole 200 mg (soln) po tid 3 days then 200 mg bid for at least 1 yr	Liposomal amphotericin
Meningitis	
Liposomal amphotericin B in dose of 5 mg/kg/day x 4-6 weeks, then itraconazole (solution) 200 mg 2-3 x /day for at least one year and until CSF analysis is normal	

Antonio Lab, 210-567-4131). This is especially important with NVP- or ETR-based ART (*AIDS* 2008;22:1885).

- Itraconazole is the azole of choice compared to ketoconazole and fluconazole (*CID* 2006;42:1289; *CID* 2001;33:1910). The liquid formulation of itraconazole is generally preferred. It may be used for initial treatment of mild to moderate histoplasmosis without CNS involvement, or it may be used for maintenance after induction with amphotericin B (*Am J Med* 1995;98:336).

- ART should not be delayed due to concern for IRIS, which is uncommon.

RESPONSE: Most patients show subjective and objective response within 1 wk. A comparison of itraconazole vs liposomal amphotericin showed similar cure rates (85-86%, but the rate of clearance of fungemia at two weeks was 50% for itraconazole compared to 15% for *AmBisome* (*AAC* 2001;45:2354). Antigen titer in blood and urine correlate with clinical response and usually decrease after 2-4 wks; blood and urine assays are recommended at 3- to 6-mo intervals during maintenance therapy to detect relapse. Clinical failure correlates with *in vitro* sensitivity test results, especially with fluconazole, which is far less active than itraconazole (*CID* 2001;33:1910). **IRIS** has been described presenting with pneumonitis, uveitis, adenitis, skin lesions, or liver abscess (*AIDS* 2006;20:119; *Am J Med* 2005;118:1038). One report indicated a large number of cases of disseminated disease during the first 6 mos following ART, suggesting activation of latent disease (*JAIDS* 2006;41:468). Another report of 4 cases included liver abscesses, lymphadenitis, intestinal obstruction, uveitis, and arthritis at a median of 45 days post-ART (*AIDS* 2006;20:119).

6 Management of Infections

MAINTENANCE

- **Preferred regimen:** Itraconazole 200 mg qd bid for at least one year (see Comment).

- **Alternative regimens:** Fluconazole 800 mg qd po for at least one year (use only if itraconazole is not tolerated).

- **Duration:** One report found that therapy can be safely stopped under the following conditions: 1) >12 mos of treatment: 2) CD4 >150 cells/mm³; 3) ART ≥6 mos and 4) urine and serum antigen <4.1 units (*CID* 2004;38:1485).

Isospora belli

Isosporiasis

PRESENTATION: The usual presentation is watery diarrhea ± fever, abdominal pain, vomiting, and wasting. Most patients have CD4 counts <50 cells/mm³ who are not receiving TMP/SMX prophylaxis (*HIV Med* 2008;8:124). The diagnosis requires detection of oocysts in stool with acid-fast stain, which is specific and reasonably sensitive, but several stool specimens may be required. There are no commercial antigen detection methods.

TREATMENT

- **Acute Infection**

   □ Preferred regimen: TMP-SMX 1 DS po bid (or equivalent IV) x 10 days

   □ Alternative regimen: Pyrimethamine 50-75 mg qd po + leucovorin acid 10-25 mg qd x 10 days

   □ Ciprofloxacin 500 mg po bid x 10 days (or other fluoroquinolone) can be used but are less effective (*Ann Intern Med* 2000;132:885)

   □ Support: Fluid and nutritional management; ART

- **Comment**

   □ CD4 count: Immunocompetent patients usually have self-limited diarrhea lasting 2-3 wks. Patients with a CD4 count >300 cells/mm³ can be managed as an immunocompetent host. AIDS patients may have severe or persistent diarrhea and are usually treated. Duration of therapy is not well defined.

   □ The response with TMP-SMX is rapid, but relapses are common with CD4 counts <200 cells/mm³ (*NEJM* 1989;320:1044; *Ann Intern Med* 2001;132:885)

   □ Pyrimethamine may be as effective as TMP-SMX, but experience is less extensive (*Ann Intern Med* 1988;109:474).

RESPONSE: AIDS patients usually respond to TMP-SMX within 2-3 days (*NEJM* 1986;315:87; *NEJM* 1989;320:1044). Stool examination may show continued shedding after clinical response.

Management of Infections

JC Virus

Progressive Multifocal Leukoencephalopathy (PML)

PRESENTATION AND DIAGNOSIS: (See *Lancet Infect Dis* 2009;9:625). Most healthy persons (70-80%) harbor JC virus as a latent virus in marrow, spleen, tonsils, etc. (*Neurol Res* 2006;28:299). PML is the only disease caused by JC virus and occurs most frequently as a devastating neurologic syndrome with insidious onset and progression over weeks or months. The disease is most commonly seen as a complication of late stage HIV, but rates in the US have decreased by over 4-fold since the beginning of the HAART era (*Neuroepidemiology* 2010;35:178). **Common features** are 1) cognitive dysfunction, dementia, seizures, aphasia, cranial nerve deficits, ataxia, hemiparesis; 2) CSF that shows no cells and normal protein; 3) no fever; 4) CD4 count that is usually <100 cells/mm^3 but may be >200 cells/mm^3 in up to one-third; 5) a head CT or MRI that shows hypodense white matter disease; and 6) a course that is inevitably progressive over weeks or months (*CID* 2003;36:1047; *CID* 2002;34: 103; *Lancet* 1997;349:1534). In a recent review of 54 cases, 36 (67%) developed PML and IRIS simultaneously and 18 (34%) had worsening of preexisting PML (*Neurology* 2009;72:1458). The former group had a lower lesion load on MRI and shorter survival (median survival of 8.5 vs. 2.5 wks in the group with worsening existing PML). In another recent review of 47 cases, the rate was 1.3/1000 patient years. CD4 count <50 cells/mm^3 was a significant risk factor, and 35 (68%) had a mean survival of 4 mos (*JID* 2009;199:77). A review of 24 PML patients who survived >5 years and were then followed a mean of 94 months found that 14 (63%) had no disability or only slight disability (*J Neurosurg Psychiatry* 2010; 81:1288). A definitive **diagnosis** requires compatible clinical history and MRI findings plus a brain biopsy positive by DFA stain for JC virus combined with either a positive CSF PCR for JC virus or typical inclusions in oligodendrocytes. PCR in CSF for JCV has a sensitivity of 75-80%, specificity of 90-99% (*J Neurol Neurosurg Psychiatry* 2000;69: 569).

TREATMENT

- **Preferred regimen:** There is no effective treatment. With ART some patients improve, some stabilize, and some progress, but ART should always be initiated in patients not already receiving it.

- **Comments**

  □ Diagnosis: Positive PCR + typical clinical and MRI findings constitute presumptive PML. If PCR is negative, consider brain biopsy depending on probability of a treatable alternative diagnosis.

  □ Prognosis: Median survival after PML diagnosis is 1-4 mos (*JAIDS* 1992;5:1030; *NEJM* 1998;338:1345; *CID* 2002;34:103; *Neurology* 2009;72:1458). See response below.

  □ Treatment trials: No antiviral or anti-inflammatory therapy is clearly effective, including cidofovir, corticosteroids, IFN-alfa, amantadine, cytarabine, adenosine, foscarnet, ganciclovir, cytosine arabinoside, 5HT2a receptor blockers (resperidone, mirtazapine, zisprasidone and cyproheptadine) (*Science* 2005;309: 381; *AIDS* 2002;16:1791; *J Neurovirol* 2001;7:364; *J Neurovirol* 2001;7: 374; *J Neurovir* 1998;4:324; *AIDS* 2002;16:1791; *NEJM* 1998; 338: 1345; *AIDS* 2000;14:517; *J Neurol 2008;255:526*). The 2008 NIH/CDC/IDSA Guidelines for OI Treatment does not advocate the use of any of these agents. The only treatment recommended is immediate ART for untreated patients; although in one report 7 patients had good neurologic recovery with steroids (*Neurology* 2009;72:1458). The presence of JCV-specific cytotoxic T-lumphocytes appears to be important in recovery (*Neurology* 2009;73:1551).

RESPONSE: The average survival is 1-6 mos, but there is great individual variation, with survival up to 19 years and spontaneous improvement without therapy (*Ann Neurol* 1998:44:341). There is no specific treatment for PML with verified merit, although ART has been associated with increased survival. In one study of 31 PML patients given ART, 18 survived. Of these, 8 improved, 6 were worse, and 4 remained stable (*J Neurovirol* 1999;5:421). In a review of 61 cases from Spain, 48% survived for 6 mos and 24% survived for 36 mos. Survival rates were similar with and without IRIS (*JAIDS* 2008;49:26). Similar variations have been noted by others (*JID* 2000;182:1077; *AIDS* 1999;13:1881; *CID* 2000;30:95; *JAIDS* 2004;37: 1268). The presence of JCV-specific cytotoxic T-lymphocytes appears to be important (*Neurology* 2009;73:1507).

PML IRIS appears to be mediated by JC virus-specific CD4 T lymphocytes. Histology may show diffuse mononuclear perivascular inflammatory infiltration throughout the cortex with positive JCV *in situ* hybridization (*J Neurol Neurosurg Psychiatry* 2003;74:1142). This is associated with contrast enhancement on MRI (*AIDS* 1999;13:1426). However, one review of 37 cases found contrast enhancement in only 21 (57%) (*Neurology* 2009;72:1458). IRIS may be associated with either clinical improvement or severe PML disease and death (*J Neuroimmunology* 2010;219:100; *Acta Neuropathol* 2005;109:449). Management of progressive neurologic deficits accompanied by signs of inflammation on neuro-imaging (edema, contrast enhancement) may include high-dose corticosteroids, or discontinuation of ART, but the 2008 NIH/CDC/IDSA Guidelines on Prevention and Treatment of Opportunistic Infection considers discontinuing ART "likely counter-productive" (*J Neuroimmunology* 2010;129:100; *Neurology* 2006; 67:1692; *Acta Neuropathol* 2005;109:449). Nevertheless, there are case reports of dramatic responses to steroids, including one report of response in 7 of 12 patients, with some dramatic improvements (*Neurologist* 2008;14:321). The 2009 IDSA/NIH/CDC Guidelines suggest that use of steroids is reasonable when PML is associated with an inflammatory response (*MMWR* 2009;58 RR4:132).

Microsporidia

Microsporidiosis (*CID* 2001;32:331)

PRESENTATION: Microsporidia are a broad group of microbes related to fungi that were implicated in 20-50% of AIDS-related chronic diarrhea in the pre-HAART era. The frequency now is much lower. The usual presentation is watery diarrhea in patients with a CD4 count <100cells/mm³. One report showed a prevalence of 11/737 (1.5%) HIV-infected patients from 10 cities in the US; the median CD4 count in these 11 patients was 33 cells/mm³ (range 3-319) (*Rev Inst Med Trop* 2007;49: 339).

DIAGNOSIS: The diagnosis is usually established by stool studies with light microscopy of stool specimens using calcofluor white, *Chromatope 2R*, or *Uvitex 2B* to detect spores (*NEJM* 1992;326:161; *Ann Trop Med Parasitol* 1993;87:99; *Adv Parasitol* 1998;40:351). These tests have sensitivity and specificity of about 100% and 80%, respectively (*JCM* 1998;36:2279). Microsporidia refers to a large group of microbes, of which only two are known to cause diarrhea: *Enterocytozoon* (*Septata*) *intestinalis*, which accounts for about 10-20% of microsporidiosis cases, and *E. bieneusi*, which accounts for 80-90%. A PCR method of detection of *E. bieneusi* has been described (*Am J Trop Meg Hyg* 2008;99:579). Non-intestinal manifestations of microsporidiosis include encephalitis, ocular infections, myositis, sinusitis, cholangiopathy and disseminated infection (*CID* 1994;19:517; *Adv Parasitol* 1998;40:321).

TREATMENT

- **Preferred regimens**

  - Optimal therapy: ART with virologic control and CD4 count increase to >100 cells/mm³

  - *E. bieneusi*: Fumagillin (20 mg tid x 14 days) based on two controlled trials showing efficacy (*AAC* 2000;44:168; *NEJM* 2002;346:1969; *AIDS* 2000;14:1341). The drug is available in the US as "*Flisint*" from Sanofi-Aventist in France.

  - Nitazoxanide (1000 mg po bid with food x 60 days) is also recommended by some but is not endorsed by the 2008 NIH/CDC/IDSA Guidelines on OIs. (Minimal effect with low CD4 count)

  - *E. intestinalis*: Albendazole (400 mg po bid until CD4 >200 cells/mm³) is recommended for initial treatment of intestinal and disseminated disease due to microspordia other than *E. bieneusi*. See also first item in comments below and pg. 189.

  - Symptomatic treatment with nutritional supplements and anti-diarrheal agents diphenoxylate/atropine (*Lomotil*), loperamide, etc.

  - Ocular: Fumagillin B 3 mg/mL in saline (fumagillin 70 mg/mL) eye drops (2 qtts q2h x 4 days then 2 qtts qid). Continue treatment

6 Management of Infections

indefinitely until patient is asymptomatic and CD4 count is >200 cells/mm³. Add albendazole 400 mg po bid for systemic infection.

- Disseminated disease due to microsporidia other than *E. bienuesi* or *V. corneae*: Albendazole course is 400 mg po bid until CD4 count is >200 cells/mm³.

- **Comments**

  - Albendazole is recommended for disseminated (non-ocular) microsporidiosis caused by any microsporidia other than *E. bienuesi* (2008 NIH/CDC/IDSA Recommendations).

  - Fumagillin proved effective in two controlled trials for microsporidiosis due to *E. bieneusi* (*NEJM* 2002;346:1963; *AIDS* 2000;14:1341).

  - Albendazole efficacy: Established only for infections involving *E. intestinalis*, which causes 10-20% of cases.

  - Anecdotal success: Reported with itraconazole, fluconazole, nitazoxanide, nitrofurantoin, atovaquone, and metronidazole (*Infect Dis Clin North Am* 1994;8:483).

  - Immune reconstitution with CD4 >100 cells/mm³: Best therapy, especially for the 80-90% of cases involving *E. bieneusi* (*Lancet* 1998;351:256; *AIDS* 1998;12:35; *JCM* 1999;37:421; *JAIDS* 2000;25:124).

  - Extraintestinal infections: *E. bellum* – sinusitis and disseminated disease; *E. cuniculi* – CNS, conjunctiva, renal, lungs; *T. hominis* – myositis; *Braciola* – myositis.

RESPONSE: Symptoms resolve with CD4 count increase to >100 cells/mm³. With fumagillin treatment of *E. bieneusi* there is response by week 4 as indicated by discontinuation of loperamide use and elimination of detectable microsporidia in stool (*NEJM* 2002;346:1963).

Molluscum Contagiosum

CAUSE: Molluscum contagiosum virus (MCV), a DNA poxvirus

PRESENTATION: Clinical presentation is with flesh-colored, pink or whitish dome-shaped papules with central umbilication (dimpling). It can occur anywhere on the body, except palms and soles. Most common areas are the face (beard area), neck, and genitals. Lesions are usually <5 mm in diameter; occasionally lesions are >1 cm (giant molluscum).

DIAGNOSIS: The diagnosis may be confirmed by KOH preparation, Tzanck smear, or biopsy that shows intraepidermal molluscum bodies. EM shows a large brick-shaped virus resembling smallpox. The virus cannot be cultivated.

TREATMENT: Standard approaches are physical destruction, topical treatment and ART. An individual lesion may be treated with curettage, cryotherapy, electrocauterization (*Sex Transm Infect* 1999;75[suppl

1]:S80), chemical cauterization (trichloroacetic acid, cantharidin, podophyllin, 5-FU, tretinoin, silver nitrate, phenol), imiquimod and topical cidofovir. Lesions usually disappear in patients responding to ART (*Eur J Dermatol* 1999;9:211). A Cochrane Library Review concluded that no single therapy was "convincingly effective" (*Cochrane Database Syst Rev* 2009;CD004767). A case report showed a dramatic response to very severe and refractory disease with IV paclitaxel (100 mg/mm², 108 mg) given every 21 days x 4 cycles (*HIV Med* 2010;18:169).

Mycobacterium avium Complex
Disseminated MAC

PRESENTATION: MAC is a ubiquitous mycobacterium found in environmental sources that is acquired by ingestion or inhalation. It is a relatively common cause of chronic pulmonary disease in otherwise healthy adults and of disseminated infection without pulmonary involvement in patients with AIDS. Person-to-person transmission is unlikely. The incidence of disseminated MAC in patients with a CD4 count <100 cells/mm³ in the absence of ART and MAC prophylaxis is 20-40%(*JID* 1992;165:1082). With ART and MAC prophylaxis, this is reduced to 2.5/1000 person years (*AIDS* 2010;24:1549).

The usual symptoms in AIDS patients are fever, night sweats, weight loss, diarrhea, and abdominal pain typically occurring in patients with a CD4 count <50 cells/mm³ (*JID* 1997;176:126; *JID* 1994;170:1601; *Lancet Infect Dis* 2004;4:557). Lab tests usually show anemia and an elevated alkaline phosphotase. The diagnosis is established by culture of MAC from a non-pulmonary, normally sterile site; blood cultures are 90-95% sensitive using Bactec 12B or 13A bottles but usually require 7-14 days. The diagnosis rarely requires biopsy of liver, bone marrow, or lymph nodes. Sputum and stool are insensitive and nonspecific culture sources (*JID* 1994;168:1045; *JID* 1994;169:289).

Pulmonary MAC (uncommon in HIV-infected patients): Infiltrate on x-ray and culture with ≥2+ growth and 1 positive AFB stain (*Am J Respir Crit Care Med* 1997;155:2041).

TREATMENT
Preferred regimens:
- Preferred: clarithromycin 500 mg po bid + ethambutol (EMB) 15 mg/kg/d po. Consider adding a third drug with CD4 count <50 cells/mm³, high MAC load (>200 CFU/mL) or absence of effective ART: rifabutin 300 mg qd po (Adjust dose for concurrent PIs or NNRTI (see www.mmhiv.com/link/CDC-TB-HIV). Therapeutic drug monitoring may be useful due to the complexity of drug interactions (*Pharmacotherapy* 2011;31:439) (see pg. 217).
- Alternative regimen: azithromycin 500-600 mg qd + ethambutol 15 mg/kg/d po +/- rifabutin (see pg. 205).

- Alternative "third drugs" are 1) levofloxacin 500 mg po qd; 2) ciprofloxacin 500-750 mg po bid; 3) moxifloxacin 400 mg qd, 4) streptomycin 1 gm IV or IM qd; 5) amikacin 10-15 mg/kg/d IV.
- ART: In treatment-naïve patients consider delay in starting ART until after 2 wks of MAC treatment to reduce drug interactions, pill burden and IRIS. The ACTG trial addressing this issue (ACTG 5164) concluded ART should begin within 2 wks of initiating treatment of a non-TB opportunistic infection (*PLoS Med* 2009;4:e5575).

Treatment failure:

Treatment failure is defined as lack of clinical response and positive blood cultures at 4-8 wks post therapy.

- Susceptibility tests should be performed and treatment should include two new drugs that are active *in vitro*. Benefit of continuing macrolide with *in vitro* resistance is unknown.
- Candidate agents are: rifabutin, amikacin and quinolones (levofloxacin, ciprofloxacin or moxifloxacin). Some recommend inclusion of an injectable agent (amikacin or streptomycin) based on data for treatment of MAC in non-AIDS patients (*Am J Respir Crit Care Med* 2007;175:367).
- Data supporting efficacy of these recommendations for management of treatment failures are poor (2008 NIH/CDC/IDSA Guidelines for Prevention and Treatment of Opportunistic Infections in Adolescents and Adults with HIV Infection). The experience is limited and not very supportive (*CID* 1999;18 Suppl 3:S237; *CID* 1999;28:1080; *JID* 1997;176:1225; *CID* 1999;29:125; *JID* 1998;178: 1446; *Ann Intern Med* 1990;113:358).

RESPONSE: Decrease in fever and in quantitative blood cultures is expected in 2-4 wks. Obtain blood cultures if there is no clinical improvement within 4-8 wks. Treatment failure is defined by positive blood cultures at 4-8 wks. Care should be taken to distinguish MAC treatment failure with MAC bacteremia from MAC IRIS, in which blood cultures are negative (discussed below).

COMMENTS

- **Severe Disease:** Use a 3-drug combination, but the best third drug is unclear (see below). Studies with rifabutin as a third drug suggest improved survival and reduced resistance (*CID* 1999;28: 1080; *CID* 2003;37:1234). Alternative third drugs are levofloxacin, moxifloxacin, ciprofloxacin, streptomycin, or amikacin, but data supporting benefit with these drugs are sparse (*NEJM* 1996;335:377; *CID* 1997;25:621; *JID* 1993;168:112). If not on ART, start ART at about 2 wks (*PLoS Med* 2009;4:e5575).
- **Clarithromycin drug interactions:** Clarithromycin AUC is increased with concurrent PIs: IDV (50%), RTV (75%), FPV (18%), LPV/r (77%), ATV (94%), TPV (19%), NVP (26%), DRV (57%) and SQV (177%). In patients with QTc prolongation, SQV is contraindicated for use with

clarithromycin. Nevertheless, no dose adjustment is thought necessary except with ATV; reduce the clarithromycin dose 50% or avoid it due to increased levels. Another concern is prolonged QTc when LPV/r or RTV are used with clarithromycin in patients with renal failure. With EFV, clarithromycin levels are decreased 39%; monitor response or use azithromycin (*NEJM* 1996;335:428). NVP AUC increases 26% and claithromycin AUC decreases 30%; monitor. With ETR the ETR AUC increases 42% and clarithromycin AUC decreases 39%; monitor response or use azithromycin (*NEJM* 1996;335: 428). With MVC use MVC 150 mg bid.

- **Rifabutin dose:** 300 mg qd, but should not exceed 300 mg qd if given with clarithromycin or fluconazole. Note interactions with PIs and NNRTIs (see Table 5-70, pg. 362 and Table 6-9, pg. 468).

- ***In vitro* susceptibility:** Should be measured routinely for clarithromycin and azithromycin. Resistance is most common in patients with prior macrolide exposure (*NEJM* 1996;335:392; *CID* 1998; 27:1369; *JID* 2000;181:1289; *NEJM* 1996;335; *JID* 1998; 178:1446; *CID* 1999;28:1080; *JID* 1997;176:1225; *CID* 1999; 29:125; *CID* 1998;27:1278; *CID* 2000;31:1245) Threshold for clarithromycin sensitivity is 32µg/mL and for azithromycin is 256 µg/mL using Bactec radiometric susceptibility testing. It is not known whether continuation of these drugs despite resistance has clinical merit.

- **Clarithromycin vs azithromycin:** In a comparative trial for MAC bacteremia, clarithromycin was superior in time to negative blood cultures (*CID* 1998;27:1278; *AAC* 1999 ; 43:2869). Nevertheless, another large trial using azithromycin 600 mg qd vs clarithromycin 500 mg bid, each combined with EMB, showed comparable results (*CID* 2000;31:1254).

- **ASA or NSAID** often effective for symptom relief.

- **Immune reconstitution:** Discontinue maintenance therapy when CD4 count >100 cells/mm³ x 6 mos + ≥12 mos treatment and asymptomatic.

MAC Immune Reconstitution Inflammatory Syndrome (IRIS)

CHARACTERISTIC FEATURES: 1) Host and timing factors: most common in the first 8 mos (usually at 1-3 mos) after initiating ART with baseline CD4 <50 cells/mm³, a good CD4 response to >100 cells/mm³ and rapid viral load response (*Lancet* 1998;351:252; *JAIDS* 1999;20:122; *Ann Intern Med* 2000;133:447; *CID* 2004;38:1159; *JAIDS* 2009;46:456). 2) The most common presentation is fever and a focal inflammatory lesion, usually cervical adenitis, but others include mediastinal adenitis, mesenteric adenitis, pericarditis, osteomyelitis, skin abscesses, CNS infections, hepatic granuloma, osteomyelitis, thoracic spine abscess, parotitis, psoas abscess, peritonitis, cholestatic liver disease, etc. (*Ann*

6 Management of Infections

Intern Med 2000;133:447; *CID* 2004;38:461; *CID* 2004;38:1159; *CID* 2005;41:1483; *Medicine* 2002;81: 213; *Lancet Infect Dis* 2005;5:361). A review of 43 cases of MAC IRIS found an incidence of 3% among ART recipients with 3 main clinical presentations: peripheral lymphadenitis, thoracic disease, and intra-abdominal disease. The median CD4 count from pre-ART baseline and at IRIS presentation were 20 cells/mm^3 and 120 cells/mm^3, respectively. Blood cultures with MAC IRIS are usually negative (*J Med Microbiol* 2010;59:1365). There was no difference in outcome in 10 patients without treatment directed at MAC, and 8 of 9 responded to prednisone (*CID* 2005;41:1483).

TREATMENT:

- Continue ART
- Continue MAC therapy
- Treat IRIS with NSAIDs; severe cases should be treated with prednisone 20-60 mg qd, with slow taper guided by symptoms.

Mycobacterium tuberculosis (TB)

EPIDEMIOLOGY AND CLINICAL FEATURES: TB is usually transmitted by inhalation from a patient with pulmonary or laryngeal TB. The immune response usually controls growth, resulting in latent TB infection. TB disease occurs as a result of progression of the initial exposure (primary disease) or activation of latent disease (*MMWR* 2003;52, RR11:1). The prevalence of latent TB in the US is 4-5% (*MMWR* 2007;56:245). The annual risk of active TB with latent infection in the pre-HAART era was increased 3- to 12-fold by HIV infection; primary TB is also relatively common and accounts for one-third of cases (*MMWR* 2003;52RR-10:1; *NEJM* 2004;350:2060). HIV promotes TB at all CD4 strata (*JID* 2005;19:150), but clinical features vary according to CD4 count. With CD4 count >350 cells/mm^3 lung lesions are "typical," with upper lobe infiltrates ± cavitation. With a CD4 count <50 cells/mm^3 extrapulmonary TB is far more common with pleuritis, pericarditis, meningitis, and disseminated disease; chest x-rays typically show lower and middle lobe and miliary infiltrates, usually without cavitation.The pathology is also different since TB with advanced HIV infection shows poorly formed granulomas. A new form of TB is TB IRIS, reflecting unmasking of active TB with immune reconstitution expressed with constitutional symptoms and focal inflammatory lesions (discussed below) (*CID* 1997;25:242; *Medicine* 1991;70:384). TB is associated with increased HIV viral load and more rapid progression of HIV infection (*Am J Respir Crit Care Med* 1995;151:129; *Am J Respir Crit Care Med* 1993;148:1293).

DIAGNOSIS: Standard tests to detect latent tuberculosis are the tuberculin skin test and the interferon-gamma release assays (IGRAs, see pg. 54). About one fourth of HIV-infected patients with active TB will have false negative tests (*Ann Intern Med* 2007;146:340). The early diagnosis and treatment of TB in patients seriously ill with HIV is a critical factor in outcome (*Lancet Infect Dis* 2009;5:e5575). The standard test for active <u>pulmonary TB</u> is AFB smear and culture on morning expectorated sputa collected over 3 days. Sputum induction and/or bronchoscopy are used if there is no sputum production. Sensitivity of AFB smear is about 50%, is similar for patients with and without AIDS, and is not better with induced sputum or bronchoscopy specimens compared with expectorated sputum (*Chest* 1992; 101:1211; *Chest* 1992;102:1040; *Am J Respir Crit Care Med* 2000; 162:2238). The most recent important new diagnostic test for *M. tuberculosis* is *Xpert*, a molecular test that will simultaneously detect this mycobacterium and rifampin resistance within 2 hrs with minimal specimen handling. Results are summarized in Table 6-5 (*NEJM* 2010; 363:1005).

■ TABLE 6-5: **Results with the *Xpert* Molecular Test to Detect *M. tuberculosis* Compared to AFB Stain and Culture**

Category	Results
■ Culture positive ■ Smear negative ■ Culture negative	■ 723/741 (97.6%) ■ 157/177 (90.2%) ■ 12/616 (2.0%)
Rifampin sensitivity ■ Resistant* ■ Sensitive	■ 200/205 (97.5%) ■ 506/506 (100%)

*   MDR-TB (Resistant INH and RIF) 200/205 (97.5%)

<u>Sensitivity tests:</u> All positive cultures should be tested for sensitivity to the 5 first-line drugs: INH, rifampin, ethambutol, PZA, and streptomycin. <u>PPD skin tests</u> and <u>interferon-gamma tests</u> have high rates of false-negative results that correlate inversely with CD4 count: up to 65% false-negatives in AIDS patients with active TB (*JID* 1992; 166:194). Positive cultures for *M. tuberculosis* approach 100% for sensitivity and 97% for specificity (*CID* 2001;31:1390).

Current recommendations for patients with untreated HIV infection and suspected active TB are early treatment of TB, and treatment of HIV dictated by the CD4 count. WHO has addressed the need for early TB treatment in high TB prevalence areas with the algorithm for "TB suspect criteria" defined as: 1) cough x 2 wks or 2) absence of cough with night sweats (T >37.5º), breathlessness due to pleural effusion or pericarditis, enlarged cervical or axillary nodes, altered mental state or abnormal chest x-ray. These patients should have an AFB smear, and if negative, a chest x-ray is done. Criteria for TB treatment are: 1) positive AFB smear; or 2) suggestive x-ray; or 3) suggestive clinical assessment (WHO 2009; www.mmhiv.com/link/2009-WHO-TB). It is emphasized that this is intended for areas with high rates of TB and HIV. Implementation in targeted areas has shown substantial benefit of algorithm management vs. standard practice in terms of 8 week survival (83% vs. 68%) (*Lancet Infect Dis* 2011;11:533). It should be emphasized that point-of-care testing for HIV provided an extraordinary advance in that diagnosis, and the molecular diagnostics for TB detection hold the same promise for tuberculosis (*PLoS One* 2011; 6:E18502).

- **Major trials to inform providers on the timing of initiating ART**
  - □ **ACTG 5221 STRIDE** (Havilar 2011 CROI;Abstr. 38)**:** The study addressed the issue of early vs. delayed ART in HIV/TB co-infection patients. Participants had CD4 counts <250 cells/mm³, were stratified by CD4 at ≥50 vs. <50 cells/mm³ and given standard TB treatment plus "immediate" ART (<2 wks) vs. "early" ART (8-12 wks). All participants received standard rifampin-containing TB treatment, TMP-SMX prophylaxis and EFV/TDF/FTC. Results at 48 weeks are summarized in Table 6-6.

  - □ **The SAPiT trial** was a comparison of outcomes for 429 untreated HIV/TB co-infection with a median baseline CD4 count of 150 cells/mm³ (2011 CROI;Abstr. 39 LB). The incidence ratio of AIDS or death among patients with a baseline CD4 count of <50 cells/mm³ was 8.5/100 person-years with early treatment (within 4 wks) vs. 26.3/100 person-years with late treatment (within 4 wks of the continuation phase). Immune reconstitution rates were 47% for early treatment and 10% for late treatment. For patients with baseline CD4 counts >50 cells/mm³ there was no statistically significant benefit to early treatment, but there was a higher rate of IRIS (HR=02.2; p=0.02). The conclusion was that patients with CD4 counts <50 cells/mm³ should start ART within 4 wks of TB treatment but delay of this until >4 wks of the continuation phase since this showed no significant risks.

  - □ **CAMELIA:** This was an open label randomized trial of early vs. late treatment of TB/HIV co-infected patients. Patients with smear positive TB received standard TB therapy and were randomized to early (2 wks after treatment of TB initiated) or late (8 wks after). The standard ART regimen was d4T/3TC/EFV. The results showed the mortality rate was 8.3/100 person years with early treatment vs. 13.8/100 persons years with late treatment, a 38% reduction with early treatment (*JID* 2007;196.S1:S46). 2010 WHO Guidelines are to start ART at 2-8 wks after initiating TB therapy. Note that the results of STRIDE, CAMELIA and SAPiT support the safety and efficacy of earlier ART despite an increased risk of IRIS.

<u>Recommendation</u> based on CAMELIA, SAPiT and STRIDE:
- **HIV-treatment already started and TB is diagnosed:**
  - □ Treat TB with the standard regimen starting immediately. The ART regimen* may need to be altered to account for drug interactions.
- **ART-naïve:** TB should be treated immediately and ART* should be initiated based on CD4 count using an appropriate regimen.

- CD4 <50 cells/mm^3: Start ART* within 2 wks
- CD4 >50 cells/mm^3: Start ART* at or shortly after week 8 of TB treatment. If symptoms of HIV are severe start ART* at week 2-4 of TB treatment
- Pregnancy: Start TB treatment immediately and ART as soon as possible (see below)
- CD4 >50 cells/mm^3 and severe HIV-associated complications: Start ART* within 2-4 wks

* ART regimen is generally EFV-based with standard TB regimen including rifampin. If PI/r-based, use rifabutin (see pg. 362).

TREATMENT: See Tables 6-7 to 6-15. Official statement of the ATS, CDC, and IDSA: Treatment of Tuberculosis (*Am J Respir Crit Care Med* 2003;167:603; www.mmhiv.com/link/2005-CDC-TB; *Lancet ID* 2007;6:710; 2008 DHHS Guidelines for Management of Opportunistic Infections).

- **Standard TB treatment:** Treatment should be started when active TB is suspected while diagnostic tests are pending. The TB regimens advocated are the same for those with or without HIV infection. All treatment should be directly observed (DOT), preferably augmented to support other medical and social support needs ("enhanced DOT"). The standard for drug susceptible strains is a 6-month course, with isoniazid (INH), rifampin (RIF), pyrazinamide (PZA) + ethambutol (EMB) for 2 mos (induction phase) followed by INH + RIF for 4 mos (maintenance phase) (Table 6-7) (*MMWR* 2005;54 RR 12:1). EMB may be stopped before 2 mos if the TB strain is susceptible to INH, RIF and PZA (*MMWR* 2003;52 RR 11:1). The maintenance phase is continued for 7 mos (total 9 mos) if there is cavitary TB, positive sputum cultures at 2 mos and for some patients with extrapulmonary TB; some authorities recommend a maintenance course of 7-10 mos (total 9-12 mos) with CNS TB or bone and joint TB (*MMWR* 2003;RR 11:1).

- TABLE 6-6: **Timing of Treatment of TB with HIV Co-infection: STRIDE**

	TB/HIV "immediate" n = 405	TB/HIV "early" n = 405
ART initiation (median)	10 days	10 weeks
Endpoint* (48 weeks)	13.0%	16.1%
CD4 ≤50 cells/mm^3	15.5%	26.6%[†]
CD4 >50 cells/mm^3	11.5%	10.3%
IRIS	11.0%	5.0%[†]

* AIDS-defining condition or death
† p=0.02

The authors recommended initiating ART with HIV/TB co-infection and a CD4 count <50 cells/mm^3.

6 Management of Infections

- □ EFV-based ART with standard anti-TB treatment including standard dose rifampin is the preferred ART regimen.
- □ DOT: Outcome is improved with enhanced directly observed therapy to provide meds and support social and other medical needs (*MMWR* 2004;53 RR-15:12).
- □ Intermittent treatment: The induction phase of DOT may be given 7 days/wk, 5 days/wk or 3 days/wk; the continuation phase may also be given intermittently including twice weekly for those with CD4 counts >100 cells/mm^3.
- □ EMB: If the isolated strain is sensitive to PZA, INH and RIF, it is appropriate to discontinue EMB.
- □ RIF: This is the only first or second line anti-TB drug that has significant interactions with antiretroviral agents.
- □ Doses: Completion should be based on the number of doses (Table 6-8) rather than the duration of treatment.
- □ Duration: Standard is 6 mos (4-drug induction phase x 2 mos followed by 2-drug continuation phase x 4 mos) (Table 6-7). The continuation phase is extended by 3 mos if the culture is positive

■ TABLE 6-7: **Treatment of Drug-susceptible TB**

Drugs	Phase 1 (8 weeks) Doses, Duration	Phase 2* Regimen, Doses, Minimum Duration
	8 weeks	16 weeks*
INH, RIF, PZA, EMB ‡	■ 7 d/wk, 56 doses, 8 wks or ■ 5 d/wk, 40 doses, 8 wks	■ INH/RIF 7 d/wk, 126 doses or 5 d/wk, 90 doses, 18 wks ■ INH/RIF 3/wk, 36 doses, 18 wks†
INH, RIF, PZA, EMB‡	■ 7 d/wk, 14 doses x 2 wks, ■ then 2x/wks* ■ 12 doses, 6 wks†	■ INH/RIF 2x/wk, 36 doses, 18 wks†
INH, RIF, PZA, EMB	■ 3x/wk, 24 doses, 8 wks†	■ INH/RIF 3x/wk, 54 doses, 18 wks†
INH, RIF, EMB	■ 7 d/wk, 56 doses or 5 d/wk, 40 doses†	■ INH/RIF 7 d/wk, 217 doses or 5 d/wk, 155 doses, 31 wks ■ INH/RIF 2x/wk, 62 doses, 31 wks†

INH = Isoniaizid, RIF = rifampin or rifabutin, PZA = pyrazinamide, EMB = ethambutol

* Duration: Pulmonary TB – 6 mo; pulmonary TB with cavity or positive culture at 2 months – 9 months; TB involving bone, joint or CNS – 9-12 mos; TB involving other extra pulmonary sites – 6-9 mos.

‡ If strain recovered is sensitive to all first line agents, discontinue EMB.

† Patients with a CD4 count <100 cells/mm^3 should receive daily therapy during the induction phase (first 8 wks) and receive daily or thrice weekly administration during the continuation phase. This is based on the observation of failure with rifamycin resistance in 5 of 156 participants in TBTC Study 23 who were treated twice weekly (*MMWR* 2002;51:214). Twice weekly treatment in the continuation phase can be done in patients with a CD4 count >100 cells/mm^3.

Drug	Daily	2x/wk	3x/wk
INH (pg. 298)	5 mg/kg (300)*	15 mg/kg (900)*†	15 mg/kg (900)*
RIF (pg. 364)	10 mg/kg (600)	10 mg/kg (600)*	10 mg/kg (600)*
PZA (wt) (pg. 350) 40-55 kg 56-75 kg 76-90 kg	1 gm 1.5 gm 2.0 gm	2.0 gm 3.0 gm 4.0 gm	1.5 gm 2.5 gm 3.0 gm
EMB (wt)‡ (pg. 265) 40-55 kg 56-75 kg 76-90 kg	800 mg 1,200 mg 1,600 mg	2,000 mg 2,800 mg 4,000 mg	1,200 mg 2,000 mg 2,400 mg

* Maximum dose in parentheses

† Twice weekly only if CD4 >100 cell/mm^3

‡ Dose adjustment with renal failure

at 2 mos or if there is cavitation. Other exceptions are CNS and bone/joint TB, which should be treated 9-12 mos.

■ **Pregnancy:** See Table 6-13.

No alterations in standard care in most cases:

- □ INH: Hepatotoxicity may be more common (*Public Health Rep* 1989;104:151) but use of prophylaxis in pregnancy is considered safe and effective.

- □ RIF: Give prophylactic vitamin K (10 mg) to neonate due to potential RIF-related hemorrhagic complications.

- □ PZA: Limited experience: recommended for use by WHO; optional in US, but if PZA is not used the duration of treatment should be 9 mos.

- □ EMB: No ocular toxicity with in utero exposure.

- □ Fluoroquinolones: Generally not recommended during pregnancy due to arthropathy in immature animals, but 1,100 cases in pregnancy registry without complications (*Obstet Gynec* 2006;107: 1120; *PEur J Obstet Gynec Reprod Biol* 2009;143:75).

- □ Aminoglycosides: Avoid streptomycin due to 10% rate of ototoxicity in neonates.

■ **Unique issues of TB with HIV co-infection**

- □ Atypical TB presentation with low CD4 count: more non-cavitary, lower- and mid-lobe involvement and extrapulmonary disease

- □ TB incidence is increased 100-fold with HIV; HIV viral loads are higher and HIV disease progresses more rapidly with active TB (*Am J Resp Crit Care Med* 1995;151:129). The increased risk of TB begins within 1 year of HIV transmission.

- □ IRIS is reported in 11-45% of patients who receive ART within 6 wks of starting TB treatment (*Int J Tuberc Lung Dis* 2006;10:946)

Management of Infections

6

- Several reports show a high rate of morbidity and mortality in the first month of TB treatment in patients with a CD4 count <100 cells/mm^3 at baseline (*JID* 2004;190:1670).

- Other differences with HIV co-infection in anti-TB therapy: 1) optimal duration is unclear; 2) CD4 <100 cells/mm^3 – continuation phase dosing should be daily or 3x/wk; 3) rifapentine is contraindicated.

- In a large trial of <u>steroids</u> for pleural TB in coinfected patients in Kampala, prednisone (50 mg qd x 2 wks, then tapered over 6 wks) was not associated with an increase in OIs or a decrease in CD4 count response (*JID* 2004;190:869).

■ TABLE 6-9: **First-line TB Agents: Adverse Reactions and Monitoring**

INH (Isoniazid) (see pg. 299)	
Formulation	50, 100, 300 mg tabs, also syrup and IM formulations
Liver	↑ ALT in 10% to 20%; clinical hepatitis 0.6%; INH/RIF 2.7%. Risk ↑ with ETOH, prior liver disease and postpartum; fatal hepatitis 0.02%
Peripheral neuropathy	Dose-related, frequency 0.2%, risk with other causes of peripheral neuropathy (diabetes, HIV, drugs, ETOH, pregnancy). Prevented with pyroxidine 25 mg/day.
Other toxicity	Rare: CNS toxicity, LE syndrome, hypersensitivity reactions, monoamine poisoning-flushing with exposure to wine, cheese, etc.
Pregnancy	Safe
Drug interaction	Levels of phenytoin and carbamazepine decreased by rifamycins
Monitoring	Usually none. Monitor LFTs monthly if pre-existing liver disease or with development of abnormal LFTs that does not require D/C therapy.
RIF (Rifampin) (see pg. 364)	
Formulation	150 mg caps
Cutaneous reactions	Pruritis ± rash
Flu syndrome	0.4-0.7% with RIF 2x/wk
Liver	Cholestatic hepatitis 0.6%; hepatotoxicity in 2.7% given INH/RIF
Orange discoloration of body fluids	Warn patients that clothing and contact lenses may be stained.
Pregnancy	Safe
Interaction: See pg. 364.	Extensive. Reduces the following to ineffective levels: oral contraceptives, methadone, warfarin, protease inhibitors; see www.mmhiv.com/link/CDC-TB (Division of Tuberculosis Elimination, CDC).
Monitoring	None

■ TABLE 6-9: **First-line TB Agents** *(Continued)*

PZA (Pyrazinamide) (see pg. 350)	
Formulation	500 mg tabs
Liver	Dose-related hepatotoxicity 1% at 25 mg/kg
Nongouty polyarthralgias	Up to 40%, rarely serious enough to D/C; treat with ASA, NSAIDs
Hyperuricemia	Expected and not consequential; gout is rare.
GI intolerance	Usually mild.
Pregnancy	Little information; use when benefit justifies an unquantified risk.
Monitoring	Uric acid levels are unnecessary but may be surrogate for adherence. LFTs when baseline liver disease and when given with RIF for latent TB.
EMB (Ethambutol)(see pg. 265)	
Formulation	100, 400 mg tabs
Ocular	Decreased acuity or decreased red-green discrimination. Risk is dose-related and minimal at 15 mg/kg; risk increases with daily administration and renal failure.
Pregnancy	Safe
Monitoring	Baseline visual acuity and Ishihara test of color discrimination. Inquire about vision changes at each monthly visit and warn patient to contact clinic immediately if change in vision. Monthly test of acuity and color discrimination with doses >15-20 mg/kg, duration >2 mos or renal failure.

- **Drug resistant TB**: Treatment is the same with and without HIV co-infection.

  □ INH resistance: Discontinue INH and give RIF/PZA/EMB x 6 mos or RIF/EMB x 12 mos preferably with PZA the first 2 mos. Add fluoroquinolone for extensive disease.

  □ RIF resistance: Discontinue RIF and give INH/EMB/PZA/FQ x 2 mos, then INH/EMB/FQ x 10-16 mos. Consider adding amikacin or capreomycin first 2-3 mos for severe disease.

  □ Multi-drug resistant (INH- and RIF-resistance)TB (MDR-TB) or extensively resistant TB (XDR-TB): consult a TB expert.

- **Risks for MDR-TB:** 1) previous history of TB; 2) exposure to MDR-TB; 3) failure to respond to standard treatment; or 4) prior residence in a country with high rates of MDR-TB.

- **XDR-TB:** The importance of this strain in patients with AIDS was initially recognized in the explosive epidemic in KwaZulu, Natal in South Africa (*Lancet* 2006;368:1575). In a review of 542 cases of TB, 221 (40%) had MDR-TB, and 53 of these had XDR-TB, which is now defined as MDR-TB (resistant to INH and RIF) that is also resistant to

6 Management of Infections

Drug	Dosing
Rifabutin	300 mg (see Table 6-8). Dose adjustment needed with PI administration.
Cycloserine	10-15 mg/kg/day, usually 500-750 mg bid
Ethionamide	15-20 mg/kg/day, usually 500-750 mg qd (max 1g/day)
Streptomycin	15 mg/kg/day, usually 1 g qd. Age >50 years: 10 mg/kg/day, usually 750 mg qd. Streptomycin is given IM or IV 5-7 d/wk x 2-4 mos, then 2-3x/wk after culture conversion.
Amikacin	10-15 mg/kg/d IV
PAS	8-12 g/day in 2-3 doses
Levofloxacin	500 mg/day
Moxifloxacin	400 mg/day

fluoroquinolones and at least one injectable anti-TB drug (*Lancet* 2006;368:1575). All patients tested had HIV infection. This appeared to be a clonal strain of TB (genotype KZN). Most were hospital acquired, and 52 of 53 (98%) patients died at a median of 16 days from the time of the first sputum collection (*Lancet* 2006;268:1575; *Science* 2006; 313:1554; *Br Med* J 2006;333:559). In a subsequent report, 29 of 48 (60%) of patients with XDR-TB without HIV co-infection responded to a 4-6 drug regimen including cycloserine, an aminoglycoside and a fluoroquinolone (*NEJM* 2008;359:563). A more recent review recommended treatment of XDR-TB with a stepwise selection of drugs in five groups based on efficacy, safety and cost (*Lancet Infect Dis* 2010;10:621): 1) first line oral drugs: high-dose INH (5 mg/kg) PZA, ETH; 2) fluoroquinolone (high dose levaquin 15 mg/kg); 3) injectables in the following order: capreomycin > kanamycin > amikacin; 4) second-line to be used in the following order: thioamides, cycloserine and PAS and 5) drugs with sparse data to be used in the following order: clofazamine > amoxicillin-clavulanate > linezolid > carabapenems > thioacetazone > clarithromycin. A report on patients with TB/HIV co-infection with newly acquired XDR-TB have this as a newly acquired strain rather than inadequate treatment of the initial TB infection (*JID* 2008; 198:1577).

■ **TB IRIS:** May occur in absence of HIV co-infection but more common with HIV and assumed to be due to immune reconstitution.

  □ Presentation: IRIS TB may be "unmasked" or may be a "paradoxical" response. The severity is variable but is clearly more common and severe with early vs. delayed ART. Most common is worsening of symptoms and x-ray changes, with fever and lymphadenopathy. In some cases there are expanding CNS lesions and/or large effusions, usually 1-3 mos after starting ART (*Arch Intern Med* 2002;162:97; *Chest* 2001;120:193; *AIDS* 2010; 24:103; *Lancet Infect Dis* 2008;8:516). Rule out other causes, especially TB treatment failure and lymphoma (see pg. 528).

a) "Unmasking" (ART-associated TB): 1) newly detected active after ART; and 2) fulfills WHO criteria for TB

b) "Paradoxical IRIS": 1) Diagnosis of TB established before ART and condition stabilized or improved on TB treatment; plus 2) at least one major or 2 minor criteria:

- Major criteria: a) new or enlarging lymph node(s) or focal tissue enlargement; b) new or worsening TB features on imaging; c) worsening TB meningitis or focal CNS defect; or d) new or worsening effusion
- Minor criteria: a) new or worsening systemic symptoms (fever, night sweats, weight loss; b) worsening pulmonary symptoms; c) abdominal conditions: hepatosplenomegaly, peritonitis, or abdominal adenopathy
- Rule out alternative causes

□ Definition from the International Network for the Study of HIV-associated IRIS (*Lancet Infect Dis* 2008;8:516)

□ Validation: One report showed good agreement with analysis of 498 patients in South Africa (*AIDS* 2010;24:103)

□ Clinical features: IRIS includes pulmonary disease (pneumonitis, effusions, lymphadenitis), ARDS, cerebritis, meningitis, parotitis, epididymitis, ascites, adenopathy (*Lancet Infect Dis* 2005;5:361; *Am J Respir Crit Care Med* 1998;158:157; *Chest* 2001;120:193).

□ Risk factors for TB IRIS: ART within 6 wks of starting TB treatment, low baseline CD4 count, high baseline VL, good CD4 and HIV response, and extrapulmonary disease (*AIDS* 2010; 24:2381; *Int. J Tuberc Lung Dis* 2006;10:946). IRIS was more common with early vs. delayed ART in SAPiT, STRIDE and CAMELIA trials but was not associated with increased mortality.

□ Treatment of Severe Cases: Prednisone 20-60 mg qd 4-8 wks with slow taper guided by symptoms. Continue TB and HIV therapy. (See above regarding corticosteroids.) Mild to moderate reaction: Treat symptomatically with NSAIDs.

- **Infection control:** New York State Department of Health AIDS Institute Guidelines (www.mmhiv.com/link/NYSD-TB).

High-risk procedures (induced sputum, aerosolized pentamidine, bronchoscopy): airborne precautions and specialized rooms

Hospitalized patients with suspected AFB smear-positive pulmonary or laryngeal TB:

6 Management of Infections

■ TABLE 6-11: **Dose Adjustment for Antiretroviral Agents when Used with Rifampin (RIF) or Rifabutin (RBT) (DHHS Guidelines 11/3/08)**

	Rifamycin dose	Comment
NNRTI		
EFV	RIF-standard	Standard EFV dose
NVP	RIF-standard	Inferior to EFV when given with RIF (*JAMA* 2008;301:530) Avoid co-administration
ETR*	RBT 300 mg/d	Avoid with ETR + DRV/r or SQV/r
PI**		
All boosted PIs‡	RBT 150 mg qod	Alternative: 150 mg 3x/wk
ATV	RBT 150 mg qod	Alternative: 150 mg 3x/wk
IDV, NFV, FPV	RBT 150 mg/d	Alternative: 300mg 3x/wk
CCR5 antagonist		
MVC	RIF 600 mg bid	MVC: 600 mg bid†
	RBT 300 mg qd	MVC: 300 mg bid†
Integrase Inhibitor		
RAL	RIF-standard	RBT-standard

*   Limited data for ETR with SQV/r, DRV/r, or TPV/r

** For the treatment of TB, most experts recommend 150 mg qd with PI/r. Consider rifabutin TDM.

†   With CYP3A inhibitor use MCV 150 mg bid with RBT and 300 mg bid with RIF

‡   Consider rifabutin TDM especially with LPV/r co-administration

■ TABLE 6-12: **Extrapulmonary TB**

Standard 4-drug regimens x 8 wks phase
followed by INH/RIF x 16 wks or 28 wks
(cavitary TB or positive sputum culture at 2 mos).

The following summarizes the duration of treatment for extrapulmonary TB.

Site	Duration	Steroids
Lymph nodes, disseminated, pleural, genitourinary,pericardial*, peritoneal pleural (not bone, joint CNS)	6-9 mos	No
Bone or joint	9-12 mos	No
CNS TB	9-12 mos	Recommended*

*   Start immediately with dexamethasone 0.3-0.4 mg/kg/d IV with taper over 6-8 wks and switch to oral treatment with discharge from hospital.

      Alternative is prednisone 1 mg/kg/d x 3 wks with taper over 3 wks.

■ TABLE 6-13: **TB in Pregnancy and Breastfeeding**

TB Regimen in pregnancy

INH/RIF/EMB x 9 mos, or standard treatment with INH/RIF/EMB/PZA x 2 mos, then INH/RIF x 4 mos.

The issue is safety of PZA, for which there is no evidence of adverse effects in pregnancy, but inadequate experience to assure safety. PZA is recommended in WHO Guidelines but not U.S. Guidelines.

Management of Infections

472

□ **Room:** code compliant with airborne precautions and AFB isolation room until: 1) TB treatment + clinical and bacterial response, as shown by 3 consecutive AFB-negative smears on different days; or 2) TB is excluded. Note: patients with smear-positive TB should receive 2 wks of anti-TB treatment before additional AFB smears are obtained.

□ **Health care workers:** upon room entry with smear-positive patient, use particulate respirators (1-5 μm filter). Surgical masks are not effective.

□ **Patient discharge criteria:** 1) Symptoms, especially cough, resolved or near resolution; 2) treatment given for TB strain known or likely to be sensitive to drugs used; 3) patient likely to adhere to regimen; 4) patient will not go to a living environment that is crowded or includes immunosuppressed persons.

MONITORING

■ **Baseline:** LFTs (ALT/AST, alkaline phosphotase, bilirubin), creatinine or BUN, platelet count, and CBC; PZA – uric acid, EMB – visual acuity.

■ **Clinical monitoring:** Clinical assessment monthly. Warn of symptoms of hepatitis to discontinue therapy and obtain medical care – nausea, vomiting, dark urine, malaise, fever >3 days. Inquire about vision in those receiving EMB.

■ **Response:** Sputum for AFB stain at 2-week intervals if baseline was positive and cultures at 4-week intervals until 2 consecutive specimens are negative. The culture at 8 wks is especially important since it usually determines the duration of the continuation phase. If culture is positive at 3 mos, repeat sensitivity tests. Positive cultures at 4 mos indicate treatment failure.

■ **Laboratory monitoring:** LFTs monthly in those with baseline tests that are abnormal and those receiving ART and in patients with symptoms of hepatitis; some recommend routine tests at 1 and 3 mos or monthly. Some recommend chest x-ray at 2 mos and at the termination of therapy.

■ **GI intolerance:** Common at initiation of treatment. Rule out hepatitis and treat symptomatically. Change time of administration or advise to take with a snack. All TB drugs may be taken with food.

■ **AST elevation:** Most asymptomatic elevations resolve spontaneously. Usual cause is hepatotoxicity due to INH, PZA >RIF; with RIF there is often disproportionate increase in alkaline phosphotase. Consider discontinuation of INH, RIF and PZA with AST >3 x ULN and symptoms or AST >5 x ULN without symptoms – substitute 3 other anti-TB drugs until AST <2 x ULN and then sequentially reintroduce RIF for 1 wk and then INH for 1 wk with AST monitoring; if tolerated assume PZA. Fluoroquinolones can be substituted for INH. Consider INH/RIF for 9 mos.

6 Management of Infections

Drug	Dose with CrCl < 30 cc/min or hemodialysis
INH	Standard; increased risk of hepatotoxicity; monitor ALT
RIF	Standard
PZA	25-35 mg/kg 3x/wk; see comment above regarding limited experience
EMB	15-25 mg/kg 3x/wk
Levofloxacin	750-1000 mg 3x/wk
Cycloserine	250 mg qd or 500 mg 3x/wk
Ethionamide	Standard
PAS	Standard
Aminoglycosides	12-15 mg/kg 2-3x/wk (monitor levels)

■ TABLE 6-15: TB **in Hepatic Insufficiency**

Criteria	Regimen
Excluding INH	RIF/PZA/EMB x 6 mos
Excluding PZA	INH/RIF/EMB x 2 mos, then INH/RIF x 7 mos
Severe liver disease	■ RIF/fluoroquinolone/cycloserine/aminoglycoside x 18 mos or RIF/fluoroquinolone/EMB ■ Streptomycin/EMB, fluoroquinolone/another second-line drug x 18-24 mos

■ **Rash:** Minor rash: treat through with antihistamines for pruritis. Severe rash: stop all drugs, then when rash has resolved reintroduce one every 2-3 days starting with RIF or rifabutin (critical drug and least likely cause of rash). If Stevens-Johnson syndrome or toxic epidermal necrolysis, request consultation and do not restart drugs.

RESPONSE: Response to therapy is similar to that in patients without HIV except for drug interactions between anti-TB and HIV drugs and the greater risk of IRIS. Most patients become afebrile within 7-14 days; persistence of fever beyond this time suggests resistance or another cause of fever (*CID* 1992;102:797). Sputum culture becomes negative ≤2 mos in 85% (*NEJM* 2001;345:189). Persistence of positive cultures at ≥4 mos suggests nonadherence or drug resistance. IRIS must be distinguished from therapeutic failure.

TREATMENT OF LATENT TB: See pg. 69-70.

Nocardia asteroides

PRESENTATION: Typically presents with a pulmonary nodule, infiltrate, or cavity that is indolent in presentation and slow to evolve. The diagnosis is based on recovery of *Nocardia* from a respiratory source.

It is important to warn the laboratory to perform modified AFB stain, use appropriate media and hold the media, because 3-5 days are required for growth. Diagnosis is based on the recovery of the pathogen along with a compatible clinical syndrome.

TREATMENT

- **Preferred regimens:** 1) slfadiazine or trisulfapyridine (not available in the US) 3-12 g qd po or IV to maintain 2-hr post-dose sulfa level at 100-150 mg/L x ≥6 mos; or 2) TMP/SMX 10 mg/kg/d TMP po or IV (pulmonary) or 15 mg/kg/d (CNS).

- **Alternative regimens**
  □ Minocycline 100 mg po bid x ≥6 mos.
  □ Other suggested regimens: Imipenem/amikacin; sulfonamide/amikacin or minocycline; ceftriaxone/amikacin.

- **Comments**
  □ Sulfonamides preferred; TMP is inactive against *Nocardia*, but TMP-SMX is often used due to the convenience of formulation.
  □ May desensitize if hypersensitive to sulfonamides (see TMP-SMX, pg. 409).
  □ Dose of sulfonamides or TMP-SMX determined by severity of illness; pulmonary or skin – low dose; CNS, severe or disseminated disease – high dose.
  □ Parenteral therapy is usually given 3-6 wks, then oral therapy.
  □ Sulfa therapy – monitor sulfa level (for therapeutic level); monitor renal function (for crystalluria and azotemia) and force fluids.

RESPONSE: Most show clinical response in 5 days. Causes of failure: 1) resistance, 2) overwhelming infection, or 3) need for drainage. May need imipenem + amikacin (*CID* 1996;22:891).

Penicillium marneffei
Penicilliosis

EPIDEMIOLOGY: *P. marneffei* is endemic in Southeast Asia, primarily northern Thailand, India, Viet Nam and southern China (*Lancet* 1994;344:110; *AIDS* 1994;8(suppl 2):35; *NEJM* 1998;339:1739; *J Med Assoc Thai* 2006;89:441; *Hong Kong Med J* 2008;14:88; *CID* 2011; 52:945).

PRESENTATION: A review of 513 cases from Viet Nam, (*CID* 2011; 52:945) from 1996-2009 for common presenting signs and symptoms showed mean age 28 years, fever (82%), cough (40%), abdominal pain (32%), diarrhea (30%), weight loss (18%), mean temperature max 39.5°C, skin lesions (71%), hepatosplenomegaly (56%) and adenopathy (26%). Lab tests showed mean hematocrit 25%, CD4 count 7 cells/mm^3 and abnormal chest 70%, (changes were reticulonidular – 50%, interstitial – 39%, consolidation – 20%). The

6 Management of Infections

diagnosis was established with blood cultures in 395/472 (84%), skin biopsies 186/195 (95%), node aspirate 17/20 (85%). This series is representative for penicillinosis complicating HIV. Most patients were treated with amphotericin or itraconazole. The case fatality rate was 20% despite therapy.

Diagnosis: The diagnosis is established by evidence of pathogen in culture, smear, PCR, or histopathology; most frequent with Wright's stain of skin scraping, node biopsy, or marrow aspirate (*Lancet* 1994;344:110; *Mycoses* 2009;52:487). Smears show elliptical yeast, some with the characteristic clear central septation (*J Med Mycol* 1993;4:195). Serum levels of galactomannan are significantly elevated and this test is suggested to facilitate an earlier diagnosis (*JCM* 2007;45:2858).

INITIAL TREATMENT (*NEJM 1993;339:1739*; 2009 NIH/CDC/IDSA Guidelines for Prevention and Treatment of Opportunistic Infections in HIV-Infected Adults and Adolescents, www.mmhiv.com/link/2009-OI-NIH-CDC-IDSA).

- **Preferred regimens**
  - Severe: Amphotericin B 0.6 mg/kg/d x 2 wks, then itraconazole oral solution 200 mg po bid x 10 wks then 200 mg qd (*CID* 1998; 26:1107).
  - Mild to moderately severe: Itraconazole 200 mg po bid x 8 wks.
  - ART: Simultaneous initiation of ART
- **Maintenance:** Itraconazole 200 mg qd for lifetime (*NEJM* 1998; 339:1739). The 2008 DHHS Opportunistic Infection Guidelines recommend treatment until the CD4 count is >100 cells/mm^3 for >6 mos (*AIDS* 2007;21:365).
- **Comments**
  - Voriconazole (400 mg bid x 1 then 200 mg bid) is effective, (*Am J Trop Med Hyg* 2007;77:350) (see pg. 208).
  - Micafungin: *In vitro* data suggests this drug might enhance activity of amphotericin or itraconazole (*JAC* 2009;63:340).
  - *In vitro* sensitivity tests: Good activity of amphotericin B, ketoconazole, itraconazole, miconazole, and 5-FC (*J Mycol Med* 1995;5:21; *AAC* 1993;37:2407).
  - Itraconazole is superior to fluconazole (*AAC* 1993;37:2407).

RESPONSE: Response rate of 93% has been reported for the recommended amphotericin/itraconazole regimen (*CID* 1998; 26:1107).One report showed no relapses with 33 cases followed a median of 18 mos after stopping itraconazole when the CD4 count was >100 cells/mm^3 x 6 mos (*AIDS* 2007;21:365). Treatment failure has not been studied extensively and options are limited. The recommendation is to repeat amphotericin and itraconazole with stress on adherence. Use aggressive ART and consider use of voriconazole.

Progressive Multifocal Leukoencephalopathy (PML) – see JC Virus, pg. 455

Pneumocystis jiroveci (P. carinii)*: (*NEJM* 2004;350:2487; *JAMA* 2009;31:2578; *Curr Opin Infect Dis* 2008;21:31; ATS Guidelines. *Am J Resp Crit Care Med* 2011;183:96)

Pneumocystis Pneumonia (PCP)

* *P. carinii* has been renamed *P. jiroveci* but the eponym PCP is retained (*Emerg Infect Dis* 2002;8:891).

CLINICAL FEATURES: Subacute onset and progression of exertional dyspnea, nonproductive cough, fever, and chest pain over days or weeks. P.E. typically shows fever, tachycardia, increased respiration rate ± rales.

LAB: Hypoxemia with reduced pO_2 or alveolar-arterial O_2 difference (A-a gradient), demonstrated at rest or post-exercise in mild cases. LDH is usually >500 mg/dL. X-ray usually shows bilateral, symmetrical interstitial infiltrates, but may be normal in up to 20% of cases (*Am J Roentgenol* 1997;169:967). Atypical findings include nodules, blebs, and cysts. Pneumothorax is relatively common and suggests this diagnosis. Thin-section CT scan shows ground glass attenuation, and gallium scan shows increased lung uptake in patients with a negative chest x-ray. A negative thin-section CT scan does not exclude PCP.

DIAGNOSIS: Initial diagnostic test is induced sputum; sensitivity averages 56% in meta-analysis of 7 reports (*Eur Respir J* 2002;20:982) or BAL with sensitivity of >95%. Because of low sensitivity of induced sputum, negative tests should be followed up with bronchoscopy. Repeat induced sputum tests do not improve the yield (*Arch Path Lab Med* 2007;131:1582). Standard stains for cysts and trophozoites are cresyl violet, Giemsa, *Diff-Quik*, Wright, and Gram-Weigert. Stains for cyst walls are Gemori-Methenamine Silver, Gram-Weigert, and toluidine blue. Some labs prefer immunofluorescent stains, which may give a higher yield (*Eur Respir J* 2002;20:982). PCR using oral wash specimens is experimental. Preliminary data show a sensitivity of 70-90% and specificity of 85%; the reduced specificity is attributed to a possible carrier state that may be corrected with a quantitative threshold (*JID* 2004;189:1697). One report of AIDS patients without PCP who underwent BAL found that 117/172 (68%) were colonized with *P. jiroveci* by PCR (*Thorax* 2008;63:329). Rates were higher with low CD4 counts and lack of PCP prophylaxis. Thus, quantitative methods such as real time PCR may be necessary to distinguish colonization and infection (*Respirology* 2009;14:203; *Thorax* 2008;63:329). One report using this technology showed what you would expect: a negative predictive value of only 53% (*JCM* 2011;49:1872). Autopsies show about 60-80% of healthy adults harbor *P. jirovecii* in the lung (*CID* 2010;50:347). Traditional stains used to

6 Management of Infections

detect PCP remain positive for weeks after treatment (*NEJM* 2004;350:2487), so treatment can be initiated before specimen collection. Serologic studies such as Low KEX-1 IgG titers may assist here (Gingo. *JAIDS* 2011:PMCID 21372726).

TREATMENT

- **Preferred regimen: Moderate or severe disease**
  - □ Trimethoprim 15-20 mg/kg/d + sulfamethoxazole 75-100 mg/kg/d po or IV in 3-4 divided doses (typical oral dose is 2 DS tid for 70 kg pt). When initial therapy is IV there should be a switch to oral TMP-SMX when improved. Total therapy is 21 days

- **Alternative: Moderate or severe disease**
  - □ <u>Pentamidine</u> 3-4 mg/kg/d IV infused over ≥ 60 minutes
  - □ <u>Primaquine</u> 15-30 mg (base) qd + <u>clindamycin</u> 600-900 mg IV q6-8h or 300-450 mg po q6-8h x 21 days

- **Adjunctive corticosteroids:** Patients with moderately severe or severe disease (defined as PaO_2 <70mm Hg at room air or A-a gradient >35 mm Hg) should receive corticosteroids (prednisone 40 mg po bid x 5 days, then 40 mg qd x 5 days, then 20 mg qd to completion of 21 day course of treatment) starting as early as possible. IV methylprednisolone can be given at 75% of prednisone dose. Efficacy of corticosteroids for hypoxemia is established (*NEJM* 1990;323:1451; *NEJM* 1990;323:1500). Cochrane library review found that use of steroids was associated with an OR of 0.56 for overall mortality according to criteria discussed above (*Cochrane Database Syst Rev* 2006;3: CD006150). The rationale for the use of steroids is that PCP prognosis correlates better with inflammatory markers than with number of organisms (*Expert Rev Mol Med* 2005;7:1). Side effects of steroids include CNS toxicity, thrush, cryptococcosis, *H. simplex* infection, tuberculosis, and other OIs (*JAIDS* 1995;8:345).

- **Preferred Regimen: Mild to moderate disease**
  - □ TMP/SMX (15-20 mg TMP/d) tid x 21 days (typical dose 2 DS tabs tid for a 70 kg patient)

- **Alternative: Mild to moderate disease**
  - □ Dapsone 100 mg po qd + TMP 5 mg/kg/d tid x 21 days
  - □ Atovaquone 750 mg po bid with food x 21 days
  - □ Primaquine 15-30 mg (base) qd + clindamycin 600-900 mg IV q6-8h or 300-450 mg po q6-8h x 21 days (Test for G6PD deficiency before giving primaquine when possible)

STARTING ART: HIV treatment should be started within 2 wks of starting PCP treatment (*PLoS One* 2009;4:e5575).

TREATMENT FAILURE: Drug failure occurs in about 10% with mild to moderate disease and can often be predicted early in the course of treatment: Poor prognostic indicators are low pO_2, older age, first episode and concurrent pulmonary KS (*CID* 2008;46:625). Response is slow, and many patients deteriorate during the first 3-5 days, possibly due to inflammation following lysis of the organism.

- **Comments**

  □ A review of 1,122 HIV-infected patients treated for PCP in London, Milan and Copenhagen from 1989-04 showed 3-month survivals of 85% for TMP-SMX, 81% for primaquine/clindamycin and 76% for pentamidine (*JAC* 2009;64:1282). The OR for death with pentamidine was 2.0.

  □ Dose: The use of 15 mg/kg/d of TMP appears to be as effective as 20 mg/kg/d and better tolerated (*NEJM* 1993;328:1521; *Ann Intern Med* 1996;124:792).

  □ ACTG 108 found that TMP-SMX, TMP-dapsone and clindamycin-primaquine were equally effective for mild-moderate PCP (*Ann Intern Med* 1996;124:792).

  □ Resistance of *P. jiroveci* to sulfonamides is suggested by mutations on the dihydropteroate synthase gene (*JID* 2000;182: 1192; *JID* 1999;180:1969; *JID* 2000;182:551), but there does not appear to be an association with treatment failure (*JID* 2000;182:551; *JAMA* 2001;286:2450; *AIDS* 2005; 19:80).

  □ Aerosolized pentamidine should not be used for therapy

  □ Adverse reactions to TMP-SMX have been noted in 25-50%, primarily rash (30-55%), fever (30-40%), leukopenia (30-40%), azotemia (1-5%), hepatitis (20%), thrombocytopenia (15%), and hypokalemia (TMP) (*JID* 1995;171:1295; *Lancet* 1991;338:431). Most can be "treated through," using antihistamines for rashes, antipyretics for fever, and antiemetics for nausea.

  □ Opinions have varied regarding initiation of ART during treatment of PCP. Some report better short-term survival (*JID* 2001; 183:1409); others report paradoxical worsening, due possibly to IRIS (*Am J Respir Crit Care Med* 2001;164:841). Immune reconstitution with acute respiratory failure has been described (*Am J Respir Crit Care Med* 2001;164:847), but is rare, possibly because steroids are used in severe PCP. ACTG5164 compared immediate vs. delayed ART in treatment-naïve patients presenting with AIDS-defining OIs. Most of the patients (63%) had PCP and the best outcome was with early ART (median 12 vs 45 days) (*PLoS One* 2009;4:e5575).

  □ Risk of PCP in virologically suppressed patients: Patients with CD4 counts 100-200 cells/mm^3 and VL <400 c/mL: Review showed only 1.2 PCP cases/1000 patient-years in absence of prophylaxis, suggesting that prophylaxis is not necessary in these patients. (*CID* 2010;51:611).

  □ Geographic clustering of cases suggests person-to-person spread (*Am J Respir Crit Care Med* 2000;162:1617; *Am J Respir Crit Care Med* 2000;162:1622; *NEJM* 2000;19:1416; *Emerg Infect Dis* 2003;

6 Management of Infections

9:132). However, isolation from other vulnerable patients is not generally advocated.

- **Prophylaxis:** See pg. 67-68, 565.

RESPONSE: Response to therapy is slow: usually 3-5 days but often up to 7-10 days. Preferred therapy (TMP-SMX) should not be changed based on an assumption of clinical failure until 8 days. Drug toxicity is common, and it may be mistaken for therapeutic non-response (*Ann Intern Med* 1996;124: 972). The mortality rate of untreated PCP is 100%; for PCP in hospitalized patients given standard regimens it is 15-20% and is 60% for those requiring ventilator support (*AIDS* 2003;17:73). An analysis of 524 cases at San Francisco General Hospital during 1997-06 showed a mortality rate of 10% with 5 predictors: increased age, recent IDU, bilirubin >0.6 mg/dL, albumin <3 gm/dL and a-A O_2 gradient >50 mm Hg (*Thorax* 2009;64:1070). One meta-analysis suggested that primaquine-clindamycin is the most effective salvage regimen (*Arch Int Med* 2001;161:1529). **PCP IRIS** has been reported with progression of pneumonia, including ARDS (*CID* 2002;35:491; *Am J Respir Crit Care Med* 2001;164:847). It must be remembered that PCP is largely the product of the inflammatory response, and severe disease is treated with steroids.

Pseudomonas aeruginosa

DIAGNOSIS: HIV infection is an established risk for *P. aerginosa* infection including bacteremia and pneumonia, usually with advanced immunosuppression and/or structural lung disease (*Infection* 2010;38: 25; *Postgrad Med* 2003;79:691; *JID* 2001;184:268). Diagnosis requires a clinically compatible case plus recovery of the organism from a normally sterile source. Caution is necessary in interpreting growth of *P. aeruginosa* in contaminated respiratory tract specimens (sputum, bronchoscopy, etc.), especially in patients with prior antibiotics use or when the organism is recovered in low numbers.

TREATMENT

- **Preferred regimen:** Preferred drugs are selected betalactams (ceftazidime, cefepime, piperacillin-tazobactam) carbapenems, aminoglycosides, colistin (multidrug resistant strains) and some fluoroquinolones. It is common practice to use two agents initially, and then one when sensitivity data are known.

- **Comments**
  - □ Antibiotic selection requires *in vitro* susceptibility data.
  - □ Reverse risk factors when feasible: neutropenia, corticosteroids, CD4 <50 cells/mm³.
  - □ The frequently quoted adage that *P. aeruginosa* requires "double coverage" is debatable. Like other pathogens it requires an agent that is active *in vitro* and, for pulmonary infections, an agent that penetrates alveolar lining fluid. Use of monotherapy with a

fluoroquinolone usually results in persistent disease with a fluoroquinolone-resistant strain (*AAC* 1999;43:1379).

Rhodococcus equi

In a review of 272 cases, patients had a subacute pulmonary infection with infiltrate on chest x-ray, cavitation in 68% the mean CD4 count was 51 cells/mm^3 and 20% had extrapulmonary involvement (*AIDS Patient Care and STDs* 2010;24:211). *R. equi* was recovered from blood cultures in 47% and from sputum or BAL specimens in 63%.

TREATMENT

- **Preferred regimen:** Vancomycin 15 mg/kg IV q12h IV or imipenem 2 g qd IV, usually combined with rifampin 600 mg qd po or ciprofloxacin 750 mg po bid or erythromycin po or IV x ≥2 wks, then oral treatment for 6 mos. ART is an important component of therapy (*Chest* 2003;123:1).

- **Comments**

  □ Sensitivity tests guide therapy: Generally sensitive to fluoroquinolones, vancomycin, macrolides; imipenem, and rifampin. Resistant *in vitro* to penicillins and cephalosporins (*CID* 2002;34:1379; *Chest* 2003;123:1; *AIDS Patient Care and STDs* 2010;4:211).

  □ Other drugs sometimes used based on *in vitro* sensitivity testing are tetracyclines, linezolid, and TMP-SMX.

  □ Duration of therapy is arbitrary, but relapses are common; most use prolonged oral maintenance therapy with macrolide or fluoroquinolone. Resistance to these agents may develop.

  □ Immune reconstitution with ART may be critical for cure.

RESPONSE: Prognosis prior to HAART era was poor (*Medicine* 1994; 73:119). The prognosis with antibacterial agents plus immune reconstitution is good; the disease is chronic or fatal in 30-40% without ART or with no response to ART.

Salmonella spp.

PRESENTATION: Typhoid fever shows little association with immunosuppression, but salmonellosis due to non-typhoid strains are substantially more common and severe in AIDS patients (*JID* 2008;56:413).The predominant strains in the U.S. are *S. enteriditis* and *S. typhimurium*. Most patients with *Salmonella* gastroenteritis are not treated because this may prolong carriage and most control their disease well. However, AIDS patients are at high risk for bacteremia, and many advocate treating all with antibiotics. A review of 5,578 HIV-infected patients with community-acquired bacteremia in Africa showed *Salmonella enterica* was the most common accounting for 1,643 (29%) of all bactermic cases cases (*Lancet Infect Dis* 2010;

6 Management of Infections

10:14). (*S. pneumoniae* and TB were the second and third most common).

TREATMENT (*CID* 2001;32:331)

- **Preferred regimen:** <u>Mild disease and CD4 count >200 cells/mm³</u>: Ciprofloxacin 500-750 mg po bid or 400 mg IV bid; total treatment is 7-14 days; 14 days with bacteremia. <u>If CD4 count <200 cells/mm³</u>: treat 2-6 wks. With <u>recurrent septicemia</u>: treat for 6 mos using agent selected by sensitivity tests. Other fluoroquinolones (moxifloxacin and levofloxacin) should be equally effective.

- **Alternative regimen:** TMP/ SMX 5-10 mg/kg/d (TMP component) IV or 1 DS bid x >2 wks (if susceptible) or ceftriaxone 1-2 g qd IV (see duration above).

- **Comments**
  - □ <u>Immunocompetent hosts</u> with salmonellosis often do well without antibiotic treatment. Most experts recommend antibiotics for all HIV-infected patients based on high rates of bacteremia. In a review of *Salmonella*-associated deaths in the US from 1990-2006, the odds ratio for a fatal outcome in patients with AIDS was 7.4. The most common food sources were chicken (48%), ground beef (28%), turkey(17%) and eggs (6%).
  - □ <u>Relapse is common</u>. Eradication of *Salmonella* carrier state has been demonstrated only with ciprofloxacin.
  - □ <u>AZT</u> is active against most *Salmonella* strains and may be effective prophylaxis (*JID* 1999;179:1553).
  - □ <u>Drug selection</u> requires *in vitro* susceptibility data, especially for ampicillin. Ciprofloxacin is preferred; ciprofloxacin resistance has been reported (*NEJM* 2001;344:1572), but is rare.
  - □ <u>Maintenance</u>: Some authorities recommend ciprofloxacin 500 mg po bid x several months or TMP-SMX 5 mg/kg/d, TMP (1 DS po bid). Need for maintenance therapy, specific regimens, and duration are not well defined.

Staphylococcus aureus

PRESENTATION: Staphylococcal infection syndromes most commonly encountered with HIV infection include:

- **Furunculosis:** There is an epidemic of infections involving "community-acquired MRSA" (USA 300 strain), which has been reported in disproportionately high numbers in MSM and other high-risk groups. One report indicated that the risk ratio for MRSA infection for MSM was 13 and was unrelated to HIV infection (*Ann Intern Med* 2008;148:409). Another review found that the risk among HIV-infected persons compared to the general population was 6-fold higher (*CID* 2010;50:979). Other studies have found significantly greater colonization in those with HIV infection (17% vs. 6%; p<0.04) (*JID* 2009;200:88). The USA 300 strain is clonal, global, and characterized by genes for production of Panton-Valentine leukocidin (which marks this strain) and *mec* IV (the mechanism of methicillin resistance, which is distinct from *mec* I-III, found in nosocomial MRSA). The most common infections associated with this strain are soft tissue infections, especially the "spider bite abscess." Rare but serious manifestations are necrotizing pneumonia, necrotizing fasciitis, and pyomyositis (*NEJM* 2006;355:666:666; *Emerg Infect Dis* 2006; 12:894; *NEJM* 2007; 30:72: *Lancet* 2007;367:751).

- **Pyomyositis:** This is classically an infection of muscle caused by *S. aureus*, usually MSSA, and sometimes called "tropical pyomyositis" due to high rates in tropical countries. Most cases present with fever and focal pain; the diagnosis is usually made by CT scan (*Radiographics* 2004;24:1029) and treatment consists of drainage + antibiotics selected by *in vitro* sensitivity tests (*Am J Med* 2004; 117:420; *J Rheumatol* 2001;28:802). Some patients respond to antibiotics without surgery (*Am Surg* 2000;66:1064).

- **Staphylococcal infections associated with injection drug use** include 1) skin and soft tissue infections, 2) vertebral disc space infections, 3) sterno-clavicular joint infections, and 4) endocarditis, especially tricuspid valve endocarditis. All of these were described well before the initial reports of HIV and none is notably different with HIV infection with respect to frequency or management recommendations.

TREATMENT

- **Preferred regimens**
  - **MSSA:** Antistaphylloccal betalactam (cephalexin/dicloxacillin, nafcillin, oxacillin, cefazolin, ceftriaxone); alternatives should be selected by *in vitro* tests. Clindamycin, fluoroquinolones, and TMP-SMX are usually active.
  - **Nosocomial MRSA:** Vancomycin 15 mg/kg q12h to achieve trough levels of 15-20 mcg/mL for serious infections (bacteremia, pneumonia, osteomyelitis, etc) (*CID* 2009;49:325). Alternatives include telavancin 10 mg/kg/d IV, ceftaroline 600 mg IV bid, linezolid 600 mg bid IV or po or daptomycin 6-8 mg/kg/d IV. Daptomycin should not be used in pulmonary infections and linezolid may be preferred to vancomycin for MRSA pneumonia (see below).
  - **Community-acquired MRSA:** Often sensitive to TMP-SMX, clindamycin or doxycycline as well as vancomycin and linezolid (*MMWR* 2003;52:993). Serious infectious requiring parenteral treatment are usually treated with vancomycin or linezolid.

- **Management recommendations of IDSA** (*CID* 2011;52:285):

Management of Infections

6

- **Cutaneous abscess:** Incision and drainage. <u>Agents for empiric use</u>: clindamycin, TMP-SMX, doxycycline/minocycline or linezolid. Indications for antibiotics: severe or extensive disease, rapid progression, co-morbidities, immunosuppression, age extremes, face or genital infections, failure to respond I & D.

- **Cellulitis:** <u>If purulent</u>, treat for *S. aureus* and *Streptococcus* with clindamycin pending culture and sensitivities. <u>If no purulent drainage</u>, betalactam for *Streptococcus* unless systemic signs or fails to respond.

- **Recurrent cutaneous abscesses:** a) <u>cover lesions</u>; b) <u>personal hygiene</u>; c) <u>consider nasal decolonization</u> with mupirocin bid x 5-10 days; and d) <u>skin decolonization</u> with dilute bleach baths (5 cc bleach/gallon or ¼ cup/¼ tub x 15 min weekly x 3 mos; e) <u>oral Abx</u>; consider rifampin + oral agent chronically only if above tactics fail and if rifampin is active; f) <u>evaluate environment and contacts</u>; evaluate, treat and/or decolonize contacts as appropriate.

- **Systemic infections with MRSA:** For serious infections (sepsis, meningitis, pneumonia, endocarditis): a) <u>IV vancomycin 15-20 mg/kg/dose</u> (actual weight), not to exceed 2 gm/dose and given over 2 hrs (to avoid red man syndrome); this assumes normal renal function; b) <u>goal</u> for serious infection is trough vancomycin level of <u>15-20 mcg/mL</u> as measured when steady state achieved (before 4th or 5th dose; c) <u>trough levels</u> should be monitored for patients who have serious infections, are obese or have renal failure; for most patients with soft tissue infections who are not obese and have normal renal function the historically recommended regimen of 1 gm IV qid is adequate; d) <u>*in vitro* activity</u> – if MRSA strain has MIC to vancomycin >2 mcg/mL; use alternative agent such as daptomycin (10 mg/kg/d) plus gentamicin or rifampin or linezolid.

Streptococcus pneumoniae

PRESENTATION: Studies of pneumococcal infections in the pre-HAART era found that the rate of community-acquired pneumococcal pneumonia is increased 8-fold with HIV infection (*Am Rev Respir Dis* 1993;148:1523) and the rate of *S. pneumoniae* bacteremia is increased 150- to 300-fold (*JAMA* 1991;265:3275). Rates of both CAP and pneumococcal bacteremia correlate with CD4 counts. Patients with pneumococcal bacteremia also have an 8-25% probability of recurrent bacteremia within 6 mos (*JAMA* 1991;265: 3275; *JID* 2002;185:1364). Most of the recurrent cases involve new strains of *S. pneumoniae* and thus do not represent relapses. In the HAART era, the rate of invasive pneumococcal infection decreased 49% (2004-5 vs. 1994-5), presumably due to ART and the herd effect of *Prevnar 7* use in pediatrics (*JAIDS* 2010;55:128). The clinical features of pneumococcal pneumonia and bacteremia are not unique in patients with HIV infection. This observation led to the large controlled trial of *Prevnar 7* vaccine in HIV-infected Malawian adults who had pneumococcal bacteremia. The recurrence rate of pneumococcal bacteremia was reduced by 74% in these patients (*NEJM* 2010;362:812). (It should be noted that *Prevnar 7* is not FDA-approved for adults). Standard diagnostic tests in hospitalized patients with community acquired pneumonia include x-rays and studies for a microbial etiology including blood culture, Gram stain, culture of sputum and urinary antigen assay for *S. pneumoniae* (*J Infect* 2007;551:300; *Am J Emerg Med* 2010;28:454). Risk factors for these infections include low CD4 count, smoking and substance abuse; low CD4 counts predict delayed response to therapy (*HIV Med* 2008;36:231). Prophylactic TMP-SMX predicts reduced antibiotic sensitivity (*AAC* 2010;54:3756).

TREATMENT

- **Preferred regimens:** Penicillin, amoxicillin, cefotaxime, ceftriaxone (see Comments), or fluoroquinolone (suspected or established penicillin resistance): Levofloxacin or moxifloxacin.

- **Alternative regimens:** Macrolide.

- **Comments:** See Pneumonia, pg. 562-566.

  □ *In vitro* susceptibility: Susceptibility of *S. pneumoniae* based on surveillance 10,000 clinical isolates from 2000-02 in the U.S.: Penicillin resistance 2%, macrolides 25%, clindamycin 6%, doxycycline 6%, levofloxacin 1% (*AAC* 2003;47:1790). More recent data based on 39,495 isolates are similar and show 30% are resistant to TMP-SMX (*Ann Clin Microbiol Antimicrob* 2008;11:7). The data on penicillin are deceptive since the breakpoint to define susceptibility has been changed. About 98% of strains are penicillin-susceptible according to the new criteria making penicillin (or amoxicillin) the drug of choice for most pneumoccal infections (*MMWR* 2008;57:1353). The macrolide data are also deceptive since only the mef A mechanism is likely to be important; this applies to approximately 18% of strains.

  □ Penicillin-resistant strains: Strains highly resistant to macrolides and penicillin (serotypes 6A, 6B, 9V, 14, 19A, 19F and 23F) are usually carried by children (*Lancet* 2008;8:785). These should be treated with fluoroquinolones quinolones (levofloxacin, or moxifloxacin). TMP-SMX is now considered inadequate for empiric therapy due to high rates of resistance. Fluoroquinolone resistance develops in adults and is uncommon (<2%) but increasing (*NEJM* 2002;346:747; *Emerg Infect Dis* 2002;8:594).

RESPONSE: Most patients respond well with clearance of bacteremia in 24-48 hrs and clinical improvement in 1-3 days. Patients with pneumococcal pneumonia may transition from IV to oral antibiotics when they are clinically better, vital signs and blood gases are improved, and they can take pills. HIV-infected patients with pneumococcal bacteremia usually respond well to treatment and actually have better survival rates than bacteremic patients without HIV infection (*Mayo Clin Proc* 2004;79:604; *CID* 2008;47:1388).

6 Management of Infections

Toxoplasma gondii
Toxoplasmic encephalitis

PRESENTATION: Toxoplasmosis in patients with HIV infection nearly always represents reactivation of latent cysts in patients with a CD4 count <100 cells/mm^3. Seroprevalence in the U.S. is about 15% but often 50-75% in some European countries and resource-limited countries. The usual clinical presentation is fever, headache, confusion, and/or focal neurologic deficits.

DIAGNOSIS: The diagnosis is based on 1) CNS imaging, 2) evidence of *T. gondii* by serology (positive IgG) and PCR of CSF, and 3) response to therapy. Typical features are ≥2 ring enhancing lesions on MRI, fever, focal neurologic defect, and positive anti-*T. gondii* IgG (>90%). PCR is an excellent diagnostic test, but in-house assays show lack of standardization (*Parasitologia* 2008;50:45). PCR becomes negative post-therapy. *T. gondii* can be demonstrated by H&E stain or immuno-peroxidase stain of a brain biopsy specimen, but this is rarely obtained or necessary. SPECT scans often help to distinguish CNS lymphoma and toxoplasmosis. Most patients respond to therapy with clinical and radiographic improvement ≤2 wks (*CID* 2001; 34:103).

TREATMENT: INITIAL

- **Preferred:** pyrimethamine (200 mg po x 1 then 50 mg (<60 kg) – 75 mg (>60 kg) po daily + sulfadiazine 1000 mg (<60 kg) – 1500 mg (>60 kg) po q6h + leucovorin 10-25 mg po qd x >6.

- **Alternative:** 1) pyrimethamine + leucovorin + clindamycin 600 mg IV or po q6h; or 2) TMP-SMX 5 mg/kg TMP and 25 mg/kg SMX IV or po bid; 3) atovaquone 1500 mg po bid with food + pyrimethamine + leucovorin; 4) atovaquone 1500 mg po bid with food + sulfadiazine 1000-1500 mg po q6h; 5) atovaquone 1500 mg po bid with food; and 6) pyrimethamine + leucovorin + azithromycin 900-1200 mg po qd.

MAINTENANCE

- **Preferred:** pyrimethamine 25-50 mg po qd + sulfadiazine 2-4 gm po qd in 2-4 doses + leucovorin 10-25 mg po qd.

- **Alternative:** 1) clindamycin 600 mg po q8h + pyrimethamine 25-50 mg po qd + leucovorin 10-25 mg po qd (+ agent to prevent PCP); and 2) atovaquone 750 mg po q6-12h +/- (pyrimethamine 25 mg po qd + leucovorin 10 mg po qd) or sulfadiazine 2-4 gm po qd.

RESPONSE: Clinical response expected in 1 wk in 60-80% and MRI response expected in 2 wks. Failure to achieve these goals should prompt consideration of alternative diagnosis, especially primary CNS lymphoma, tuberculous, or brain abscess. Stereotatic biopsy is usually required, and yields a definitive diagnosis in 98% of cases (*CID* 2000;30:49).

■ Comments

- □ There is no <u>parenteral form of pyrimethamine</u>. For patients who need IV treatment: TMP-SMX or pyrimethamine po + clindamycin IV.

- □ <u>Pyrimethamine + sulfadiazine is preferred</u>; pyrimethamine + clindamycin is less effective but better tolerated (*CID* 1996;22:268). All other regimens listed have been less well studied.

- □ <u>Leucovorin dose</u> can be increased to 50-100 mg qd to reverse pyrimethamine marrow toxicity: anemia, neutropenia and/or thrombocytopenia.

- □ <u>Atovaquone regimens</u>: May wish to confirm serum level ≥18 µg/mL due to variable absorption. (*Lancet* 1992; 340; 637; *AIDS* 1996; 10:1107; *CID* 1997;24:422)

- □ <u>Alternative regimens</u> (Limited data): Minocycline or doxycycline + clarithromycin, pyrimethamine or doxycycline combined with pyrimethamine (and leucovorin), sulfadiazine or clarithromycin (*AAC* 1995;39:276; *Scand JID* 1993;25;157). Azithromycin (*AIDS* 2001; 15:583); clarithromycin (*AAC* 1991;35: 2049); atovaquone (*CID* 2002;34:1243); TMP-SMX (*AAC* 1998;42:1346).

■ TABLE 6-16: **Treatment of CNS Toxoplasmosis** (2009 NIH/CDC/IDSA Guidelines for Prevention and Treatment of Opportunistic Infections in HIV-Infected Adults and Adolescents www.mmhiv.com/link/2009-OI-NIH-CDC-IDSA)

Initial Treatment: 6 weeks
Preferred:
■ Pyrimethamine 200 mg po x 1, then 50 mg (<60 kg) or 75 mg (>60 kg) po/d plus sulfadiazine1000 mg (<60/kg) or 1500 mg (>60 kg) po q6h plus leucovorin 10-25 mg po/d
Alternatives:
■ Pyrimethamine/leucovorin (above doses) plus clindamycin 600 mg IV or po q6h ■ TMP-SMX (5 mg/kg TMP) IV or po bid ■ Pyrimethamine/leucovorin (above doses) plus Atovaquone 1500 mg po with food bid ■ Atovaquone 1500 mg po with food bid ■ Atovaquone 1500 mg po with food bid + sulfadiazine 1000-1500 mg po q6h ■ Pyrimethamine/leucovorin (above doses) plus azithromycin 900-1200 mg po/d
Maintenance
Preferred:
■ Pyrimethamine 25-50 mg po/d plus sulfadiazine 2-4 gm po/d (in 2-4 daily doses) plus leucovorin 10-25 mg po/d
Alternatives:
■ Pyrimethamine/leucovorin (above doses) plus clindamycin 600 mg po q 8h ■ Atovaquone 750 mg po q 6-12 h +/- either (pyrimethamine 25 mg po plus leucovorin 10 mg po/d) or (sulfadiazine 2-4 gm po/d)

6 Management of Infections

- Adjunctive corticosteroid therapy only for mass effect on imaging.
- Brain biopsy: Strongly consider if there is failure to respond clinically and by imaging.
- PCP prophylaxis: Pyrimethamine-sulfadiazine, TMP-SMX and atovaquone + pyrimethamine provide effective PCP prophylaxis; pyrimethamine-clindamycin does not.
- *In vitro* activity: Tests of pyrimethamine and atovaquone show consistent activity, but there is more variation with sulfadiazine (*AAC* 2008;52:1269). Meaning for clinical care is unclear.

IMMUNE RECONSTITUTION: Discontinue maintenance therapy when CD4 count >200 cells/mm^3 x 6 mos, initial therapy completed + asymptomatic.

PROPHYLAXIS: See pg. 70-71.

Treponema pallidum

Syphilis: CDC Recommendations (*MMWR* 2010;59:RR-12)

STAGES – CLASSIFICATION

- **Primary:** genital ulcer
- **Secondary (2-8 wks):** macular, papular, or maculopapular rash that is generalized including palms and soles, generalized lymphadenopathy ± constitutional symptoms or aseptic meningitis
- **Tertiary:** cardiac, neurologic, ocular, auditory, or gummatous
- **Latent:** early latent <1 year; late latent >1 year or duration unknown

DIAGNOSIS: See pg. 50.

- **Primary:** painless nodule → ulcer (chancre) at site of contact – with HIV there may be multiple chancres

TREATMENT

- **Primary and secondary:** benzathine penicillin 2.4 million units IM x 1; penicillin allergy: doxycycline 100 mg po bid x 14d
- **Early latent:** (<1 year and normal CSF exam): benzathine penicillin 2.4 million units IM x 1; penicillin allergy: doxycycline 100 mg po bid x 14d
- **Late latent:** >1 year or unknown duration and normal CSF exam: benzathine penicillin 2.4 million units qw x3; penicillin allergy: doxycycline 100 mg po bid x 4 wks
- **Neurosyphilis:** aqueous penicillin G 18-24 million units IV/d (3-4 million units IV q4h) x 10-14d. Alternative: procaine penicillin 2.4 million units IM/d + probenecid 500 mg po 4 x/d x 10-14d. Penicillin allergy: desensitize (Table 6-17) or (with non-IgE mediated allergy) ceftriaxone 2 gm q24h IM or IV/d x 10-14d (see below)
- **CNS syphilis:** meningitis, hearing loss, ocular disease (uveitis, iritis, neuroretinitis, optic neuritis) acute or chronic altered mental status, loss of vibration sense. Diagnosis is established by CSF changes

showing mononuclear pleocytosis (>WBC/mL), mild elevation or protein +/- positive VDRL. The CSF VDRL is specific but not sensitive; the CDF FDT ABS is sensitive but not specific.

- **Follow-up for late syphilis:** (secondary, tertiary and latent). Non-treponemal test titers correlate with disease activity. Changes in RPR or VDRL titers are significant if ≥4-fold (2 dilutions), and changes reflect disease activity and treatment. Treponemal tests usually remain positive for life and do not change with disease activity or treatment. The RPR or VDRL titer should be repeated at 6 and 12 months after treatment using the same test and same lab. Patients with symptoms that persist or reoccur or have a sustained 4-fold increase in titer either failed treatment or were reinfected. If the titer does not decline (about 15%), there should be continued follow-up, CDF exam and consideration of retreatment.

■ TABLE 6-1 /: **Penicillin Allergy Skin Test and Desensitization (*MMWR* 2002;51[RR-6]:28)**

Penicillin Skin Test:

- Reagents: benzylpenicilloyd poly-L-lysine (*Pre-Pen*) + minor determinant if available. If minor determinant is not available, use *Pre-Pen* only.
- Positive control for epicutaneous test is commercial histamine (1 mg/mL).
- Negative control is diluent, usually saline.
- Sequence: epicutaneous test→ positive (wheal >4 mm at 15 min) = penicillin allergy; negative histamine control + negative prick test − unreliable; positive histamine test + negative prick test = do intradermal test.
- Epicutaneous (prick) test: drops on forearm pierced with #26 needle without blood wheal >4 mm at 15 min is positive.
- Intradermal test: 0.02 mL intradermal injection forearm with #26 or #27 needle; at 15 min a wheal >2 mm larger than negative controls and the initial wheal = positive

Desensitization:

- Indication: positive skin test.
- Route: oral or IV; oral is safer and easier.
- Site: hospital setting.
- Time: requires 4 hours.
- Schedule: administer every 15 minutes using the following amount in 30-mL aliquots for oral administration.

Dose	Units/mL	mL	Units	Dose	Units/mL	mL	Units
1	1,000	0.10	100	8	10,000	1.20	12000
2	1,000	0.20	200	9	10,000	2.40	24000
3	1,000	0.04	400	10	10,000	4.80	48000
4	1,000	0.80	800	11	80,000	1.00	80000
5	1,000	1.60	1600	12	80,000	2.00	160000
6	1,000	3.20	3200	13	80,000	4.00	320000
7	1,000	6.40	6400	14	80,000	8.00	640000

Management of Infections 6

INDICATIONS FOR LP: 2010 CDC guidelines* recommend that all HIV-infected patients with syphilis and neurologic symptoms undergo lumbar puncture (LP) for CSF examination. The need for LP in patients without neurologic signs or symptoms remains controversial, but CDC guidelines do not recommend routine LP in such patients. Some experts have suggested that LP be performed in patients with CD4 counts <350 cells/mm^3 and RPR titer ≥1:32 (*Sex Transm Dis* 2007;34:145, *Clin Infect Dis* 2009;48:816). LP is indicated in patients who do not have an appropriate fall in RPR titer over 12 to 24 mos.

* www.mmhiv.com/link/2010-CDC-STD

Management of Infections

CARDIAC COMPLICATIONS

Dilated Cardiomyopathy

Note that the prior classic study (*NEJM* 1998;339:1092) has been withdrawn for reasons that are not clear.

CAUSE: Unknown, but hypotheses include: 1) mitochondrial toxicity from AZT (*Ann Intern Med 1992*;116:311; *Cardiovasc Res* 2003;60: 147; *CID* 2003;37:109; *JAIDS* 2004;37:S30; *Chem Res Toxicol* 2008; 21:990), 2) HIV infection of myocardial cells (*NEJM* 1998;339:1093; *Cardiovas Toxicol* 2004;4:97), 3) L-carnitine deficiency (*AIDS* 1992; 6:203), 4) selenium deficiency (*Curr HIV Res* 2007;5:129; *NEJM* 1999; 340:732), 5) Proinflammatory cytokines: TNF-alfa, IL-1and IL-6, (*Int J Cardiol* 2007;120:150), 6) Autoimmunity (*J Am Coll Cardiol* 1993;22: 1385; *Eur Heart J* 1995;16:50) and 7) opportunistic infections (*Wien Klin Wocheuschr* 2008;120:77).

FREQUENCY: The frequency depends to a large extent on the definition and the sensitivity of the test method. A rate of 6-8% for symptomatic cardiomyopathy was noted in longitudinal studies in the pre-HAART era (*Eur Heart J* 1992;13:1452; *Clin Immunol Immunopathol* 1993;68:234). Incidence in a prospective study was 16/1000 patient years (*NEJM* 1998;339:1093). Rates of left ventricular diastolic dysfunction with routine ECHO are much higher and correlate with stage of immunosuppression (*Heart* 1998;80:184). Rates are thought to have decreased during the HAART era by as much as 7-fold (*Wein Klin Wocheuschr* 2008;120:77; *Am Heart J* 2006;151:1147). Nevertheless, the SUN study, with echocardiographs in 656 unselected HIV infected patients with average age of 41 years and median CD4 count of 462 cells/mm^3, found that 18% had left ventricular dysfunction, 40% had left atrial enlargement and 57% had pulmonary hypertension (*CID* 2011;52:378). These changes correlated with elevated hsCRP.

SYMPTOMS: CHF, arrhythmias, cyanosis, and/or syncope

DIAGNOSIS: Echocardiogram showing ejection fraction <50% normal ± arrhythmias on EKG, not otherwise explained. Criterion for dilated cardiomyopathy in the major study was an EF <45% and end diastolic volume index >80 mL/M^2 (*NEJM* 1998;339:1093). Myocardial biopsies in 76 patients in this study showed myocarditis with inflammatory cells in 63; culture yielded coxsackie B in 15 and CMV in 4.

7 Systems Review

TREATMENT (*Am J Cardiol* 1999;83:1A)

- **ART:** use non-AZT-containing regimen. One study found that ART reduced rates of cardiomyopathy but did not clearly reverse cardiomyopathy (*J Infect* 2000;40;282).

- **ACE inhibitor:** enalapril 2.5 mg bid; titrate up to 20 mg bid.

  Alternatives: captopril 6.25 mg tid up to 50 mg tid or lisinopril 10 mg qd titrated up to 40 mg qd

- **Persistent symptoms:** add diuretic: hydrochlorothiazide 25-50 mg qd, furosemide 10-40 mg qd (up to 240 mg bid) or spironolactone 25 mg qd (up to 50 mg bid)

- **Refractory:** consider digoxin 0.125-0.25 mg qd

- **Other options:** treat hypertension, treat hyperlipidemia, discontinue alcohol, cocaine, AZT and smoking. Some recommend supplemental antioxidants such as carnitine and/or selenium (200 µg/d) if deficient (*NEJM* 1999;340:732).

Cardiovascular Complications of Antiretroviral Agents: See pg. 136-145.

DERMATOLOGIC COMPLICATIONS

OVERVIEW: A review of 897 patients with HIV-infection referred for a dermatology consult in Baltimore from 1996-2002 found that the most frequent diagnoses were folliculitis (18%), condyloma accuminatum (12%), seborrhea (11%), xerosis cutis (10%), dermatophytic infection (7%), warts (7%), hyperpigmentation (6%) and purigo nodularis (6%) (*J Am Acad Dermatol* 2006;54:581). Most of these conditions were associated with low CD4 counts (folliculitis, idiopathic pruritis, prurigo nodularis, molluscum and seborrhea). Pruritis was especially common and often unexplained ("idiopathic pruritis"); this is thought to result from immune dysregulation and is sometimes accompanied by eosinophilia (*JID* 1996;54:266).

Papular Pruritic Eruption (PPE)

Typical presentation is pruritic darkened papules 0.2-1.0 cm diameter most common on extremities. One report implicates a hypersensitivity to insect bites as the cause (*JAMA* 2004;292:2614). The diagnosis can usually be established by a skin biopsy. The differential diagnosis includes eosinophilic folliculitis and pruritis nodularis. The best treatment is ART, but this usually requires >16 weeks for a good response. Other treatments include topical steroids or topical capsaicin (*Top HIV Med* 2010;18:16).

Bacillary Angiomatosis: See *Arch Intern Med* 1994;154:524; *Dermatology* 2000;21:326; *CID* 2005;40:S154; and pg. 423.

The usual <u>presentation</u> is papular, nodular, pedunculated and/or verrucous lesions that start as red or purple papules and gradually expand to nodules or pedunculated masses. They appear vascular and may bleed extensively with trauma. There are usually one or several lesions, but there may be hundreds. The <u>differential diagnosis</u> includes Kaposi's sarcoma, cherry angioma, hemangioma, pyogenic granuloma and dermatofibroma. The diagnosis is based on skin biopsy showing lobular vascular proliferation with inflammation and Warthin Starry silver stain showing typical organisms as small black clusters. Serology is available (IFA and EIA); IFA titers >1:256 usually indicates active infection. See *Bartonella* pg. 423.

Cryptococcosis: (see *CID* 2000;30:652 and pg. 455-439).

The typical <u>presentation</u> is nodular, papular, follicular, or ulcerative skin lesions; may resemble molluscum. Usual locations are face, neck, scalp. The diagnosis is made with the cryptococcal antigen assay and biopsy with Gomori methenamine silver stain to show typical encapsulated, budding yeast, and positive culture. <u>Perform LP</u> in any patient with a positive serum cryptococcal antigen or culture for *C. neoformans* (if positive, see pg. 433). <u>Treatment</u>, if negative LP, fluconazole 400 mg qd po x 8 wks, then 200 mg qd. If positive LP, see pg. 433.

Dermatophytic Fungal Infections

Fungal infection of skin, hair, and nails is caused by *Tinea rubrum, T. mentagrophytes, M. canis, E. floccosum, T. tonsurans, T. verrucosum* and *T. soudanense* (*Candida* causes typical nail and skin lesions, and *Malassezia furfur* causes tinea vesicolor. Note: *Candida* and *M. furfur* are not dermatophytes). The usual <u>presentations</u> include:

- **T. pedis:** Interdigital pruritis, scaling, fissures and maceration. Concomitant nail dystrophies, plantar and moccasin variants may include interdigital involvement, pruritic and red lesions between toes ± interdigital fissures, extension to adjacent skin and nails, scaling is always present ("athlete's foot").

- **Onychomycosis** starts with discoloration and thickening, usually on distal nail at one side and spreads toward the other side and toward the cuticle, leaving heaped-up keratinous debris.

- **T. corporis:** Circular erythematous scaling that spreads with central clearing (ringworm).

- **T. cruris:** Red scaly patch on inner thigh with sharply demarcated borders.

DIAGNOSIS: Scrapings of skin lesion or discolored nail bed for KOH preparation. This may be supplemented with culture of scraping on Sabouraud's medium. The <u>treatment</u> is agent and location specific:

- **Onychomycosis:** Topical therapy is usually not effective.

  □ Preferred treatment: <u>Terbinafine</u> (*Lamisil*) 250 mg qd x 6 wks (fingernails) or 12 wks (toenails). Terbinafine is hepatotoxic and is expensive but has better long-term results than itraconazole (*Brit J Dermatol* 1999;141[Suppl 56]:15). <u>Itraconazole</u> "pulse therapy," 400 mg/d for 1 wk/mo x 2 mos (fingernails) or x 3 mos (toenails). Main concerns are hepatotoxicity, drug interactions, cardiotoxicity, and cost of treating a benign infection.

- **Tinea corporis, tinea cruris, tinea pedis:** Topical agent for 2 wks (T. cruris) to 4 wks (T. pedis): clotrimazole (*Lotrimin*)* 1% cream or lotion bid; econazole (*Spectazole*) 1% cream qd or bid; ketoconazole (*Nizoral*) 2% cream qd; miconazole (*Monostat-Derm*)* 2% cream bid; butenafine (*Mentax*) 1% cream; terbinafine (*Lamisil*)* 1% cream or gel qd or bid; Tolnaftate (*Tinactin*)* 1% cream, gel, powder, solution, or aerosol bid.

  ───────────
  * Available over-the-counter.

- **Refractory, chronic, or extensive disease:** Terbinafine 250 mg qd x 2-4 wks; itraconazole 100-200 mg qd x 2-4 wks. Grise-ofulvin microsized 250-500 mg bid. Griseofulvin should be last of treatment options.

Drug Eruptions: (*J Allergy Clin Immunol* 2008;121:826)

Most common are antibiotics, especially sulfonamides (TMP/SMX), beta-lactams, anticonvulsants, NNRTIs, and FPV and DRV, both of which include sulfa moieties.

The usual <u>presentation</u> is a morbilliform, erythematous, usually pruritic ± low grade fever, usually within 2 wks of new drug or days after reexposure. Most common is a maculopapular rash that starts on the chest, face and arms. Less common and more severe forms include: <u>urticaria</u> (intensely pruritic, edematous, and circumscribed); <u>anaphylaxis</u> (laryngeal edema, nausea, vomiting ± shock); <u>hypersensitivity syndrome</u> (severe reaction with rash and fever ± hepatitis, arthralgias, lymphadenopathy, and hematologic changes with eosinophilia and atypical lymphocytes, usually at 2 to 6 weeks after drug is started) (*NEJM* 1994;331:1272). (See abacavir pg. 179 and nevirapine pg. 330); <u>Stevens Johnson syndrome (SJS)</u> (fever, erosive stomatitis, disseminated erosions ± blisters dark red macules, ocular involvement; mortality 5%); and <u>toxic epidermal necrolysis (TEN)s</u> (epidermal necrosis with scalded skin appearance ± mucous).

In severe symptomatic reactions, discontinue implicated agent (for TMP-SMX, see pg. 409) and <u>treatment</u>: <u>pruritic uncomplicated drug</u>

rashes (antihistamines, topical antipruritics, and topical corticosteroids); SJS and TEN (severe cases are managed as burns with supportive care; corticosteroids are not indicated (*Cutis* 1996;57:223) and avoidance required for ABC, NVP hepatotoxicity and any other drug implicated in SJS or TEN). Desensitization protocol is available for TMP-SMX (see pg. 411).

Folliculitis

A review of 897 HIV-infected patients referred for a dermatology consultation found that folliculitis was the most common diagnosis, accounting for 161 (18%) (*J Am Acad Derm* 2006;54:581). *Staphylococcus aureus* is the most common cause. Other causes include *Pityrosporum ovale* (intrafollicular yeast), *Demodex folliculorum* (intrafollicular mite), and eosinophilic folliculitis, in which biopsy shows eosinophilic inflammation without a detectable infectious agent. The presentation with *S. aureus* is folliculitis that usually involves skin follicles in the upper arms, upper trunk, upper legs and buttocks (see pg. 482). This may resemble PPE, may be pruritic and may present with pustules. Eosinophilic folliculitis presents with very pruritic lesions that may resemble acne or PPI but are preferentially located n the upper body including the neck, head and upper chest. These lesions are distinguished from acne by intense pruritis and from PPE by less discoloration. The cause is unknown. The diagnosis is made by the presentation and biopsy: follicular inflammation ± follicular destruction and abscess formation. Special stains such as PAS and B+B may show infectious agent. Multiple eosinophils destroying the hair follicle wall and eosinophilic abscesses are seen in eosinophilic folliculitis. Culture of pustule may grow *S. aureus*. The treatment: *S. aureus*: topical erythromycin or clindamycin or systemic antistaphylococcal antibiotic; *P. ovale*: topical or systemic antifungal agents; *D. folliculorum*: permethrin cream or topical metronidazole; eosinophilic: topical steroids, phototherapy with UVB and/or PUVA (*NEJM* 1988;318:1183; *Arch Dermatol* 1995;131:360); general: antihistamines (high dose, mixed classes together) for symptomatic relief.

Furunculosis: See *Staphylococcus aureus*, pg. 482.

Herpes Simplex: See *CID* 2005;40:S167 and pg. 44.

Herpes Zoster: See pg. 449.

Kaposi's Sarcoma (KS): See pg. 532.

7 Systems Review

Prurigo Nodularis (*Int J Dermatol* 1999;37:401)

Most common with CD4 <200 cells/mm³. The cause is unknown. The presentation is intense pruritis with excoriated nodules >1 cm diameter that are hyperpigmented. The lesions are generally symmetric, start on the arms and then spread to the upper trunk. Unreachable areas such as the mid back are usually spared. This may be a variant of PPE or other primary dermatologic condition. The major treatment modality is symptomatic to prevent vicious cycle pruritis: pruritis → scratch trauma → lichenification → increased pruritis. Treatment includes occlusive dressings, high potency steroids, hydroxyzine 10-25 mg hs or doxepin 10-25 mg hs, or mirtazipine 15-30 mg hs. Phototherapy may help. Thalidomide has reported benefit in refractory cases (*Arch Dermatol* 2004;140:845).

Scabies (*MMWR* 2002;51[RR-6]:68)

This is caused by a mite. The <u>presentation</u> is small red papules that are intensely pruritic, especially at night. There may be a "burrow," a 3- to 15-mm line which represents the superficial tunnel the female mite digs at 2 mm/d to lay eggs. Usual locations are the interdigital webs of the fingers, volar aspect of the wrist, periumbilical area, axilla, thighs, buttocks, genitalia, feet, and breasts. Scabies crostosus (crusted or "Norwegian" scabies) is a severe form seen in compromised hosts, including AIDS patients. There is uncontrolled spread to involve large areas, sometimes the total skin surface with scales and crusts that show thousands of mites. The <u>diagnosis</u> is made by detecting the mite which is 0.4 x 0.3 mm, 8-legged, and shaped like a turtle. It is visible to the naked eye but burrowing precludes detection. Scrape infected area, place on a slide with a coverslip, and examine under 10x magnification to demonstrate mites or eggs. Many authorities have abandoned the standard scalpel scrape in favor of packing tape left on the skin for 30 seconds (*Arch Dermatol* 2011;147:468 and 147:494). The treatment should include family members and close contacts treated at the same time using:

- **Permethrin cream** (5%) applied to total body, from the head to the feet, and washed off at 8-14 hours. Re-treat at 1-2 wks. All household members must be treated simultaneously even if asymptomatic. A 30-g tube is usually adequate for an adult.

- **Lindane** (1%) 1 oz lotion or 30 g cream applied as a thin layer to total body, from the neck down, and washed off at 8 hours is an alternative. Lindane is less expensive than permethrin, but there is rare resistance and more side effects.

- **Ivermectin** 200 µg/kg po repeated at 2 wks (*NEJM* 1995;333:26). Not recommended as first-line treatment in uncomplicated cases.

- Note that the rash and pruritis may persist up to 2 wks post-treatment – warn patients. <u>Bedding and clothing</u> that has been used recently must be decontaminated. Machine wash in hot water and machine dry with high heat, or dry clean. For itching: hydroxyzine or diphenhydramine. For scabies crustosus (crusted scabies): isolate immediately and use strict barrier precautions. Treat with ivermectin 200 μg/kg po followed by a second dose 1-2 wks later, plus permethrin topically until scales and crust have resolved. Topical karolytics such as salicylic acid gel or urea creams are also recommended.

Seborrheic Dermatitis

The usual <u>cause</u> is the yeast, which can be recovered from lesions, but may not play a central role in HIV-associated seborrhea (*J Am Acad Dermatol* 1992;27:37). The <u>presentation</u> is erythematous plaques with greasy scales and indistinct margins on located on the scalp, central face, post-auricular area, presternal, axillary, and occasionally pubic area. <u>Treatment</u> consists of ART, mild potency steroid such as triamcinolone 0.1% or weaker (desonide 0.05%), hydrocortisone 2.5% for the face ± ketoconazole 2% cream applied twice per day for the duration of the flare only, and tar-based shampoos (*Z-tar, Pentrax, DHS tar, T-gel, Ionil T plus*), selenium sulfide (*Selsun, Exelderm*), or zinc pyrithione (*Head & Shoulders, Zincon, DHS zinc*) applied daily, or ketoconazole shampoo applied twice per week. Leave lather on for five minutes before rinsing.

GASTROINTESTINAL COMPLICATIONS

Anorexia, Nausea, Vomiting

MAJOR CAUSES: Medications (especially ARVs, antibiotics, opiates, and NSAIDs), depression, intracranial pathology, GI disease, hypogonadism, pregnancy, lactic acidosis, acute gastroenteritis

ART: Nausea ± vomiting and/or abdominal pain are reported in 2-17% of patients given PIs (*JAIDS* 2004;37:1111). The most common agents, in rank order, are RTV, IDV, LPV/r, TPV/r, FPV, SQV, DRV and ATV. The effect is dose-related and most common with boosted PIs with ≥200 mg RTV/d. Similar symptoms are frequent with AZT.

EVALUATION: If relationship to medication unclear, consider medication change, morning testosterone level, GI evaluation (endoscopy, CT scan), intracranial evaluation (head CT scan or or MRI) or empiric treatment.

TREATMENT: Treat underlying condition.

- **Anorexia**
  - Megestrol (*Megace*) 400-800 mg qd. Weight gain is mostly fat. May decrease testosterone level or increase blood sugar. Consider megestrol (pg. 324) + testosterone (pg. 394).

7 Systems Review

- Dronabinol (*Marinol*) 2.5 mg po bid; active ingredient of marijuana. Weight gain is mostly fat.

- **Nausea and vomiting**

  - Prochlorperazine (*Compazine*) 5-10 mg po q6-8h; trimetho-benzamide (*Tigan*) 250 mg po q6-8h; metoclopramide (*Reglan*) 5-10 mg po q6-8h; dimenhydrinate (*Dramamine*) 50 mg po q6h-q8h; lorazapam (*Ativan*) 0.025-0.05 mg/kg IV or IM; haloperidol (*Haldol*) 1-5 mg bid po or IM; dronabinol 2.5-5 mg po bid; ondansetron (*Zofran*) 0.2 mg/kg IV or IM.

  - Note: Phenothiazines (haloperidol, metoclopramide, prochlor-perazine, trimethobenzamide) may cause dystonia. Metoclo-pramide is preferable to dimenhydrinate, oxazepam, and ondansetron.

  - PEG: May require percutaneous endoscopic gastrostomy (PEG) to deliver nutrition and medications, including ART regimen.

ORAL LESIONS

Aphthous Ulcers

CAUSE: Unknown

The lesions appear as single or multiple white or yellow circumscribed ulcer with a red halo. The differential include HSV, CMV, drug-induced ulcers; biopsy recommended for non-healing ulcers. Often recurrent.

CLASSIFICATION

- **Minor:**<0.5 cm diameter, usually self-limiting with healing in 7-10 days.

- **Major:**>0.5 cm, deep, prolonged, heals slowly, causes pain, especially with eating, and may prevent oral intake (*AIDS* 1992;6:963; *Oral Surg Oral Med Oral Pathol* 1996;81:141)

TREATMENT

- **ART:** Response of aphthous ulcers may be dramatic (*Int J Infect Dis* 2006;11:278).

- **Topical treatment with applications 2x to 4x/d**

  - Lidocaine solution before meals

  - Triamcinolone hexacetonide in *Orabase* – preferred (*J Am Dent Assoc* 2003;134:200)

  - Fluocinonide gel (*Lidex*) 0.05% ointment mixed 1:1 with *Orabase* or covered with *Orabase*

  - Amlexanox (*Aphthasol*) 5% oral paste (*J Oral Maxillofac Surg* 1993;51:243).

■ TABLE 7-1: **Oral Lesions (Classification of the ACTG Subcommittee Oral HIV/AIDS Research Alliance) (***J Oral Pathol Med* **2009;38:481)**

Lesion	Character	Location	Pain	Biopsy required?
Candidiasis	White or yellow plaques	Palate, tongue, Buccal mucosa	None or mild	No
Hairy leukoplakia	White, corrugated	Lateral tongue	None	No
Herpes simplex	Vesicular ulcers	Vermillion border (Gingiva), palate	Mild-moderate	No
Aphthous ulcers	White, yellow ulcers	Soft palate mucosa	Severe	No
Necrotizing gingivitis	Yellow ulcers necrotic	Anywhere	Severe	Yes
Bacterial gingivitis	Necrotic, putrid	Local or generalized	Severe	No
Kaposi's sarcoma	Red, purple nodule	Anywhere, especially palate	None-moderate	Yes
Squamous cell cancer	Red, white indurated	Anywhere, especially tongue	None-severe	Yes

- **Oral and intralesional therapy (refractory cases)**
  - Prednisone 40 mg qd po x 1-2 wks then taper (*Am J Clin Dermatol* 2003;4:669)
  - Colchicine 1.5 mg qd (*J Am Acad Dermatol* 1994;31:459)
  - Dapsone 100 mg qd
  - Pentoxifylline (*Trental*) 400 mg po tid with meals
  - Thalidomide 200 mg qd po x 4-6 wks ± maintenance with 200 mg 2x/wk. Note: Thalidomide is "experimental" for aphthous ulcers. See pg. 398 for purchase instructions. Thalidomide has strict requirements for use, but is very effective (*NEJM* 1997;337: 1086; *CID* 1995;20:250; *JID* 1999;180:61; *Arch Dermatol* 1990; 126:923; *Spec Care Dentist* 2005;25:236).

Gingivitis

CAUSE: Anaerobic bacteria

PHASES: Linear gingival erythema → necrotizing gingivitis → necrotizing periodontitis → necrotizing stomatitis

TREATMENT

- **Routine dental care:** Brush and floss ± topical antiseptics: *Listerine* swish x 30-60 seconds bid, *Peridex*, etc.
- **Dental consultation:** Curettage and debridement
- **Antibiotics** (necrotizing stomatitis): metronidazole; alternatives – clindamycin and amoxicillin-clavulanate

7 Systems Review

Herpes Simplex: See pg. 447.

Kaposi's Sarcoma: See pg. 532.

Oral Hairy Leukoplakia (OHL)

CAUSE: Intense replication of EBV (*CID* 1997;25:1392)

PRESENTATION: Unilateral or bilateral adherent white/gray patches on lingual lateral margins ± dorsal or ventral surface of tongue. Patches are irregular folds and projections.

DIFFERENTIAL: Candidiasis: OHL does not respond to azoles and cannot be scraped off, unlike *Candida*; Others: squamous cell carcinoma or traumatic leukoplakia.

DIAGNOSIS: Diagnosis is usually clinical; biopsy is sometimes advocated for lesions that require therapy and don't respond, but is rarely necessary.

IMPLICATIONS: Found almost exclusively with HIV, indicates low CD4 count, predicts AIDS, and responds to ART.

TREATMENT (*CID* 1997;25:1392): Rarely symptomatic and rarely treated, but occasional patients have pain or have concern about appearance. The options include:

- **ART** (preferred)
- **Anti-EBV treatment:** Acyclovir 800 mg po 5x/d x 2-3 wks, then 1.2-2 gm/d. Other effective antivirals include famciclovir, valacyclovir, foscarnet, ganciclovir, and valganciclovir. Lesions recur when treatment is discontinued.
- **Other:** topical podophylline

Salivary Gland Enlargement

CAUSE: The most common cause is diffuse infiltrative lymphocytosis syndrome (DILS), a condition associated with HIV and with Sjögren's syndrome (*Arthritis Rheum* 2006;55:466; *Ann Intern Med* 1996;125:494). May be seen with IRIS (*Int J STD AIDS* 2008;19:305).

PRESENTATION: Parotid enlargement, cystic, unilateral or bilateral, non-tender, usually asymptomatic; may be painful, cosmetically disfiguring, or cause xerostomia (*Ear Nose Throat J* 1990;69:475; *Arthritis Rheum* 2006;55:466; *Rheumatology* 2008;47:952).

DIFFERENTIAL: Must differentiate cystic from solid lesion with CT scan (*Laryngoscope* 1998;98:772) and/or fine needle aspiration (FNA). FNA useful for microbiology and cytology and decompression. May require biopsy to exclude tumor, especially lymphoma. Biopsy usually shows histology resembling Sjögren's syndrome; characteristic features are severe salivary duct atypia and foci of lymphocytes, predominantly

Systems Review

CD8+ lymphocytes (*Arch Pathol Lab Med* 2000;124:1773; *J Oral Pathol Med* 2003;32:544); alternatively, there may be "non-specific chronic sialadenitis" (*Oral Dis* 2003;9:55). The most common pathogens when there is infection are mycobacteria and CMV. The frequency of this complication has decreased substantially during the HAART era (*Arthritis Rheum* 2006;55:466).

TREATMENT

- FNA for decompression of fluid-filled parotid cysts; may require large-bore needle for aspiration.

- **Xerostomia:** Sugarless chewing gum, artificial saliva, pilocarpine

Candidiasis, Oropharygeal (thrush): See pg. 425.

Diarrhea

Note that most studies of acute and chronic diarrhea were done in the pre-HAART era when this complication was often associated with advanced immunosuppression and high rates of "AIDS enteropathy" and OI complications (MAC, CMV and cryptosporidiosis), which are now far less common (*AIDS* 2005;18:107).

Acute diarrhea (defined as ≥3 loose or watery stools/d for 3-10 days)

INCIDENCE AND CAUSE: A review in 44,778 HIV-infected persons followed at >100 medical facilities in the U.S. from 1992-2002 found an annual incidence of 7.2 cases of bacterial diarrhea per 1000 patient-years and yielded bacterial pathogens in 1,115 (*CID* 2005;41: 1621). The most common bacterial pathogens, in rank order, were *C. difficile* (598 cases; 54%) *Shigella* (156, 14%), *C. jejuni* (154; 14%), Salmonella (82; 7%); *S. aureus* (43, 4%),and MAC (22; 2%).

DIAGNOSTIC EVALUATION

Medication-related

- Main antiretroviral agents: All PIs, especially LPV/r, SQV, and ddl (buffered formulation)
- Management (*CID* 2000;30:908)
  - □ Loperamide 4 mg, then 2 mg every loose stool, up to 16/d
  - □ Calcium 500 mg bid; psyllium 1 tsp qd-bid or 2 bars qd-bid; oat bran 1500 mg bid
  - □ Pancreatic enzymes 1-2 tabs with meals

Pathogen detection (*CID* 2001;32:331; *Arch Pathol Lab Med* 2001;125: 1042)

- Blood culture: MAC, *Salmonella* (see pg. 481-482)
- Stool culture: *Salmonella, Shigella, C. jejuni, Vibrio, Yersinia, E. coli* 0157

7 Systems Review

- Stool assay for *C. difficile* toxin A and B by EIA, PCR or a combination test for toxin and *C. difficile*.

- O&P examination + modified acid-fast stain (*Cryptosporidia, Cyclospora, Isospora*), trichrome or other stain for microsporidia, and antigen detection (*Giardia*)

Radiology: : CT scan with contrast – *C. difficile* colitis, CMV colitis and lymphoma.

Endoscopy: Most useful for CMV, Kaposi's sarcoma, and lymphoma

CAMPYLOBACTER JEJUNI: 4-8% of HIV-infected patients with acute diarrhea; rates are increased up to 39-fold in MSM (*CID* 1997;24:1107; *CID* 1998;26:91; *CID* 2005;40:S152). HIV-Infected persons with low CD4 counts are at increased risk for enteric infection and for bacteremia with non-jejuni species of campylobacter including *Campylobacter coli, cineadi, fennelliae, laridis, fetus* and *upsaliensis*. Most labs cannot recover these agents in stool cultures but can usually detect them in blood cultures. Clinical features of *C. jejuni* enteric infection: watery diarrhea or bloody flux, fever, fecal leukocytes variable; any CD4 count. *C. jejuni,* warn lab if suspect other campylobacter species in stool. Blood cultures give the highest yield with these non-*C. jejuni* species. Treatment (*CID* 2001;32:331): ciprofloxacin 500 mg po bid or azithromycin 500 mg po qd. Modify according to in vitro activity. With bacteremia: consider adding an aminoglycoside. Duration for mild or moderate disease is 7 days; for bacteremia it is ≥ 2 wks.

CLOSTRIDIUM DIFFICILE: See pg. 430.

ENTERIC VIRUSES: Account for >30% of HIV-infected patients with acute diarrhea. Clinical features: Watery diarrhea, acute, but one-third become chronic; any CD4 cell count. The major agents: norovirus, adenovirus, astrovirus, picornavirus, calicivirus (*NEJM* 1993;329:14); clinical laboratories cannot detect these viruses.

NOROVIRUS: This virus is the major cause of infectious diarrhea in the world. It is also the leading cause of outbreaks of diarrhea associated with foodborne disease, residents of healthcare facilities, passengers on cruise ships, travelers and immunocompromised patients (*Discov Med* 2010;10:61; *CID* 2009;49:1061). It is expressed with vomiting and diarrhea, often in the winter ("winter vomiting disease"). The diagnosis can be established with RT-PCR of stools or emesis. The classic diagnostic criteria are "*Kaplan's Criteria*": 1) duration of 12-60 hrs; 2) incubation period of 24-48 hrs; 3) >50% of affected persons have vomiting; and 4) there is no bacterial pathogen found. Management is infection control and symptomatic treatment of patients.

IDIOPATHIC: 25-40% of HIV-infected patients with acute diarrhea have noninfectious causes; rule out medications, dietary, irritable syndrome etc. Infectious causes should be excluded if symptoms are severe or chronic and include culture, O & P examination and *C. difficile* test.

EMPIRIC TREATMENT, SEVERE ACUTE IDIOPATHIC DIARRHEA

- Empiric lomotil or loparamide. Note that some consider *C. difficile* infection to be a contraindication to these anti-peristaltic agents, but supporting evidence is slim (*CID* 2009;48:598).

- Empiric antiobiotic treatment for severe diarrhea may include: ciprofloxacin 500 mg po bid; ofloxacin 200-300 mg po bid or other fluoroquinolone x 5 days ± metronidazole (*Arch Intern Med* 1990;150:541; *Ann Intern Med 1992;117:202; CID* 2001;32:331).

HIV enteropathy

Described in the pre-HAART era as a diarrheal syndrome associated with advanced immunosuppression (CD4 <100 cells/mm^3) with no identified pathogen and characterized by non-specific pathologic changes in the small bowel (*Infect Dis Clin Pract* 2010;5:293; *AIDS* 2005;19:107). Postulated mechanisms included defective transport (*AIDS* 1998;12:43), changes in intestinal microtubule cytoskeleton (*AIDS* 2001;15:123) or HIV infection of the GI epithelial cells (*J Biomed Sci* 2003;10:156). There was no concensus, but the condition has nearly disappeared in the HAART era.

CRYPTOSPORIDIA: See pg. 439.

CYTOMEGALOVIRUS: See pg. 441.

ISOSPORA BELLI: See pg. 454.

MICROSPORIDIA: *ENTEROCYTOZOON BIENEUSI* **or** *ENTEROCYTOZOON* **(SEPTATA) INTESTINALIS:** See pg. 457.

MYCOBACTERIUM AVIUM **COMPLEX (MAC):** See pg. 459.

Esophagitis: See Table 7-2, pg. 504.

DIFFERENTIAL: Consider non-HIV-related causes, especially if CD4 is >200 cells/mm^3. Most common are medication- or food-related esophagitis and GERD. With CD4 <200 cells/mm^3: most common is *Candida*; less common are aphthous ulcers or CMV; HSV is infrequent; rare causes include TB, *M. avium*, histoplasmosis, PCP, cryptosporidia, Kaposi's sarcoma and lymphoma.

7 Systems Review

	Candida	Cytomegalovirus (CMV)	Herpes Simplex Virus	Aphthous Ulcers
See also:	pg. 425	pg. 441	pg. 447	pg. 498
Frequency	50-70%	10-20%	2-5%	10-20%
Clinical features				
Dysphagia	+++	+	+	+
Odynophagia	++	+++	+++	+++
Thrush	50-70%	<25%	<5%	<10%
Oral ulcers	Rare	Uncommon	Often	Uncommon
Pain	Diffuse	Focal	Focal	Focal
Fever	Infrequent	Often	Infrequent	Infrequent
Diagnosis				
Endoscopy	■ Usually treated empirically ■ Pseudo-membranous plaques; may involve entire esophagus	■ Biopsy required for diagnosis ■ Erythema and erosions/ulcers, single or multiple discrete lesions, often distal.	■ Biopsy required for diagnosis ■ Erythema and erosions/ulcers, usually small, coalescing, shallow	■ Similar in appearance and location to CMV ulcers ■ Biopsy required to rule out CMV and HSV
Micro-biology	■ Brush: Yeast and pseudo-mycelium on KOH prep or PAS ■ Culture with sensitivities may be useful with suspected resistance	■ Biopsy: Intra-cellular inclusions and/or positive culture. ■ Highest yield with histopath of biopsy and culture. Culture not recommended false positives.	■ Brush/biopsy: Intracyto-plasmic inclusions + multinucleate giant cells, FA stain, and/or positive culture.	■ Negative studies for *Candida*, HSV, CMV, and other diagnoses.

Notes:

1. One-third of AIDS patients in pre-HAART era developed esophageal symptoms (*Gut* 1989;30:1033). Esophageal ulcers are usually due to CMV (45%), or they are idiopathic aphthous ulcers (40%); HSV accounts for only 5% (*Ann Intern Med* 1995;122:143).

2. With endoscopy a diagnosis is established in about 70-95% (*Arch Intern Med* 1991;151:1567). Response to empiric treatment often precludes need for endoscopic diagnosis of *Candida* esophagitis. Yield with barium swallow 20-30%.

3. Other considerations: Drug-induced dysphagia (*Am J Med* 1988;88:512), including AZT (*Ann Intern Med* 1990;162:65) *M. avium*, TB, cryptosporidia, *P. jirovecii*, primary HIV infection, histoplasmosis, KS or lymphoma (*BMJ* 1988;296:92; *Gastrointest Endosc* 1986;32:96).

4. Fluconazole is the preferred treatment for *Candida* because of established efficacy, more predictable absorption, and fewer drug interactions compared with alternative azoles.

Systems Review

LIVER AND PANCREATIC DISEASE

Liver disease is now the most common non-AIDS-associated disease cause of death in persons with HIV infection (*Arch Intern Med* 2006;166:1632; *AIDS* 2010;24:1537). Major contributing factors are hepatitis B and C co-infection, alcohol abuse and, possibly, hepatic injury from ART agents (*JID* 2008;197 Suppl 3:S279). The liver may also play a very central role in immune activation reflecting the role of Kupffer cells to control microbial translocation (*AIDS* 2009;23:2397): The following is a brief review of management issues dealing with liver disease in the patient with HIV infection. The role of ART and ART-associated complications is reviewed (see pg. 145-147).

Hepatitis

Hepatitis A, B (see pg. 507), **and C** (see pg. 513)

Alcohol toxicity or other substance abuse (*JAIDS* 2001;27:4426)

Chronic nonviral: Alcoholic, nonalcoholic steatohepatitis (see below), autoimmune hepatitis, hemochromatosis, sarcoidosis

Drug toxicity: Acetaminophen (*CID* 2004;38:565), INH, statins, ART agents: 1) steatohepatitis (ddI, d4T, AZT); 2) hepatic necrosis (NVP) (see pg. 335) and ABC hypersensitivity (see pg. 145, 164); 3) severe hepatic disease (TPV) (FDA warning 2007, www.aptivus.com) and transaminitis (PIs) (*AIDS* 2004;18:2277) (see pg. 145-146).

Hypersensitivity: Phenytoin, ABC, TMP-SMX, NVP, ABC

Opportunistic infections including MAC and CMV: See pgs 459 and 441.

ART-associated Liver Disease: See pg. 147t.

- Immune reconstitution inflammatory syndrome (*JAIDS* 2001;27:426; *CID* 2004;38:S65) (see pg. 525).
- HBV may also flare with IRIS.
- NVP hepatitis; may also note rash and other symptoms of a hypersensitivity reaction. Most common in females with baseline CD4 >250 cells/mm^3 or men with baseline CD4 >400 cells/mm^3 (see pg. 335).
- PI/NNRTI transaminitis: 15-30% rate is increased 2-fold with HCV coinfection (*CID* 2002;34:831; *JAMA* 2000;283:74; *Hepatology* 2002; 35:182). Other risks for drug-related hepatotoxicity are renal failure and thrombocytopenia (*JAIDS* 2006;43:320). TPV/r is the most hepatotoxic PI.
- Increased indirect bilirubin due to ATV and IDV.

Type	Seroprevalence* Transmission	Incubation Period	Diagnosis	Course
A	Fecal-oral; food; unknown source in 50% ■ Gen. population: 40-50% immune ■ Acute hepatitis: 50%	15-50 days	■ Acute: IgM ■ Prior infection or vaccination: Total HAV antibody (IgG)	■ Fulminant and fatal in 0.6%; fulminant in 15% with HCV ■ Very high ALT/AST ■ Self limited in >99% ■ No chronic form
B	Sex, blood, and perinatal ■ Seroprevalence of HbsAb: vaccinated <10 years previously 90%; general population 3-14%; IDU 60-80%; MSM 35-80% ■ Seroprevalence of HbsAg (chronic HBV): general population 0.1-0.2%; MSM 6-17%; IDU 7-10%; immigrants from high-risk areas 13%; HIV-infected (US) 7-10%	45-160 days	■ Acute: HBsAg + anti-HBc IgM ■ Chronic: HBsAg x 6 mos + anti-HBc IgG ■ Vaccinated: HBsAb	■ Fulminant and fatal in 1.4% ■ Chronic hepatitis in 6% of general population; 10-15% of patients with AIDS
C	Blood (>sex and perinatal) ■ General population: 1.8% ■ IDU: 60-90% ■ Hemophilia: 60-90% ■ MSM: 2-8%	15-50 days	■ EIA Ab + quantative HCV RNA	■ Chronic hepatitis after acute HCV in 80% ■ Cirrhosis in 10-15% in 20 years but increased risk of progression with HIV coinfection or ETOH ■ HCV has little or no effect on rate of HIV infection progression

* Seroprevalence for adults in the U.S.

Steatosis

The term refers to fatty liver disease with intracytoplasmic accumulation of triglyceride fat that may be associated with inflammation (steatohepatitis). It can be a component of alcoholic liver disease (alcoholic steatosis) or non-alcoholic liver disease (NASH). The diagnosis is suspected by elevated ALT and AST combined with risk factors. The diagnosis is established by biopsy or with imaging by US, CT or MRI. The cause is multifactorial, but with HIV infection the dominant issues are ART agents and HCV co-infection (*CID* 2006; 43:365; *Gastroenterology* 2011;140:809). Contributing factors are obesity, alcoholism, diabetes and hyperlipidemia). The major HIV medications implicated are the tymidine analogs (d4T, AZT) and ddI, which are now infrequently used in the US. A major contemporary cause is HCV co-infection which is associated with significant hepatic fibrosis (*AIDS* 2005;19:585; *Hepatology* 2008;47:1118; *JID* 2005;192:1943). A review of 28 patients with HIV/HCV co-infection, and had sequential biopsies showed 74% had significant regression of hepatic steatosis with ART and increased CD4 counts (*Gastroenterology* 2011;140:809). The authors urged attention or prevention with attention to the dominant co-morbidities of obesity and alcohol intake.

Cholangiopathy, AIDS: (*Dig Dis* 1998;16:2025)

Cause: *Cryptosporidium* is the most common identified microbial cause (see pg. 439). Other causes: microsporidia, CMV and *Cyclospora*. About 20-40% are idiopathic. Frequency: relatively rare and seen primarily in late stage AIDS. Presentation: right upper quadrant pain, LFTs show cholestasis. Late stage HIV with CD4 count <100 cells/mm^3. Diagnosis: alkaline phosphatase levels are high, often >8 x ULN. Level predicts prognosis. Usual method to establish the diagnosis is ERCP (preferred); ultrasound is 75-95% specific. Treatment: ART is the most important treatment. Treat pathogen when possible – CMV and *Cyclospora*. Usual treatment is mechanical and based on lesion. ERCP is used for both diagnosis and treatment.

Viral Hepatitis
Hepatitis B (*Hepatology* 2007;45:507)

DIAGNOSIS: Positive serology for HBsAg for ≥26 wks indicates chronic infection (see pg. 57).

PREVALENCE: HBV is transmitted like HIV by blood, sex and childbirth. Primary HBV infection in adults is usually subclinical and self-limited, but about 6% develop chronic HBV infection defined by persistent HBsAg x 6 mos. The seroprevalence of HBsAg in US adults is about 0.2%; it is higher in MSM, IDUs, persons with multiple sex partners and immigrants from areas where HBV is endemic (Africa, Southeast Asia and Eastern Europe). The prevalence of HBsAg in patients with HIV infection in the US and Europe is 7-10% (*JAIDS* 1991;4:416; *JID* 2003;188:571; *Topics HIV Med* 2007;15:163). These rates of co-infection are much higher in some countries where HBV is endemic (*AF J Med Sci* 2006;35:337).

NATURAL HISTORY: The natural history of chronic HBV monoinfection is highly variable. About 25% have persistent active viral replication with HBeAg and high levels of HBV DNA in serum (usually >20,000 IU/mL) associated with progressive liver injury with cirrhosis and a risk of hepatocellular carcinoma. Others have spontaneous remission with a spontaneous decrease in HBV DNA levels and seroconversion from HBeAg pos to HBeAg neg and anti-HBe. This transition occurs at a rate of about 10%/yr in monoinfected patients, but less often with HIV/HBV co-infection *(Ann Intern Med* 1981;94:744; *Clin Gastroenterol Hepatol* 2006;4:936). Levels of HBV DNA are lower in HBeAg negative patients, but some of these patients have progressive liver disease with HBV levels >2,000 IU/mL or there may be progressive severe HBeAg negative liver disease. Uncommon extrahepatic complications of HBV infection include glomerulonephritis, polyarteritis nodosa and vasculitis.

The impact of HIV on HBV infection is substantial: (Hepatology 2009;49 Suppl 5: S138)

- HIV confers an increased risk of chronic HBV after acute infection (10-15%) especially with low CD4 count.

- Decreased HBeAg clearance

- Decreased hepatic inflammatory response with lower ALT levels

- Higher levels of HBV DNA and rates of HBeAg positivity with the associated risks of HBV-associated liver disease and hepatocellular carcinoma (*JAMA* 2006; 295:65; *CID* 2003;37:1678; *Lancet* 2002;360;1921; *JAIDS* 1991; 416). This is the presumed explanation for the 19-fold increase in the risk of hepatic deaths associated with HIV co-infection in the MACS cohort (*Lancet* 2002;360:1921).

- Treatment of both infections is confounded by overlapping activities and risk of resistance with nucleosides including 3TC, FTC, TDF and ETV (entecavir).

LAB TESTING AND MONITORING

- **HBV screening:** HBsAg, HBsAb, HBcAb (see Table 7-4)
- **Neg HBSAb HBsAg:** Vaccinate
- **Baseline testing** (HBsAg pos):
  - HBV replication: HBeAg, HBeAb and HBV DNA (HBV DNA indicates active HBV infection)
  - Liver function: ALT, albumin, bilirubin, prothrombin time, CBC with platelet count
  - Assess co-infection: Anti-HCV and anti-HAV
- Note: HBsAb may disappear with reappearance of HBs especially with low CD4 counts. May need to repeat screening test with otherwise unexplained increase in LFTs.
- Isolated anti-HBe without HBSAg is unclear – screen for HBV DNA before vaccinating.

■ TABLE 7-4: **Diagnostic Tests for Hepatitis B**

Status	HBs Ag	HBs Ab	HBc Ab	HBe Ag	HBe Ab	Viral load
Incubation	+	−	−	+/−	−	Low
Acute HBV	+	−	+	+	−	High
Inactive	+	−	+	−	+	Low
Chronic	+	−	+	+/−	−	High/Low
Resolved	−	+	+	−	+	Negative
Vaccinated	−	+*	−	−	−	Negative
Occult	−	−	+	−	−	High/Low

* Ab titer >= 10 IU/L required for immunity

- **Monitoring in absence of HBV treatment:** LFTs every 6 mos incuding ALT, albumin, bilirubin, prothrombin time and CBC with platelet count. For hepatocellular carcinoma risk, some advocate AFP or ultrasound evaluations every 6 mos (*Hepatology* 2001;34: 1225), but the effectiveness of this strategy is unknown and the best screening method is not known; this monitoring is not recommended in the 2009 NIH/CDC/IDSA Guidelines for Prevention and Treatment of Opportunistic Infections in HIV-Infected Adults and Adolescents (www.mmhiv.com/link/2009-OI-NIH-CDC-IDSA).

TERMS (Tables 7-5 and 7-6)

- Chronic HBV infection: HBsAg positive 2x separated by 6 mo

- Inactive carrier state: HBsAg positive with negative HBeAg, low level plasma HBV DNA (<20,000 IU/mL) and normal ALT. Prognosis is good but there is risk of reactivation and hepatocellular carcinoma (*J Med Virol* 2005;77:173; *Semin. Liver Dis* 2005;25:143).

- HBeAg seroreversion: Indicates loss of HBeAg and development of HBeAb. This occurs spontaneously at about 10% per year in mono-infected patients; data for co-infected patients are not available but probably lower (*Ann Intern Med* 1981;94:744)

- Reactivation or HBV flare: This may occur spontaneously, with immunosuppression or with chemotherapy and is usually expressed with increased ALT. The differential includes drug-related hepatotoxicity and hepatitis co-infection (HAV, HCV or HDV), withdrawal of anti-HBV agents (3TC, FTC, TDF), HBV resistance to 3TC/FTC, or TDF etc), alcohol, etc. (*CID* 1999;28:1032; *JAMA* 2000;283:2526).

MANAGEMENT (Tables 7-5 to 7-9)

- **Negative screening tests:** Patients with negative HBsAg and anti-HBs should receive HBV vaccine (see pg. 75).There is controversy in

7 Systems Review

patients with anti HBc only, but some recommend HBV vaccine if no evidence of chronic infection (negative HBV DNA) (*JID* 2005;191:1435).

- **Patients with chronic HBV co-infection** should 1) be advised to avoid or limit alcohol consumption; 2) receive HAV vaccine, preferably when CD4 count is >200 cells/mm^3; 3) be evaluated for HBV treatment, 4) choose antiretroviral regimens for HIV based on anti-HBV activity of the nucleoside analog components (see below), 5) be counseled on the risks of HBV transmission, including the need for barrier protection of sexual partners and 6) be advised that contacts should be evaluated for HBV vaccine.

- **Treatment of HBV (Table 7-5):** Indications to treat HBV. <u>Goal of treatment</u>: Prevent progression of HBV-related morbidity and mortality. With HBeAg positive patients the goal of treatment is seroconversion of anti-HBe combined with undetectable HBV DNA. With HBeAg-negative patients with elevated HBV DNA the treatment is usually Indefinite or lifelong to achieve sustained viral suppression. <u>Indications</u>: (2009 NIH/CDC/IDSA Guidelines for Prevention and Treatment of Opportunistic Infections in HIV-Infected Adults and Adolescents www.mmhiv.com/link/2009-OI-NIH-CDC-IDSA).

1. HBeAg pos + HBV DNA >20,000 IU/mL and elevated ALT
2. HBeAg neg + HBV DNA >2,000 IU/mL and elevated ALT
3. Most experts recommend treatment of HBV in all patients with HIV co-infection plus detectable HBV DNA since this combination is associated with more rapid progression of HBV. This

■ TABLE 7-5: **Management of HBV with HIV Co-infection Based on 2008 NIH/CDC/IDSA Guidelines**

HIV/HBV Category	HBV Treatment
On ART	<u>3TC and FTC naïve</u> 3TC 300 mg/d or FTC 200 mg/d + TDF 300 mg/d <u>3TC or FTC-experienced + detectable HBV DNA</u> 1. Not on TDF: Add TDF to 3TC or FTC or 2. Adefovir 10 mg/d + 3TC or FTC or 3. Entecavir 1 mg/d if HIV <50 c/mL + HBV does not show YMDD mutation <u>Duration</u>: Indefinite
No ART; HBV treatment only	<u>HBeAg neg and HBV DNA >2000 c/mL</u> Adefovir 10 mg/d or Peg-IFN <u>HBeAg pos, ALT , HBV DNA >20,000 c/mL</u> Peg-IFN 2a 180 mg SQ/wk x 48 wks
ART without HBV treatment indications	TDF/FTC or TDF/3TC, but do not use TDF, FTC or 3TC without second active against HBV

Systems Review

recommendation is stronger if the ALT is elevated or if there is evidence of hepatic fibrosis or inflammation on biopsy.

- **Monitoring response:** ALT and HBV DNA level q3mos. Detectable HBV DNA at 6 mos usually indicates treatment failure and the need to modify therapy (*AIDS Rev* 2007;9:40).

■ TABLE 7-6: **Management of HIV/HBV Co-infection Based on Guidelines from NYS AIDS Institute** (www.mmhiv.com/link/NYSD-HIV-HBV)

Indications to Treat
HBV DNA level >2000 IU/mL
Consider treatment with detectable HBV DNA <2000 IU/mL and elevated ALT or fibrosis or inflammation.

Treatment
Treat HIV regardless of CD4 count with two drugs active against HBV

Caveats
Discontinuing treatment of HBV or HIV: Avoid; if necessary monitor ALT carefully
Change ART: Continue agents active against HBV
Drugs: Use TDF/FTC or TDF+3TC (usually TDF/FTC) unless contraindicated by renal insufficiency or fulminant hepatic disease
HBV treatment without ARV: PegIFN 2a 180 mg/wk x 48 weeks. Avoid monotherapy with 3TC, FTC, telbivudine, entecavir or adefovir
Cirrhosis: Risk of life threatening hepatitis with immune reconstitution and baseline CD4 <200/mm³. Consider adding adefovir, but this is controversial
Hepatocellular carcinoma: If risk is increased: Screen with alfafetoprotein (AFP) every 3-6 mos or image annually (CT, MRI, US); with cirrhosis image q6mos.

Monitoring	
Test	**Frequency**
HBeAg & HBeAb	Baseline and q3-6mos if HBeAg +
ALT	Every 3-6 months
HBV DNA	Serial measurements if <2000 IU/mL + HBeAg + ALT increased. Measure q3-6mos with therapy.
PT, INR, AST, Platelets	Baseline and q6mos
AFP	Baseline and q3-6mos with risk for HCC
Liver Biopsy	Patients who consider deferring HBV treatment and those with HIV/HBV/HCV

7 Systems Review

■ TABLE 7-7: **Indications for Treatment of HBV without HIV Treatment**

Source*	eAg†	Recommendation
AASLD	+	HBV DNA >20,000 IU/mL + ALT >2 x ULN
	–	HBV DNA 2,000 IU/mL + ALT >2 x ULN
AGA	+	HBV DNA >20,000 IU/mL + elevated ALT
	–	HBV DNA >2,000 IU/mL + elevated ALT
EASL	+	HBV DNA >2,000 IU/mL and/or elevated ALT + liver bx showing necroinflammation or fibrosis‡
	–	HBV DNA >2,000 IU/mL and/or elevated ALT + liver bx as above
DHHS	+	CD4 >350 + HBV DNA >20,000 IU/mL + ALT >2 x ULN
	–	CD4 >350 + HBV DNA >2,000 IU/mL + ALT > 2 x ULN

* AASLD = Am Asoc Study of Liver disease; AGA = Amer Gastroenterology ASSOC; EASL = European Assoc Study of Liver Disease; DDHS = Dept of Health and Services 2008

† eAg = eAntigen

‡ Non-invasive markers could also be used

■ TABLE 7-8: **Treatment of HBV with HIV Co-infection: Recommendations of the 2011 DHHS Guidelines and Thio (*Hepatology* 2009;49 Suppl 5: S 138)**

HIV and HBV Treatment
HIV treated concurrently
Preferred: TDF/FTC (standard dose) monitor HBV DNA levels q6-12mos to detect HBV resistance
Alternative: If TDF cannot be used
1. Entecavir (0.5-1.0 mg/d): can be added but only with complete HIV suppression since entecavir has low level activity against HIV with risk of 184V mutation (*AIDS* 2008;22:947; *NEJM* 2007;356:2614). If HBV strain is known to be resistant to 3TC, there is concern for the increased likelihood of entecavir resistance by HBV; increase entecavir dose to 1.0 mg/d and monitor HBV DNA levels q3mos.
2. Peginterferon alfa 2a (180 ug SC weekly): may be given for HBV since there is no issue with resistance.
3. Adefovir (10 mg/d): note that this has relatively poor activity vs. HBV (Lancet 2001;358:718; Antivir Ther 2008;13:895).
4. Telbivudine: resistance rates are 25% at 2 years with monotherapy, and there must be complete HIV suppression. This agent may have activity against HIV (*AIDS* 2009;23:546) although other reports did not confirm this (*AAC* 2010;54:2670; *Antivir Ther* 2009;14:869).
Alternatives if HBV is resistant to 3TC
1. TDF (preferred)
2. Adofovir, entecavir or telbivudine
HBV treatment only
Avoid 3TC, FTC, TDF, and entecavir in patients not receiving ART

■ TABLE 7-9: HBV/HIV Co-infection

Drug Dose	Activity vs. HIV	Activity vs. HBV	Comment
3TC 300 mg/d	+ +	+ +	YMDD mutants with HBV resistance emergence rate with monotherapy: 21% at 1 yr, 94% at 4 yrs (*AIDS* 2006;20:863; *CID* 2004:37:1678): Give with TDF
FTC 200 mg/d	+ +	+ +	Assumed to be nearly identical to 3TC except longer T½
TDF 300 mg/d	+ +	+ +	Good activity, especially when combined with 3TC or FTC vs. HBV (*NEJM* 2003:348:177)
Telbivudine 600 mg/d	–	+	Shares resistance mutation with 3TC. No HIV activity in vitro but limited clinical experience with co-infection. Cumulative resistance 34% at year 3 (Seto WK. *J Hepatol* 2010;PMID 2114718)
Peginterferon 5 MU/d or 10 MU 3x/wks 16-48 wks	+	+	No resistance issues. Only drug shown to cause HBsAg conversion (*J Gen Intern Med* 2011;26:326) – Disadvantage is toxicity and CD4 decrease with HIV
Entecavir 0.5-1.0 mg/d	+	+ +	Resistance requires 3 mutations: (AAC 2004:48:3498). Resistance more common with 3TC resistance – Weak HIV activity can lead to 184V mutation if HIV not fully suppressed (*NEJM* 2007;356:2614)
Adefovir	+ /–	+ +	Active against HIV but not at doses used. Resistant strains partially resistant to TDF and 3TC. Reduce this risk with concurrent 3TC (*Gastroenterology* 2007;133:1445); Inferior to entecavir for HBV (*Hepatology* 2011;54:91)

Hepatitis C

DIAGNOSIS: Test for HCV includes: 1) screen, usually with EIA for anti-HCV; 2) confirm positives with HCV RNA; 3) determine genotype if treatment is anticipated because this predicts response to therapy and 4) quantitative HCV RNA to monitor response to HCV treatment. If seronegative HCV is suspected based on elevated transaminases or risk factors, then a test for HCV RNA should be performed (*Clin Liver Dis* 2003;7:179). False-negative screening serology is most common with CD4 cell counts <100 cells/mm³. Unlike HIV, HCV viral load does not correlate with progression.

EPIDEMIOLOGY: A national survey for HCV prevalence in the US (NHANES) conducted in 1999-2002 (*Ann Intern Med* 2006; 144:705) showed a prevalence rate of 1.6%, or about 4 million, includ-ing 3.2 million with chronic HCV. The most recent survey showed a seroprevalence rate of 1.68% (*Clin Gastroenterol Hepatol* 2011;9:524). The greatest risk was among IDUs, who account for 54% of cases (*CID* 2005;40:951) and have a seroprevalence of 35% in the CIDUS III survey in the US in 2002-04 (*CID* 2008;46:1852). The rate correlates with years of drug use with an OR of 1.09 for each year after year 2.

Systems Review

7

Since 2004 there has been a substantial increase in HCV rates in MSM in Europe, Australia and the US (*Curr Infect Dis Rep* 2010;12:118; *AIDS* 2011;25:1083). The global prevalence is 3% with 170 million persons. About 15-30% of people with HIV are co-infected with HCV (*CID* 2001;33:562). Co-infection with HIV is common because both viruses are transmitted by the same mechanisms: contaminated blood, sex and perinatal transmission.(*J Hepatol* 2006;44:Suppl. S6; *AIDS* 2005;19: 969; *CID* 2007;44:1123). However, the rates of transmission in these categories are very different, as summarized below:

Transmission rates (in absence of treatment or prophylaxis)

	HIV	HCV
Needle stick injury	0.3%	3%
Discordant couples	13%/yr	3%/yr
Perinatal transmission	20-30%	2-5%

NATURAL HISTORY: Acute HCV infection occurs 2-12 wks after HCV transmission with ALT levels usually 10-20 x ULN at 2-8 wks, HCV-RNA at 1-2 wks and anti HCV at 6-8 wks (*Am J Gastroenterol* 2008;103:1283). About 20-30% develop symptoms, usually at 6-8 wks. Spontaneous resolution occurs in 20-40%; HCV-RNA detected ≥6 mos after infection is defined as chronic HCV.

With chronic HCV the natural history shows progression to cirrhosis in 5-25% in 20 years; after cirrhosis, the rate of progression to liver failure is 1-2%/year and to hepatocellular carcinoma 1-7%/year (*NEJM* 1995;332:1463; *NEJM* 1992;327:1906; *NEJM* 1999; 340:1228; *Gastroenterology* 1997;112:463). Co-infection with HIV in 15-30% of US patients with HIV (*Sex Trans Infect* 2004;80:326; *World J Gastroenterol* 2007;13:2436) is generally associated with lower rates of spontaneous clearance, higher HCV RNA levels and a 3-fold increase in rates of progression to cirrhosis, liver failure, and hepatocellular carcinoma (*CID* 2001;33:240; *Lancet* 1997;350:1425; *JID* 1996;174:690; *Blood* 1994;84:1020; *JID* 2000;181:844; *JAIDS* 1993;6: 602; *JID* 1999;179:1254; *CID* 2001;22:562; *JID* 2001;183: 1112); *CID* 2004;38:128). Other factors associated with more rapid progression of HCV are male sex, alcohol use >50 g/d, age >35 years, and low CD4 count (*Lancet* 1997;349:825; *CID* 2004;38:128). HCV has little or no effect on HIV-related disease progression or on HIV response to ART (*JAMA* 2002;288:199). Multiple studies have demonstrated a significant increase in mortality with HCV coinfection compared to HIV alone, but some of this effect is due to injection drug use, which is often present (*JAIDS* 2003;33:365). A Veterans Administration review found that the rate of cirrhosis with HCV/HIV co-infection was increased 10-fold compared to HCV monoinfection; the rate of hepatic cancer was increased 5-fold (*Arch Intern Med* 2004;164:2349). The rate of cirrhosis was increased 19-fold in the HAART era. However, multiple other reports suggest ART reduces the rate of hepatic fibrosis with HCV (*J Hepatol* 2006;44:47; *CID* 2006;42:262; *Antivir Ther* 2006;

11:839; *Lancet* 2003;362:1708). One report noted the 3-year survival with HCV/HIV and cirrhosis is relatively good (87%), but it is poor with hepatic decompensation (*AIDS* 2011;25:899). It does not appear that HCV alters the rate of HIV progression (*JAMA* 1998;280:544; *JAMA* 1998;279:35).

ART-ASSOCIATED HEPATOTOXICITY (WITH HEPATITIS C): See pg. 145-146. Antiretroviral agents are associated with increased risk of asymptomatic elevations of transaminase levels with HIV-HCV co-infection (*JAMA* 2000;283:74; *AIDS* 2000;14:2895; *JAIDS* 2001;27: 426). Nevertheless, one large cohort of co-infected patients found that that these changes were often self-limited even when the PI was continued, and there were no cases of irreversible liver failure (*JAMA* 2000;283:74). A retrospective review of 5272 patients with HIV including 48% with chronic HBV or HCV co-infection found that the frequency of transaminase elevations was the same with or without ART (*AIDS* 2007;21:599). There are no clear guidelines for modifying ART for antiretroviral therapy with co-infection, although a common recommendation is to discontinue these agents if patients are symptomatic or have transaminase levels over 5x ULN or over 3.5x baseline levels. Most patients with grade 3/4 toxicity are asymptomatic (*JID* 2002;186:23). In these cases there should be an investigation for other causes of liver disease (hepatitis A or B, OIs, alcohol or other hepatotoxic medications). Consider a change in antiretroviral agents if no reversible cause can be found. If the ALT level does not change or if it increases, consider liver biopsy and HCV treatment. If the ALT decreases, resume ART with a new drug regimen and monitor ALT closely. NVP is the only antiretroviral agent that is often considered to be contraindicated with baseline hepatic disease including HCV coinfection, but there is no evidence that the hepatic necrosis seen with this drug has any association with HCV (*Lancet* 2004;363:1253; *JAIDS* 2004;36:772). The rate of grade 3/4 adverse reactions for ALT/AST elevations for TPV/r in phase II/III clinical trials was 11.1%, but 85% were asymptomatic (*BMC Infect Dis* 2009;9:203). Use TPV/r with caution in patients with baseline hepatic disease.

MANAGEMENT: ART plays an unclear role in reducing the rate of progression of HCV, and HCV treatment plays an unclear role in reducing the rate of progression of HIV (2011 DHHS Guidelines for ART and the NIH/CDC/DSA Recommendations for the Prevention and Treatment of Opportunistic Infections in HIV-Infected Adults and Adolescents)

- All HCV/HIV co-infected patients should: 1) be advised to abstain from alcohol use or at least limit consumption to <20-50 gm alcohol/wk (2-5 drinks); 2) hepatotoxic drugs should be avoided including iron supplements in the absence of iron deficiency and acetaminophen in doses >2 gm/d; 3) they should be informed

7 Systems Review

about methods to prevent transmission of both infections (use condoms and avoid needle sharing); 4) they should receive vaccinations for HBV and HAV if susceptible; 5) they should be evaluated for HCV disease severity and treatment; 6) consider ART for all HCV infected patients with HIV regardless of CD4 count; and 7) consider evaluation for hepatocellular carcinoma by ultrasound or alphafetoprotein (AFP) every 6-12 mos.

■ **Evaluation**

□ Quantitative HCV RNA by RT-PCR or bDNA: This test does not predict prognosis but predicts response to treatment and is used to monitor therapy

□ Genotype analysis of HCV: This predicts response to therapy and dose of ribavirin

□ Hepatic transaminases: Note that ALT and AST values fluctuate and may be normal with advanced liver disease (*Gastroenterology* 2003;124:97)

□ CT scan or ultrasound to detect heptocellular carcinoma

□ Test to evaluate the fibrosis stage include liver biopsy, which is invasive but also the only FDA-approved staging method and considered the gold standard. The concern is sampling error. Other methods to stage liver disease include the *FibroScan*, which is new, not readily available and not FDA-approved for liver staging. The third method is laboratory test formulas, which are readily available, but variable in sensitivity and specificity (*Hepatology* 2006;41:175; *AIDS* 2003;17:721; *JAIDS* 2005; 40:538; *JAIDS* 2006;41:175; *J Clin Gastroenterol* 2008;42:827; *Liver Int* 2008;28:486; *Clin Chim Acta* 2007;381:119; *Intervirology* 2008;51 Suppl 1:11 and 27; *J Hepatol* 2008;48:835). One of the popular noninvasive liver fibrosis scoring formulas is the **FIB-4**, which predicts significant fibrosis based on age and three variables (AST, ALT and platelet count). This was used to calculate the Ishak fibrosis score based on correlates with liver biopsies in 832 patents. The derived formula based on this analysis: age (years) x AST (UI/L) x PLT (10^9/L) x ALT (IU/L). The corresponding scores were fibrosis class 1: <1.45; class 2: 1.46-3.25 and class 3: >3.25 (*Hepatology* 2006;43:1377). A second fibrosis scoring system is the **APRI index** based on the AST-to-platelet ratio: AST (with ULN 40 IU/L/platelet count (platelets x 10^9/L) x 100. The corresponding scores are APRI class 1 = <0.5, class 2 = 0.51-1.5. and class 3 = >1.5 (*JAIDS* 2005;40:538). An advantage to these systems is the ability to avoid liver biopsy in many cases (*CID* 2011;52:1164). \

■ **Indications to treat:** The goals of therapy are to eradicate HCV as indicated by a "Sustained Viral Response" (SVR), the elusive cure that cannot be achieved with HIV or HBV. The success of treatment (SVR rate) has historically been judged largely by the experience with genotype type 1, since this is the most refractory to therapy and the dominant genotype in the US, Europe and Japan. Initial studies with genotype infection using interferon for 6 mos yielded a cure rate of 5%; the addition of ribavirin and prolongation to 48 weeks increased the SVR to 25%. Pegylated interferon was associated with an SVR of 40% (*Lancet* 2001;359:958; *NEJM* 2002;347:975). The advent of multiple new agents (designated direct-acting antivirals, or DAAs) began in 2011 with testing and FDA approval of telapravir and bocepravir. These are orally-administered protease inhibitors, which, when combined with peginterferon/ribavirin, can achieve cure rates of 55-75% (*Lancet* 2010;376:705; *NEJM* 2009;360:1827). With these new treatment options there are several important caveats that impact decision making for the HCV/HIV co-infected patient:

- At the time of FDA approval (May, 2011) the only new agent with available data for HIV/HCV co-infection was telaprevir (TVR).

- It appears that peginterferon and ribavirin will still be required (*Lancet* 2010;376:705).

- The new PIs remind us of the initial PI-based regimens for HIV with extensive drug interactions, side effects, resistance and multiple daily doses.

- Patients receiving TVR requiring ART will need to be on ATV/r-, EFV- or RAL-based ART due to drug interactions or lack of data with other HIV agents.

- The new agents will be expensive, especially when adding in the cost of peg-IFN/ribavirin.

- The pipeline is extremely dense with multiple classes: interferon lamba, protease inhibitors, polymerase inhibitors, NS5A inhibitors and cyclophilin inhibitors. These agents are expected to reach the marketplace by 2013-14. Like the experience with ART, it is expected that treatment will be much easier and more effective at that time, so those patients who can wait should wait. Prioritization may be made on the basis of fibrosis score using liver biopsy and contraindications for peg-IFN (pg. 342) and ribavirin (pg. 360).

RECOMMENDATIONS FOR EVALUATION AND TREATMENT

- **Pre-therapy: General evaluation for use of peg-IFN/ribavirin**
  - Lab: CBC, ALT, AST, creatinine
  - Assess comorbidities: substance abuse, psychiatric disease, cardiopulmonary disease, renal disease
  - Evaluate HIV status: CD4 count, VL, active OIs
  - Evaluate HCV status: HCV genotype, HCV viral load, ALT
  - Consider liver biopsy or *FibroScan*; if contraindicated, unavailable, or refused, may elect to treat without biopsy. (Liver biopsy is most important when SVR is less likely, as with genotype 1.)

7 Systems Review

- □ Counsel patient on benefits and risks
- □ Consider modification of ART. Avoid ddI, which is contraindicated with ribavirin and AZT (exacerbates treatment-related anemia).

TELAPREVIR (preliminary recommendations made at the time of FDA approval and the 2011 CROI meeting) (see pg. 383): TVR is metabolized by CYP3A4 so AUC levels are significantly reduced by DRV/r, FPV/r, LPV/r ($\downarrow$35-54%) and to a lesser extent by ATV/r ($\downarrow$20%). There is also a reduction in TVR levels with concurrent EFV that can be offset with higher doses of TVR (1125 mg q8h). The favored concurrent ART regimens to give with telaprevir based on trial data are ATV/r, EFV and (presumably) RAL (Sulkowski M. 2011 CROI;Abstr. 147LB). Criteria for use and recommended regimens are summarized on pg. 386. Points to emphasize are that candidates for telaprevir therapy with HIV/HCV co-infection should have: 1) genotype 1 infection; 2) controlled HIV infection (VL <50 c/mL using ATV/r, EFV or RAL-based ART; 3) meet all the criteria for peg-IFN and RBV and 4) have compensated liver disease but sufficient disease to predict substantial consequences if treatment is delayed until there are additional anti-HCV options available by expanded access (2012) or FDA approval (2013).

MONITORING (PEG-IFN/RBV) See IFN (pg. 343), RBV (pg. 360)

- **Reinforce:** birth control now and for 6 mos after completion of treatment
- **Lab:**
  - □ <u>CBC, ALT</u> at wks 2 and 4, then at 4- to 8-wk intervals

    ANC <750 cells/mm^3 use G-CSF or reduce interferon

    ANC <500 cells/mm^3 discontinue interferon; consider G-CSF
  - □ <u>Hgb</u> <10 g/dL consider EPO or reduce ribavirin 200 mg/d

    <8 g/dL discontinue ribavirin; consider EPO
  - □ <u>HIV VL + CD4</u> count at 12-wk intervals
  - □ <u>Thyroid</u>: TSH at 3- to 6-mo intervals
- **Neuropsychiatry:** evaluate monthly; consider antidepressants (SSRI) ± consult
- **HCV:** quantitative HCV RNA at 12 wks. If positive or HCV decrease of <2 log$_{10}$ with genotype 1, most experts discontinue therapy probability of SVR is <3%). Repeat HCV RNA at 24 wks; if undetected, continue treatment to 48 wks; obtain an HCV RNA level.
- **Post-therapy:** HCV RNA PCR at 6 mos

LIVER TRANSPLANTATION WITH HIV INFECTION

United States (www.hivtransplant.com) accessed June 1, 2011

Source: HIV + Solid Organ Transplant: Multisite study; sponsors: University of California, San Francisco and NIH (21 sites)

Systems Review

Inclusion criteria:

- CD4 count >200/uL at any time during 16 weeks before transplant
- HIV VL: <50 c/mL (*Amplicor*) or <75 c/mL (*bDNA Versant*) within 16 weeks before transplant
- Meet standard listing criteria for placement on waiting list

Exclusion criteria:

- History of PML
- Chronic cryptosporidiosis >1 month
- Primary CNS lymphoma

Note: history of hepatocellular carcinoma is not an exclusion

Experience: (AIDS 2011;25:777): A review of 15 series with 686 HIV-infected patients followed a median of 42 mos showed: 1) survival at one year was 84.5% and at 5 years was 63%; 2) HIV viral suppression was 89% at 5 years and 3) recurrance of active HCV disease was noted in 95/184 (52%) with a median time to recurrence of two months.

Pancreatitis (*Am J Med* 1999;107:78)

INCIDENCE: A review of EuroSIDA data for 2001-06 found a pancreatitis rate of 1.3 cases/1000 person years (*AIDS* 2008;22:47). Another report from Kaiser Permanente Medical Care Program for 2001-06 found a rate that was 5-fold higher than the general population and noted no decline in rates from the pre-HAART era (*AIDS* 2008;22:145). The difference is possibly explained by a different definition with lipase >4x ULN in the Kaiser report vs. individual case reviews in the EuroSIDA report (*AIDS* 2008;22:997).

MAJOR CAUSES

- **Drugs**, especially ddI or ddI + d4T ± hydroxyurea. May be complication of lactic acidosis (NRTI-associated mitochondrial toxicity) or secondary to PI-associated hypertriglyceridemia with elevated triglyceride levels – usually >1000 mg/dL. **Less common drugs:** d4T, 3TC (pediatrics), LPV/r, RTV, INH, rifampin, TMP-SMX, pentamidine, corticosteroids, sulfonamides, erythromycin, paromomycin. A recent report from EuroSIDA found no association between cummulative exposure to ddI or d4T and risk of pancreatitis (*AIDS* 2008;22:47).

- **Opportunistic infections:** CMV. Less common: MAC, TB, cryptosporidium, toxoplasmosis, cryptococcus

- **Conditions that cause pancreatitis in general population**, especially alcoholism. Less common: Gallstones, hypertriglyceridemia (avg level is 4500 mg/dL), post ERCP (3-5% of procedures), trauma. **Note:** Despite association between hypertriglyceridemia and PIs, other medications appear to account for >90% of cases (*Pancreas* 2003;27:E1)

7 Systems Review

DIAGNOSIS

- **Amylase** >3x ULN; p-isoamylase is more specific but not usually measured (*Mayo Clin Proc* 1996;71:1138). Other causes of hyperamylasemia: other intra-abdominal conditions, diseases of salivary gland, tumors (lung and ovary) and renal failure.
- **Other tests**
  - Lipase: As sensitive as amylase but more specific. Need for amylase plus lipase is arbitrary.
  - CT Scan: Best method to image (*Radiology* 1994;193:297). Used to 1) exclude other serious intra-abdominal conditions, 2) stage pancreatitis, and 3) detect complications.

TREATMENT: Supportive – IV fluids, pain control, and NPO

PROGNOSIS: Best predictor of outcome is APACHE II score (*Am J Gastroenterol* 2003;98:1278)

HEMATOLOGIC COMPLICATIONS

GENERAL: Hematologic abnormalities include neutropenia, anemia and thrombocytopenia. These were major issues in HIV care in all areas of the world in the pre-HAART era but are now major concerns primarily in resource-limited settings. The ACTG PEARLS (Prospective Evaluation of Antiretrovirals in Resource-Limited Settings) has reviewed prevalence data for these complications among 1,571 ART-naïve patients in Brazil, Haiti, India, Malawi, South Africa, Thailand, Zimbabawe and the US from 2005 to 2007. Participants had CD4 counts <300 cells/mm^3 and no acute illness (*Internal J Infect Dis* 2010;14:e1088). The main findings:

- Neutropenia (ANC <1,300/mL): prevalence 4.3%; greatest in Africa, Haiti and US
- Anemia (Hgb ≤10 gm/dL): prevalence 11.9%; 50% macrocytic; highest rates in Africa and Haiti
- Thrombocytopenia (platelet count <120,000/mL): prevalence 7.2% with highest rates in India, Brazil, Malawi and US

Anemia

SYMPTOMS: Oxygen delivery becomes impaired with activity when the hemoglobin levels are <8-9 g/dL and becomes impaired at rest with hemoglobin levels <5 g/dL (*JAMA* 1998;279:217). Symptoms of chronic anemia include exertional dyspnea, fatigue, and a hyper-dynamic state (bounding pulses, palpitations, roaring in ears). Late complications include confusion, CHF, angina.

CAUSES

- **HIV and immune activation:** HIV infection of marrow progenitor cells

(*CID* 2000;30:504). Incidence correlates with immune state: 12% with CD4 count <200 cells/mm³, 37% with AIDS-defining OI (*Blood* 1998;91:301). Anemia predicts death independent of CD4 count and VL (*Semin Hematol Suppl* 4;6:18; *AIDS* 1999;13:943; *AIDS Rev* 2002;4:13; *JAIDS* 2004;37:1245; *Antir Ther* 2008;13:595; *HIV Med* 2010;11:143). More recent studies suggest the anemia, like hsCRP and IL-6, is an expression of immune activation.

◻ Findings: Normocytic, normochromic, low reticulocyte count, low erythropoeitin (EPO) level.

◻ Factors that correlate with anemia are: CD4 <200 cells/mm³, high VL, female sex, use of AZT, reduced BMI and black race (*CID* 2004; 38:1454; *JAIDS* 2004;37:1245) and biomarkers of immune activation.

◻ Treatment: ART. With immune reconstitution, prior reports show increases in Hgb of 1.0-2.0 gm/dL at 6 mos (*JAIDS* 2001;28:221; *AIDS* 1999;13:943), but results are inconsistent (*CID* 2000;30:504). Consider EPO (starting at 40,000 units/wk or 50-100 units/kg TIW) with symptomatic and refractory cases (see pg. 264). Note the average wholesale price (AWP) cost of EPO is about $550/wk. It should also be noted that this would not address the issue of immune activation.

- **Marrow-infiltrating infection or tumor** (lymphoma, especially non-cleaved cell type, or Kaposi's sarcoma, rare) or infection (MAC, tuberculosis, CMV, histoplasmosis). Findings include: normocytic, normochromic, low platelet count, evidence of etiologic mechanism.

- **Parvovirus B19:** Infects erythroid precursors; symptoms reflect marginal reserve (sickle cell disease, etc.) and inability to eradicate infection due to immune deficiency. More recent studies suggest that Parvovirus B19 is a very rare cause of anemia in patients with HIV Infection (*CID* 2010;50:115).

  ◻ Findings: Normocytic, normochromic anemia, without reticulocytes, positive IgG and IgM serology for parvovirus, positive serum dot blot hybridization or PCR for parvovirus B19. The diagnosis is most likely with severe anemia, i.e., hematocrit <24%, no reticulocytes and CD4 count <100 cells/mm³ (*JID* 1997;176:269).

  ◻ Treatment: May eradicate pathogen with ART (*CID* 2001;32: E122). Standard treatment with persistent parvovirus B19 and immunosuppression is IVIG 400 mg/kg/d x 5 days (*Ann Intern Med* 1990;113:926)

- **Nutritional deficiency:** Common in late stage HIV, including B12 deficiency in 20% of AIDS patients (*Eur J Haematol* 1987;38:141) and folate deficiency due to folic acid malabsorption (*J Intern Med* 1991;230:227).

  ◻ Findings: Megaloblastic anemia (MCV >100 not ascribed to AZT or

7 Systems Review

521

d4T) ± hypersegmented polymorphonuclear cells, low reticulocyte count with serum B12 (cobalamin) level <125-200 pg/mL (*Semin Hematol* 1999;36:75) or a serum folate level <2-4 ng/mL (<2 ng/mL is more definitive). Note: A single hospital meal may significantly increase the serum folate level.

- □ Treatment: Folate deficiency – folic acid 1-5 mg qd x 1-4 mos. B12 deficiency – cobalamin 1 g IM qd x 7 days, then every week x 4, then every month or 1-2 g po qd (*Blood* 1998;92:1191).

- **Iron deficiency:** Usually indicates blood loss, especially from GI tract.

  - □ Findings: Most studies to detect iron deficiency show the likely cause is anemia of chronic disease with decreased Fe (<60 µg/dL), low transferrin (<300 µg/dL), and normal or increased ferritin. Ferritin level <40 ng/mL suggests iron deficiency and a level <15 ng/mL is 99% sensitive for this diagnosis but only 50% specific (*J Gen Intern Med* 1992;7:145).

  - □ Treatment: Identify and treat source of loss + ferrous sulfate 325 mg tid.

- **Drug-induced marrow suppression ± red cell aplasia:** Most common with AZT; less common with AZT, ganciclovir, valganiciclovir, sulfonamides, dapsone, antineoplastic drugs, amphotericin, ribavirin, pyrimethamine, interferon, TMP-SMX, phenytoin (also seen with HIV *per se*, parvovirus B19, and non-Hodgkin's lymphoma).

  - □ Findings: Normocytic, normochromic anemia (macrocytic with AZT or d4T), low or normal reticulocyte count.

  - □ Treatment: Discontinue implicated agent ± EPO (see pg. 263).

- **Drug-induced hemolytic anemia:** Most common with dapsone, primaquine, and ribavirin. Hemolytic anemia is also seen with TTP. The risk with dapsone and primaquine is dose-related and most common with G6PD deficiency. See pg. 61.

  - □ Findings: Reticulocytosis, increased LDH, increased indirect bilirubin, methemoglobinemia, and reduced haptoglobin. The combination of a haptoglobin <25 mg/dL + elevated LDH is 90% specific and 92% sensitive for hemolytic anemia (*JAMA* 1980; 243:1909). The peripheral smear may show spherocytes and fragmented RBCs. Note: Coombs test is commonly positive.

  - □ Treatment: Consists of oxygen, transfusion, and discontinuation of implicated drug. Severe cases in absence of G6PD deficiency are treated with IV methylene blue (I mg/kg) (*JAIDS* 1996;12:477). Activated charcoal may be given to reduce dapsone levels (see pg. 221).

DIAGNOSTIC EVALATION

- **Laboratory tests:** MCV, peripheral smear, reticulocyte count, bilirubin (total and direct), iron studies (ferritin, iron, transferrin, TIBC), stool hemocult, consider bone marrow biopsy.
- **Suggested algorithm AETC** (www.mmhiv.com/link/AETC-anemia)

  Reticulocyte >2%
  - □ Indirect bilirubin high
    1. Autoimmune Coombs – positive
    2. Oxidant drugs and G6PD deficiency
    3. Fragmented RBC's and low platelets: DIC
  - □ Indirect bilirubin normal
    1. Acute blood loss
    2. Replacement of iron, folate or B12

  Reticulocyte count <2%
  - □ Indirect bilirubin high: B12 or folate deficiency
  - □ Indirect bilirubin normal or low
    1. MCV low: chronic blood loss
    2. MCV normal: anemia of chronic disease, drug induced, HIV, marrow infiltrate disease
    3. MCV high: AZT, chemotherapy, d4T, ganciclovir, other drugs.

Idiopathic Thrombocytopenia Purpura (ITP)

DEFINITION: Unexplained platelet count <100,000/mL

CAUSES

- **Most cases** are ascribed to HIV infection of multi-lineage hematopoietic progenitor cells in the marrow (*CID* 2000;30:504; *NEJM* 1992;327:1779). A case of immune reconstitution TTP has been reported (*AIDS* 2007,21.2559).
- **Drug induced:** Review of 561 reports showed the best supporting data for a causal role for drugs in patients without HIV infection were for heparin, quinidine, gold, and TMP-SMX (*Ann Intern Med* 1998;129:886). Others with "level 1 evidence" that are used in HIV-infected patients: rifampin, amphotericin, vancomycin, ethambutol, sulfisoxazole, and lithium. It appears that HIV-infection increases the risk of heparin-induced thrombocytopenia (*CID* 2007; 45:1393).

TREATMENT (*CID* 1995;21:415; *NEJM* 1999;341:1239) (Table 7-10, pg. 524)

- **ART:** Two reports showed that with viral suppression and CD4 count rebound, median platelet count increase was 18,000/mL and 45,000/mL at 3 mos (*CID* 2000;30:504; *NEJM* 1999;341:1239). One report noted an inverse relationship between the platelet count and HIV VL (*AIDS Res Human Retroviruses* 2007;23:256).

7 Systems Review

Clinical Status	Treatment
Asymptomatic	■ HAART ■ Discontinue implicated drug and monitor response.
Persistent symptomatic or required for procedure	■ Above ■ Prednisone 30-60 mg/day with rapid taper to 5-10 mg/day. Risk of OI. Only 10% to 20% have sustained response. ■ IVIG 400 mg/kg days 1, 2 and 14, then every 2 to 4 weeks. Raises platelet count within 4 days; median peak response time is 3 weeks. Very expensive. ■ Rho(D) immune globulin (*WinRho*) 25-50 μg/kg over 3 to 5 minutes in Rh(+) patients, repeat day 3 to 4 prn, then at 3 to 4 week intervals as needed. Similar to IVIG but rapid infusion and less expensive (10% cost of IVIG). Hemolysis may occur peaking at day 6; response at 1-3 days, peaks at day 8. ■ Splenectomy: experience is variable; some good (*Arch Surg* 1989;124:625), some bad (*Lancet* 1987;2:342).
Hemorrhage	Packed red cells/platelet transfusions plus prednisone 60-100 mg/day or IVIG 1 g/kg days I, 2, and 14.

* Frequency in HIV-infected patients with Kaposi's sarcoma at any anatomical site.

■ **Drug-induced:** Median time to recovery with discontinuation of the implicated agent is 7 days (*Ann Intern Med* 1998;129:886).

■ **Standard treatments of ITP** (prednisone, IVIG, splenectomy, etc.): Response rates are 40-90%; the main problem is durability (*CID* 1995;21:415).

Neutropenia

DEFINITION: Absolute neutrophil count <750/mm³ (Some use thresholds of 500/mm³ or 1000/mm³)

CAUSE: Usually due to HIV *per se* or to drugs such as AZT, ganciclovir, valganciclovir, foscarnet, ribivirin, flucytosine, pyrimethamine, TMP-SMX, interferon and cancer chemotherapy.

SYMPTOMS: Reported risk of bacterial infections is variable, but the largest review shows an increase in hospitalization with an ANC <500 /mm³ (*Arch Intern Med* 1997;157:1825). Other reviews show that few HIV-infected patients have excessive neutropenia-associated infections (*CID* 2001;32:469).

TREATMENT

■ **HIV-associated:** ART – ANC increase with immune reconstitution is variable (*CID* 2000;30:504; *JAIDS* 2001;28:221). Severe and persistent neutropenia may respond to G-CSF or GM-CSF (see pg. 291).

■ **Drug-associated:** Most common causes are AZT, ganciclovir, or valganciclovir; other causes include flucytosine, amphotericin, sulfonamides, pyrimethamine, pentamidine, antineoplastic drugs, and interferon. Treatment is to discontinue the implicated drug and/or give G-CSF or GM-CSF (see pg. 291).

- **G-CSF or GM-CSF:** See pg. 291. Usual initial dose is 150-300 mcg qd or 3x/wk. Dose can be titrated to lowest dose necessary to maintain ANC >1000/mm^3. (*NEJM* 1987;371:593). Monitor CBC during cytokine treatment 2x/wk.

Thrombotic Thrombocytopenia Purpura (TTP)

DEFINITION: Thrombotic microangiopathy, hemolytic uremic syndrome (HUS), and TTP represent syndromes characterized by hemolytic anemia, thrombocytopenia, and renal failure, often with fever and neurologic changes (*CID* 2006;42:1488).

CAUSE: Platelet thrombi in selected organs

FREQUENCY: Unclear, may be early or late in course (*Ann Intern Med* 1988;109:194)

LAB DIAGNOSIS: 1) anemia; 2) thrombocytopenia (platelet count 5,000-120,000/mL); 3) peripheral smear shows fragmented RBCs (schistocytes, helmet cells) ± nucleated cells; 4) increased creatinine; 5) evidence of hemolysis: increased reticulocytes, indirect bilirubin, and LDH and low haptoglobin; and 6) normal coagulation parameters

TREATMENT: The usual course is progressive with irreversible renal failure and death. Standard treatment is plasma exchange until platelet count is normal and LDH is normal (*NEJM* 1991;325:393). An average of 7-16 exchanges are required to induce remission. With poor response, add prednisone 60 mg qd; other interventions include IVIG, antiplatelet drugs, vincristine, and splenectomy. A review of 24 cases found prompt initiation of ART and plasma exchange ± steroids led to prompt remission. Rituximab was used in some refractory cases (*Brit J Haematol* 2011;153:515).

IMMUNE RECONSTITUTION INFLAMMATORY SYNDROME (IRIS)

DEFINITION: A practical definition is a paradoxical worsening of a preexisting infection or the presentation of a previously undiagnosed condition in HIV-infected patients soon after commencement of ART (French. *CID* 2009;48:101). Most cases occur in the first few weeks or months of ART. Paradoxical IRIS applies to patients with a known infection who improve with pathogen-specific treatment but deteriorate with ART. In this case, the pathogens may not be cultivable at the time of IRIS. Unmasking IRIS refers to the detection of a previously unknown pathogen that can be cultured and usually shows a prominent clinical expression that accompanies immune recovery (*Curr Opin HIV AIDS* 2010;5:504).

"Official definitions"

- **M.A. French:** (*AIDS* 2004:18:1615) Must have major criteria A and B, or major A criteria and any two minor criteria.
  - □ **Major criteria**

    A. Atypical presentation of opportunistic infection or tumors in patients responding to ART

    - □ Localized disease (e.g., severe fever or painful lesion)
    - □ Exaggerated inflammatory response (e.g., severe fever or painful lesions)
    - □ Atypical inflammatory response (e.g., necrosis, granulomas, suppuration, or perivascular lymphocytic inflammatory cell infiltrate)
    - □ Progression or organ dysfunction or enlargement of preexisting lesion after definite clinical improvement with pathogen-specific therapy prior to ART and exclusion of treatment toxicity and new diagnoses

    B. Decrease in VL >1 $\log_{10}$ copies/mL
  - □ **Minor criteria**
    - □ Increased CD4 cell count
    - □ Increase in an immune response specific to the relevant pathogen (e.g., DTH response to mycobacterial antigens)
    - □ Spontaneous resolution of disease without specific antimicrobial therapy or tumor chemotherapy with continuation of ART

- **Robertson, et al.** (*CID* 2006;42:1639)
  - □ New onset or worsening symptoms of an infection or inflammatory condition after start of ART
  - □ Symptoms not explained by:
    - □ Newly acquired infection
    - □ Predicted course of previously diagnosed infection
    - □ Adverse effects of drug therapy
  - □ Decrease in VL >1 $\log_{10}$ copies/mL

PATHOGENESIS AND RATES: The presumed mechanism is severe CD4 lymphopenia and a dysregulated immune response in terms of qualitative and quantitative recovery of pathogen-specific cellular and humoral responses to multiple opportunistic pathogens including primarily mycobacteria, fungi and viruses: *M. tuberculosis*, MAC, CMV, EBV, HBV, HCV and *C. albicans* (*Science* 1997;277:112; *CID* 2000;30:882; *AIDS* 2002;616:2129; *JID* 2002;185:1813; *Drugs* 2008;68:191; *Curr Opin HIV AIDS* 2009;22:651; *Clin Microbiol Rev* 2009;22:651). IRIS may target viable or dead microbial pathogens, host

Systems Review

antigens (with autoimmune disease) or tumor antigens. The most frequently reported cases of IRIS are with tuberculosis, disseminated MAC and cryptococcal meningitis. One retrospective review found rates of 30-34% for each of these three conditions (*AIDS* 2005;19: 399). Others report rates of 10-23% (*CID* 2006;42:418; *HIV Med* 2005;6:140; *AIDS* 2006;20:2390; *CID* 2009;49:1424). The rate in the US in ACTG 5164 was 7.6%, but that may be deceptively low since PCP was the most common OI, and steroid treatment may have reduced rates in that subset (*PLoS One* 2009;4:e5575).

CLINICAL FEATURES: Nearly any pathogen can cause IRIS, but the most common are mycobacteria (TB and MAC) and fungi (especially *Cryptococcus*) The interval from ART to IRIS is 60% within 60 days with a reported range of 3-658 days (*Curr Opinion Infact Dis* 2006; 19:20). Risk factors with OI pathogens include: CD4 count <50-100 cells/mm^3 at initiation of ART, high VL at baseline, rapid fall in HIV VL, treatment-naïve at time of OI treatment and short interval between ART and OI treatment (*AIDS* 2005;19:399, *CID* 2006;42:418; *HIV Med* 2000;1:107; *AIDS Res Ther* 2007; 4:9). There are two patterns: 1) ART given at the time of OI treatment with IRIS complicating the response to treatment with paradoxical worsening of a treated OI, and 2) ART given to a clinically stable patient with new expression of a dormant and previously unrecognized condition ("unmasked IRIS"). The differential diagnosis usually includes: 1) paradoxical worsening of a treated OI, 2) initial expression of a previously unrecognized complication of HIV, 3) therapeutic failure of a treated OI or 4) adverse drug reaction.

PRINCIPLES FOR PREVENTION AND TREATMENT: Prevention refers to methods of managing opportunistic infections that are likely to cause IRIS when treating both the OI and HIV.

■ **When to start ART:** The 2011 DHHS guidelines identify three scenarios for initiating ART in HIV treatment-naïve patients who present with an OI:

1) The complication has no specific therapy: ART should be given immediately. Examples are cryptosporidiosis, microsporidiosis, HIV-associated dementia and PML.

2) The complication has specific therapy and is known to have IRIS as a common feature, and a brief delay in ART is appropriate. Examples are disseminated MAC, PCP and cryptococcal meningitis. There is no consensus on what "brief" means. ACTG 5164 randomized 282 patients in this category to "immediate ART" (within 14 days) or "deferred ART" (>28 days). Results favored "immediate treatment" in terms of rates of death/AIDS progression (14% vs. 24%; p=NS). There were no significant differences in grade 3 or 4 adverse events, adherence, hospitalizations or risk of IRIS (*PLoS One* 2009;4:e5575). The median delay of ART in the "immediate" group was 12 days. On the basis

of these data the recommendation is to initiate ART rapidly with a delay of no more than 2 weeks when immediate therapy risks IRIS, polypharmacy and adverse reactions and drug interactions.

3) Tuberculosis: The recommendations for this co-infection are separate because of the complexity of the issue due to the high incidence of IRIS , the high risk of death with low CD4 counts and the consequences of treatment with 7 drugs that have overlapping toxicities and complex interactions (with rifampin). However, as above, the greatest concern here is delayed ART in patients with late stage HIV (CD4 <50 cells/mm^3) resulting in early mortality, which is usually attributed to delayed ART and rarely to IRIS TB (*JAIDS* 2007;44:229). ACTG 5221 (STRIDE) found that immediate ART (within 2 wks of TB treatment) was associated with a better survival rate in patients with CD4 counts <50 cells/mm^3 compared to starting ART at 8-12 wks, when the baseline CD4 count was <50 cells/mm^3, although the rate of IRIS was higher (Havlir. 2011 CROI:Abstr. 38). See pg. 464-465 for specific recommendations.

- **Treatment of IRIS** usually consists of continued drugs for the OI and HIV with use of NSAIDS and/or corticosteroids for symptomatic treatment of IRIS. There are no controlled trials of NSAIDs or steroids, but anecdotal reports show benefit. NSAIDS are obviously preferred, but systemic symptoms that are severe or cases with large inflammatory masses usually require steroids using prednisone 1-2 mg/kg/d for 1-2 wks followed by tapering based on symptoms. Most patients show improvement within 3 days (*Thorax* 2004;59:704; *CID* 2005;41:1483). In some cases it is necessary to give prolonged courses, surgically resect masses, or drain abscesses, or even stop treatment of HIV and/or OI due to life-threatening IRIS.

SPECIFIC IRIS FORMS:

- **TB IRIS:** The frequency is strongly correlated with the interval between initiation of ART after treating TB, but the risk of death is far greater if ART is delayed in patients with late stage HIV with CD4 counts <50 cells/mm^3 (*JAIDS* 2007;44:229). The most common presentations include fever, adenopathy, worsening pulmonary infiltrates and/or pleural effusions (*Lancet Infect Dis* 2005;5:361). Extrapulmonary expression includes expanding CNS lesions, meningitis, cord lesions and cervical adenopathy. Most cases occur within 8 weeks of initiating ART; extrapulmonary TB often occurs later – often 5-10 mos later (*CID* 1998;26:1008; *CID* 1994;19: 793). The recommended course of corticosteroids is variable, but often reported at 20-80 mg qd for 5-12 wks (*AIDS Res Ther* 2007;4:9). See pg. 470.

- **MAC:** The most common presentation is pulmonary disease or lymphadentis with abscess formation (*Lancet* 1998;351:252; *Lancet*

Pathogen/Condition	Clincal expression
Infectious Diseases	
Aspergillosis (pg. 421)	Pulmonary disease with mucous impaction (case report)
Bartonellosis (pg. 423)	Lymphagangitis, splenic inflammation
Chlamydia trachomatis	Reiter syndrome
Herpes simplex (pg. 447)	Erosive lesions
Histoplasmosis (pg. 451)	Pulmonary disease; adenitis; skin lesions
HHV-8 (pg. 532)	Worsening of Kaposi sarcoma; Castleman disease
Human papillomavirus	Warts
JC virus (pg. 455)	Inflammatory PML with enhancement or MRI
Leishmaniasis	Increased skin disease, visceral disease, uveitis
Molluscum contagiosum	Increased skin lesions
M. tuberculosis (pg. 462)	Fever, lymphadenopathy (abdominal, mediastinal, cervical), pneumonitis, pleural effusions, lung abscesses, expanding CNS lesions
Mycobacteria – other	
BCG	Skin abscess; adenitis
M. leprae	Skin ulcerations; neuritis
M. xenopi	Pneumonia
M. genavense	Adenitis
M. scrofulaceum	Adenitis, parotitis
M. kansasii	Pneumonia
P. jiroveci (pg. 477)	Progressive pneumonia; ARDS; granulomatous pneumonia
Parvovirus B19	Encephalitis
Strongyloides stercoralis	Disseminated disease
Toxoplasmosis (pg. 486)	Encephalitis
Non-infectious Diseases	
Autoimmune disorder	Hyperthyroidism; SLE, rheumatoid arthritis, Graves disease
Malignancy (pg. 530)	Kaposi sarcoma with inflammatory skin and mucosal lesions, pneumonitis, adenopathy Non-Hodgkins lymphoma – relapse
Miscellaneous	Guillain Barré syndrome, tattoo ink inflammatory response, interstitial lymphoid pneumonitis and sarcoidosis; parotid gland enlargement

7 Systems Review

Inf Dis 2005;5:361). This usually occurs at 1-3 wks after initiation of ART but can be up to 84 days (*JAIDS* 1999;20:122). Large abscesses may require excision, drainage or needle aspiration; post-operative healing is often poor (*CID* 2004; 38:461). Other presentations include pneumonitis, osteomyelitis or septic arthritis. See pg. 461-462.

- **CMV:** IRIS after CMV retinitis with vitritis is reported in 18-63% of cases (*HIV Med* 2000;1:107; *JID* 1999;179:697; *Ophthalmology* 2006;113:684). This can occur rapidly and cause blindness. The usual therapy is intra-ocular cortiscosteroids (*Retina* 2003;23:495; *Br J Ophth* 1999;83:540). See pg. 446.

- **Cryptococcal meningitis:** *C. neoformans* IRIS meningitis is not dissimilar from AIDS-related *C. neoformans* meningitis (*CID* 2005; 40:1049). The most common presentation is worsening meningitis symptoms (*CID* 2005;40:1049). Other presentations include adenitis and mediastinitis (*J Infect* 2002;45:173). Treatment of the IRIS meningitis form includes anti-cryptococcal agents, LPs to control intracranial pressure and systemic corticosteroids (*Int J STD AIDS* 2002;13:724). See pg. 437-438.

- **Hepatitis B or C:** Elevated transaminase is usually mild but can cause liver decompensation with cirrhosis.

- **PML:** New or worsening CNS disease (*J Neurovirol* 2005;11 Suppl 2:16; *CID* 2002;35:1250). See pg. 456.

- **Miscellaneous forms:** See Table 7-11, pg. 529.

MALIGNANCIES

HIV infection is a well-established risk factor for several tumors designated AIDS-defining cancers. Compared to the general population the rate with HIV infection is magnified 3,640-fold for Kaposi's sarcoma (HHV-8) 77-fold for non-Hodgkin's lymphoma (EBV) and 8-fold for cervical cancer (HPV). These tumors are caused by the designated viruses and presumably reflect risk associated with immune surveillance (*J Nat Cancer Instit* 2011;103:753). The availability of HAART and the increasing age of patients living with HIV infection have been associated with a dramatic decrease in the frequency of AIDS-defining cancers and total cancers (Table 7-12), although non-AIDS-defining malignancies now account for about 10% of deaths in all patients with HIV infection, and some cancers (anal, liver, lung, breast, prostate, Hodgkin disease) are increasing without explanation in this population (*AIDS* 2010;24:1537).

The data in Table 7-12 are based on the HIV/AIDS Cancer Match Study, which links 15 HIV and cancer registries in the US. The conclusion is that the increase in non-AIDS associated malignancies was driven primarily by aging in the HIV population. There may be some contamination in the separation of microbe-mediated vs. no microbe since Hodgkin's lymphoma, anal cancer and hepatoma are usually

■ TABLE 7-12: **Estimated Cancers in Persons with AIDS in the US in the pre-HAART Era and the post-HAART Era***

Cancer	1991-95	2001-05
AIDS-defining		
Kaposi's sarcoma	21,483	3,827[†]
Non-Hodgkin's lymphoma	12,778	5,968[†]
Cervical cancer	327	530
Total	34,587	10,325[†]
Non-AIDS-defining		
Oral	181	503[†]
Colon	108	438[†]
Anal	206	1,564[†]
Liver	116	583[†]
Lung	875	1,882[†]
Breast	36	337[†]
Prostate	87	759[†]
Hodgkin's lymphoma	426	897[†]
Total	3,193	10,059[†]
Total Cancers	38,922	20,821[†]

* Adapted from *J Nat Cancer Instit* 2010;103:753
† p <0.001

microbial-mediated. Similar results were reported from Germany (*Eur J Med Res* 2011;16:101). An unexplained enigma is the 2- to 3- fold increased rate of lung cancer even when adjusted for smoking (*CID* 2007;45:203; *JAIDS* 2010;55:510)

Cancer prevention strategies include:

- ART:(reduces KS and non-Hodgkin's lymphoma
- Smoking cessation. see Table 7-28, pg. 567
- Safe sex and IDU rehabilitation to prevent oncogenic viruses: HBV, HCV, HPV and HHV8; condoms shown to reduce HPV transmission (only)
- HCV and HBV therapy
- HPV vaccination (*Lancet* 2011;377:2085)
- Cancer screening at age >50 yrs: colonoscopy; repeat every 5-10 yrs; fecal occult blood annually
- Females >40-50 yrs: mammogram yearly; MRI if high risk
- Males >50 yrs: rectal exam and PSA screening (benefit is unclear)
- Anal Pap smear: MSM, but no clear guidelines form authoritative sources (see pg. 55)

7 Systems Review

- Cervical Pap smear (see pg. 55)

- Cirrhosis: semi-annual alpha-fetoprotein (AFP) or ultrasound, but unclear cost-effectiveness

In terms of prognosis, outcome is largely dictated by the tumor type and response to standard intervention, but there are also data showing that low CD4 count and high VL (>400 c/mL) strongly influenced outcome (*AIDS* 2011;25:691). The highest morality rates in this series of 650 ART recipients with cancer showed two-year mortality rates of 91% for CNS lymphoma, 84% for hepatic carcinoma and 68% for lung cancer.

RISK: A review of AIDS and cancer registries for 1981-96 involving 8,828 AIDS patients >60 years of age found the following relative risks compared to controls without AIDS: Kaposi's sarcoma, 545; NHL, 24.6; Hodgkin's lymphoma, 13.1; anal cancer, 8.2; leukemia, 2.4; and lung cancer, 1.9. There was no significant difference for cervical cancer (*JAIDS* 2004;36:861). A review of data from MACS found 75% decrease in the rate of AIDS diagnosing cancers (ADC) with ART (*JAIDS* 2008;48:485). The strong relationship between CD4 count and ADC was shown in the multicenter US Military Study (Crum-Cianflone NF. 5th IAS;Abstr. WEPEB250). A review of the Moore Clinic database found that ART was associated with a decrease in AIDS-associated malignancies, but also found an increase in other cancers, especially lung and liver (*AIDS* 2008;22:489). This increase of other types of cancers has been reported by others (*Ann Intern Med* 2008;148:728). Review of the Dutch ATHENA data with 11,459 patients showed 232 non-AIDS cancers, primarily lung (44), anal (37), Hodgkin's lymphoma and laryngeal (20).

Anal cancer: See pg. 55-57.

Kaposi's Sarcoma

CAUSE: HHV-8. Mechanism of infection is thought to be by HHV-8 in saliva (*JAIDS* 2006;42:420; *Sex Transm Infect* 2006;82:229; *Nat Rev Cancer* 2010;10:707)).

FREQUENCY: Rate is up to 3,640-fold higher with HIV compared with general population and 300-fold higher than other immunosuppressed patients (*Lancet* 1990;335:123; *J Natl Cancer Inst* 2002;94:1204). The incidence is 10-20x higher in MSM, but is increased >200-fold in women as well (*JAIDS* 2004;36:978). The postulated mechanism is upregulation of cytokines that regulate angiogenesis and lymphangiogenesis by HIV (*Lancet* 2004;364:740). The rate has decreased about 5- to 6-fold in the HAART era (*JAMA* 2002;287:221; *J Nat Cancer Instit* 2010;103:753; *JAMA* 2011;305:1450).

Systems Review

PRESENTATION: Firm purple to brown-black macules, patches, nodules, papules that are usually asymptomatic – neither pruritic nor painful, and usually on legs, face, oral cavity, and genitalia. Complications include lymphedema (especially legs, face, and genitalia) and visceral involvement (especially mouth, GI tract, and lungs). ART reduces the frequency of KS (*JAIDS* 2003;33:614), and when it develops during antiretroviral therapy the course is less aggressive (*Cancer* 2003;98: 2440).

DIFFERENTIAL: Bacillary angiomatosis (biopsy with silver stain to show organisms); hematoma, nevus, hemangioma, B-cell lymphoma, and pyogenic granuloma. Biopsy should be performed on at least one lesion to confirm the diagnosis; this is especially important with rapidly growing lesions.

PROGNOSIS: CD4 count plus tumor burden staging (ACTG – *J Clin Oncol* 1989;7:201). TIS: Extent of Tumor (T), Immune status (I), Severity of systemic illness (S). TIS predicts survival (*J Clin Oncol* 1997; 15:385). Good prognosis – lesions confined to skin, CD4 count >150 cells/mm^3, no "B" symptoms.

DIAGNOSIS (NYS AIDS Institute Guidelines)

- **Skin and oral cavity:** Inspection plus biopsy of one typical lesion
- **Lung:** Suspect with cutaneous lesion plus unexplained dyspnea, wheezing or hemoptysis. Evaluation: X-ray or CT scan shows bilateral perihilar/lower zone reticulonodular infiltrates. These are

■ TABLE 7-13: **Frequency, Presentation, and Diagnosis of Kaposi's Sarcoma**

Site	Frequency*	Presentation	Diagnosis
Skin	>95%	Purple or black-brown nodular skin or oral lesions ± edema	Appearance and biopsy
Oral	30%	Usually palate or gums	Appearance and biopsy (skin biopsy preferred)
GI	40%	Pain, bleeding, or obstruction ■ Most are asymptomatic ■ Most have skin lesions ■ May occur at any level	Endoscopy to see hemorrhagic nodule; biopsy is often negative (*Gastroenterology* 1988;89: 102). Assume diagnosis if skin biopsy is positive
Lung	20-50%	Dyspnea, cough, wheezing, and/or hemoptysis. may cause parenchymal or endobronchial lesions or pleural effusion. Pleural effusion: serosanguinous, cytology negative. X-ray: infiltrates diffuse or nodular.	CT scan and bronchoscopy. Endobronchial TB – red raised lesions – biopsy often negative.

7 Systems Review

often flame-shaped (*Ann Thorac Med* 2010;5:201). Diagnosis: Bronchoscopy to detect typical red raised or flat lesions, usually at bronchial branch points. Diagnosis is established by inspection; biopsy is unnecessary and may cause bleeding.

- **GI:** Suspect with cutaneous lesion plus unexplained GI symptoms. usually pain, bleeding or obstruction. Diagnosis: Upper and lower endoscopy to detect typical raised, red mucosal lesion.

TREATMENT

- **ART:** Associated with lesion regression, decreased incidence, and prolonged survival (*J Clin Oncol* 2001;19:3848; *J Med Virol* 1999;57:140; *AIDS* 1997;11:261; *Mayo Clin Proc* 1998;73:439; *AIDS* 2000;14:987).

- **Antiviral therapy:** Foscarnet, cidofovir, and ganciclovir are active against HHV-8 (*J Clin Invest* 1997;99:2082), but these drugs do not appear to cause tumor regression (*JAIDS* 1999;20:34)

- **Chemotherapy:** Vinblastine injections, topical cisretinoic acid gel (*Panretin* gel), liquid nitrogen, radiation (low dose), cryosurgery, or laser therapy.

- **Systemic therapy:**

  □ Indications: 1) Pulmonary KS; 2) visceral KS; 3) extensive cutaneous lesions (arbitrarily >25 skin lesion); 4) rapidly progressive cutaneous KS; or 5) KS associated lymphedema.

  □ Systemic treatment: 1) Optimize ART management and OI prophylaxis first; 2) Agents: liposomal anthracyclines: liposomal doxorubicin (*Doxil*) or liposomal daunorubicine (*DaunoXome*); paclitaxel (*Taxol*)

RESPONSE: Kaposi's sarcoma cannot be cured; goals of therapy are to reduce symptoms and prevent progression. ART is associated with reduced tumor burden. Antiviral drugs directed against HHV-8 have no established benefit (*JAIDS* 1999;20:34).

- **Local therapy:** Local injections of vinblastine cause reduced lesion size but not elimination in most patients (*Cancer* 1993;71:1722).

- **Systemic therapy:** Liposomal anthracyclines usually show good results with few side effects. Paclitaxel is as effective but more toxic due to neutropenia and thrombocytopenia; side effects are dose related; lower doses appear as effective with less marrow suppression. See pg. 232-234.

- **Immune reconstitution KS:** In a review of 150 treatment-naïve patients with KS who started ART, 10 (6.6%) developed progressive KS (*J Clin Oncol* 2005;23:5224). Clinical presentation consists of worsening KS with lymphadenopathy, more skin lesions, skin lesions that are more violaceous and associated with more edema (*CID* 2004; 39:1852).

HIV-associated lymphomas

Most are B cell lymphomas. Histologic types include B cell diffuse large cell lymphoma, primary effusion lymphoma, primary B cell CNS lymphoma, Burkitt's lymphoma, and Hodgkin's disease. In an analysis of 6,788 NHL cases, 96 (1.4%) were T-cell lymphomas; the relative risk in AIDS patients vs the general population was 15. T-cell lymphomas include mycosis fungoides, peripheral lymphomas, cutaneous lymphomas, and adult T cell lymphoma (*JAIDS* 2001;26:371). Most HIV-associated lymphomas increase in frequency with declining CD4 counts. Hodgkin's lymphoma is an exception, which presumably explains the increasing rate of Hodgkin's disease during the HAART era (*Blood* 2006;108:3788; *J Natl Cancer Instit* 2011;103:753). A review of 187 HIV-associated cases of Hodkin's disease found strong correlations with low CD4 count (50-100 cells/mm³) and onset within 1-3 mos after starting ART, suggesting a form of immune reconstitution (*Blood* 2011;178:44; *AIDS* 2011;25:1395).

Non-Hodgkin's Lymphoma (NHL)

CAUSE: Immunosuppression (CD4 count <100 cells/mm³) and EBV (50-80%)

FREQUENCY AND TYPE: NHL is 200-600 times more common among HIV-infected patients compared with the general population (*Int J Cancer* 1997;73:645; *JAIDS* 2004;36:978). The rate is about 3% for patients with AIDS (*JAIDS* 2002;29:418). Most (70-90%) are high-grade diffuse large cell or Burkitt-like lymphomas (*Am J Med* 2001; *Brit J Haematol* 2001;112:863). The incidence of NHL has decreased substantially during the HAART era (*CID* 2009;48:633). A review of cancer and HIV registries in the US showed the number of NHL cases decreased from 12,778 in 1991-95 to 5,968 in 2001-05 (*J Natl Cancer Instit* 2011;103:753). A recent review of 61 cases of NHL in AIDS patients in France showed the median age at diagnosis of NHL was 40 years. The median CD4 count was 237 and the major independent risks were time below a CD4 count of 350 cells/mm³ and VL >500 c/mL (Bruyand M. 5th IAS 2009;Abstr. WEPEB243; *CID* 2009;49:1109).

PRESENTATION: Compared with NHL in the general population, HIV-infected patients have high rates of stage IV disease with "B" symptoms and sparse node involvement. Common sites of infection and forms of clinical presentation are fever of unknown origin, hepatic dysfunction, marrow involvement, lung disease (effusions, multi-nodular infiltrates, consolidation, mass lesions, or local or diffuse interstitial infiltrates, hilar adenopathy), GI involvement (any level – pain and weight loss), and CNS (aseptic meningitis, cranial nerve palsies, CNS mass lesions).

DIAGNOSIS: Lymph nodes that are >2 cm or progressively enlarging should be biopsied. Imaging of nodes is recommended for unexplained

7 Systems Review

constitutional symptoms such as fever, weight loss or night sweats ≥ 2 wks. Biopsy new, enlarged (>2 cm) or enlarging nodes. The diagnostic yield of fine-needle aspiration (FNA) in patients with HIV infection and adenopathy is reported at 65-75% (*Internat J STD AIDS* 2008;19:553; *ACTA Cytol* 2001;45:589; *Acta Cytol* 2000;44;960). The major differential diagnosis is PGL; malignancies account for 10-20%.

EVALUATION: 1) blood tests: CBC, liver function tests, creatinine, calcium, phosphorus, LDH; 2) marrow aspiration and biopsy; 3) contrast enhanced brain MRI; 4) LP for cells, protein and EBV RNA test. PET/CT scans are commonly used to help diagnose lymphomas, localize the tumor and evaluate response to chemotherapy (*Cancer* 2005;104:1066), but there is still a need to confirm the diagnosis with biopsy and a considerable clinical skill for interpreting disseminated disease as well as response to treatment (*Transfus Apher Sci* 2011;44:167).

TREATMENT

- **ART:** Patients receiving ART should continue it during chemotherapy. Use caution with discontinuation of NNRTI-based ART because of the long half-life of EFV and NVP (see pg. 117-118). AZT should be avoided during chemotherapy.

- **OI Prophylaxis:** Should be based on CD4 count. If >400 cells/mm³ use prophylaxis dictated by immunosuppression of the chemotherapy regimen.

- **Chemotherapy:** Full dose if possible.

  □ **CHOP** (Cyclophosphamide, doxorubicin vincristine and prednisone) (*J Clin Oncol* 2001;19:2171; *Cancer* 2001;91:155) or

  □ **CDE** (Cyclophosphamide, doxorubicin and etoposide (*J Clin Oncol* 2004;22:1491)

  □ **Rituximab** may improve tumor response but may risk infectious death with CD4 <50 cells/mm³ (*Blood* 2005;105:1891; *Br J Haematol* 2008;140:411; *Cancer* 2008;113;117)

- **CNS prophylaxis:** Predicted by CSF EBV DNA (*J Clin Oncol* 2000;18: 3325)

- **Peripheral stem cell transplant** in HIV infection with lymphomas is feasible in the HAART era; about 100 cases have been reported with complete remission in 48-90% (*Cell Transplant* 2011;20:351).

RESPONSE: Initial response to chemotherapy rates are 50-60%, but relapse rates are high and the long-term prognosis is poor with median survival <1 year. With relapse in patients with HIV clinical stability, consider investigational chemotherapy with stem cell support (*Blood* 2001; 98:3857). The usual cause of death is progressive lymphoma or progressive HIV with OIs (*Semin Oncol* 1998;25:492). The prognosis is significantly better with ART; one report showed an 84% 1 year survival with ART + chemotherapy (*AIDS* 2001;15:1483). The prognosis with lymphoma plus HIV infection in the HAART era is significantly worse than for lymphoma alone. A review of 259 HIV infected and 8,230 HIV uninfected incident NHL patients showed a 2-year mortality rate of 59% for the HIV-infected group compared to 30% in the HIV-uninfected group. Poor prognostic correlates were CD4 count <200 cells/mm^3, prior AIDS-defining diagnosis or Burkitt's subtype (*AIDS* 2010;24:1765). Nevertheless, one report found that patients who achieve complete remission with chemotherapy had a 3-year survival (74%) that was comparable to that of HIV-negative patients with NHL (*CID* 2004;38:142). Another report found that ART is associated with reduced chemotherapy-related toxicity as well as improved survival (*J Clin Oncol* 2004;22:1491).

Burkitt's lymphoma

Standard therapy used in patients without HIV

Plasmablastic lymphoma

Use standard regimens (No successful regimens known)

Hodgkin's disease

Classical Hodgkin's lymphoma is associated with immunosuppression and includes three categories: HIV-associated; iatrogenic (chronic corticosteroids, etc.); and post-transplant. All forms are treated with ABVD – adriamycin, bleomycin, vinblastine and dacarbazine (*Am J Hematol* 2011;86:170). Use of ART has enabled more aggressive treatment, including high-dose chemotherapy and stem cell rescue for patients who fail initial therapy (Spina M. *Adv Hematol* 2011;PMCID PMC2948898).

Primary CNS Lymphoma (PCNSL): See pg. 551.

Primary Effusion Lymphoma (PEL)

CAUSE: HHV-8 and EBV (*NEJM* 1995;332:1186; *Clin Microbiol Rev* 2002;15:439; *CID* 2008;47:1209)

FREQUENCY: Rare: tumor registries crossed with AIDS registries show a frequency of 0.004% or 0.14% of non-Hodgkin's lymphoma in patients with AIDS (*JAIDS* 2002;29:418)

PRESENTATION: Serous effusions (pleural, peritoneal, pericardial, joint spaces) with no masses (*Hum Pathol* 1997;28:801). Development of solid tissue lymphomas is rare (*Acta Hematol* 2010;123:237).

DIAGNOSIS: Effusions are serous, contain high-grade malignant lymphocytes and HHV-8

7 Systems Review

TREATMENT

- **ART** plus rituximab, corticosteroids and cyclophosphphamide (*Acta Haemtol* 2010;123:237).

- **Alternatives:** Pegylated liposomal doxorubicin or liposomal daunorubicin. Recent reports have shown benefit, even complete regression, of Castleman's disease with rituximab and/or thalidomide (*AIDS* 2008;22:1232; *Am J Hematol* 2004;73:176; *Am J Hematol* 2008;22: 498).

RESPONSE: This tumor usually does not extend beyond serosal surfaces, but prognosis is poor, with median survival of 2-6 mos (*JAIDS* 1996;13:215; *J Clin Oncol* 2003;21:3948; *AIDS* 2008;22:1685; *AM J Hematol* 2008;83:804). Most patients show temporary response to therapy with decrease in effusion size. The CD4 count is the most important predictor of progression (*CID* 2005;40:1022). A case report showed complete regression of PEL with ART *(AIDS* 2008;22:1236).

NEUROLOGIC COMPLICATIONS:
Peripheral nervous system

HIV-Associated Neuromuscular Weakness Syndrome (HANWS)

CAUSE: Postulated to be caused by mitochondrial toxicity attributed to deoxy NRTIs, primarily d4T (*NEJM* 2002;346:811; *CID* 2003; 15:131; *AIDS* 2004;18:1403).

CLINICAL FEATURES: A review of 19 probable cases showed a median lactic acid level of 4.9 mmol/L; 88% had taken d4T for a median duration of 10.5 months (*AIDS* 2004;18:1403). The only treatment is d4T withdrawal. Pathology studies and EMG showed involvement of peripheral nerves, muscles or both. Clinical features include ascending paresis, areflexia and cranial neuropathies. CPK levels are often elevated. The diagnosis is based on the finding of new onset limb weakness ± sensory involvement that is acute (1-2 wks) or subacute (>2 wks) involving legs or legs and arms and the absence of alternative confounding illnesses: Guillain-Barré syndrome, myasthenia gravis, myelopathy, hypokalemia, stroke. This complication has nearly disappeared due to concerns about d4T, although it is occasionally seen in some resource-limited countries (*J Med Assoc Thai* 2011;94:501).

Cytomegalovirus radiculitis: See pg.445.

Inflammatory Demyelinating Polyneuropathy

CAUSE: Unclear; immunopathogenic mechanism with inflammation and breakdown of peripheral nerve myelin is suspected.

FREQUENCY: Uncommon

DIAGNOSIS: There are two forms: acute demyelinating neuropathy (AIDP, Guillain-Barré Syndrome), which occurs early in the course of HIV, and a more chronic relapsing motor weakness, CIDP, which usually occurs in late-stage HIV. Both present with a progressive ascending paralysis with mild sensory involvement. CSF shows increased protein and mononuclear pleocytosis; EMG and nerve conduction studies are critical for diagnosis. Nerve biopsy may be needed; should show mononuclear, macrophage infiltrate, and internodal demyelination (*Ann Neurol* 1987;21:3240).

TREATMENT

- **AIDP:** Plasmapheresis: five exchanges with maintenance as needed; or, as alternative, IVIG 0.4 g/kg/d x 5 days (monitor renal function).

- **CIDP:** Oral prednisone (1 mg/kg/d) or intermittent plasmapheresis or IVIG; each continued until there is a therapeutic response.

RESPONSE: Treatment usually halts progression; CIDP may require prolonged courses (*Ann Neurol* 1987;21:3240).

Peripheral Neuropathy and Sensory Peripheral Neuropathy

Peripheral neuropathy is defined as loss of vibratory sensation of both great toes or absent/hypoactive ankle reflexes bilaterally. This form is asymptomatic and detect by neurologic exam. Sensory peripheral neuropathy (SPN) includes two forms: HIV-associated distal sensory polyneuropathy (HIV-DSP) and ART toxic neuropathy (ATN). These sensory neuropathies resemble the neuropathies that occur with diabetes and alcoholism. The diagnosis is based on the history of numbness, paresthesias or burning pain in the feet; exam shows reduced or absent ankle jerks.

A review of 2,141 patients in ACTG trials from 2000-2007 showed the frequency of the peripheral neuropathy was 32%, and for SPN it was 8.6% (*AIDS* 2011;25:919). Drugs implicated in ATN are ddI and the thymidine analogues, primarily d4T. These are rarely used now except in resource-limited countries (*Neurology* 1988;38:794; *Neurology* 2006;66:1679). The major findings of the ACTG review were:

- The prevalence of asymptomatic PN was 22.6% and 4.3% for symptomatic PN.

- The findings persist regardless of HIV treatment and treatment response in terms of viral suppression and immune recovery.

- The frequency of symptomatic PN increased with increasing age, baseline CD4 <200 cells/mm^3, high baseline VL, history of diabetes and use of a statin (*Neurology* 2002;58:1333).

- Patients who stopped receiving neurotoxic ART drugs showed 54% had these symptoms persist, and 18% cleared these symptoms.

Syndrome	Symptoms	Clinical Features	Ancillary Studies/ Treatment
Distal sensory neuropathy (DSN)	■ Pain and numbness in toes and feet; ankles, calves, and fingers involved in more advanced cases ■ CD4 cell count <200/mm³, but can occur at higher CD4 level	■ Reduced pinprick/vibratory sensation ■ Reduced or absent ankle jerks ■ Contact allodynia (hypersensitivity) present in most cases	■ Skin biopsy shows epidermal denervation ■ Electromyography/ nerve conduction velocities (EMG/NCV) show a predominantly axonal neuropathy ■ Quantitative sensory testing or thermal thresholds may be helpful
Antiretroviral toxic neuropathy (ATN)	■ Same as DSN (above), but symptoms occur after initiation of ddl, d4T. ■ Any CD4 cell count. ■ More common in older patients and patients with diabetes	■ Same as DSN (above)	■ EMG/NCVs show a predominantly axonal neuropathy ■ Discontinuation of presumed neuro-toxic medication if severe ■ Symptoms may worsen for a few weeks (coasting) before improving
Tarsal tunnel syndrome	■ Pain and numbness predominantly in anterior portion of soles of feet	■ Reduced sensation over soles of feet ■ Positive Tinel's sign at tarsal tunnel	■ Infiltration of local anesthetic in tarsal tunnel may provide symptomatic relief
HIV-associated neuromuscular weakness syndrome	■ Ascending paresis with areflexia ± cranial nerve or sensory involvement ■ Usually associated with prolonged d4T use	■ Lactate and CPK levels usually ↑ ■ EMG/nerve conduction studies – axonal neuropathy and myopathy	■ Discontinue NRTIs, especially d4T ■ Prognosis for survival is poor
HIV-associated myopathy/AZT myopathy	■ Pain and aching in muscles, usually in thighs and shoulders. ■ Weakness with difficulty when rising from a chair or reaching above shoulders ■ Any CD4 cell count	■ Mild/moderate muscle tenderness ■ Weakness, predominantly in proximal muscles (i.e., deltoids, hip flexors) ■ Normal sensory exam/normal reflexes	■ CPK ↑ ■ EMG shows irritable myopathy ■ Discontinue AZT and follow CPK every 2 weeks. Symptoms/signs/ CPK should improve within 1 month

continued on next page

Systems Review

Syndrome	Symptoms	Clinical Features	Ancillary Studies/ Treatment
Polyradiculitis	■ Rapidly evolving weakness and numbness in legs (both proximally and distally), with bowel/bladder incontinence ■ May occur at high or low CD4 cell count	■ Diffuse weakness in legs ■ Diffuse sensory abnormalities in legs and buttocks ■ Reduced/absent reflexes at knees and ankles	■ EMG/NCV show multilevel nerve root involvement ■ Spinal fluid helpful in determining CMV or HSV as cause ■ Treat CMV polyradiculopathy with ganciclovir or foscarnet
Vacuolar myelopathy	■ Stiffness and weakness in legs with leg numbness. ■ Bowel/bladder incontinence in advanced cases ■ CD4 count <200 cells/mm^3	■ Weakness and spasticity, mainly in hip, knee, and ankle flexors ■ Brisk knee jerks, upgoing toes ■ If sensory neuropathy coexists, then distal sensory loss and reduced/ absent jerks	■ Spinal fluid may show elevated protein 0-10 cells/mm^3 ■ Exclude B-12 deficiency and HTLV-1 co-infection ■ Thoracic spinal imaging normal ■ No established therapy, but physical therapy or methionine (3 g bid) and ART may be helpful (*Neurology* 1998;51:266)
Inflammatory demyelinating polyneuropathies	■ Predominantly weakness in arms and legs, with minor sensory symptoms. ■ CD4 count: may occur at any level	■ Diffuse weakness including facial musculature, asymmetric in early cases, with diffuse absent reflexes ■ Minor sensory signs	■ EMG/NCVs show a demyelinating polyneuropathy ■ Spinal fluid shows a very high protein with mild to moderate lymphocytic pleocytosis, but all cultures are negative ■ Treatment: Plasmapheresis. IVIG and/or ART
Mononeuritis or mononeuritis multiplex	■ Mix of motor and sensory defects ■ Asymmetric ■ Evolves over weeks ■ CD4 count is variable	■ EMG and nerve conduction – asymmetric and multifocal defects ■ R/O CMV (CSF or sural nerve biopsy) and HCV	■ CD4 count >200 cells/mm^3 – possible steroids ■ CD4 counts <50 cells/mm^3 and severe – treat for CMV

7 Systems Review

Distal sensory peripheral neuropathy (DSPN) and antiretroviral toxic neuropathy (ATN) (*AIDS* 2002;16:2105).

CAUSE: HIV infection *per se*, usually with CD4 count <200 cells/mm³ and/or dideoxy NRTIs: ddI and d4T, (*AIDS* 2000;14:273). DSN and ATN are indistinguishable by clinical features or biopsy.

TREATMENT

- **Contributing drugs and conditions to address:** ddI, d4T, metronidazole (long term), B6 overdose, INH (but incidence only 0.07%) (*AIDS* 2010;24 Suppl 5:S29), elevated triglycerides (*AIDS* 2009;23:2317; *AIDS* 2011;25:F1), vincristine, thalidomide, B12 deficiency, alcoholism, diabetes and uremia). Hepatitis C does not appear to play a role here (*Neurology* 2009;73:309).

- **Literature review:** A review through 2010 of controlled clinical trials of pharmacologic agents used to treat painful HIV-associated sensory neuropathy concluded efficacy vs. placebo for smoked cannabis, topical capsaicin (8%) and recombinant nerve growth factor. (Note that the latter is not available and smoked cannabis cannot be generally recommended (*PLoS One* 2010;5:e14433).

- **Pharmacologic treatment:**

  □ Gabapentin (*Neurontin*) 300-1200 mg PO tid. One placebo-controlled trial showed modest benefit (*J Neurol* 2004;251:1260).

  □ Lamotrigine (*Lamictal*) 25 mg bid increasing to 300 mg/d over 6 wks; one of the few treatments with confirmed benefit in clinical trials (*Neurology* 2000;54:2115) but results are inconsistent and there is a high incidence of rash. Longer trial confirmed efficacy but only in patients who were receiving neurotoxic ARTs (*Neurology* 2003;60:1508-14). Another study, a placebo-controlled trial in 220 patients using lamotrigine doses of 200, 300, or 400 mg/d vs placebo added to gabapentin, a tricyclic antidepressant or a nonopoid analgesic, showed no benefit for lamotragine (but was well tolerated) (*J Pain Symptom Manage* 2007;34:446). A Cochrane Library analysis reviewed 11 controlled trials with 2,622 participants and concluded there was no evidence of benefit at doses of 200-400 mg/d and 10% developed a rash (*Cochrane Database Syst Rev* 2011;2:CD006044).

  □ Tricyclic antidepressants nortriptyline 10 mg hs increased by 10 mg q5d to maximum 75 mg hs or 10-20 mg po tid; other tricyclics (amitriptyline, desipramine, or imipramine) are considered comparable. One trial failed to show response to tricyclics (*JAMA* 1998;280:1590). A more recent review showed limited pain improvement with antidepressants (*Pain* 2010;150:575). A high-concentration patch (8%) has been tested with a 30- or 60-min application repeated every 90 days effectively reduced neuropathic pain for up to one-year (*Drugs* 2010;70:1831).

- Ibuprofen: 600-800 mg tid
- Gabapentin (400 mg bid to ceiling 3600 mg/d) ± nortriptiline (10 mg bid to ceiling target of 100 mg/d (*Lancet* 2009;374:1252). Participants had diabetic or post herpetic neuraligia. At maximum tolerated doses, both drugs showed significant reductions in pain scores, but optimal results with the combination with both.
- Capsaicin-containing ointments (*Zostrix,* etc.): often not well tolerated. A high-concentration patch (8%) has been tested with a 30- or 60-min application repeated every 90 days effectively reduced pain for up to one year (*Drugs* 2010;70:1831)
- Lidocaine 20-30% ointment (lidocaine gel) was not effective in a controlled trial (*JAIDS* 2004;37:1584))
- Phenytoin 200-400 mg qd
- Marijuana: a placebo-controlled trial in 50 patients found that smoked marijuana, 3 cigarettes/d, was associated with a significant reduction in pain (*Neurology* 2007; 68:515). A review of use of medicinal marijuana showed therapeutic benefit but major barriers to treatment access (*J Opioid Manag* 2009;5:257).
- Severe pain: methadone – up to 20 mg qid; fentanyl patch 25-100 mcg/hour q72h or morphine (note: drug interactions between fentanyl and protease inhibitors).
- Acupuncture failed in one reported trial (*JAMA* 1998;280;1590).
- Miscellaneous: avoid tight footwear, limit walking, bridge at foot of the bed, use foot soaks.

RESPONSE: Sensory neuropathy due to NRTIs is usually reversible if the implicated agent is discontinued early, e.g., within 2 wks of the onset of symptoms. If continued, the pain eventually becomes irreversible and may be incapacitating. Response with drug discontinuation is often delayed for several weeks and then shows gradual improvement that may require up to 12 wks after discontinuing nucleosides (*JAIDS* 1992;5:60; *Neurology* 1996;46:999). Treatment of sensory neuropathy, beyond discontinuing implicated medications and addressing contributing conditions, is medication directed at pain control. Placebo-controlled trials have shown benefit with gabapentin, nortriptyline, topical capsaicin, cannabis and lamotrigine.

Central Nervous System: See Table 7-15.

Cytomegalovirus Encephalitis: See pg. 446.
CAUSE: CMV + CD4 count <50 cells/mm^3
FREQUENCY: <0.5% of AIDS patients
PRESENTATION: Rapidly progressive delirium, cranial nerve deficits, nystagmus, ataxia, headache with fever ± CMV retinitis

DIAGNOSIS: MRI shows periventricular confluent lesions with enhancement. CMV PCR in CSF is >80% sensitive and 90% specific; and cultures of CSF for CMV are usually negative.

TREATMENT: Ganciclovir (pg. 288), foscarnet (pg. 286), or both IV.

RESPONSE: Trial of foscarnet plus ganciclovir showed a median survival of 94 days compared with 42 days in historic controls (*AIDS* 2000;14:517).

HIV-associated neurocognitive defects (HAND)

HISTORIC CONTEXT: The impact of HIV infection on cognitive function was recognized early in the epidemic which was profound and led to the term "AIDS dementia complex" (ADC) in 1986. In 1991 the American Academy of Neurology proposed two categories: 1) HIV-associated dementia; and 2) a milder form with minor cognitive or motor impairment (*Neurology* 1991;41:778). More recently there was an alternative classification with three categories: 1) asymptomatic neurocognitive impairment (ANI); 2) HIV-associated mild neuro-cognitive disorder (MND); and HIV-associated dementia (HAD) (*Neurology* 2007;69:1789). Specific criteria for the 2007 definition are:

- HIV-associated asymptomatic neurocognitive impairment (ANI):
  - □ 1) acquired impairment in cognitive function that is >1 SD below a demographically corrected mean using neuropsychological testing that assesses seven cognitive areas; 2) cognitive loss does not impair daily function and 3) no evidence of delirium or dementia or preexisting cause.

- HIV-associated mild neurocognitive disorder (MND):
  - □ 1) acquired impairment of cognition, 2) cognitive impairment causes at least mild interference of mental acuity and inefficiency in work, homemaking or social observation and 3) no evidence of delirium or dementia.

- HIV-associated dementia (HAD):
  - □ 1) acquired cognitive impairment of at least 2.0 SD below demographically-corrected mean, 2) cognitive impairment causes substantial interference with work, homemaking or social functioning.

This classification with three levels of HIV-related neurocognitive impairment is referred to as the "Frascati Criteria" (*Neurology* 2007;69:1789) and has been used by CHARTER to evaluate 1551 HIV-infected persons from six US HIV programs. This included comprehensive neuropsychological testing, review of other relevant issues and CSF exam (*Neurology* 2010;75:2087). Results with 1,316 who did not have severe comorbidities showed 53% were considered normal, 38% had ANI, 12% had MND and 2.4% had HAD. This indicates a substantial decrease in the 10-15% prevalence of HAD in

■ TABLE 7-15: **Central Nervous System Conditions in Patients with HIV Infection**

Agent/Condition Frequency (All AIDS Patients)	Clinical Features	CT Scan/MRI	Cerebrospinal Fluid (CSF*)	Other Diagnostic Tests
Toxoplasmosis (2-4%) (pg 486)	■ Fever, reduced alertness, headache,focal neurological deficits (80%), seizures (30%) ■ Evolution: <2 wks ■ CD4 count <100 cells/mm³	■ Location: Basal ganglia, gray-white junction ■ Sites: Usually multiple ■ Enhancement: prominent; Usually ring lesions (1-2 cm) ■ Edema/mass effect: Usually not as great as lymphoma	■ Normal: 20-30% ■ Protein: 10-50 mg/dL ■ WBC: 0-40 (monos) ■ Experimental: Toxo Ag (ELISA) or PCR	■ *Toxoplasma* serology (IgG) false-negative in <5% ■ Response to empiric therapy: >85%; most respond by day 7 (*NEJM* 1993;329:995) ■ MRI: Repeat at 2 wks ■ Definitive diagnosis: Brain biopsy
Primary CNS Lymphoma (2%) (pg 551)	■ Afebrile, headache, focal neurological findings; mental status change (60%), personality or behavioral; seizures (15%) ■ Evolution: 2-8 wks ■ CD4 count <100 cells/mm³	■ Location: Periventricular, anywhere, 2-6 cm ■ Sites: One or many ■ Enhancement: Prominent; usually solid, irregular ■ Edema/mass effect: Prominent	■ Normal: 30-50% ■ Protein: 10-150 mg/dL ■ WBC: 0-100 (monos) ■ EBV PCR pos in 50-80%	■ Suspect with negative *Toxoplasma*. IgG, single lesion, or failure to respond to empiric toxoplasmosis treatment (MRI and clinical evaluation at 2 wks) ■ Thallium 201 SPECT scan (90% sensitive and specific)
Cryptococcal meningitis (8-10%) (pg 433)	■ Fever, headache, alert (75%); less common are visual changes, stiff neck, cranial nerve deficits, seizures (10%); no focal neurologic deficits ■ Evolution: <2 weeks ■ CD4 count <100 cells/mm³	■ Usually normal or shows increased intracranial pressure ■ Enhancement: Negative or meningeal enhancement ■ Edema mass effect: Ventricular enlargement/ obstructive hydrocephalus	■ Protein: 30-150 mg/dL ■ WBC: 0-100 (monos) ■ Culture positive: 95-100% ■ India ink pos: 60-80% ■ Cryptococcal Ag: >95% sensitive and specific	■ Cryptococcal antigen in serum – sensitivity 95% ■ Definitive diagnosis: CSF antigen sensitivity and specificity >99% and/or positive culture

continued on next page

545

7 Systems Review

Agent/Condition Frequency (All AIDS Patients)	Clinical Features	CT Scan/MRI	Cerebrospinal Fluid (CSF*)	Other Diagnostic Tests
CMV (>0.5%) (pg 441)	■ Fever ±, delirium, lethargy, disorientation; headache; stiff neck, photophobia, cranial nerve deficits; no focal neurologic deficits ■ Evolution: <2 wks ■ CD4 <100 cells/mm³	■ Location: Periventricular, brainstem ■ Site: Confluent ■ Enhancement: Variable, prominent to none.	■ CSF may be normal ■ Protein: 100-1000 mg/dL ■ WBC: 10-1000 (polys)/mL ■ Glucose usually decreased ■ CMV PCR positive >80% ■ CSF cultures usually negative for CMV	■ Definitive diagnosis: Brain biopsy with histopathology and/or positive culture ■ Hyponatremia (reflects CMV adrenalitis) ■ Retinal exam for CMV retinitis
HIV Dementia (7%) (pg 544)	■ Afebrile; triad of cognitive, motor, and behavioral dysfunction. ■ Early: Decreased memory, concentration, attention, coordination; ataxia ■ Late: Global dementia, paraplegia, mutism ■ Evolution: Weeks to months ■ CD4 <200 cells/mm³	■ Location: Diffuse, deep white matter hyperintensities ■ Site: Diffuse, ill-defined ■ Enhancement: Negative ■ Atrophy: Prominent ■ No mass effect	■ Normal: 30-50% ■ Protein: Increased in 60% ■ WBC: Increased in 5-10% (monos) ■ Beta-2 micro-globulin elevated (>3 mg/L)	■ Neuropsycho-logical tests show subcortical dementia ■ HIV dementia scale for screening (see pg. 549)
Neurosyphilis (0.5%) (pg 488)	■ Asymptomatic meningeal: headache, fever, photo-phobia, meningismus ± seizures, focal findings, cranial nerve palsies ■ Tabes dorsalis: Sharp pains, paresthesias, decreased DTRs, loss of pupil response	■ Aseptic meningitis: May show meningeal enhancement ■ General paresis: Cortical atrophy, sometimes with infarcts ■ Meningo-vascular syphilis: strokes	■ Protein: 45-200 mg/dL ■ WBC: 5-100 (monos) ■ VDRL positive: Sensitivity 65%, specificity 100% positive ■ Experimental: PCR for *T. pallidum*	■ Serum VDRL and FTA-ABS are clue in >90%; false-negative serum VDRL in 5-10% with tabes dorsalis or general paresis

continued on next page

Systems Review

Agent/Condition Frequency (All AIDS Patients)	Clinical Features	CT Scan/MRI	Cerebrospinal Fluid (CSF*)	Other Diagnostic Tests
Neurosyphilis (0.5%) *continued* (pg 488)	■ General paresis: Memory loss, dementia, personality changes, loss of pupil response ■ Meningo-vascular: Strokes, myelitis ■ Ocular: Iritis, uveitis, optic neuritis ■ Any CD4 cell count			■ Definitive diagnosis: Positive CSF VDRL (found in 60-70%) ■ Note: Most common forms in HIV-infected persons are ocular, meningeal, and meningo-vascular.
PML (1-2%) (pg 455)	■ No fever; no headache; impaired speech, vision, motor function, cranial nerves ■ Evolution: Weeks to months ■ CD4 <100 cells/mm³; some >200 cells/mm³	■ Location: White matter, subcortical, multifocal ■ Sites: Variable ■ Enhancement: Negative ■ No mass effect	■ Normal CSF ■ PCR for JC virus: 80%	■ Brain biopsy: Positive DFA stain for JC virus
Tuberculosis (0.5-1.0%) (pg 462)	■ Fever, reduced alertness, headache, meningismus, focal deficits (20%) ■ CD4 <350 cells/mm³	■ Intracerebral lesions in 50-70% (*N NEJM* 1992;326:668; *Am J Med* 1992;93:524)	■ Normal: 5% to 10% ■ Protein: normal (40%) 500/mL ■ WBC: 5-2000 (average is 60-70% monos) ■ Glucose: CSF/serum <50% ■ AFB smear positive: 20%	■ Chest x-ray: active TB in 50%; PPD positive: 20-30% ■ Definitive diagnosis: positive CSF culture

* **Normal values:** Protein: 15-45 mg/dL; traumatic tap: 1 mg/1000 RBCs; glucose: 40-80 mg/dL or CSF/blood glucose ratio >0.6; leukocyte counts: <5 mononuclear cells/mL, 5-10 is suspect, 1 PMN is suspect; bloody tap: 1 WBC/700 RBC; opening pressure: 80-200 mm H_2O.

CSF analysis in asymptomatic HIV-infected persons shows 40-50% have elevated protein and/or pleocytosis (>5 mononuclear cells/mL); the frequency of pleocytosis decreases with progressive disease.

Systems Review

7

the pre-HAART era (*Neurology* 2992;42:472). A major risk factor for HAD was a nadir CD4 count <200 cells/mm³. This analysis found no significant or favorable relationship between the use of drugs that have high CNS penetration scores (pg. 550), although others have found a correlation (*Neurology* 2011;76:693; *Ann Neurol* 2004;56:416).

CAUSE: Chronic encephalitis with progressive or static encephalopathy due to CNS HIV infection with prominent immune activation. Some work suggests that there is an up-regulation of endogenous antioxidant defenses in the brain. The failure of this neuroprotective mechanism causes accumulation of sphingomyelin and cognitive function. Co-morbidities that play a role are aging, hepatitis C and drug abuse (*Int Rev Psychiatry* 2008;20:25; *Neurology* 2008;70:1753).

INCIDENCE: Prior reports suggested the incidence of HAD was 7% after AIDS in pre-HAART era and 2-3% in the early HAART era (*Neurology* 2001;56:257). More recent work with sensitive neurocognitive testing and imaging indicates about half of patients with HIV infection have neurocognitive defects (*J Neurovirol* 2009;15:187).

PRESENTATION: Prior studies showed high rates of subcortical dementia in late stage HIV with CD4 count <200 cells/mm³ and subcortical dementia. See Table 7-16. Early symptoms: apathy, memory loss, cognitive slowing, depression, and withdrawal. Motor defects include gait instability and reduced hand coordination. Late stages show global loss of cognition, severe psychomotor retardation, and mutism. There may be seizures, which are usually easily controlled. The rate of progression is highly variable, but the average from first symptoms to death in the pre-HAART era was 6 mos (*Medicine* 1987;66:407). Physical examination in early disease shows defective rapid eye limb movement, and generalized hyperreflexia. In late stages, there is tremor, clonus, and frontal release signs. The more recent studies noted above (*J Neurovirol* 2009;15:187) showed high rates of cognitive impairment even in early stage HIV infection that correlated with central white matter damage demonstrated with diffusion tensor imaging. Changes were seen at all stages of HIV but were more widespread in patients with AIDS. Cognitive changes correlated with white matter injury in the internal capsule, corpus callosum and superior longitudinal fasciculus.

DIAGNOSIS: History, physical examination, and screening with HIV Dementia Scale. Formal testing includes Trail Making B, Digital Symbol, Grooved Pegboard, and the HIV Dementia Scale (Table 7-16). MRI shows cerebral atrophy (which can be present without symptoms), typically with rarefaction of white matter (*J Neurol Neurosurg Psych* 1997;62:346). CSF shows increased protein with 0-15 mononuclear cells; pleocytosis is absent in 65%. Main goal is to exclude alternative diagnosis because no test is specific for HAD.

TREATMENT: The HIV Dementia Scale (see Table 7-16) can be used to follow response to ARV treatment. ART has reduced the frequency of

HAD, but there are sparse data to show efficacy of ART for reversing established HAD (*J Neurovirol* 2002;8:136; *J Neurol* 2004;10:350). Some studies suggest that CNS penetration antiretrovirals is an important correlate with neurologic improvement (*Arch Neurol* 2004; 61:1699), but others do not (*AIDS* 23;23:1359; *J Neurovirol* 2009;15: 187). CNS penetration was studied in CHARTER, that included an analysis of 374 patients who were receiving ART and had simultaneous serum and CSF level measurements. Antiretroviral agents with the best CNS penetration based on CSF levels are AZT, ABC, NVP, LPV/r, ATV/r and IDV/r (see Table 7-18) (HIV *Med* 2008;16:15; *AIDS* 2009;23:83; *JAIDS* 1998;235:238; *AIDS* 2009; 23:83). Some patients who have progressive dementia despite good virologic control by conventional monitoring have resistant virus in the CNS suggesting that genotypic resistance tests of HIV isolated in CSF could facilitate regimen selection (*J Virol* 2004; 78:10133). There are no specific treatments for HIV dementia (*Int Rev Psychiatry* 2008;20.25).

■ TABLE 7-16: **HIV Dementia Scale** (*AIDS Reader* 2002;12:29)

Maximum Score	Test*
See below	**Memory registration:** 4 words given (hat, dog, green, peach) and have the patient repeat them.
6	**Psychomotor speed:** Record the time, in seconds, that it takes the patient to write the alphabet. Score: <21 sec = 6, 21.1-24 sec = 5, 24.1-27 sec = 4, 27.1-30 sec = 3, 30.1-33 sec = 2; 33.1-36 sec = 1, >36 = 0
4	**Memory recall:** Ask for the four words from above. For words not remembered give semantic clue, e.g. "animal" (dog), "color" (green), etc. 1 point for each correct answer.
2	**Construction:** Copy a cube and record time. Score: <25 sec = 2, 25-35 sec = 1, >35 = 0

* ≤7/12 is threshold for dementia but is non-specific requiring additional neurologic evaluation.

RESPONSE: ART is associated with significant increases in survival (*AIDS* 2003;17:1539) and reduced incidence of HAD, but its role in treatment of HAD specifically is less clear (*Brain Path* 2003;13:104). Severe progressive dementia similar to the course seen in the pre-HAART era is sometimes seen. The issue of response of HAD to ART is obviously a key issue. This was addressed by the HIV Imaging Consortium, which did proton magnetic resonance spectroscopy in 124 patients with HIV dementia (*AIDS* 2011;25:625). Results showed the brain injury persists. There is also evidence that clinically-stable patients may have progressive cognitive impairment (*JAIDS* 2005;38:3; *AIDS* 2010;24:983).

7 Systems Review

■ TABLE 7-17: **AIDS Dementia Complex Staging**

Stage	Description
Stage 0	**Normal**
Stage 0.5	**Subclinical:** Minimal – equivocal symptoms; no work impairment.
Stage 1.0	**Mild:** Minimal intellectual or motor impairment; able to do all but more demanding work or ADL.
Stage 2.0	**Moderate:** Cannot work or perform demanding ADL; capable of self care.
Stage 3.0	**Severe:** Major intellectual disability; unable to walk unassisted.
Stage 4.0	**End stage:** Nnear vegetative stage; paraplegia or quadriplegia.

CNS Penetration Effectiveness Ranks 2011 Scoring System

The CNS Penetration Effectiveness (CPE) score is a method to estimate CNS penetration of antiretroviral drugs (*Arch Neurolog* 2008; 65:65) provided by the CNS HIV Anti-Retroviral Therapy Effects Research (CHARTER) study, a multicenter, prospective observational study cohort based in six North American locations. Penetration of ART drugs is estimated based on CSF pharmacology, chemical characteristics and effectiveness in CNS infections. Validation was done by assessing antiviral effect with simultaneous measurement of CSF and plasma HIV viral load in 833 patients receiving these drugs (*Arch Neurol* 2008;65:65). The ranking is 1-4, with 4 indicating the best penetration and 1 indicating the poorest (Table 7-18). The metric used to analyze changes with standardized tests with periodic testing is the NPZ3 score – Neurocognitive Z (standardized T score) converted to Z by averaging three measurements.

Several studies have demonstrated the relevance of the CPE score, including a multicenter analysis of 2,636 patients (median CD4 244 cells/mm^3) who underwent standardized neurologic testing. Patients

■ TABLE 7-18: **CNS Penetration Effectiveness Rankings Scoring System**

Class	Ranking			
	1	2	3	4
NRTI	TDF	ddl 3TC d4T	FTC ABC	AZT
NNRTI		ETR	EFV	
PI	NFV RTV SQV/r TPV/r	ATV ATV/r FPV	DRV/r FPV/r LPV/r	IDV/r
Integrated Inhibitor			RAL	

Systems Review

taking ART regimens with better CPE scores performed better with sequential neurocognitive testing (*AIDS* 2011;25:357). There are two points of concern in these analysis. First, analysis of 22,356 patients who initiated ART between 1996 and 2008 in the UK collaborative HIV Cohort (CHIC) Study found that the median CPE score (Table 7-18) increased from 7 in 1996-97 to 9 in 2000-01 but then declined to 6 in 2006-08 (*Neurology* 2011;76:693). Of note, this analysis also found a correlation between the CPE score and CNS complications. The second concern is the previously cited ACTG (ALLRT) cohort, which demonstrated the positive correlation between the CPE score and neurocognitive function (*AIDS* 2011;25:357), also found that more than 3 antiretrovirals may be required to treat HIV in the CNS.

Primary CNS Lymphoma (PCNSL)

CAUSE: Virtually all are EBV-associated (*Lancet* 1991;337:805).

FREQUENCY: The prevalence in the period 1985-90 was over 1000 times higher than in the general population (*Lancet* 1991;338:969). The incidence has declined in the HAART era but not as much as other HIV complications (*JAIDS* 2000;25:451). HIV infection now accounts for 27% of CNS lymphomas; rates have dereased about 10-fold during the HAART era: 297/100,000 to 26/100,000 (*JAMA* 2011;305:1450).

PRESENTATION: A review of 248 cases of immunocompetent patients showed 43% had neuropsychiatric signs, 33% had increased intracranial pressure, 14% had seizures and 4% had ocular symptoms (*Arch Neurol* 2010;67:291). The "B symptoms" (fever, weight loss, night sweats) are rare. CD4 count is usually <50 cells/mm^3.

DIAGNOSIS: The CD4 count is usually <50 cells/mm^3. MRI with contrast usually shows a single enhancing lesion, but there may be multiple lesions and MRI sometimes shows ring forms (*Am J Neuroradiol* 1997;18:563). These lesions usually involve the corpus callosum, periventricular area, or periependymal area; they are often >4 cm in diameter and usually show a mass effect (*Neurology* 1997;48:687; *J Neuroncol* 2005;72:169). The diagnosis is established with brain biopsy, positive CSF cytology and possibly by EBV DNA in CSF (see below). Major differential diagnosis is toxoplasmosis.

Factors favoring CNS lymphoma are: 1) typical neuroimaging results (above), 2) negative anti-*Toxoplasma* IgG serology, 3) failure to respond to empiric treatment of toxoplasmosis within 1-2 wks, 4) lack of fever, and 5) thallium SPECT scan with early thallium uptake. CSF EBV PCR is >94% specific and 50-80% sensitive (*CID* 2002;34:103; *J Natl Cancer Inst* 1998;90:364; *Lancet* 1992;342:398).Others report much lower specificity of CSF EBV DNA and suggest quantitation with a 10,000 c/mL threshold (*J Clin Virol* 2008;42:433). Stereotactic brain biopsy is definitive and usually reserved for patients who fail to respond to toxoplasmosis treatment (*AIDS* 1995;9:1243; *CID* 2002;34:103). A

7 Systems Review

review of five reports with 486 AIDS patients undergoing stereotactic brain biopsy showed a 4% morbidity rate (*CID* 2002;34:103).

THERAPY

- **Standard:** Radiation plus corticosteroids (*J Neuro Sci* 1999;163:32) or methotrexate (*J Clin Oncol* 2003;21:1044). A comparison of 41 patients with HIV-associated CNS lymphomas and 45 without HIV showed the latter group had a much better treatment response and survival (*J Neuroncol* 2011;101:257).

- **Chemotherapy:** May be combined with radiation plus corticosteroids. Usually reserved for patients with elevated CD4 counts. Possible benefit is recently reported with methotrexate plus ifosfamide (*Ann Hematol* 2009;88:133) and with intra-arterial chemotherapy with methotrexate plus IV etoposide and cyclophosphomide (*J Neuroloncol* 2008;90:329).

RESPONSE: Response rates to radiation therapy plus corticosteroids is 20-50%, but these results are temporary, and the average duration of life following the onset of symptoms was only about 4 mos in the pre-HAART era (*Crit Rev Oncol* 1998;9:199; *Semin Oncol* 1998;25:492). One report concerning 22 cases seen from 1996-2009 showed a 2 year survival of 16% (*AIDS* 2011;25:691). A trial with methotrexate showed a 74% radiographic response rate with modest toxicity (*J Clin Oncol* 2002;31:171).

Toxoplasmosis: See pg. 486.

OPHTHALMIC COMPLICATIONS

Historic perspective: CMV was the dominant ocular complication in the pre-HAART era with a 30% lifetime risk (*Arch Ophthal* 1996;114:821; *Arch Ophthal* 1996;114:23). HAART brought a dramatic decrease in this complication that exceeded that seen with all other OIs (*Am J Ophth* 1997;124:227; *AIDS* 1998;12:1931). However, some late presenters still develop this complication, and some patients relapse despite high CD4 counts (*CID* 2001;32:815; *Ann Intern Med* 2002;137:239). The major academic group that has provided research and epidemiologic data on ocular complications of HIV in the HAART era is LSOCA (Longitudinal Study of the Ocular Complications of AIDS). This prospective observational database involving multiple ophthalmology centers is funded by the National Eye Institute. Data for 1998-2003 is based on 1,632 patients. Note that this population is not representative of contemporary patients with HIV infection since they are enrolled after referral to an ophthalmologist. Baseline data showed that 88% were receiving ART, median CD4 count at entry was 164 cells/mm^3 and median nadir CD4 count was 30 cells/mm^3 (*Ophth* 2007;114:780). Ocular complications of AIDS patients at enrollment are shown in Table 7-19.

Systems Review

■ TABLE 7-19: **Ocular Complication of HIV Infection**

	Prevalence (%) (1,632 patients)	Incidence/1000 patient-years
Adnexa		
Kaposi's sarcoma	0.4	1.1
Zoster	0.1	0.1
Molluscum	0.6	1.4
Retina		
CMV	22.1	56
Necrotizing herpes	0.4	1.0
Toxoplasmosis	0.3	0.7
Arterial occlusion	0.2	2.0
Retinal vein occlusion	0.2	0.4
Choroiditis		
Choroid	0.4	0.8
Pneumocystis	0.1	0.1
Other		
Syphilitic uveitis	0.1	0.1

CMV Retinitis: See pg. 441.

Microangiopathy

HIV microangiopathy may present with cotton wool spots, intraretinal hemorrhages, and/or microaneurysms. These are more common with low CD4 counts; they are inconsequential and require no treatment. Microaneurysms associated with anemia often respond to increased hematocrit. Other findings may respond to ART.

Microsporidial Keratoconjunctivitis

The cause is usually *Encephalitozoon hellem*; diagnosis by ophthalmologist with slit lamp plus conjunctival scrapings or biopsy. Treatment is fumagillin and ART.

Pneumocystis jiroveci Choroidopathy

Diagnosis – yellow or orange lesions at posterior pole of retina; treatment – standard PCP regimens.

Toxoplasma Retinitis

Diagnosis is based on multiple white or cream-colored retinal lesions without hemorrhages (as commonly seen with CMV) and without pigmented lesions (as seen with toxoplasmosis retinitis in immunocompetent hosts). Treatment is similar to regimens for CNS toxoplasmosis.

Syphilis: See pg. 488.

Ocular forms include uveitis, optic neuritis, and chorioretinitis. Standard treatment is the same as CNS syphilis using aqueous penicillin G 18-24 million units/d IV x 10-14 days (see pg. 488-489).

Zoster Ophthalmicus

Diagnosis is presumptive based on typical dermatomal rash in the distribution of the first branch of the trigeminal nerve. Treatment should be in conjunction with an ophthalmologist as described on pg. 449-451.

ORAL COMPLICATIONS: See pg. 498.

OSTEOPOROSIS

Multiple studies show increased rates of bone disease in patients with HIV infection. A meta-analysis of reports found that patients with HIV infection had a 6.4 relative risk (RR) of decreased bone density and a 3.7 RR of osteoporosis compared to controls. These observations are accompanied by increased rates of fragility fractures defined as fractures with less trauma than a fall from the upright position (*J Clin Endocrinol Metabol* 2008;93:3499). Several groups have shown that HIV-infected patients with and without ART have increased rates of fractures compared to age-matched controls in the HOPS study (*CID* 2011;52:1061; the VA Aging study (2010 CROI;Abstr. 130); and the VA study (*J Clin Endocron* 2008;93:3499).

DIAGNOSIS: Diagnostic testing, definitions and indications for DXA scans: See pg. 62.

CAUSE: The cause of osteopenia, osteoporosis and fragility fractures in patients with HIV infection is multifactorial: immune activation, HIV treatment (especially TDF) and many co-morbidities. Major conditions listed in a 2010 comprehensive review (*CID* 2010;51:651) include estrogen or testosterone deficiency, adrenal deficiency, hyperthyroidism, malabsorption, hemophilia, sickle cell disease, emphysema, alcoholism, dietary calcium deficiency, methadone, opiates, sedentary lifestyle, smoking, chronic metabolic acidosis, chronic infection, chronic renal disease, depression, vitamin D deficiency and multiple medications: glitazones, ART, steroids and

PPIs. For a diagnostic evaluation, the following showed a 92% success rate in defining a cause (*J Clin Endocrinol Metabol* 2002;87:443) (see pg. 62).

- History and physical exam that focuses on causes of osteoporosis
- CBC, chemistry profile, metabolic panel
- Serum 25-hydroxyvitamin D
- Parathyroid and thyroid stimulating hormone
- Total and free testosterone (men)
- Estradiol, FSH, LH and prolactin in young amenorrheic women
- Simultaneous spot urine and serum phosphate and creatinine to calculate fractional excretion of phosphate (patients on TDF)

TREATMENT

- **Indications:** 1) Men or women >50 years with T score total hip, femoral neck or lumbar spine >-2.5 or a fragility fracture; 2) osteopenia with a risk of a fracture of the hip, shoulder or spine of >3% (hip) or >20% (all 3 combined) based on the WHO Fracture Risk Assessment (FRAX) (www.mmhiv.com/link/FRAX). Note that these figures are based on cost effectiveness of treatment in the US, and there is concern that FRAX may underestimate the risks of osteoporosis with HIV infection (*HIV Med* 2008;9:72). See pg. 62.

- **Treatment based on cause**

  □ Vitamin D deficiency: 1) vitamin D3 ergocalciferol 50,000 IU qw x 8-12 wks then monthly; 2) vitamin D2 (cholecalciferol) 2,000 IU/d x 12 wks, then 1000-2000 IU/d; preferred to dose for levels >15 ng/mL and a goal of >32 ng/mL.

  □ Phosphate wasting: TDF treated patients with fragility fracture or 1) 2 scores exceeding -2.0; discontinue TDF if urinary phosphate wasting and hypophosphatemia; 2) significant hypophatemia: calcium (1-2 gm/d) and phosphorus (1-2 gm/d)

  □ Bisphosphonates (preferred): 1) ibandronate q3mos.; 2) zolendronic acid yearly

  □ Second line: 1) postmenopausal women – estrogen replacement; 2) intranasal calcitonin (relatively low efficacy); 3) teriparatide (analog of PTH)

PSYCHIATRIC COMPLICATIONS

DIFFERENTIAL: Nonpsychiatric conditions that are often mistaken as psychiatric include:

- Infection: HIV-associated dementia; neurosyphilis
- Deficiencies: vitamin B6, B12 or A; zinc
- Endocrine disorder: thyroid disease, adrenal insufficiency or hypogonadism

7 Systems Review

- Medication adverse reactions: EFV, corticosteroids, interferon
- Substance abuse

Bipolar Disorder (Manic Depression)

FREQUENCY: 9% of AIDS patients are referred for psychiatric evaluation (*JAMA* 2001;86:2849)

DIAGNOSIS: Manic episodes, depressive episodes, and mixed episodes. Differential includes familial bipolar disorder and AIDS mania (no family history, no episodes prior to late stage HIV, co-morbid cognitive impairment). Mania is defined as a period of abnormal mood that is elevated, expansive or irritable with >3 of the following: 1) grandiosity; 2) decreased sleep (<3 hrs/d); 3) excessive talking; 4) psychomotor agitation; 5) racing thoughts; 6) distractability; 7) excessive pleasurable activities; and/or 8) psychomotor agitation.

TREATMENT

- **AIDS Mania:** ART (acute management); valproic acid (*Depakoke, Depakene*); gabapentin (*Neurontin*); quetiapine (*Seroquel*); aripiprazole (*Abilify*); ziprasidone (*Geodon*); risperidone (*Risperdal*)
- **Favored agents** to control symptoms: valproic acid, gabapentin and other anticonvulsants
- Care should be directed by a psychiatrist

Delirium

DIAGNOSIS: Impaired consciousness, inability to focus or sustain interest, cognitive changes, global derangement of brain function, acute onset, altered consciousness, or disorganized thinking. Reported frequency in HIV-infected patients is 12-29% (*Psychosomatics* 1996;37:469; *Psychosomatics* 1998;39:214).

TREATMENT: Correct underlying condition, which may be infection- or medication-related.

- **Agitation:** Neuroleptics such as haloperidol, chlorpromazine or risperidone
- **Agitation that puts others at risk:** Neuroleptics + low dose of lorazepam for sedation

Demoralization

FREQUENCY: 20% of AIDS patients referred for psychiatric evaluation

DIAGNOSIS: Exaggerated grief state, sadness, hopelessness, often precipitated by life circumstances. Often mistaken for depression, but unlike depression, patients often can enjoy some facets of life, feel best in the mornings, and do not respond to antidepressants.

TREATMENT: Psychotherapy and support

Systems Review

RESPONSE: Responds to psychotherapy; usually not to anti-depressants

Grief (Normal state of low mood focused on loss)

Treatment is psychological rather than pharmacological (support groups, buddy systems).

Major Depression

FREQUENCY: 20% of AIDS patients referred for psychiatric evaluation (*JAMA* 2001;286:2849)

PRESENTATION: Depressed mood, loss of pleasure from activities (anhedonia), anorexia, morning insomnia or hypersomnia, difficulty concentrating, thoughts of suicide. Depression is a major contributor to medication nonadherence (Grenard JL. *J Gen Intern Med* 2011; PMID 21533823).

DIFFERENTIAL: Dementia, delirium, demoralization, intoxications or withdrawal, neurologic diseases

PATIENT HEALTH QUESTIONNAIRE: PH Q-9 (www.mmhiv.com/link/PHQ-9)

Screening test:

- *Do you feel sad, depressed or hopeless?*
- *Have you lost interest/pleasure in things that you usually enjoy?*

If yes to both: recommend PHQ-9 (see Table 7-20)

■ TABLE 7-20: **Patient Health Questionnaire PHQ-9***

PHQ-9: In last 2 weeks have you had –	No	Several days	Most days	Nearly every day
1. Little interest or pleasure in doing things				
2. Felt down, depressed or hopeless				
3. Trouble sleeping – too little or too much				
4. Feeling tired or having little energy				
5. Poor appetite or overeating				
6. Feeling bad about yourself				
7. Trouble concentrating				
8. Moving or speaking slowly or being restless				
9. Thought that you would be better off dead				

* Ask: "In the last 2 weeks, how often have you had _____."
   "No" = 0, "several days" = 1, "most days" = 2, and "nearly every day" = 3.
  Score ≥20:   1) Refer to psychiatrist (suicidal, violent or psych history), or
                 2) Give an antidepressant
  Score 15-20: Consider antidepressant
  Score 10-14: Supportive counseling
  Score <10:   Reassure and educate

7 Systems Review

TREATMENT: Antidepressants (Table 7-21 and 7-22) starting with low doses and titrating slowly ("start low and go slow") with appropriate attention to side effects and serum levels.

RESPONSE: Response rates to antidepressants is 85%; cure rate >50% (*Psychosomatic* 1997;38:423).

Commonly used agent by class

- SSRIs: citalopram (*Celexa*); sertraline (*Zoloft*) fluoxetine (*Prozac*), paroxetine (*Paxil*), escitalopram (*Lexapro*)
- Tricyclics: nortriptyline (*Aventyl, Pamelor*), desipramine (*Norpramin*), doxepin (*Adapin, Sinequan*), imipramine (*Tofranil*)
- Novel antidepressants: bupropion (*Wellbutrin*), venlafaxine (*Effexor*), mirtazapine (*Remeron*)
- Psychostimulants: methylphenidate (*Concerta, Ritalin,* etc), dextroamphetamine (*Adderall*)

■ TABLE 7-21: **Depression: Drug Selection**

Agent	Advantages	Disadvantages
SSRIs	■ Relatively safe and well tolerated ■ Compared with tricyclics: Fewer drug interactions and side effects ■ Safety with overdose	■ ADRs: Sexual dysfunction, substrate and inhibitor of P450 enzymes ■ Use with PI or NNRTI may increase level of SSRI
Tricyclics	■ Equally effective compared with SSRIs ■ Also useful for neuropathy insomnia and diarrhea	■ ADRs: Anticholinergic effects, dry mouth, blurred vision, orthostasis ■ Use with PI or NNRTI may increase tricyclic level ■ Refractory arrhythmia with overdose

■ TABLE 7-22: **Specific Antidepressant Recommendations**

Drug Regimen	Comment
Paroxetine (*Paxil*) 10-40 mg/day	May sedate: If insomnia – give hs; may cause sexual dysfunction, headache or nausea
Sertraline (*Zoloft*) 50-100 mg/day	Use lower doses with PIs due to drug interactions; may cause insominia, agitation,, sexual dysfunction, headache; note long half life
Fluoxetine (*Prozac*) 10-40 mg/day	Rarely sedating, not fatal with overdose, no anticholinergic effects, may cause insomnia agitation, sexual dysfunction; note long half life
Citalopram (*Celexa*) 10-60 mg/day	Fewer drug interactions compared to other SSRIs; may cause nausea & sedation
Venlafaxine XR (*Effexor* XR) 75-375 mg/day	Less drug interactions; may cause headache, nausea, sexual dysfunction
Mirtazapine (*Remeron*) 15-45 mg/day	Start with 15 mg hs and then increase to 15 mg at 7 days; may cause weight gain & dry mouth

Systems Review

Obsessive-Compulsive Disorder

DIAGNOSIS: Recurrent obsessions (preoccupying thoughts that the patient finds irrational and tries to resist) and/or compulsions (actions driven by obsessions to reduce anxiety)

TREATMENT: Refer to psychiatrist or a mental health specialist.

Panic Attacks

DIAGNOSIS: Recurring anxiety attacks with fear plus somatic symptoms of excitation lasting <1 hour

TREATMENT: SSRI and refer to a psychiatrist

Sleep Disturbance

Medications with FDA approval for insomnia have potential for reinforcement and habituation. Evaluate patient for cause (major depression, mania, substance use disorder, demoralization) and refer for appropriate treatment. Insomnia temporally related to a specific stress (pre-op, grief, etc.) may be treated with sedatives or hypnotics up to 1 wk or with trazodone 25-150 mg hs for up to 4 wks.

Substance Use Disorders

DIAGNOSIS: Use of substances despite clear evidence of negative consequences. Dependence: Persistent use or seeking use, withdrawal, tolerance, and physical dependence.

TREATMENT: (NYS AIDS Institute – Jan. 2008)

www.mmhiv.com/link/NYSD-Substance-Abuse

Opioide dependency:

1. Methadone treatment: Usually started with mandated visits 5-6 days/wk with gradual reduction to weekly attendance at 1 year. Initial dose usually 30-40 mg/d with increases to maintenance doses of 80-120 mg/d.

2. Buprenorphine treatment: Provider requirements: 1) 8 hr course, 2) registration with DEA and 3) limit to 30 patients/physician. Usual starting dose is 12-24 mg qd with maximum 32 mg/d.

3. Naltrexone: Only if methadone or buprenorphine cannot be used.

Cocaine dependence: No drug is approved for cocaine dependency. Non-pharmacologic treatments include the 12-step program and acupuncture.

Benzodiazepines: Detoxification

Methamphetamine: Possible benefit from bupropion, modafinil and baclofen.

7 Systems Review

Agent	Treatment
Sedative/hypnotic EtOH, benzodiazepines, and barbiturates	■ Long acting benzodiazepines (chlordiazepoxide, diazepam
Alprazolam (*Xanax*)	■ Substitute clonazepam and taper
Cocaine	■ Suicidal symptoms common; may need brief hospitalization
Opioids	■ Clonidine for autonomic instability. Buprenorphine or methadone tapers; dicyclomine for GI distress

PULMONARY COMPLICATIONS

The major study of lung disease in the pre-HAART era was the six-center Pulmonary Complications of HIV Infect Study – a prospective observational analysis of 1,130 HIV-infected patients and 167 risk-matched HIV-negative controls (*Am Rev Resp Dis* 1990;141:1356; *NEJM* 1995;333:845; *CID* 1999;29:536). Rates of *Pneumocystis* pneumonia and bacterial pneumonia were approximately the same (5.5 vs. 5.1/100 person-years, respectively). With respect to the 252 cases of bacterial pneumonia: 1) the major identified pathogens were *S. pneumoniae* (36), *S. aureus* (13), *H. influenzae* (12) and *P. aeruginosa* (6); 2) rates of bacterial pneumonia were reduced 67% with PCP prophylaxis; and 3) the rates correlated with CD4 count, but 33% had counts >200/mm^3.

A more recent retrospective review (1999-2007) is an analysis from the Veterans Aging Cohort Study Virtual Cohort consisting of 33,420 HIV-infected US Veterans compared to 66,840 without HIV infection matched by age, sex, race and ethnicity (*Am J Respir Crit Care* 2011;183:388). Baseline data for the HIV-infected patients were: median age 45 years; median CD4 count 264 cells/mm^3; male 98%; VL <400 c/mL 14%; IDU 23%; HCV infection 30%; ART 65%; and ever smoked 80%. The baseline pulmonary issues are summarized in Table 7-24.

■ TABLE 7-24: **Baseline Pulmonary Lesions in 33,420 HIV-infected Patients**

	HIV-infected n = 33,420	Controls n = 66,840
Lung cancer	0.55%	0.38%*
Pulmonary hypertension	0.20%	0.16%
Pulmonary fibrosis	0.37%	0.10%*
Bacterial pneumonia	7.5%	1.1%*
Pneumocystis pneumonia	5.3%	0*
Tuberculosis	2.0%	0.14%*

p = <0.001

Systems Review

	Incidence rate/1000 patient years*	
	HIV +	**HIV –**
Bacterial pneumonia	28.0	5.8
Pneumocystis pneumonia	9.9	0.02
Tuberculosis	4.5	0.6
COPD	20.3	17.5
Pulmonary hypertension	1.2	0.8
Pulmonary fibrosis	0.9	0.6

* All differences are significantly different (p = <0.01)

The incidence rates of bacterial pneumonia, COPD, tuberculosis, pulmonary hypertension and pulmonary fibrosis were all significantly increased with HIV infection after adjustment for confounders (Table 7-25). The authors emphasized that the risk for these pulmonary complications also correlated with age and smoking suggesting age over 45 years, smoking and HIV each contribute to immunosenescence which is clinically expressed with the complications found.

Pulmonary Hypertension: (*Adv Cardiol* 2003;40:197; *Am J Resp Crit Care Med* 2008;177:108)

CAUSE: Possible genetic predisposition (*Ann NY Acad Sci* 2001;946:82)

FREQUENCY: Infrequent (0.5%), but risk is 2500-fold higher with HIV based on low rates in the general population (1-2 million) (*Expert Rev Respir Med* 2011;5:257; *Chest* 1991;100:1268). A review of the Veterans Cohort Study with 33,420 US Veterans found that the rate of pulmonary hypertension was 1.2/1000 PY compared to 0.8/1000 age-matched controls (*Am Respir Crit Care Med* 2011;183:388). The rate of pulmonary hypertension in this and other reports does not correlate with CD4, and results with ART are variable (*Clin Microbiol Infect* 2011;17:25).

SYMPTOMS: Major symptom is dyspnea. In a review of 154 case reports, the average CD4 count at diagnosis was 352 ± 304 cells/mm^3, average duration of known HIV infection was 4.3 years, mean age was 35 years and main symptoms were dyspnea (93%), pedal edema (18%), syncope (13%) and fatigue (11%) (*HIV Med* 2010;11:620).

DIAGNOSIS: X-ray shows enlarged pulmonary trunk or central pulmonary vessels (early), massive right ventricular and right atrial enlargement (late). ECHO shows dilated right atrium and ventricle ± tricuspid insufficiency. Doppler ECHO shows pulmonary arterial

7 Systems Review

systolic BP >30 mm Hg. The best test is cardiac catheterization to demonstrate increased pulmonary artery pressure (>25 mm Hg), increased right atrial pressure, and normal pulmonary capillary pressure. Lung scan and pulmonary function tests are normal.

TREATMENT (*Clin Microbiol Infect* 2011;17:25; *HIV Med* 2010;11:620)

- **ART:** Some reports show impressive improvement with ART (*CID* 2004;38:1178), but others do not (*CID* 2004;39:1549; *Heart* 2006;92:1164).

- **Iloprost:** 2.5-5 mcg inhalations 6-9x/d (*Eur Repir J* 2004;23:321).

- **Epoprostenol**: Initiate at 2 ng/kg/min (mean dose 8 ng/kg/min), infusions at 8-24 ng/kg/min (*Am J Respir Crit Care Med* 2003;167: 1433)

- **Sildenafil** 25 mg qd. Increase by 25 mg every 3-4 days up to 25 mg qid (*AIDS* 2001;15:1747; *AIDS* 2002;16:1568; *NEJM* 2000;343: 1342). Note drug interactions with antiretroviral agents.

- **Other:** There are no studies showing benefit of diuretics, anticoagulants, calcium channel blockers or phosphodiesterase V inhibitors (*HIV Med* 2010;11:620)

Pneumonia: See *S. pneumoniae*, pg. 484-485.

PRESENTATION: Cough, dyspnea, and fever ± sputum production

CAUSE: The single major prospective study of pulmonary complications of HIV was discontinued in the pre-HAART era – 1995 (*Am J Respir Crit Care Med* 1997;155:72). Data from 3 years (1992-1995) showed 521 infections: PCP 45%, common bacteria 42%, tuberculosis 5%, CMV 4%, *Aspergillus* 2%, and cryptococcosis 1%. The risk of bacterial pneumonia was increased 7.8-fold higher than in the general population (*Am Rev Respir Dis* 1993;148:1523). The most recent large comprehensive review was the VA Aging Virtual Cohort Study consisting of 33,420 HIV-infected veterans and 66,840 age, sex, race and ethnicity controls (1999-2007) (*Am J Resp Crit Care Med* 2011; 183:388). The rate of bacterial pneumonia was 5-fold greater in the HIV group compared to veterans without HIV. The most common bacterial pathogen associated with HIV is *S. pneumoniae*; other bacteria that are disproportionately represented are *S. aureus* and *P. aeruginosa* (*NEJM* 1995;333:845; *Ann Intern Med* 1986;104:38; *Crit Care Med* 2001;29:548; Akgun KM. *J Intensive Care Med* 2011;26:151).

Influenza does not appear to be unusually common or severe in patients with HIV infection. A combination of reported case series in the 2009 H1N1 epidemic showed one death among 88 hospitalized patients with HIV infection (*JAIDS* 2011;56:e111). Data from California showed that HIV-infected patients accounted for 22 of 1,088 (3%) hospitalized patients and 4 of 110 (4%) deaths (*JAMA* 2009;302:1896).

- **HIV stage** based on CD4 count (see Table 7-27, pg. 564).

- **Time course:** Pyogenic infections and influenza evolve rapidly. PCP develops slowly in HIV-infected patients, with an average duration of 3 wks prior to presentation.
- **Imaging:** chest x-ray is adequate for most pulmonary complications of HIV. One blinded trial of HIV-infected patients showed accurate detection in 64% of bacterial pneumonias, 75% of PCP cases and 84% of tuberculosis cases (*Thor Imaging* 1997;12:47). High resolution CT scan is more expensive, sensitive and accurate, including accurate detection for 90% of KS and 94% of PCP and a 93% negative predictive value for excluding active pulmonary disease (*Ann Thor Med* 2010;5:201). Specific conditions:
  - Bacterial pneumonia: same as changes in immunocompetent hosts, especially lobar or segmental consolidation and rapid progression.
  - Influenza: typical changes are bilateral with multiple lobe involvement, predominance in perihilar and peripheral areas with ground glass, consolidation or nodular opacities (*Radiology* 2010;255:252).

- TABLE 7-26: **Correlation of Chest X-ray Changes and Etiology of Pneumonia (*Ann Thorac Med* 2010;5:201)**

Change	Common	Uncommon
Consolidation	Pyogenic bacteria, Kaposi's sarcoma, cryptococcosis	*Nocardia, M. tuberculosis, M. kansasii, Legionella, B. bronchiseptica*
Reticulonodular infiltrates	*P. jiroveci, M. tuberculosis,* histoplasmosis, coccidioidomycosis	Kaposi's sarcoma, toxoplasmosis, CMV, leishmania, lymphoid interstital pneumonitis
Nodules	*M. tuberculosis,* cryptococcosis	Kaposi's sarcoma, *Nocardia,* PCP
Cavity	*M. tuberculosis, S. aureus* (IDU), *Nocardia, P. aeruginosa,* cryptococcosis, coccidioidomycosis, histoplasmosis, aspergillosis, anaerobes	*M. kansasii,* MAC, *Legionella, P. carinii,* lymphoma, *Klebsiella, Rhodococcus equi*
Hilar nodes	*M. tuberculosis,* histoplasmosis, coccidioidomycosis, lymphoma, Kaposi sarcoma	*M. kansasii,* MAC
Pleural effusion	Pyogenic bacteria, Kaposi sarcoma, *M. tuberculosis* (congestive heart failure, hypoalbuminemia	Cryptococcosis, MAC, histoplasmosis, coccidioidomycosis, aspergillosis, anaerobes, *Nocardia,* lymphoma, toxoplasmosis, primary effusion lymphoma
Adenopathy	*M. tuberculosis*	*Cryptococcus,* cancer

7 Systems Review

- PCP: x-rays lag clinical symptoms. Classic changes: bilateral symmetric perihilar or diffuse infiltrates appearing as reticular or ground glass infiltrates. Cysts and pneumothoraces are common. Normal chest x-rays in 10% (*CID* 2010;30:S5).

- Tuberculosis: with CD4 count >200 cells/mm³ the changes with TB are typical for an immunocompetent host with reactivation with upper lobe cavitary disease. With lower CD4 counts there are often lower lobe involvement, patchy consolidation, effusions, adenopathy, cavities and/or nodules. About 15% are normal on the chest x-ray, but high resolution CT will show abnormalities with adenopathy and "tree-in-bud" pattern, which is asymmetric (*NEJM* 1999;340:367; *J Thorac Imaging* 2002;17:28).

- Kaposi's sarcoma: bilateral, perihilar and lower zone reticulonodular infiltrates, sometimes with the classical flame-shaped nodules. Pulmonary effusions are common (*J Comput Assist Tomogr* 1993;17:60; *Ann Intern Med* 1985;102:471).

- Lymphoma: well-defined single or multiple nodules that are often large and peripheral (unlike KS) (*Chest* 1996;110:729).

■ TABLE 7-27: **Etiology Correlated with CD4 Count**

CD4 cell count	Etiology
>200 cells/mm³	*S. pneumoniae, M. tuberculosis, S. aureus* (IDU), influenza, Non-Hodgkin lymphoma
50-200 cells/mm³	Above + *P. jiroveci*, cryptococcosis, histoplasmosis, coccidioidomycosis, *Nocardia, M. kansasii*, Kaposi sarcoma
<50 cells/mm³	Above + *P. aeruginosa, Aspergillus*, MAC, CMV

- **Prophylaxis:** TMP-SMX (see Figure 7-3) effectively reduces incidence of PCP and bacterial pneumonia including cases involving *S. pneumoniae, Legionella, H. influenzae*, and *S. aureus*. Influenza vaccine appears to decrease the risk of influenza (*Arch Intern Med* 2001;161:441). *Pneumovax* shows variable results (*Br Med J* 2002; 325:292), and a systematic review of 15 reports concluded "moderate support" and the need for more data (Pederson R. *HIV Med* 2011;12:323). INH substantially reduces the risk of TB (*JAMA* 2005; 293:2719).

- **Bacteria:** The most common bacterial causes of pneumonia are, in rank order: *S. pneumoniae, H. influenzae, P. aeruginosa,* and *S. aureus* (*CID* 2006;43:90; *CID* 1996;23:107; *Am J Respir Crit Care Med* 1995;152:1309; *NEJM* 1995;333:845; *JID* 2001;184: 268; *AIDS* 2002;16:2361; *JAIDS* 1994;7:823; *AIDS* 2003;17: 2109). The risk of pneumococcal bacteremia is increased 150- to 300-fold with HIV. *H. influenzae* pneumonia usually involves non-typeable strains (*JAMA* 1992;268:3350). *P. aeruginosa* is a cause of pneumonia in late stage HIV infection and often causes bacteremia and relapses (*JAIDS* 1994;7:823; *NEJM* 2010;362:812).

Systems Review

■ FIGURE 7-3: **PCP Prophylaxis**

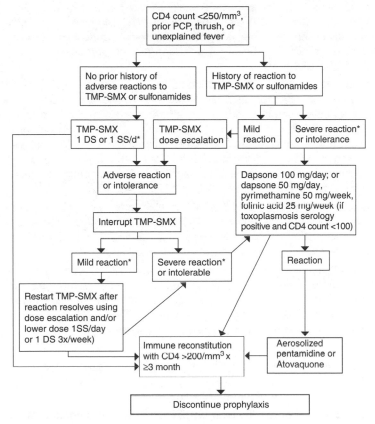

* **Severe:** Urticaria, angioedema, Stevens-Johnson reaction, or fever.
Intolerance: GI symptoms, rash/pruritis.
Mild: Tolerable with aggressive supportive care and/or dose reduction.

■ **Atypical:** Pneumonia due to *M. pneumoniae, C. pneumoniae,* and *Legionella* appear to be relatively uncommon in patients with HIV infection (*Eur J Clin Microbiol Infect Dis* 1997;16:720; *NEJM* 1997; 337:682; *NEJM* 1995;333:845; *Am J Resp Crit Care Med* 1995;152: 1309; *CID* 1996;23:107; *Am J Resp Crit Care Med* 2000;162:2063; *CID* 2004;40[suppl 3]:S150); *AIDS Patient Care STDS* 2008;22:473). A comparison of HIV-infected patients with legionellosis (n=15) or PCP (n=46) found that most cases had other predisposing conditions and higher CD4 counts (*Scand J Infect Dis* 2007;39:122)

DIAGNOSTIC SPECIMENS

■ **Expectorated sputum:** Controversial, due in part to poor technique in collecting, transporting, and processing specimens.

7 Systems Review

- **Expectorated sputum for *M. tuberculosis*:** The yield with three specimens is 50-60% for AFB stain (*Am J Respir Crit Care Med* 2001;164:2020). PCR methods provide an diagnosis with 98% sensitivity and 99% specificity compared to conventional culture and should rapidly replace that antiquated process (*NEJM* 2010;383:1005).

- **Induced sputum:** Recommended as an alternative to expectorated sputum for detection of AFB in patients who cannot produce an expectorated sample and as an alternative to bronchoscopy for detection of PCP. Sensitivity for detection of TB by AFB smear is about the same as it is for expectorated sputum; for PCP sensitivity averages 56% (*Eur Resp J* 2002;20:982). PCR methods are sensitive, but asymptomatic carriage of *P. jiroveci* limits specificity (*Proc Am Thorac Soc* 2011;8:17; *JCM* 2011;49:1872).

- **Bronchoscopy:** The yield for PCP is 95% or comparable to open-lung biopsy (*JAMA* 2001;286:2450). For *M. tuberculosis*, sensitivity is similar to that for expectorated sputum (above). For other bacteria, bronchoscopy is no better than expectorated sputum.

- **Miscellaneous:** tests to consider in atypical or nonresponsive pulmonary infections include *Legionella* urinary antigen, *H. capsulatum* serum and urinary antigen, serum cryptococcal antigen, CT scan and bronchoscopy with biopsy.

EMPIRIC TREATMENT for BACTERIAL PNEUMONIA (2007 IDSA/ATS Guidelines) (*CID* 2007;44 Suppl 4:S27)

- **Outpatient:** doxycycline or macrolide (azithromycin or clarithromycin) (IDSA Guidelines for Community-Acquired Pneumonia; *CID* 2007;44 Suppl 2:S27).

- **Co-morbidity or antibiotics within 90 days of hospitalization:** respiratory fluoroquinolone (levofloxacin or moxifloxacin)

- **Hospitalized patient:** Respiratory fluoroquinolone (moxifloxacin of levofloxacin) or a combination of a betalactam (cefotaxime or ceftriaxone or ampicillin-sulbactam) plus a macrolide (usually azithromycin)

- **ICU admission:** Betalactam plus either a macrolide or betalactam + respiratory fluoroquinolone

- **Suspected PCP:** Add TMP-SMX or alternative PCP treatment. Note that TMP-SMX is inadequate for empiric use for common bacterial causes of CAP so this should be combination therapy and aggressive diagnostic studies: bronchoscopy and/or induced sputum, sputum culture and gram-stain, urinary antigen for *S. pneumoniae* and *Legionella*.

Systems Review

Smoking: Cessation Guidelines: See Table 7-28.

■ TABLE 7-28: **Smoking Cessation**

Product	Regimen	Duration	Side effects	Comment
Varenicline tabs (*Chantix*)	Day 1-3: 0.5 mg QD Day 4-7: 0.5 mg BID Day 8+: 1 mg BID	12-24 wks	Nausea, Sleep problems, Constipation and/or Headaches	Treat 12 wks, continue to wk 24 if stopped smoking at 12 wks to improve long-term abstinence
Non-nicotine therapy				
Bupropion (*Wellbutin SR, Zyban*)	150 mg/d x 3 d, then 150 mg qd*	7-12 wks up to 6 mo for abstinance	Insomnia, dry mouth, agitation	Start 1 wk before quit date; easy to use
Nortriptyline	75-100 mg/d	12 wk	Sedation, dry mouth. dizziness	Start 10-28 days before quit date at dose of 25 mg/d with increase as tolerated
Clonidine	0.1-0.3 mg bid	3-10 wks	Dry mouth, sedation. dizziness	Side effects common
Nicotine-replacement				
Transdermal patch	7, 14, or 21 mg patch x 24 h or 15 mg patch 16 hr	8-10 wks	Insomnia, skin irritation	Start with 21 mg x 4 wks. No prescription needed; steady dose but user cannot adjust dose.
Nicotine gum	2 mg <25 cig/d 4 mg >25 cig/d	8-12 wks	Dammage teeth, dyspepsia	Available without prescription. User controls dose; proper chewing required.
Nicotine lozenge	2 mg <25 cig/d 4 mg >25 cig/d	3-6 mo	Headache, nausea, cough	1 lozenge q1-2h x 6 wks then q2-4h x 3 wks, then q4-8h x 3 wks, then prn
Vapor inhaler (*Nicotrol* inhaler)	6-16 cartridges/d with 4 mg/cartridge	3-6 mo	Mouth irritation, cough	User controlled; need frequent puffing.
Nasal spray (*Nicotrol* NS)	1-2 doses/hr 0.5 in each nostril	3-6 mo	Nasal irritation, cough	User controlled; rapid delivery of high nicotine levels

* Adapted from New York State Department of Health AIDS Institute, "Smoking Cessation in HIV-Infected Patients," www.mmhiv.com/link/NYSD-Smoking)

Multiple studies show that 40-70% of HIV-infected adults are current smokers, summarized in (*HIV Med* 2011;12:412). The Veterans Administration Study of HIV infection (n=1034) found that mortality correlated with smoking (incident risk ratio 2.3 for current smokers) (*AIDS Educ Prev* 2009; Suppl A:40). Thus, smoking cessation is associated with substantial health benefits for anyone, but especially for those with HIV infection.

RENAL COMPLICATIONS

OVERVIEW

- Screening for renal disease risk: Race, family history, CD4 count, HIV VL, nephrotoxic drug (current and prior use), co-morbidities (hypertension, diabetes, hepatitis C)

- Recommendations for routine serum creatine (with basic chemistry) at entry to care q6-12mos before ART, at ART baseline, at 2-8 wks and then q6-12mos, and urinalysis at entry to care and at ART initiation and then every 6 mos if receiving TDF and every 12 mos if not (2011 DHHS Guidelines) (*CID* 2004;40:1559). The importance of screening is increased in those with a risk for HIVAN or other renal disease.

  □ Urinalysis at entry to care, at baseline for ART and then q6mos if receiving TDF or q12mos if not

  □ Annual screening if high risk (African American, CD4 <200 cells/mm^3, or HIV RNA >4000 c/mL) or high-risk disease (diabetes, hypertension, HCV) or receiving TDF (*CID* 2004;40:1559).

  □ Proteinuria >1 + by dipstick: Quantitate proteinuria with "spot" urine protein:creatinine ratio. A protein:creatinine ratio ≤ 0.2 is normal, a ratio of 1 equates to 1 gm protein and a ratio of 2-3 indicates nephrosis and presumed glomerular disease.

  □ Chronic kidney disease – defined as renal disease >3 mos.

  □ Cockcroft-Gault equations for calculating creatine clearance (online calculation available):

  Male: $$\frac{(140 - age) \times weight\ (kg)}{72 \times serum\ creatinine\ (mg/dL)}$$

  Female: $$\frac{(140 - age) \times weight\ (kg)}{72 \times serum\ creatinine\ (mg/dL)} \times 0.85$$

  □ Chronic kidney disease: ultrasound to detect stones and assess renal size.

  small: <9 cm – often severe kidney disease
  large: HIVAN (but nonspecific)

  □ Other studies: HBV, HCV, complement, ANA, cryoglobulin, quantitative immunoglobulin, blood glucose, protein electrophoresis

Systems Review

- **Renal transplantation:** A consortium of 19 US transplant centers have reported three year results for renal trransplantation in patients with HIV infection (2003-09) (*NEJM* 2010;363:2004).

  □ Criteria: 1) CD4 count >200 cells/mm³; 2) HIV viral load <50 c/mL (*Amplicor HIV-1*, Roche) or <75 c/mL (*bDNA Versant 3.0*, Bayer) while receiving stable ART 16 wks prior to transplant; 3) no history of PML, cryptospordiosis, CNS lymphoma or visceral KS and 4) patients with HBV or HCV were required to have a liver biopsy to exclude cirrhosis.

  □ Baseline data for 150 patients: Median age 46 years, median CD4 count 534 cells/mm³, HCV 19%, HBV 3%; Cause of renal failure: HBP 25%, HIVAN 24%.

  □ Results
    □ Patient survival: 1 yr – 94%; 3 yrs – 88%
    □ Graft survival: 1 yr – 90%; 3 yrs – 74%
    □ Rejection incidence: 31%
    □ Progression of HIV: 5 AIDS defining complications

  □ Conclusions: Renal transplantation is "highly feasible" in this population. The rates of patient and graft survival were between the rate for transplant recipients without HIV and recipients >65 years. There was an unexpectedly high rate of rejection (by a factor of 2-3).

- **Acute kidney injury (AKI):** This is defined as an increase in serum creatinine by 0.3 mg/dL within 48 hrs or decrease in urine output to <0.5/mL/kg/hr for 6 hrs. Incidence is reported at 6 cases per 100 patient-years (*Kidney Int* 2005;67:1526). Most common HIV-associated causes are HIVAN, HCV cryoglobulinemia, and drug-related (*CID* 2006;42:1488). Predictors include concurrent diabetes, chronic renal or liver disease, and hepatitis (*AIDS* 2006;20:561) One review of 2,274 patients found that the risk is much higher with CD4 counts <100 cells/mm³ (OR 7) and decreases by >10-fold with HIV treatment >3 mos (*CID* 2008;47:242). Drugs most likely to cause ARF in this population are aminoglycosides, amphotericin, cidofovir, foscarnet, pentamidine, TMP-SMX, and high-dose acyclovir. Antiretroviral drugs implicated are IDV with indinavir crystalluria (*JAIDS* 2003;32:135) and TDF with acute tubular necrosis (*CID* 2006;42:283). More recent reports of AKI in outpatients found that the causes were diverse, including prerenal azotemia (38%), acute tubular necrosis (20%) or drug related (15%) (*HIV Ther* 2010;4:589; *Kidney Int* 2010;78:478). A review of 29 patients with AKI who had acute interstitial nephritis found that most had drug toxicity due to NSAIDs or TMP-SMX (*Clin J Am Soc Nephrol* 2010;5:798). ARV agents were implicated in only three, and none had the classic triad of fever, rash and pyuria.

7 Systems Review

- **Chronic kidney disease (CKD):** Proteinuria is detected in 5% of patients with HIV (*AIDS* 2007;21:1003), and 2-10% have reduced eGFR. In black patients, HIVAN is a common cause (discussed below). In non-blacks, a common cause is immune complex mediated kidney disease (HIVICK) (*Kidney Int* 1993l44L1327); other common causes include diabetes, hypertension, IgA nephropathy, hepatitis C membrane, proliferative glomerulonephritis, etc.

- **HIV medication-associated renal injury:** Most common and important is TDF, which can cause AKI or CKD (see pg. 392). IDV may cause AKI due to IDV crystallization and interstitial nephritis (*AIDS* 1998;12:2433; *Ann Pharmacother* 1998;32:843) (see pg. 296). There have also been associated with renal crystallization and interstitial nephritis with ATV (*Antivir Ther* 2011;16:119; *AIDS* 201;24:2239) (see pg. 200). In a EuroSIDA cohort study with 6,843 patients found CKD was associated with use of TDF, IDV, ATV and LPV/r, each additional year of use increased the rate of CKD by 16% for TDF and 22% for ATV; when ATV and TDF were combined the increase in CKD was 41%/year (*AIDS* 2010;24:1667).

- **Racial differences:** Chronic renal disease defined as a GFR <60/mL/min/1.7 mm^3 (*Ann Intern Med* 2003; 139:137) is relatively common in patients with HIV, with an incidence rate of 11 cases/1000 person years in one report (*JID* 2008;197:1548). However, once chronic renal disease develops, the risk of progression to ESRD is far greater in blacks with a hazard ratio of 17.7 and a GFR decline that is 6-fold more rapid (*JID* 2008;197:1548). This racial disparity appears to be independent of underlying etiology, although HIVAN appears to be nearly exclusively seen in patients of African descent (see below). It should be noted that the association of black race with ESRD in patients with AIDS was noted early in the epidemic (*NEJM* 1984;310:669). It has been noted in the US Veterans Affairs Medical System (*J Am Soc Nephrol* 2007;18:2968) that ESRD is relatively rare in European whites (*AIDS* 2007;21:1119; *JID* 2008;197:1490). A report from Zimbabwe on 3,316 African patients given ART found that 52 (1.6%) developed a GFR <30 mL/min/1.7 m^2 by week 96 (*CID* 2008;46:1271). There was no significant association with any ART regimen, although 74% received TDF.

Hepatitis C Coinfection: (*J Am Soc Nephrol* 1999;10:1566)

CAUSE: Mixed cryoglobulinemia

SYMPTOMS: Palpable purpura, decreased complement, and renal disease with hematuria and proteinuria; may present with acute renal failure and/or nephrotic syndrome (*J Hepatol* 2008;49:613).

DIAGNOSIS: 1) evidence of hepatitis C (positive EIA and HCV RNA); 2) renal disease (hematuria and proteinuria) that may be in the nephrotic range; 3) low complement; 4) renal biopsy evidence of HCV-immune complexes; and 5) circulating cryoglobulins ± skin biopsy of purpuric lesion.

TREATMENT: Pegylated interferon + ribavirin is preferred (see pg. 517), but ribavirin is not recommended with creatinine clearance <50 mL/min due to increased risk of toxicity (e.g., hemolytic anemia). During acute disease, some recommend corticosteroids and plasmapheresis. With progressive renal failure and/or nephrotic range proteinuria, some recommend cyclophosphamide or rituximab (*Kidney Int* 2006;69:436).

Heroin Nephropathy (HAN) (*CID* 2005;40:1559)

CAUSE: Unknown, possibly glomerular epithelial cell injury from toxin contaminant (*Am J Kidney Dis* 1995;25:689)

FREQUENCY: Unknown, but decreasing with increasing purity of street heroin. Frequency is increased in African Americans, who account for 94% of renal failure cases in one series of 98 patients (*JAMA* 1983;250:2935).

DIFFERENTIAL: Main differential is HIVAN. Characteristics of HAN: 1) hypertension, 2) small kidneys by ultrasound, 3) less rapid progression to end-stage renal disease (20-40 mos vs 1-4 mos), 4) less proteinuria, and 5) differences on renal biopsy (*Semin Nephrol* 2003;23:117).

HIV-Associated Nephropathy (HIVAN)

CAUSE: Unknown, but most likely HIV infection of glomerular endothelial and mesangial cells (*NEJM* 2001;344:1979; *Nat Med* 2002; 8:522). HIVAN is found almost exclusively in patients of African descent (*Kidney Int* 2004;66:1145; *Am Kidney Dis* 2000;35:884;*JID* 2008;197:1548).

FREQUENCY: An analysis of 3,976 HIV-infected patients in Baltimore, including 3,332 (78%) African Americans, found an incidence rate for ESRD due to HIVAN in African Americans to be about 1/1000 patient-years (*JID* 2008;197:1548); a review in the UK showed an incidence rate of 0.6/1000 patient years for black patients (*CID* 2008:46:1288). A review of HIV-infected patients with reduced baseline GFR found that 100/284 (35%) progressed to ESRD, of whom 99 were African American. Renal biopsies in 73 showed HIVAN in 37 (37%). Risk factors for HIVAN in African Americans include AIDS and VL >100,000 c/mL, male sex and family history of renal disease (*CID* 2006;42:1488; *Am J Kidney Dis* 1999;34:254; *Am J Kidney Dis* 2000;35:884) and injection drug use (*Kidney Int* 1987;31:1678; *Kidney Int* 1990;37:1325; *NEJM* 1987;316:1062). ART has a protective effect, with a 60% reduction in incidence in one large study (*AIDS* 2004;18:541). However, another review of 61 cases showed that viral suppression

7 Systems Review

with ART had a survival benefit but no benefit with respect to renal outcome (*CID* 2008;46:1282) (see below).

DIAGNOSIS: Baseline proteinuria is a sensitive predictor of chronic renal disease (*Clin Nephrol* 2004;61:1; *JAIDS* 2003;32:2003). Characteristic features are: 1) nearly all patients are of African descent; 2) there is a rapid rise in creatinine, 3) nephrotic range proteinuria (> 3 gm/d) and 4) detectable HIV VL (*Topics HIV Med* 2007;14:164). Other common features are normal blood pressure, large echogenic kidneys, lack of peripheral edema despite hypoalbuninemia, late stage HIV infection and rapid progression to ESRD in 1-4 mos. (*Kidney Int* 1995;48:311; *Am J Roentgenol* 1998;171:713; *NEJM* 1987;316:1062; *Semin Dialy* 2003;16:233). Thus, typical clinical features are GFR <60 mL/min for >3 mo, proteinuria >1.5 gm/24 hr, typical echogenic kidneys and absence of alternative causes (*CID* 2008;46:1282). A definitive diagnosis requires renal biopsy. Renal biopsy shows a collapsing focal glomerulosclerosis with tubulo-interstitial injury. Renal biopsy is recommended to establish this diagnosis according to an NIH review of HIV-associated renal disease (*Ann Intern Med* 2003; 139:214). A review of 55 HIV-infected patients with >3 gm/d proteinuria plus renal biopsy found that only 29 (53%) had HIVAN, emphasizing the need for renal biopsy (*Am J Med* 2006;118: 1288). Collapsing glomerulopathy, the hallmark of HIVAN, has now been described in patients with autoimmune diseases without HIV (*Lupus* 2011;20:866).

TREATMENT

- **ART:** All patients should be treated with ART regardless of CD4 count. ART also appears to protect against HIVAN. A 12-year study found HIVAN in 7% of African Americans with AIDS who were receiving ART and 26% in those who were not treated (*AIDS* 2004; 18:541). Initial data based on biopsy results indicate benefit with ART (*Lancet* 1998;352:783; *Clin Nephrol* 2002;57: 335; *NEJM* 2001;344:1979). Some show dramatic improvement (*NEJM* 2001;344:1979), but this may be only temporary (*AIDS Patient Care STD* 2000;14:657) as another report found that once HIVAN is established, the use of ART has little impact on progression of HIVAN to ESRD (*CID* 2008;46:1282).

- **Dialysis** (*Am J Kidney Dis* 1997;29:549) One report found that one-third of HIVAN patients required dialysis within one month of the diagnosis (*Nephrol Dial Transplant* 2006; 21:2809)

- **ACE Inhibitors** Treatment with captopril (6.25-25 mg po tid) and other ACE inhibitors has beneficial results, and should be used in patients who do not respond to ART (*Kidney Int* 2003;64:1462; *J Am Soc Nephrol* 1997;8:1140; *Am J Kidney Dis* 1996;28:202).

- **Corticosteroids** Prednisone (60 mg qd x 2-11 wks, followed by 2-26 wk taper) shows variable results in terms of renal function and proteinuria (*Am J Med* 1994;97:145; *Kidney Int* 2000;58:1253; *Semin Nephrol* 1998;18:446). Supporting data are considered limited (*Clin Nephrol* 2002;57:336).

HIV-Associated Immune-Mediated Glomerulonephritides

DEFINITION: Includes postinfectious glomerulonephritis, membranous nephritis, IgA nephritis, fibrillary glomerulonephritis, immunotactoid glomerulopathy, and membranoproliferative glomerulonephritis (*Ann Intern Med* 2003; 139:214; *Kidney Int* 2005;67:1381; *Nephrol Dial Transplant* 1993;8:11; *CID* 2006;42:1488).

FREQUENCY: Estimated at 15-80% in HIV-infected patients with chronic renal disease (*CID* 2006;42:1488). Unlike HIVAN, there is no predisposition in persons of African descent.

TREATMENT: ART, ACE inhibitors, and/or corticosteroids (*Clin Nephrol* 2003;60:187; *Nephrol Dial Transplant* 1997;12:2796).

Nephrotoxic Drugs: (ATV see pg. 193, IDV see pg. 294, TDF see pg. 388).

Thrombotic Thrombocytopenia Purpura: See pg. 525.

Abbreviations Used in This Guide

3TC: Lamivudine

3TC/ZDV: Lamivudine + Zidovudine

Ab: Antibody

ABC: Abacavir

ACTG: AIDS Clinical Trials Group

ADC: AIDS-Defining Conditions

ADR: Adverse Drug Reaction

AFB: Acid-fast Bacillus

AFP: Alphafetoprotein

Ag: Antigen

AIDP: Acute Inflammatory Demyelinating Neuropathy

AKI: Acute Kidney Injury

ALC: Absolute Lymphocyte Count

ALT: Alanine aminotransferase

ANC: Absolute Neutrophil Count

ANRS: French National Agency for AIDS Research (Agence National de recherché sur le SIDA)

APRI: AST-to-Platelet Ratio Index

APV: Amprenavir

ART: AntiRetrovial Therapy

ART-CC: ART Cohort Collaboration

ARV: AntiRetroViral

ATN: ART Toxic Neuropathy

ATV: Atazanavir

ATV/r: Atazanavir/ritonavir

AUC: Area Under the Curve

AZT: Zidovudine

BA: Bacillary Angiomatosis

bDNA: branched DNA

bid or BID: Twice daily

BMD: Bone mineral densitivity

BUN: Blood Urea Nitrogen

cART: Combination AntiRetroviral Therapy

CBC: Complete Blood Count

CCR5: A chemokine receptor on lymphocytes

CDC: Center for Disease Control

CF: Complement Fixation

CFR: Circulating Recombinant Forms

CHARTER: CNS HIV Anti-Retroviral Therapy Effects Research

CI: Confidence Interval (usually 95%)

CIDP: Chronic Inflammatory Demyelinating Neuropathy

CKD: Chronic Kidney Disease

Cmax: maximum Concentration

CME: Continuing Medical Education

Cmin: minimum Concentration

CMV: Cytomegalovirus

CNS: Central Nervous System

C-P: Child-Pugh (severity of liver disease)

CPE: CNS Penetration score

CPK: Creatine PhosphoKinase

CrCl: Creatinine Clearance

CRP: C-Reactive Protein

CSF: CerebroSpinal Fluid

CT: Computerized Tomography

CVD: CardioVascular Disease

CVL: Community Viral Load

CYP 450: Cytochrome P450 (enzymes that catalyze metabolism of drugs)

D/M: Dual/Mixed tropic

D:A:D: Data on Adverse events of HIV Drugs

d4T: Stavudine

ddC: Zalcitabine

ddI: Didanosine

DEXA: Dual Energy X-RAY

8

Abbreviations (*continued*)

Absorptiometry

DHHS: Department of Health and Human Service

DILS: Diffuse Infiltrative Lymphocytosis Syndrom

DLV: Delavirdine

DM: Diabetes Mellitus

DOT: Directly Observed Therapy

DRV: Darunavir

DRV/r: Darunavir/ritonavir

DSPN: Distal Sensory Peripheral Neuropathy

DXA: Dual energy X-ray Absorptiometry

EBV: Ebstein Barr Virus

EC: Enteric Coated

EFV/TDF/FTC: Efavirenz/ Tenofovir/Emtricitabine

EIA: Enzyme ImmunoAssay

EMB: Ethambutol

ENF: Enfurvirtide

EPO: Erythropoietin

Epub: In press - but available on PubMed

ERCP: Endoscopic Retrograde Cholangiopancreatography

ESRD: End Stage Renal Disease

ETR: Etravirine

FBS: Fasting Blood Sugar

FDA: Federal Drug Administration

FIB-4: Hepatic Fibrosis score (F0-F4)

FNA: Fine Needle Aspiration

FPV: Fosamprenavir

FRAX: Fracture Risk Assessment

FTC: Emtricitabine

G6PD: Glucose-6-Phosphate Dehydrogenase

GALT: Gut Associated Lymphoid Tissue

HAART: Highly Active Anti-Retroviral Therapy

HAD: HIV-Associated Dementia

HAN: Heroin Associated Nephropathy

HAND: HIV-associated Neurocognitive Defects

HANWS: HIV-Associated Neuromuscular Weakness Syndrome

HAV: Hepatitis A Virus

HBcAg: Hepatitis B core Antigen

HBeAg: Hepatitis B e Antigen

HBsAb: Hepatitis B virus surface antibody

HBsAg: Hepatitis B surface Antigen

HBV: Hepatitis B Virus

HCV: Hepatitis C Virus

HCW: Health Care Workers

HDL-C: High-Density Lipoprotein Cholesterol

HHV 1-8: Human Herpes Viruses 1-8

HIV-1: Human Immunodeficiency Virus type 1

HIV-2: Human Immunodeficiency Virus type 2

HIVAN: HIV-Associated Nephropathy

HPV: Human Papilloma Virus

HRA: High Resolution Anoscopy

hsCRP: Hypersensitive C Reactive Protein

HSR: HyperSensitivity Reaction

HSV: Herpes Simplex Virus

HTLV-1: Human T-cell Leukemia Virus type 1

IAS-USA: International Antiviral Society – USA

Abbreviations (*continued*)

ICL: Idiopathic CD4 Lymphopenia

ICP: IntraCranial Pressure

IDSA: Infectious Diseases Society of America

IDU: Injection Drug Use

IDV: Indinavir

IDV/r: Indinavir/ritonavir

IFN: Interferon

IFN-gamma: Interferon gamma

IGRA: Interferon-Gamma Release Assay

IL-2: Interleukin-2

IL-6: Interleukin-6

IL-7: Interleukin-7

INH: Isoniazid

InSTI: Integrase strand transfer inhibitor (integrase inhibitor)

IOM: Institute of Medicine

IRB: Institutional Review Board

IRIS: Immune Reconstitution Inflammatory Syndrome

ITP: Idiopathic Thrombocytopenia Purpura

IVIG: IntraVenous Immune Globulin

JC Virus: John Cunningham Virus

KS: Kaposi Sarcoma

LDL-C: Low-Density Lipoprotein Cholesterol

LFT: Liver Function Test

LPV: Lopinavir

LPV/r: Lopinavir/ritonavir

LSOCA: Longitudinal Study of the Ocular Complications of HIV

LTBI: Latent Tuberculosis Infection

MAC: *Mycobacterium Avium* Complex

MACS: Multi-AIDS Cohort Study

MDR: Multi-Drug Resistant

MMR: Measles, Mumps, Rubella (vaccine)

MND: HIV-associated Mild Neurocognitive Disorder

MRSA: Methicillin-Resistant *Staphylococcus aureus*

MSM: Men who have Sex with Men

MSSA: Methicillin-Sensitive *Staphylococcus aureus*

MTB: *Mycobacterium Tuberculosis*

MTCT: Mother-To-Child Transmission

MVC: Maraviroc

NA-ACCORD: North American AIDS Cohort Collaboration on Research and Design

NAAT: Nucleic Acid Amplification Test

NASH: Non-Alcoholic Steatosis

NFV: Nelfinavir

NHANES: National Health and Nutrition Examination Survey

NHL: Non-Hodgkins Lymphoma

NIH: National Institutes of Health

NNRTI: Non-Nucleoside Reverse Transcriptase Inhibitor

nPEP: non-occupational Post Exposure Prophylaxis

NRTI: Nucleoside Reverse Transcriptase Inhibitor

NVP: Nevirapine

OHL: Oral Hairy Leucoplakia

OI: Opportunistic Infection

OR: Odds Ratio

PAH: Pulmonary Arterial Hypertension

PCNSL: Primary CNS Lymphoma

PCP: *Pneumocystis* Pneumonia

PCR: Polymerase Chain Reaction

pegIFN: Pegylated Interferon

Medical Management of HIV Infection: Index

8

Abbreviations (*continued*)

PEP: Post Exposure Prophylaxis

PHQ: Patient Health Questionnaire

PI: Protease Inhibitor

PI/r: Protease Inhibitor boosted with ritonavir

PML: Progressive Multifocal Leukoencephalopathy

PN: Peripheral Neuropathy

PO: By mouth (per oral)

PPE: Papular Pruritic Eruption

PrEP: PreExposure Prophylaxis

PZA: Pyrazinamide

qd or QD: Once daily

qid or QID: Four times daily

QTc: Time from the beginning of the Q wave to the end of the T wave

R5: HIV strains that bind the CCR5 co-receptor

RAL: Raltegravir

RBV: Ribavirin

RIF: Rifampin

RPR: Rapid Plasma Reagin

RPV: Rilpivirine

RR: Relative Risk

RT: Reverse Transcriptase

RT-PCR: Reverse Trancriptase Polymerase Chain Reaction

RTV: Ritonavir

SJS: Stevens Johnson Syndrome

SMART: Strategies in Management of Anti-Retroviral Therapy

SOCA: Study of the Ocular Complications of AIDS

SQV: Saquinavir

SQV/r: Saquinavir/ritonavir

STD: Sexually Transmitted Disease

STI: Sexually Transmitted Infection

SVR: Sustained (Hepatitis C) Viral Response

T1/2: Half Life

T20: Enfuvirtide

TAM: Thymidine Analog Mutation

TC: Total Cholesterol

TDF: Tenofovir DF

TDM: Therapeutic Drug Monitoring

TEN: Toxic Epidermal Necrolysis

TG: Triglyceride

tid or TID: Three times daily

TLOVR: Time to Loss of Virologic Response

TMP/SMX: Trimethoprim-Sulfamethoxazole

TPV: Tipranavir

TPV/r: Tipranavir/ritonavir

TST: Tuberculin Skin Test

TTP: Thrombolic Thromboycytopenia Purpura

TVR: Telaprevir

ULN: Upper Limit of Normal

US: Ultrasound

UVB: Phototherapy

VA: Veterans Administration

VL: Viral Load (usually HIV)

VZV: Varicella Zoster Virus

WB: Western Blot

X4: HIV strains that bind to the CXCR4 co-receptor

XDR: Extremely Drug Resistant

ZDV: Zidovudine

ART Agents – Standard Abbreviations

3TC: Lamivudine

ABC: Abacavir

APV: Amprenavir

ATV: Atazanavir

AZT: Zidovudine

d4T: Stavudine

ddC: Zalcitabine

ddI: Didanosine

DLV: Delavirdine

DRV: Darunavir

EFV: Efavirenz

ENF: Enfurvirtide

ETR: Etravirine

FPV: Fosamprenavir

FTC: Emtricitabine

IDV: Indinavir

LPV/r: Lopinavir/ritonavir

MVC: Maraviroc

NFV: Nelfinavir

NVP: Nevirapine

RAL: Raltegravir

RPV: Rilpivirine

RTV: Ritonavir

SQV: Saquinavir

T20: Enfuvirtide

TDF: Tenofovir DF

TPV: Tipranavir

ZDV: Zidovudine

Non-standard Journal Abbreviations used in this guide

AAC: Antimicrob Ag Chemother

CID: Clin Infect Dis

JAC: J Antimicrob Ther

JAIDS: J AIDS

JCM: J Clin Microbiol

JID: J Infect Dis

MMWR: Morb Mort Wkly Report

NEJM: N Engl J Med

Index of Trials

Bold entries indicate primary reference.
Page numbers followed by "t" indicate table entries.

Index of Trials (*continued*)

Medical Management of HIV Infection: Index

8

Index of Tables

Index of Tables (*continued*)

Index of Tables (*continued*)

Medical Management of HIV Infection: Index

8

Index of Tables (*continued*)

Index

*Page numbers followed by "t" indicate table entries. **Bold** entries indicate primary reference.*

#

3TC (Lamivudine): **304-308**; CNS penetration 550t; convenience 103t; FDA approval 81t; fold change cutoffs 47t; as initial regimen 88-90, 91t; PEP 170t; in pregnancy 152t, 154t, 155t, 157t, 163t, 165t; in renal and hepatic failure 148t; resistance mutations 38t, 112, 116

A

Abacavir (ABC, *Ziagen*): **179-186**; CNS penetration 550; convenience 103t; FDA approval 81t; fold change cutoffs 47t; hypersensitivity 61-62; initial regimen 89, 91t; pregnancy 152, 153t, 157t; PEP 170t, 175t; resistance mutations 38t

Abacavir hypersensitivity: **61-62, 184-185**; 99t, 146, 147t, 170t, 180, 182t, 494, 505

ABC (Abacavir): **179-186**; CNS penetration 550; convenience 103t; FDA approval 81t; fold change cutoffs 47t; hypersensitivity 61-62; initial regimen 89, 91t; pregnancy 152, 153t, 157t; PEP 170t, 175t; resistance mutations 38t

Abelcet (Amphotericin B): **190-193**; for Aspergillis 422-423; for Coccidioidomycosis 432, for *C. neoformans* 433-438; for esophagitis 427; for histoplasmosis 453t; for penicilinosis 476

Acute retroviral syndrome: 1, 15, 3t, 169

Acyclovir (*Zovirax*): **186-189**

Adherence: **101-105**; TB 299; virologic failure 110-113

Adverse drug reactions (ADRs): **109t, 127**; *see also specific drugs*

Agenerase (Amprenavir, APV): discontinued; see Fosamprenavir

AIDS case definition: **4t, 5t**

AIDS defining conditions: 5t

Albendazole (*Albenza*): **189-190**; for microsporidia 457-458

Alinia (Nitazoxanide): 440, 457

AmBisome (Amphotericin B): **190-193**; for Aspergillis 422-423; for Coccidioidomycosis 432; for *C. neoformans* 433-438; for esophagitis 427; for histoplasmosis 453t; for penicilinosis 476

Amphotec (Amphotericin B): **190-193**; for Aspergillis 422-423; for *C. neoformans* 433-438; for Coccidioidomycosis 432; for esophagitis 427; for histoplasmosis 453t; for penicilinosis 476

Amphotericin B (*Abelcet, Amphotec, AmBisome*): **190-193**; for Aspergillis 422-423; for *C. neoformans* 433-438; for Coccidioidomycosis 432; for esophagitis 427; for histoplasmosis 453t; for penicilinosis 476

Amprenavir (APV, *Agenerase*): discontinued; see Fosamprenavir

Anal cancer: **55t**; 3t, 56-57; HPV vaccine 78; 531t

Anal Pap smear: **56-57**; 531

Ancobon (Flucytosine): **279-280**

Androderm (Testosterone): **394-397**; lab tests 63-64; treatment 130, 394-397

AndroGel (Testosterone): **394-397**; lab tests 63-64; treatment 130, 394-397

Anemia: **520-523**; 3t; AZT 417-419; dapsone 222-223; EPO 263-265; G6PD deficiency 61; primaquine 349-350; TTP 525

Anorexia: **497-498**; dronabinol 242

Antidepressants: **407-408**; for major depression 557-558; for peripheral neuropathy 542; *see also specific drugs*

Antiemetics: *see specific drugs*

Antimycobacterial therapy: *see specific drugs*

Antiretroviral agents: **81-176**; advantages / disadvantages 96-100t; adverse effects 127-151; convenience factor 103t; dose adjustments 125-127; FDA-approved 81t; guidelines recommendations 91t; hepatic and